ADHD in Adults

Characterization, Diagnosis, and Treatment

ADHD in Adults

Characterization, Diagnosis, and Treatment

Edited by
Jan K. Buitelaar
Cornelis C. Kan
Philip J. Asherson

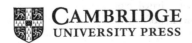

CAMBRIDGE UNIVERSITY PRESS
Cambridge, New York, Melbourne, Madrid, Cape Town,
Singapore, São Paulo, Delhi, Mexico City

Cambridge University Press
The Edinburgh Building, Cambridge CB2 8RU, UK

Published in the United States of America by Cambridge University Press, New York

www.cambridge.org
Information on this title: www.cambridge.org/9780521864312

First published 2011

A catalogue record for this publication is available from the British Library

Library of Congress Cataloguing in Publication data
ADHD in adults : characterization, diagnosis, and treatment /
edited by Jan K. Buitelaar, Cornelis C. Kan, Philip Asherson.
    p.   cm.
Includes bibliographical references and index.
ISBN 978-0-521-86431-2 (hardback)
1. Attention-deficit disorder in adults.   I. Buitelaar, Jan K.,
1953–   II. Kan, Cornelis C., 1964–   III. Asherson, Philip, 1960–
IV. Title.
RC394.A85A343   2010
616.85′89 – dc22   2010046160

ISBN 978-0-521-86431-2 Hardback

Contents

Contents

Contributors

Leonard A. Adler
Departments of Neurology and Psychiatry, New York University Medical Center, New York, NY, USA

Henrik Anckarsäter
Senior Consultant, Forensic Psychiatry, Universities of Gothenburg and Lund, Hisings Backa, Sweden

L. Eugene Arnold
Professor Emeritus of Psychiatry, Ohio State University, Sunbury, OH, USA

Philip J. Asherson
MRC Social, Genetic and Developmental Psychiatry Centre, Institute of Psychiatry, King's College London, London, UK

Russell Barkley
Department of Psychiatry, Medical University of South Carolina, Charleston, South Carolina, USA

Joseph Biederman
Department of Psychiatry, Massachusetts General Hospital, Boston, MA, and Department of Psychiatry, Harvard Medical School, Boston, MA, USA

Andrew D. Blackwell
University Department of Psychiatry, Addenbrookes Hospital, Cambridge, UK

Jessica Bramham
Clinical Psychologist, Adult ADHD Service, The Maudsley Hospital, London, UK

Thomas E. Brown
Associate Director of the Yale Clinic for Attention and Related Disorders, Department of Psychiatry, Yale University School of Medicine, New Haven, CT, USA

Richard Bruggeman
University Centre of Psychiatry, University Medical Centre, University of Groningen, Groningen, The Netherlands

Jan K. Buitelaar
Radboud University Nijmegen Medical Centre, Department of Cognitive Neuroscience Nijmegen, The Netherlands

C. Keith Conners
Duke University Medical Center, Durham, NC, USA

Jonathan H. Dowson
University Department of Psychiatry, Addenbrookes Hospital, Cambridge, UK

Steve V. Faraone
Department of Psychiatry, Harvard Medical School at Massachusetts Mental Health Center, Boston, MA, USA

Christopher Gibbins
Psychologist and Fellow, ADHD Clinic, Children's and Women's Health Centre, British Columbia, Canada

Christopher Gillberg
Department of Child and Adolescent Psychiatry, Göteborg University, Göteborg, Sweden

I. Carina Gillberg
Institute of Child and Youth Psychiatry, University of Uppsala, and Department of Child and Adolescent Psychiatry, University of Göteborg, Sweden

Ylva Ginsberg
Psychiatry Southwest, Karolinska University Hospital, Huddinge, Sweden

Laurence L. Greenhill
Division of Child and Adolescent Psychiatry, Columbia University and New York State Psychiatric Institute, New York, NY, USA

Julia D. Hunter
Fellow, ADHD Clinic, Children's and Women's Health Centre, British Columbia, Canada

Cornelis C. Kan
Radboud University Nijmegen Medical Centre, Department of Psychiatry, Nijmegen, The Netherlands

Ronald C. Kessler
Department of Health Care Policy, Harvard Medical School, Boston, MA, USA

Scott H. Kollins
Assistant Professor and Director, Duke ADHD Program, Department of Psychiatry and Behavioral Science, Duke University School of Medicine, Durham, NC, USA

J. J. Sandra Kooij
PsyQ, Programme Adult ADHD, The Hague, The Netherlands

Johanna Krause
Outpatient Clinic for Psychiatry and Psychotherapy, Ottobrunn, Germany

Jonna Kuntsi
MRC Social, Genetic and Developmental Psychiatry Centre, Institute of Psychiatry, King's College London, UK

Florence Levy
Head of Child and Family East, Prince of Wales Hospital and Sydney Children's Community Centre, School of Psychiatry, University of New South Wales, Sydney, Australia

Stephen P. McDermott
Cognitive Therapy Institute, Cognitive Therapy and Research Program, Massachusetts General Hospital, Harvard Medical School, Boston, MA, USA

Gráinne McLoughlin
MRC Social, Genetic and Developmental Psychiatry Centre, Institute of Psychiatry, King's College London, UK

Mitul A. Mehta
Institute of Psychiatry at King's College London, and Division of Neuroscience and Mental Health, Imperial College, London, UK

Asko Niemela
Oulu University Hospital, Department of Psychiatry, Finland

Eleni Paliokosta
Consultant Child and Adolescent Psychiatrist, Adult ADHD Service, The Maudsley Hospital, London, UK

Yannis Paloyelis
MRC Social, Genetic and Developmental Psychiatry Centre, Institute of Psychiatry, King's College London

Vangelis Pappas
Consultant Psychiatrist, Ioannina District General Hospital, Ioannina, Greece

Patricia Quinn
Developmental Pediatrician, Washington, DC, and Clinical Assistant Professor of Pediatrics, Georgetown University Medical Center, Washington, DC, USA

Maria Råstam
Department of Child and Adolescent Psychiatry, Göteborg University, Göteborg, Sweden

Doris Ryffel
Psychiatrist, Bern, Switzerland

David Shaw
Department of Psychiatry, New York University School of Medicine and Psychiatry Service, New York VA Harbor Healthcare System, New York, NY, USA

Seija Sirviö
Spanga Psychiatric Unit for Adults, Stockholm, Sweden

Thomas Spencer
Associate Chief, Pediatric Psychopharmacology Unit, Massachusetts General Hospital, and Associate Professor of Psychiatry, Harvard Medical School, Boston, MA, USA

Lacramioara Spetie
Child and Adolescent Psychiatrist, Nationwide Children's Hospital Division of Child and Adolescent Psychiatry, Columbus, OH, USA

Siegfried Tuinier
The late Siegfried Tuinier was formerly at Vincent van Gogh Institute, Venray, The Netherlands

Fiona E. van Dijk
Radboud University Nijmegen Medical Centre, Department of Psychiatry, Nijmegen, The Netherlands

Anne M. D. N. van Lammeren
University Centre of Psychiatry, University Medical Centre, Groningen, The Netherlands

Wim J. C. Verbeeck
Vincent van Gogh Institute, Venray, The Netherlands

Margaret Weiss
Clinical Head, ADHD Clinic, Children's and Women's Health Centre, British Columbia, Canada

Timothy E. Wilens
Director, Substance Abuse Services, Pediatric Psychopharmacology Clinic, Massachusetts General Hospital, and Associate Professor of Psychiatry, Harvard Medical School, Boston, MA, USA

Kiriakos Xenitidis
Consultant Psychiatrist, Adult ADHD Service, The Maudsley Hospital, London, UK

Preface

Reviewing adult ADHD: Reintegration after differentiation

Originally, attention-deficit hyperactivity disorder (ADHD; formerly called minimal brain damage/dysfunction) was considered to be a childhood disorder and was therefore not diagnosed in adults. This concept that ADHD was a child-only disorder began to change in the 1970s. For the first time, two preliminary reports in 1976 on the nature of ADHD symptoms and psychosocial impairments in adults with a past history of childhood ADHD argued that ADHD might not always be outgrown in adulthood. The authors emphasized many similarities between ADHD in children and in adults in patterns of core symptoms and comorbidity, association with impairments and cognitive performance measures, and response to medication (Hechtman et al., 1976; Wood et al., 1976).

Subsequently, in 1980, the category of attention deficit disorder (ADD), residual type, was defined in *DSM-III* (American Psychiatric Association, 1980); this category provided the first opportunity to make a formal diagnosis of ADHD in adults with a past history of ADD and persisting attention and concentration problems, without a requirement of persisting hyperactivity symptoms. This diagnostic possibility must have served a purpose in practice, because its removal in the *DSM-III-R* (American Psychiatric Association, 1987) led to a request from a number of researchers and clinicians to restore it (Shaffer, 1994); efforts followed to define appropriate diagnostic criteria for ADHD in adults (Ward, Wender, & Reimherr, 1993; Wender, 1987). Although the category of ADD, residual type, was not restored in the *DSM-IV*, the *DSM-IV* ADHD criteria were modified in such a way that they could be applied more easily to adults (American Psychiatric Association, 1994).

Since then, the acceptance of adult ADHD by the professional community and the general public has been growing (Jaffe, 1995). Several longitudinal follow-up studies convincingly showed that ADHD symptoms persist in a significant proportion of adults with a history of childhood ADHD (Mannuzza et al., 1993, 1997, 1998; Weiss & Hechtman, 1993; Weiss et al., 1985). These studies were important in establishing that ADHD often persists into adulthood, with age-related changes in the way that the characteristic symptoms of the disorder present in adults.

The importance of diagnosing ADHD in adults was further supported by studies on treatment efficacy. Studies undertaken to investigate whether psychostimulant treatments were effective in adults with ADHD reported comparable effect sizes to those seen in children (Arnold, Strobl, & Weisenberg, 1972; Mattes, Boswell, & Oliver, 1984; Wender, Reimherr, & Wood, 1981; Wender, Wood, & Reimherr, 1985; Wood et al., 1976).

A landmark in the recognition of adult ADHD was the study that demonstrated significant differences in the cerebral glucose metabolism of adults with ADHD compared to control subjects (Zametkin et al., 1990). This study was innovative in two ways: it applied the new neuroimaging research paradigm to ADHD, and it did so in a sample of adults instead of children. The fMRI study of Bush et al. in 1999 – the first to demonstrate the absence of inhibitory activity of the anterior cingulate in ADHD – was carried out in adults as well.

In addition to its recognition in clinical practice, adult ADHD has developed into a research field of interest in its own right. In the last decade, the number of scientific reports on adult ADHD has increased exponentially, as shown in Figure 1.

In this exponential growth we also witness an increasing differentiation. Investigators are increasingly focusing and making progress on specific subtopics with respect to adult ADHD, and it is no longer easy to oversee the entire body of knowledge on ADHD in adulthood.

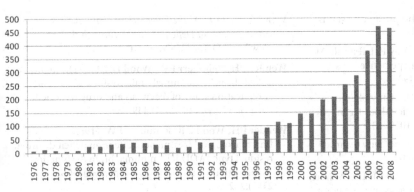

Figure 1 Number of hits in Pubmed using the keywords "ADHD" and "adult."

Therefore, the time has come to integrate many of the new insights that have been achieved during recent years. Because adult ADHD is no longer exclusively an American issue, we requested experts in different fields of adult ADHD from Europe, as well as the United States, to make a contribution to an up-to-date handbook on ADHD in adulthood. From their efforts we have assembled the present collaborative transatlantic overview.

This book is divided into the following sections:

- development of adult ADHD as an epidemiological concept
- insights into the pathophysiology of adult ADHD derived from modern research methods (genetics, neuroimaging, electrophysiology)
- proper methods to assess and diagnose adult ADHD
- the most prevalent comorbid disorders of adult ADHD
- evidence-based pharmacological treatments of adult ADHD
- the most promising psychological and social treatment strategies for adult ADHD
- alternative biological treatments for adult ADHD

The final chapter anticipates the way in which the criteria for adult ADHD might change in *DSM-V*. Probably more attention will be paid to formulating separate adult criteria, thereby acknowledging the differences between the juvenile and the adult phenotype and building on the progress made in our understanding of ADHD in adults. It appears that adult ADHD has finally grown up into a mature entity with its own adult-specific challenges.

We wish to thank all of the authors who have contributed to this book and shared their present state of knowledge, which we consider of great value, with all of the potentially interested readers. We hope that the readers will share our opinion on this book's value.

Jan K. Buitelaar
Cornelis C. Kan
Philip J. Asherson

References

American Psychiatric Association. (1980). *Diagnostic and Statistical Manual of Mental Disorders.* 3rd ed. Washington, DC: American Psychiatric Association.

American Psychiatric Association. (1987). *Diagnostic and Statistical Manual of Mental Disorders.* 3rd ed. rev. Washington, DC: American Psychiatric Association.

American Psychiatric Association. (1994). *Diagnostic and Statistical Manual of Mental Disorders.* 4th ed. Washington, DC: American Psychiatric Association.

Arnold LE, Strobl D, Weisenberg A. (1972). Hyperkinetic adult. Study of the "paradoxical" amphetamine response. *JAMA* **222**(6):693–4.

Bush G, Frazier JA, Rauch SL, Seidman LJ, Whalen PJ, Jenike MA, et al. (1999). Anterior cingulate cortex dysfunction in attention-deficit/hyperactivity disorder revealed by fMRI and the counting Stroop. *Biol Psychiatry* **45**(12):1542–52.

Hechtman L, Weiss G, Finklestein J, Werner A, Benn R. (1976). Hyperactives as young adults: preliminary report. *Can Med Assoc J* **115**(7):625–30.

Jaffe P. (1995). History and overview of adulthood ADD. In: **Nadeau KG,** ed. *A Comprehensive Guide to Attention Deficit Disorder in Adults: Research, Diagnosis, and Treatment.* New York: Brunner/Mazel: 3–17.

Mannuzza S, Klein RG, Bessler A, Malloy P, Hynes ME. (1997). Educational and occupational outcome of hyperactive boys grown up. *J Am Acad Child Adolesc Psychiatry* **36**(9):1222–7.

Mannuzza S, Klein RG, Bessler A, Malloy P, LaPadula M. (1993). Adult outcome of hyperactive boys. Educational achievement, occupational rank, and psychiatric status. *Arch Gen Psychiatry* 50(7):565–76.

Mannuzza S, Klein RG, Bessler A, Malloy P, LaPadula M. (1998). Adult psychiatric status of hyperactive boys grown up. *Am J Psychiatry* 155(4):493–8.

Mattes JA, Boswell L, Oliver H. (1984). Methylphenidate effects on symptoms of attention deficit disorder in adults. *Arch Gen Psychiatry* 41(11):1059–63.

Shaffer D. (1994). Attention deficit hyperactivity disorder in adults. *Am J Psychiatry* 151(5):633–8.

Ward MF, Wender PH, Reimherr FW. (1993). The Wender Utah Rating Scale: an aid in the retrospective diagnosis of childhood attention deficit hyperactivity disorder. *Am J Psychiatry* 150(6):885–90.

Weiss G, Hechtman L. (1993). *Hyperactive Children Grow Up*. 2nd. ed. New York: Guilford.

Weiss G, Hechtman L, Milroy T, Perlman T. (1985). Psychiatric status of hyperactives as adults: a controlled prospective 15-year follow-up of 63 hyperactive children. *J Am Acad Child Psychiatry* 24(2):211–20.

Wender PH. (1987). *The Hyperactive Child, Adolescent and Adult: Attention Deficit Disorder Through the Lifespan*. New York: Oxford University Press.

Wender PH, Reimherr FW, Wood DR. (1981). Attention deficit disorder ('minimal brain dysfunction') in adults. A replication study of diagnosis and drug treatment. *Arch Gen Psychiatry* 38(4):449–56.

Wender PH, Wood DR, Reimherr FW. (1985). Pharmacological treatment of attention deficit disorder, residual type (ADD,RT, "minimal brain dysfunction," "hyperactivity") in adults. *Psychopharmacol Bull* 21(2):222–31.

Wood DR, Reimherr FW, Wender PH, Johnson GE. (1976). Diagnosis and treatment of minimal brain dysfunction in adults: a preliminary report. *Arch Gen Psychiatry* 33(12):1453–60.

Zametkin AJ, Nordahl TE, Gross M, King AC, Semple WE, Rumsey J, et al. (1990). Cerebral glucose metabolism in adults with hyperactivity of childhood onset. *N Engl J Med* 323(20):1361–6.

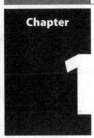

Chapter

The course and persistence of ADHD throughout the life-cycle

Joseph Biederman

An important step in understanding the significance and therapeutic needs of psychiatric syndromes is documenting the course of the disorder. Those individuals who have chronic forms of disorder generally suffer greater consequences as a result, have more severe forms of disorder, and require the most aggressive intervention. Over time, the perception that attention-deficit hyperactivity disorder (ADHD) is a syndrome of childhood misbehavior that wanes throughout puberty and adolescence has been challenged by volumes of research and a continual refinement of standardized diagnostic criteria.

Attempting to understand the burden of psychiatric illness across the life span is often complicated by the fact that, with the progression of time and parallel developmental maturation, the core features of a disorder may present differently. Thus the study and treatment of childhood psychopathology often require an interpretation of symptom expression that takes into account normal development. Examining ADHD across the life span presents unique challenges because the diagnostic criteria require that the disorder be evident by 7 years of age. Natural development leads to many behavioral changes throughout childhood, adolescence, and adulthood, requiring that clinically relevant research have a nuanced interpretation of symptom expression of ADHD in older subjects.

This chapter describes the history of the disorder and the current longitudinal studies of ADHD children into adulthood, with a special focus on the changing operational definition of the disorder, the reliance on the presence of hyperactivity in diagnosis, the impact of normal developmental maturation on recognizing problem behaviors at different ages, and the clinical significance of the diagnosis in older or adult subjects.

Definition and diagnostic criteria

ADHD has long been considered a behavioral disorder of childhood even if under different names. In the 1930s, hyperkinesis, impulsivity, learning disability, and short attention span were described as minimal brain damage and later as minimal brain dysfunction because these symptoms mimicked those seen in patients with frank central nervous system (CNS) injuries. In the 1950s, this label was modified to hyperactive child syndrome, with the eventual inclusion of hyperkinetic reaction of childhood in *DSM-II* in 1968 (American Psychiatric Association, 1968). Each of these labels and sets of criterion was focused exclusively on children and placed the most importance on hyperactivity and impulsivity as hallmarks of the disorder. Although the section of *DSM-II* dedicated to hyperkinetic reaction of childhood was very brief and unstructured, it remained the prevailing standard until publication of *DSM-III* in 1980 (American Psychiatric Association, 1980).

DSM-III represented a significant change in the description of the disorder and was the first to formally recognize inattention as a significant component of the disorder. Its definition also recognized developmental variability and indicated that this variability may play a role in the presentation of the disorder in individuals of different ages. Most importantly for this discussion, *DSM-III* included a residual type of ADHD that could be diagnosed in individuals with a history of meeting full criteria for the disorder, but who presented with a reduced set of symptoms, if the remaining symptoms continued to cause significant levels of impairment. Although the revision of *DSM-III* published in 1987 (American Psychiatric Association, 1987) eliminated the residual type of ADHD, this type returned in 1994 with the publication of *DSM-IV* (American Psychiatric Association, 1994), which also offered

ADHD in Adults: Characterization, Diagnosis and Treatment, ed. Jan Buitelaar, Cornelis Kan and Philip Asherson.
Published by Cambridge University Press. © Cambridge University Press 2011.

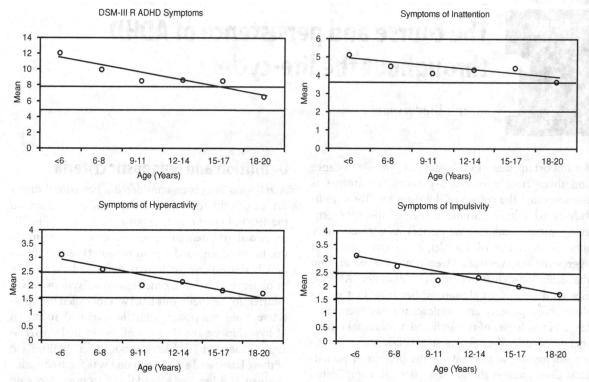

Figure 1.1 Age-dependent decline of ADHD symptoms.

criteria for specific subtypes of ADHD marked by inattention, hyperactivity/impulsivity, or both core features of the disorder.

As the field has struggled with how to characterize ADHD for the past several decades, there has been a consistent underlying notion that ADHD is not a completely remitting condition in all cases. The emphasis on hyperactivity in earlier years has also been shown to affect the rates of persistence of the disorder in prospective follow-up studies with the longest duration.

Age-dependent symptom decline

Much of the difficulty in making the diagnosis of ADHD in children arises from the fact that many of its symptoms are similar to developmentally appropriate behavior in young children. It is natural for a 4-year-old child to exhibit hyperactivity and impulsivity, for example. The diagnosis of ADHD in very young children then relies on the extent to which reported symptoms are more pronounced or prevalent than in other children of the same age. This may affect estimates of duration and definitions of chronic ADHD because as children normally outgrow much of the hyperactivity

and impulsivity, the degree to which these symptoms continue to be of primary concern in making the diagnosis may also decline.

My colleagues and I specifically addressed the relative rate of decline of the core symptoms of ADHD from childhood into early adulthood to offer a developmental perspective on symptom decline (Biederman et al., 2000). ADHD subjects who returned for 4-year follow-up study were examined at multiple time points to estimate the prevalence of different symptomatic categories in different age groups. For each of the ADHD subjects (N = 128), we had five time points of symptom observations: (1) symptoms that had occurred at the disorder's onset as reported retrospectively during the baseline assessment; (2) symptoms that were currently active at baseline; (3) symptoms that were currently active at the Year One follow-up assessment; (4) symptoms that were active at the beginning of the interval covered by the 4-year follow-up based on subject recall; and (5) symptoms that were currently active at the Year Four follow-up assessment.

The mean number of ADHD symptoms in our sample of ADHD children and adolescents was

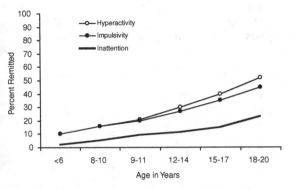

Figure 1.2 Prevalence of symptomatic remission with increasing age.

modeled as a function of age. In Figure 1.1 the predicted regression lines are plotted and horizontal lines are darkened at the value corresponding to full or subthreshold diagnoses. Age was significantly associated with symptom decline for total ADHD symptoms, as well as for each of the symptom subtypes (all Wald $\chi_{(1)}^2 > 22.9$, all p values <0.001). However, the mean number of symptoms did not fall below the subthreshold level for any of the symptom summations of any age group studied. On average, symptoms of inattention did not fall below the full threshold level by 20 years of age, whereas symptoms of hyperactivity and impulsivity did fall below the full threshold level between 9 and 11 years of age.

However, group averages do not indicate the actual prevalence of remission in each age group. Figure 1.2 presents the prevalence of symptomatic remission (having less than half of the symptoms required for the full diagnosis) for all ADHD symptoms and for each of the subtypes. We found a different rate of symptomatic decline for inattention and hyperactivity/impulsivity. Whereas symptoms of inattention declined at a very modest rate, those of hyperactivity and impulsivity remitted much more abruptly. This work demonstrated that, even in a sample of ADHD children with a high rate of symptom persistence (Biederman et al., 1996), overt symptoms of hyperactivity and impulsivity tend to decline with increasing age. Hart et al. (1995) documented a similar pattern of ADHD-subtype specific persistence: the mean number of hyperactive/impulsive symptoms declined with age, whereas the mean number of inattentive symptoms remained stable from age 8 to 15 years. Thus, it seems that the persistence of ADHD is contingent on continued inattention more than on overt hyperactivity or impulsivity.

Impact of symptom decline patterns on rates of persistence

A relatively large number of studies have been published that estimate the persistence of ADHD throughout adolescence and adulthood. Table 1.1 presents the pertinent results from each these studies. Clearly, the rate of ADHD at follow-up varies considerably from one study to the next. For example, Mannuzza et al. (1998) reported that at follow-up 4% of previously hyperactive boys continued to have ADHD, whereas Hart et al. (1995) found that 85% of ADHD cases met criteria for ADHD at follow-up. However, these divergent findings should not be surprising considering the significant heterogeneity between these studies in diagnostic criteria employed, duration of follow-up, and age of the sample at follow-up.

Table 1.1 also indicates that the changing diagnostic classification of ADHD over the years has influenced estimates of persistence of the disorder. The studies listed in Table 1.1 are categorized by the diagnostic system that was used to ascertain the samples. Samples in studies initiated under *DSM-II* had the lowest rate of persistence, whereas the rate of persistence in samples identified under *DSM-III-R* was the highest. This finding is consistent with our earlier work showing the increased rate of remission from hyperactive and impulsive symptoms relative to symptoms of inattention.

Perhaps one of the most important variables is age at follow-up – certainly a 5-year follow-up of 12-year-olds will result in a higher prevalence of ADHD than a 5-year follow-up of 25-year-olds. Hill and Schoener (1996) used this level of heterogeneity in age to estimate the expected rate of ADHD in older populations. They conducted a secondary data analysis of a subset of the studies presented in Table 1.1, selecting those in which the original diagnoses were made concurrently with the creation of the studies' baseline in childhood and in which the follow-up reported the persistence of standardized assessments of ADHD. Hill and Schoener fit a model to these data that predicted an exponential decline in the rate of ADHD and estimated the rate of adult ADHD to range from about 0.8% at age 20 to 0.05% at age 40. At first glance, these results seem to provide strong support for the idea that ADHD is essentially a remitting disorder.

Alternatively, the explanation for these discrepant findings may be that the use of different methods to determine diagnostic status at follow-up led to

Table 1.1 Published studies estimating the persistence of ADHD throughout adolescence and adulthood

	Age range or mean at baseline (years)	Age at follow-up (years)	ADHD persistence		Follow-up ADHD diagnosis
***DSM-II* diagnosis at baseline**					
Mendelson et al. (1971)	9.9	13.4	42	50	*DSM-II*
Borland & Heckman (1976)	7.5	30.4	10	50*	*DSM-II*
Mannuzza & Gittelman (1984)	7.9	17.4	12	33	*DSM-III*
Mannuzza (1984)	7.9	17.4	13	36*	*DSM-III*
Gittelman & Mannuzza (1985)	9.3	18.3	31	31	*DSM-III*
Gittelman (1985)	9.3	18.3	40	40*	*DSM-III*
Mannuzza et al. (1991)	7.3	18.5	21	22	*DSM-III*
Mannuzza et al. (1991)	7.3	18.5	41	43*	*DSM-III*
Mannuzza et al. (1993)	9.3	25.5	7	8	*DSM-III, III-R*
Mannuzza et al. (1993)	9.3	25.5	10	11*	*DSM-III, III-R*
Mannuzza et al. (1998)	7.3	24.1	3	4	*DSM- III-R*
Mannuzza et al. (1998)	7.3	24.1	3	4*	*DSM- III-R*
Lambert et al. (1987)	7.7	14.3	25	43	*DSM-III*
Lambert (1988)	9.3	18.3	47	80*	*DSM-III*
Feldman et al. (1979).	10.0	15.5	35	43	*DSM-II*
August et al. (1983)	10.7	14.2	19	86*	*DSM-III*
Weiss et al. (1985)	6–12	25.1	42	66*	*DSM-III*
Yan (1996)	10.0	25.5	140	70*	*DSM- III-R*
Combined estimate			39 ± 21%		
***DSM-III* diagnosis at baseline**					
Cantwell & Baker (1989)	5.5	9.7	28	80	*DSM-III*
Offord et al. (1992)	4–12	8–16	16	34	*DSM-III*
Claude & Firestone (1995)	7.3	19.7	26	50	*DSM- III-R*
Rasmussen & Gillberg (2000)	7	22	28	56*	*DSM-IV*
Rasmussen & Gillberg (2000)	7	22	24	48	*DSM-IV*
Combined estimate			53 ± 41%		
***DSM-III-R* diagnosis at baseline**					
Barkley et al. (1990)	4–12	14.9	88	72	*DSM- III-R*
Barkley et al. (1990)	4–12	14.9	102	83*	*DSM- III-R*
Barkley et al. (2002)	4–12	21.1	78	58	*DSM-IV*
Barkley et al. (2002)	4–12	21.1	89	66*	*DSM-IV*
Har et al. (1995)	9.4	10.4	89	84	*DSM-III-R*
Hart et al. (1995)	9.4	11.4	90	85	*DSM-III-R*
Hart et al. (1995)	9.4	12.4	92	77	*DSM-III-R*
Biederman et al. (1996)	10.5	14.5	109	85*	*DSM-III-R*
Biederman et al. (1996)	10.5	14.5	78	61	*DSM-III-R*
Biederman (2006)	10.5	22.8	63	58*	*DSM-IV*
Biederman (2006)	11.2	16.4	101	82*	*DSM-IV*
Combined estimate			73 ± 27%%		

*Residual ADHD diagnosis.

different results. Because the number of symptoms present determines diagnostic status, different ways of interpreting symptom decline could lead to drastically different results. Focusing only on those subjects who continue to meet full diagnostic criteria may inflate the rate of remission by requiring a threshold that is too high because one still expects older subjects to present with significant rates of hyperactivity or impulsivity.

In our previous analysis of symptom decline (Biederman et al., 2000), we also assessed three levels of remission: syndromatic, symptomatic, and functional. *Syndromatic* remission refers to the loss of full diagnostic status, *symptomatic* remission refers to the loss of partial diagnostic status, and functional remission refers to the loss of partial diagnostic status plus functional recovery (full recovery). In our data, the rate of remission from the full disorder (syndromatic remission) was quite high, with 60% of our subjects aged 18 to 20 years old no longer meeting criteria for ADHD (Biederman et al., 2000). However, nearly one-third of subjects were still experiencing some ADHD symptoms (a symptomatic remission rate of 30%), and the majority of ADHD subjects continued to report low levels of functioning despite remission of the full diagnostic criteria (a functional remission rate of only 10%).

Therefore, Hill and Schoener (1996) may have been far too optimistic in declaring that the prevalence of ADHD in adult samples was nearly nonexistent. An expanded analysis of the literature supports the notion that in many studies subjects fail to reach symptomatic remission. Faraone et al. (2006) revisited Hill and Schoener's analyses by including studies that reported the follow-up rate of ADHD-residual type (analogous to symptomatic persistence). It should not be surprising that the inclusion of the less stringent definition of persistence resulted in higher rates in older subjects (see Fig. 1.3). Their meta-analysis found that, of children diagnosed with ADHD during childhood, 62% will continue to be symptomatic although only 19% would continue to meet full diagnostic criteria at age 25.

Although high rates of syndromatic remission indicate that individuals with ADHD frequently lose full diagnostic status, these figures may be misleading because they cannot distinguish individuals who fall just below the diagnostic threshold from those with very few active symptoms of the disorder. It is technically correct that those diagnosed with

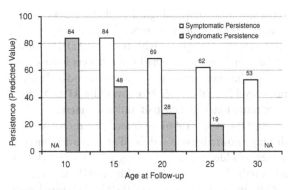

Figure 1.3 Predicted rate of persistence in follow-up studies of ADHD children.

ADHD in childhood who reach adulthood with one less symptom of the disorder may no longer satisfy criteria for ADHD, but it is clinically dubious to equate the absence of full syndromatic status with full recovery.

Thus, as expected from the work of Fischer (1997) and Biederman et al. (2000), the apparent prognosis of ADHD depends on what definition of persistence one uses. Our work examining differential rates of decline of ADHD symptom cores indicates that the choice of definition should be influenced by an individual's age and developmental expectations regarding hyperactivity, impulsivity, and inattention.

Clinical significance of ADHD in adults

If adult ADHD is a clinically significant disorder, then adults with ADHD should show functional impairments in multiple domains. Several studies suggest this to be the case. In an early study, Borland and Heckman (1976) compared ADHD adults with their non-ADHD siblings. The ADHD adults had lower socioeconomic status, more work difficulties, and more frequent job changes. Morrison (1980a, 1980b) compared ADHD adults with psychiatric controls matched for age and sex. The ADHD adults had fewer years of education and lower rates of professional employment. Similarly, others have shown that, among patients with substance use disorders, ADHD predicts social maladjustment, immaturity, fewer social assets, lower occupational achievement, and high rates of separation and divorce (Alterman et al., 1982; Eyre et al., 1982; De Obaldia & Parsons, 1984; Tarter, 1982; Wilens et al., 1998).

Murphy and Barkley (1996) compared 172 ADHD adults with 30 non-ADHD adults. The ADHD adults reported more psychological maladjustment, more speeding violations, and more frequent changes in employment. Compared with the non-ADHD adults, more ADHD adults had had their drivers license suspended, had performed poorly at work, and had quit or been fired from their job. Moreover, the ADHD adults were more likely to have had multiple marriages.

Barkley et al. (1996) evaluated the motor vehicle driving knowledge and skills and negative driving outcomes of older teens and young adults with ADHD. Although the young adults with ADHD showed no deficits in driving knowledge, they had elevated rates of speeding citations, suspended licenses, crashes, and accidents causing bodily injury compared to those without ADHD. They were more likely to be rated by themselves and others as having poorer driving habits. In addition, on a computer-simulated driving test, young adults with ADHD had more crashes, scrapes, and erratic steering.

Given that academic underachievement is a well-known correlate of ADHD in childhood (Hinshaw, 1992), ADHD adults ought to have histories reflecting school problems. Several studies have shown this to be so. Our work demonstrated that, compared with control adults, ADHD adults had significantly higher rates of repeated grades, tutoring, placement in special classes, and reading disability. Similarly, Murphy and Barkley (1996) showed that adults with ADHD had histories marked by poorer educational performance and more frequent school disciplinary actions against them. Notably, in addition to showing an increased likelihood of having a history of school failure, Seidman et al. (1998) demonstrated that this history could not be accounted for by age, learning disabilities, psychiatric comorbidity, or gender.

We recently conducted a survey of 1000 ADHD and non-ADHD adults in the United States (Biederman et al., 2006). This survey, which had the largest sample of community-diagnosed adults with ADHD ever studied, showed that adults with self-reported ADHD in the community suffer from significant impairments across multiple domains of functioning. We found adult ADHD to be associated with histories of school failure, occupational impairment, substance use, traffic violations, arrests, decreased quality of life, and sexual problems. Taken together, these findings support the idea that, even in those adults diagnosed in the community, ADHD is a clinically significant and highly disabling disorder (Biederman et al., 2006).

Impact of treatment on course

Although there is a wealth of research on the efficacy of pharmacotherapy in treating symptoms of ADHD (Spencer et al., 1996, 2002), we do not know if treatment during childhood has an impact on the symptomatic or functional remission from the disorder as described here. In fact we are unable to assess the impact of treatment in the short or long term in naturalistic studies because exposure to therapy is not randomly assigned (Faraone et al., 1992). Observational research of treatment efficacy is often misleading because of confounding by indication: a situation in which severely ill patients are more likely to receive treatment so that aggressive therapy appears to be inversely associated with improvement solely due to the inability to control the allocation of treatment.

For example, subjects likely to be among remitters may be likely to receive therapy for a shorter duration because their symptoms have remitted, whereas those with persistent symptoms are more likely to have been exposed to a longer period of treatment. Under this reasonable assumption, naturalistic studies would clearly show that treatment is inversely associated with rates of remission. Research is needed that examines both the motivation for continued treatment in naturalistic follow-up studies and the impact of therapy in subjects treated in a randomized clinical trial over the long term.

Summary

At any age, ADHD may be considered a chronic disorder because its symptoms may persist for a long period of time and over a wide range of settings. The use of more developmentally appropriate measures of ADHD in adolescents and adults reveals that a sizable proportion of children with the disorder will continue to exhibit impairing symptoms of the disorder into adulthood. The impact of ADHD on society is enormous in terms of financial cost, stress to families, impact on academic and vocational activities, as well as negative effects on self-esteem. Because the disorder is not episodic but frequently chronic, ADHD may be a relatively common psychiatric disorder of adulthood in reference to other disorders.

References

Alterman AI, Petrarulo E, et al. (1982). Hyperactivity and alcoholism: familial and behavioral correlates. *Addict Behav* 7:413–21.

American Psychiatric Association. (1968). *Diagnostic and Statistical Manual of Mental Disorders*. 2nd ed. Washington, DC: American Psychiatric Association.

American Psychiatric Association. (1980). *Diagnostic and Statistical Manual of Mental Disorders*. 3rd ed. Washington, DC: American Psychiatric Association.

American Psychiatric Association. (1987). *Diagnostic and Statistical Manual of Mental Disorders*. 3rd ed. rev. Washington, DC: American Psychiatric Association.

American Psychiatric Association. (1994). *Diagnostic and Statistical Manual of Mental Disorders*. 4th ed. Washington, DC: American Psychiatric Association.

August GJ, Stewart MA, et al. (1983). A four-year follow-up of hyperactive boys with and without conduct disorder. *Br J Psychiatry* 143:192–8.

Barkley RA, Fischer M, Edelbrock CS, Smallish L. (1990). The adolescent outcome of hyperactive children diagnosed by research criteria: I. An 8-year prospective follow-up study. *J Am Acad Child Adolesc Psychiatry* 29(4):546–57.

Barkley RA, Fischer M, Smallish L, Fletcher K. (2002). The persistence of attention-deficit/hyperactivity disorder into young adulthood as a function of reporting source and definition of disorder. *J Abnorm Psychol* 111(2):279–89.

Barkley R, Murphy K, Kwasnik D. (1996). Motor vehicle driving competencies and risks in teens and young adults with attention deficit hyperactivity disorder. *Pediatrics* 98(6):1089–95.

Biederman J, Faraone SV, Milberger S, Curtis S, Chen L, Marrs A, et al. (1996). Predictors of persistence and remission of ADHD: results from a four-year prospective follow-up study of ADHD children. *J Am Acad Child Adolesc Psychiatry* 35(3): 343–51.

Biederman J, Faraone SV, Spencer TJ, Mick E, Monuteaux MC, Aleardi M. (2006). Functional impairments in adults with self-reports of diagnosed ADHD: a controlled study of 1001 adults in the community. *J Clin Psychiatry* 67(4):524–40.

Biederman, J, Faraone SV, Spencer T, Wilens T, Mick E, Lapey KA. (1994). Gender differences in a sample of adults with attention deficit hyperactivity disorder. *Psychiatry Research* 53(1):13–29.

Biederman J, Mick E, Faraone SV. (2000). Age-dependent decline of symptoms of attention deficit hyperactivity disorder: Impact of remission definition and symptom type. *Am J Psychiatry* 157(5):816–8.

Biederman J, Monuteaux MC, Mick E, Spencer T, Wilens TE, Klein KL, et al. (2006). Psychopathology in females with attention-deficit/hyperactivity disorder: a controlled, five-year prospective study. *Biol Psychiatry* 60(10):1098–105.

Biederman J, Monuteaux MC, Mick E, Spencer T, Wilens TE, Silva JM, Snyder LE, Faraone SV. (2006). Young adult outcome of attention deficit hyperactivity disorder: a controlled 10 year prospective follow-up study. *Psychol Med* 36(2):167–79.

Borland BL, Heckman HK. (1976). Hyperactive boys and their brothers: a 25-year follow-up study. *Arch Gen Psychiatry* 33:669–75.

Cantwell DP, Baker L. (1989). Stability and natural history of DSM-III childhood diagnoses. *J Am Acad Child Adolesc Psychiatry* 28(5):691–700.

Claude D, Firestone P. (1995). The development of ADHD boys: a 12-year follow-up. *Can J Behav Sci* 27(2): 226–49.

De Obaldia R, Parsons O. (1984). Relationship of neuropsychological performance to primary alcoholism and self-reported symptoms of childhood minimal brain dysfunction. *J Stud Alcohol* 45(5):386–91.

Eyre S, Rounsaville BJ, Kleber HD. (1982). History of childhood hyperactivity in a clinical population of opiate addicts. *J Nerv Ment Dis* 170(9):522–29.

Faraone, S., J. Biederman, Mick E. (2006). The age dependent decline of attention-deficit/hyperactivity disorder: a meta-analysis of follow-up studies. *Psychol Med* 36(2):159–65.

Faraone SV, Simpson JC, Brown WA. (1992). Mathematical models of complex dose-response relationships: implications for experimental design in psychopharmacologic research. *Stat Med* 11: 685–702.

Feldman S, Denhoff E, et al. (1979). The attention disorders and related syndromes: Outcome in adolescent and young adult life. In: Denhoff E, Stern L, eds. *Minimal Brain Dysfunction: A Developmental Approach*. New York: Masson: 133–48.

Fischer M. (1997). The persistence of ADHD into adulthood: it depends on whom you ask. *ADHD Rep* 5:8–10.

Gittelman R, Mannuzza S, Shenker R, Bonagura N. (1985). Hyperactive boys almost grown up: I. Psychiatric status. *Arch Gen Psychiatry* 42:937–47.

Hart EL, Lahey BB, Loeber R, Applegate B, Frick PJ. (1995). Developmental change in attention-deficit hyperactivity disorder in boys: a four-year longitudinal study. *J Abnorm Child Psychol* 23(6):729–49.

Hill J, Schoener E. (1996). Age-dependent decline of attention deficit hyperactivity disorder. *Am J Psychiatry* 153(9):1143–6.

Hinshaw SP. (1992). Externalizing behavior problems and academic underachievement in childhood and adolescence: causal relationships and underlying mechanisms. *Psychol Bull* 111(1):127–55.

Lambert NM. (1988). Adolescent outcomes for hyperactive children: perspectives on general and specific patterns of childhood risk for adolescent educational, social and mental health problems. *Am Psychol* **43**(10):786–99.

Lambert NM, Hartsough CS, Sassone D, Sandoval J. (1987). Persistence of hyperactivity symptoms from childhood to adolescence and associated outcomes. *Am J Orthopsychiatry* **57**(1):22–32.

Mannuzza S, Gittelman R. (1984). The adolescent outcome of hyperactive girls. *Psychiatry Res* **13**:19–29.

Mannuzza S, Klein RG, Bonagura N, Malloy P, Giampino TL, Addalli KA. (1991). Hyperactive boys almost grown up: V. Replication of psychiatric status. *Arch Gen Psychiatry* **48**(1):77–83.

Mannuzza S, Klein RG, Bessler A, Malloy P, LaPadula M. (1993). Adult outcome of hyperactive boys: educational achievement, occupational rank and psychiatric status. *Arch Gen Psychiatry* **50**:565–76.

Mannuzza S, Klein RG, Bessler A, Malloy P, LaPadula M. (1998). Adult psychiatric status of hyperactive boys grown up. *Am J Psychiatry* **155**(4):493–8.

Mendelson W, Johnson N, Stewart MA. (1971). Hyperactive children as teenagers: a follow-up study. *J Nerv Ment Dis* **153**(4):273–9.

Morrison JR. (1980a). Adult psychiatric disorders in parents of hyperactive children. *Am J Psychiatry* **137**:825–7.

Morrison JR. (1980b). Childhood hyperactivity in an adult psychiatric population: social factors. *J Clin Psychiatry* **41**(2):40–3.

Murphy K, Barkley RA. (1996). Attention deficit hyperactivity disorder adults: comorbidities and adaptive impairments. *Compr Psychiatry* **37**(6): 393–401.

Offord DR, Boyle MH, Racine YA, Fleming JE, Cadman DT, Blum HM, et al. (1992). Outcome, prognosis and risk in a longitudinal follow-up study. *J Am Acad Child Adolesc Psychiatry* **31**(5):916–23.

Rasmussen P, Gillberg C. (2000). Natural outcome of ADHD with developmental coordination disorder at age 22 years: a controlled, longitudinal, community-based study." *J Am Acad Child Adolesc Psychiatry* **39**(11):1424–31.

Seidman LJ, Biederman J, Weber W, Hatch M, Faraone SV. (1998). Neuropsychological function in adults with attention-deficit hyperactivity disorder. *Biol Psychiatry* **44**(4):260–8.

Spencer TJ, Biederman J, Wilens TE, Faraone SV. (2002). Novel treatments for attention-deficit/hyperactivity disorder in children. *J Clin Psychiatry* **63**(suppl 12):16–22.

Spencer T, Biederman J, Wilens T, Harding M, O'Donnell D, Griffin S. (1996). Pharmacotherapy of attention deficit hyperactivity disorder across the lifecycle: a literature review. *J Am Acad Child Adolesc Psychiatry* **35**(4):409–32.

Tarter RE. (1982). Psychosocial history, minimal brain dysfunction and differential drinking patterns of male alcoholics. *J Clin Psychol* **38**(4):867–73.

Weiss G, Hechtman L, Milroy T, Perlman T. (1985). Psychiatric status of hyperactives as adults: a controlled prospective 15-year follow-up of 63 hyperactive children. *J Am Acad Child Adolesc Psychiatry* **24**(2):211–20.

Wilens TE, Biederman J, Mick E. (1998). Does ADHD affect the course of substance abuse? Findings from a sample of adults with and without ADHD. *Am J Addict* **7**:156–63.

Yan W. (1996). An investigation of adult outcome of hyperactive children in Shanghai. *Chin Med J* **109**(11):877–80.

Chapter

2

The prevalence and correlates of adult ADHD

Ronald C. Kessler, Leonard A. Adler, Russell Barkley, Joseph Biederman, C. Keith Conners, Laurence L. Greenhill, and Thomas Spencer

It has long been known that attention-deficit/hyperactivity disorder (ADHD) is one of the most common psychiatric disorders among children (Bird et al., 1988; Shekim et al., 1985). However, there is much less agreement about the extent to which ADHD persists into adulthood. Indeed, some authors state that adult ADHD is very rare (Shaffer, 1994), whereas others report that it is quite common (Barkley, 1997). The claim that adult ADHD is rare can be traced to theoretical discussions about the role of maturation in resolving childhood impulsivity (Cantwell, 1985). The empirical study that is consistently cited to support this claim is the influential meta-analysis carried out by Hill and Schoener (1996) of nine prospective studies of children who were diagnosed with ADHD and then followed between 4 and 16 years. The aim of the meta-analysis was to develop a mathematical model of the extent to which ADHD prevalence decreases with age. The nonlinear model developed by Hill and Schoener to fit the data in these nine studies estimated that ADHD prevalence decreases by approximately 50% every 5 years. Based on the assumption that ADHD prevalence is 4% in childhood, this model predicted that prevalence at age 40 would only be a fraction of 1%.

Subsequent critiques have argued that several methodological factors (e.g. small number of studies, nonrepresentative studies, inappropriate statistical model, sample attrition, reporting bias) introduced imprecision and potential bias into the Hill and Schoener estimates of ADHD persistence (Mannuzza, Klein, & Moulton, 2003; Sawilowsky & Musial, 1988). Leaving aside issues of change in diagnostic criteria and sample selection bias, which are endemic to adult follow-up studies of children diagnosed with ADHD in the past, the key issue in these critiques is whether to require adults to meet full diagnostic criteria or to

have only some symptoms to be counted as cases. In their meta-analysis Hill and Schoener required adults to meet full diagnostic criteria, resulting in adults who had ADHD as children being classified as "remitted" even if they continued to have seriously impairing symptoms. An indication of how critical this distinction is can be seen in a subsequent short-term follow-up study of an ADHD patient sample, which found that, although only 38% of cases continued to meet full criteria for ADHD at age 19, 90% continued to have clinically significant impairment associated with remaining symptoms (Biederman, Mick, & Faraone, 2000).

Uncertainty about diagnostic criteria

It is important to note in this regard that diagnostic criteria for ADHD have never been developed specifically for adults, making it unclear what it means to meet "full criteria" for adult ADHD. In *DSM-III*, the category of residual attention-deficit disorder was defined to include adults who met full criteria for the disorder as children and have a partial syndrome as adults, but this category was removed from *DSM-III-R*. Meanwhile, a number of clinical research groups have proposed that the distribution of the three cardinal symptom clusters found among children – inattention, hyperactivity, and impulsivity – shifts in adulthood so that inattention becomes the most prominent symptom cluster, and other symptoms, such as affective lability, explosive temper, inability to tolerate stress, and dysphoria, emerge as more prominent than in childhood (Riccio et al., 2005; Wender et al., 1985). Based on this change in symptom presentation, experts agree that more research is needed to develop valid diagnostic criteria for adult ADHD (Adler & Cohen, 2004; McGough & Barkley, 2004; Wender, Wolf, & Wasserstein, 2001).

ADHD in Adults: Characterization, Diagnosis and Treatment, ed. Jan Buitelaar, Cornelis Kan and Philip Asherson.
Published by Cambridge University Press. © Cambridge University Press 2011.

In light of this uncertainty about diagnostic criteria, a legitimate question can be raised whether adult ADHD is a genuine disorder. The data are quite compelling that it is. This conclusion is based both on (1) clinical evidence that diagnosis, albeit fettered with the conceptual problems described in the last paragraph, is of considerable value in predicting symptom persistence and progression, severity, and treatment response, and on (2) evidence of genetic transmission and abnormalities in brain structure and function (Resnick, 2005; Seidman, Valera, & Makris, 2005; Wilens, Faraone, & Biederman, 2004).

Indirect assessments of prevalence

Given that ADHD is a genuine adult disorder, how common is ADHD in adulthood? The answer is clouded by the uncertainty associated with diagnostic issues. Because of this uncertainty, none of the many adult community psychiatric epidemiological surveys carried out over the past two decades with either the Diagnostic Interview Schedule (Robins et al., 1981) or the Composite International Diagnostic Interview (CIDI; Robins et al., 1988) included an assessment of adult ADHD. As a result, little is known about the general population epidemiology of adult manifestations of this disorder. Attempts to estimate prevalence by extrapolation from childhood prevalence estimates in conjunction with adult persistence estimates (Barkley et al., 2002; Biederman et al., 2000; Mannuzza et al., 1988; Weiss et al., 1985) or by direct estimation from small sample of adults (Murphy & Barkley, 1996) or of college students (Heiligenstein et al., 1998) have yielded prevalence estimates ranging from 1–6%. However, these estimates are all based on convenience samples.

One way to obtain a more accurate prevalence estimate would be to build on a more firm set of estimates from previous studies that linked information about prevalence in childhood with information about persistence into adulthood. Faraone and his colleagues recently reported the results of a comprehensive meta-analysis of all published follow-up studies of ADHD; it provides the best currently available estimate of persistence into adulthood (Faraone, Biederman, & Mick, 2006). This study, which was carried out along the same lines as the Hill and Schoener meta-analysis (1996), deviated from the earlier approach in distinguishing between syndromal and subsyndromal persistence of adult ADHD. The analysis showed that,

whereas only a relatively small proportion of cases (approximately 15%) in the studies examined continued to meet full criteria for ADHD in adulthood, a majority (approximately two-thirds) continued to have enough symptoms and impairment to qualify for a *DSM-IV* diagnosis of ADHD in partial remission.

The population prevalence of broadly defined ADHD at age 25, then, might be expected to be roughly two-thirds as high as the prevalence in childhood, although caution is needed in making this extrapolation based on the fact that the follow-up studies examined by Faraone et al. (2006) included clinical samples in which the most serious childhood cases are presumably overrepresented. This factor is important because severity of childhood symptoms strongly predicts adult ADHD persistence (Kessler, Adler, Barkley, et al., 2005). A further complication in using this indirect way to estimate the prevalence of adult ADHD is that prevalence estimates of childhood ADHD have an extremely wide range – from as low at 1.5% to as high as 19.8% (Cuffe et al., 2001; Cuffe, Moore, & McKeown, 2005; Faraone et al., 2003; Pastor & Reuben, 2005). If we take the median of the range, which is 7–9%, we would predict that the prevalence of adult ADHD would be roughly 5–6%, but this could be an overestimate for the reason described in the first part of this paragraph.

Screening assessments of prevalence

Two recent reports described the results of general population surveys that attempted to screen for adult ADHD (Faraone & Biederman, 2005; Kooij et al., 2005). Faraone and Biederman (2005) carried out a telephone survey with 966 adults in the United States that used semi-structured research clinical interviews to assess adult ADHD using *DSM-IV* criteria. The authors estimated that 2.9% of respondents met full *DSM-IV* criteria for ADHD and that 16.4% met subthreshold criteria. Kooij et al. (2005) carried out a self-report survey of a representative sample of 1813 adults selected from an automated general practitioner registry in the Netherlands. They used a fully structured questionnaire to estimate the prevalence of adult ADHD. No clinical follow-up interviews were carried out to validate these self-reports. The authors estimated the prevalence of adult ADHD to be 1.0% when full *DSM-IV* criteria were required and 2.5% when the diagnosis was relaxed to require four rather than six current symptoms.

A direct assessment of prevalence

The NCS-R

The only published adult ADHD prevalence study that was based on a nationally representative general population sample with clinical calibration was carried out in conjunction with the US National Comorbidity Survey Replication (NCS-R; Kessler & Merikangas, 2004). A fully structured retrospective assessment of childhood ADHD and a fully structured screen for adult ADHD were both developed for use in the NCS-R as part of the revised WMH-CIDI (World Mental Health-CIDI; Kessler & Ustun, 2004). These assessments were administered face-to-face to a nationally representative sample of 3,199 people in the age range of 18–44 as part of the larger NCS-R interview. In addition, blinded clinical reappraisal follow-up interviews to diagnose adult ADHD were carried out with a probability subsample of 154 NCS-R respondents, thereby oversampling those who met criteria for adult ADHD in the fully structured assessment (Kessler, Adler, Ames, et al., 2005). Other *DSM-IV* diagnoses made in this sample with the CIDI included anxiety disorders (panic disorder, generalized anxiety disorder, agoraphobia without panic disorder, specific phobia, social phobia, post traumatic stress disorder, obsessive-compulsive disorder), mood disorders (major depressive disorder, dysthymia, bipolar disorder I or II), impulse-control disorders (oppositional-defiant disorder, conduct disorder, intermittent explosive disorder), and substance use disorders (alcohol and drug abuse and dependence).

Multiple imputation

An innovative method was used in the NCS-R to estimate the prevalence of clinician-assessed *DSM-IV* adult ADHD in the total US population aged 18–44; it took into consideration the prevalence estimate in the small clinical reappraisal, the strength of the association between the fully structured assessment and the clinical assessment in the clinical reappraisal subsample, and the distribution of responses to the structured questions in the full sample. This method, known as multiple imputation (MI; Rubin, 1987), first assigned predicted probabilities of meeting *DSM-IV* criteria for a diagnosis of adult ADHD to each respondent in the sample who did not participate in the clinical reappraisal study, based on the results of logistic regression analysis carried out in the clinical reappraisal subsample that linked responses to the fully structured questions with clinical diagnoses. After these predicted probabilities were assigned, the probability was transformed to a dichotomous case classification separately for each respondent by random selection from the binomial distribution for the predicted probability.

Estimated prevalence

A strong predictive association was found in the clinical reappraisal subsample between responses to the structured questions and the clinical diagnoses of adult ADHD (with a 0.86 area under the receiver operator characteristic curve [AUC]), thereby justifying the use of the imputation method described earlier. However, this method clearly leads to errors in classification because the AUC is less than 1.0. Although the imputation nonetheless yields an unbiased estimate of prevalence and generally conservative estimates of associations, this imprecision increases the standard error of the prevalence estimate. The MI method deals with this problem by using simulation to estimate standard errors of parameter estimates. This is done by repeating the entire imputation process a number of times (10 times in the NCS-R application), beginning with the selection of a new pseudo-sample of size 154 for each replicate from the clinical reappraisal subsample and reestimation of parameter values for the prediction equation. All substantive analyses of the data were then replicated 10 times, once for each set of imputations, and the standard errors of descriptive statistics were calculated empirically by combining information about the average within-replicate variance in the parameter estimates with information about between-replicate variance in the parameter estimates.

The vast majority of NCS-R respondents in the age range 18–44 (Table 2.1, Column I) reported that they had no clinically significant problems with inattention, hyperactivity, or impulsivity during their childhood (85.8%). Smaller percentages reported either sub-threshold childhood symptoms of ADHD (7.5%), full childhood criteria but no current symptoms (4.0%), or full childhood criteria in addition to current symptoms (2.6%). A strong monotonic relationship was found between this four-category WMH-CIDI classification scheme and blind clinical diagnoses of adult ADHD in the clinical calibration sample (Table 2.1, Column II). The MI-estimated prevalence of adult ADHD based on the 10 imputed case classifications of adult ADHD (standard error in parentheses) is 4.4%

Table 2.1 Distribution of adult ADHD imputation classes in the NCS-R[1] and conditional prevalence of clinician-rated adult ADHD in the clinical reappraisal subsample

ADHD risk	Total sample distribution		Conditional prevalence of adult ADHD in the clinical reappraisal subsample	
	%	(se)	%	(se)
None	85.8	(0.8)	0.0	–
Low	7.5	(0.5)	7.3	(6.4)
Medium	4.0	(0.4)	36.6	(8.9)
High	2.6	(0.4)	84.8	(7.7)
Total	100.0		4.4	(0.6)
(n)	(3199)	(154)		

[1] Part II respondents aged 18–44.

Table 2.2 Impairments in 30-day functioning associated with adult ADHD in the NCS-R[1]

	%[2]	(se)[2]	OR[3]	(95% CI)[3]
I. Basic functioning				
Self-care	7.6	(2.7)	2.2*	(1.0–4.8)
Mobility	26.7	(4.7)	3.9*	(2.3–6.8)
Cognition	29.9	(5.3)	2.6*	(1.5–4.5)
II. Instrumental functioning				
Time out of role	38.3	(4.9)	2.7*	(1.8–4.1)
Productive role functioning	35.0	(4.6)	2.1*	(1.4–3.2)
Social role functioning	18.6	(3.5)	3.5*	(2.1–5.9)

* Significant at the 0.05 level, two-sided design-based MI tests.
[1] Part II respondents aged 18–44.
[2] Percent (standard error) of adults with ADHD who have the impairment.
[3] Based on bivariate logistic regression analysis using MI to estimate odds ratios (ORs) and 95% confidence intervals (95% CI).

(0.6). It is noteworthy that exactly the same estimated prevalence and standard error are obtained by using a more conventional two-stage sampling adjustment.

Socio-demographic correlates

As the NCS-R sample is quite large, it was possible to go beyond simple estimation of prevalence to consider correlates of adult ADHD. ADHD was estimated to be significantly more prevalent among men than women, people with low compared to high education and family income, unmarried compared to married people, and unemployed compared to employed people (Kessler, Adler, Barkley, et al., 2006). The odds ratios (ORs) associated with these predictors were all found to be moderate in size (1.7–2.4). The strongest socio-demographic correlate of adult ADHD in the NCS-R was race-ethnicity, with non-Hispanic Blacks having significantly lower odds of the disorder than non-Hispanic Whites (0.3). No significant associations were found with age (in the 18–44 age range), region of the country, or urbanicity. The absence of an association with age is especially striking in light of the suggestion based on the Hill and Schoener (1996) meta-analysis that the prevalence of ADHD decreases by 50% every 5 years. The nationally representative NCS-R results show clearly that no such decline exists in the general population.

Comorbidity with other DSM-IV disorders

Statistically significant comorbodities were found in the NCS-R between adult ADHD and a wide range of other *DSM-IV*/CIDI anxiety, mood, impulse-control, and substance use disorders (Kessler, Adler, Barkley, et al., 2006). ORs were generally somewhat larger for comorbidities with 12-month than with lifetime disorders, suggesting indirectly that adult ADHD is associated with these disorders being somewhat more persistent than otherwise. ORs with 12-month disorders were in the range of 3.3–6.1 for mood disorders, 2.6–5.3 for anxiety disorders, 2.1–14.9 for substance disorders, and 3.8–9.8 for impulse-control disorders. Very strong ORs with 12-month drug dependence (14.9) and oppositional-defiant disorder (9.8) were especially noteworthy.

Associations with basic and instrumental functioning

Adult ADHD was found in the NCS-R to be significantly associated with serious difficulties in all three areas of basic functioning assessed in the WHO Disability Assessment Schedule (WHO-DAS; Chwastiak & Von Korff, 2003): self-care, mobility, and cognition (Table 2.2). ORs of these impairments for people with adult ADHD versus without adult ADHD were in the range of 2.2. Adult ADHD was also found in the NCS-R to be significantly related to all three WHO-DAS measures of disability in instrumental functioning: elevated odds of high days out of role (2.7), high impairment in productive role functioning (2.1), and high impairment in social role functioning (3.5).

Table 2.3 Twelve-month treatment among respondents with adult ADHD in the NCS-R[1]

	%	(se)
Specialty	25.9	4.4
General medical	18.8	3.4
Human services	7.4	1.5
CAM[2]	18.4	5.1
Any treatment	42.4	4.4

[1] Part II respondents aged 18–44
[2] Complementary and alternative medicine.

Associations with work performance

The NCS-R analysis also examined associations of adult ADHD with work performance (Kessler, Adler, Barkley, et al., 2005). The prevalence of ADHD among employed people (4.2) was found to be roughly comparable to prevalence in the total population, although it was higher among male than female workers and among blue-collar than white-collar workers. An analysis of work performance based on the WHO Health and Work Performance Questionnaire (Kessler, Ames, et al., 2004; Kessler, Barber, et al., 2003) showed that ADHD was associated with an enormous amount of work role impairment. At the individual level, workers with ADHD were estimated to have an annual average of 35 more lost work performance days than comparable (in terms of socio-demographics and job requirements) workers without ADHD. This negative impact of ADHD on work performance was especially pronounced among blue-collar workers, who had an annual average excess of 56 lost work performance days). At the population level, these adverse workplace effects of ADHD were projected to total 120 million lost work days and $19.5 billion lost human capital annually in the United States.

Treatment

Of respondents with adult ADHD in the NCS-R, 42.4% reported that they received treatment for problems with their mental health or substance problems at some time in the 12 months before the NCS-R interview (Table 2.3). The majority of these respondents (25.9% of all respondents with the disorder) were seen in the mental health specialty sector. A significantly higher proportion of females than males with adult ADHD received treatment for mental or substance problems in the 12 months before the interview (53.1% vs. 36.5%, $z = 2.6, p = 0.014$). However, comparison of reports about disorder-specific and overall treatment showed that only 25.2% of treated cases were receiving treatment for their symptoms of ADHD (22.8% of females vs. 27.7% of males, $z = 0.5, p = 0.598$). Because of this low proportion, only 10.9% of respondents with adult ADHD received treatment for ADHD in the 12 months before the interview (12.1% of females vs. 10.1% of males, $z = 0.4, p = 0.657$).

Is adult ADHD more prevalent in the United States than elsewhere in the world?

The vast majority of clinical and community epidemiological research on ADHD has been carried out in the United States, leading to an impression that ADHD is more common in the United States than in other countries (Taylor & Sandberg, 1984). However, comparative studies of the factor structure of self-reported ADHD symptoms among children in several English-speaking countries (United States, Canada, United Kingdom, Australia, and New Zealand) have found both comparable factor structures and comparable symptom prevalence estimates (Taylor, 1986; Taylor & Sandberg, 1984). A recent comprehensive review of the estimated prevalence of childhood ADHD in 50 published studies from around the world (20 in the United States and 30 in all other countries combined) concluded that the prevalence of ADHD is at least as high in some other countries as in the United States (Faraone et al., 2003).

But what of the worldwide prevalence of adult ADHD? The evidence is too scant to make an informed statement. Indeed, the only published community prevalence study of adult ADHD outside the United States is the Kooij et al. (2005) study from the Netherlands that we cited earlier. However, additional information will soon be available from the WHO WMH Survey Initiative (Demyttenaere et al., 2004), which is a series of nationally representative general population epidemiological surveys of mental disorders that were carried out in nearly 30 countries around the world (see www.hcp.med.harvard.edu/wmh). The same assessment of adult ADHD as in the NCS-R was included in a number of the WMH surveys. Although most of these surveys are still in progress, plans exist to replicate the NCS-R analyses once data become available from all of them.

Future directions

As demonstrated in this review, the epidemiological literature on adult ADHD is very limited. Only one nationally representative general population survey (the NCS-R) ever included a rigorous clinical assessment of adult ADHD. Even in that one study, the assessment did not consider ADHD in partial remission despite other evidence that that type might be considerably more common than syndromal adult ADHD (Faraone & Biederman, 2005; Faraone et al., 2006). The anticipated publication of results from the WHO World Mental Health surveys will go a long way in addressing the first of these problems, but will still not provide data on subsyndromal cases.

A more serious limitation of the existing literature is that uncertainties exist about the appropriate criteria for adult ADHD. The criteria for ADHD were developed with children in mind and offer only limited guidance regarding diagnosis of adults. This lack of guidance is of considerable concern because clinical studies make it clear that symptoms of ADHD are more heterogeneous and subtle in adults than in children (DeQuiros & Kinsbourne, 2001; Wender et al., 2001). As a result, many experts believe that the valid assessment of adult ADHD might require either an increase in the variety of symptoms assessed (Barkley, 1995), a reduction in the severity threshold for considering a symptom clinically significant (Ratey et al., 1992), or a reduction in the *DSM-IV* six-of-nine symptom requirement (McBurnett, 1997). This matter of appropriate diagnostic criteria needs to be settled before much progress can be made in epidemiological research.

Another important unresolved issue in the assessment of adult ADHD concerns the mode of assessment. Childhood ADHD is diagnosed largely on the basis of parent and teacher reports rather than self-reports because parents and teachers are both in good positions to observe child behavior and because children with ADHD often have little insight into the severity of their symptoms (Jensen et al., 1999). The situation is different for adults, for whom there is great variability in the extent to which other people observe their behavior and where access to reliable informants varies with the respondent's marital status, occupational status, and social networks; as a practical matter it is therefore necessary to base assessment largely on self-reports (Wender et al., 2001). As a result, epidemiological studies of adult ADHD have relied almost entirely on self-reports. This reliance might be problematic in that some methodological studies comparing adult self-reports versus informant reports of ADHD symptoms have documented a similar pattern of disagreement as in studies of child self-reports versus informant reports, with informants reporting higher symptom levels than focal respondents (Gittelman & Mannuzza, 1985; Zucker et al., 2002). This finding suggests that self-report scales might underestimate the true prevalence of adult ADHD. If so, a new paradigm for assessing adult ADHD might need to be developed.

This last issue could be very difficult to address because of the practical impossibility of obtaining informant reports on adult emotional functioning in representative community epidemiological surveys other than through reports provided by spouses; this difficulty is exacerbated by the fact that a comparatively high proportion of people with adult ADHD seem to be either separated or divorced. However, this concern has been somewhat lessened by the fact that the one methodological study of adult self versus informant ADHD symptom reports carried out in a nonclinical sample found fairly strong associations between the two reports and no self–informant difference in reported symptom severity (Murphy & Schachar, 2000).

This problem is presumably greater in obtaining retrospective adult assessments of childhood ADHD, which are required for a diagnosis of adult ADHD. There is good evidence, based on prospective studies that compare adult retrospective reports with baseline evaluations made in childhood, that such retrospective reports are often inaccurate in their particulars even when they are based on clinical interviews (Shaffer, 1994). Nonetheless, it is important to note that follow-up studies show that the vast majority of adults who were diagnosed with ADHD as children retrospectively report at least some symptoms of childhood ADHD (Mannuzza et al., 2002). A more serious problem might be that a meaningful minority of adults known not to have had hyperactivity in childhood retrospectively recalled that they had childhood symptoms of ADHD (Mannuzza et al. 2002). Methodological research is needed to sort out these uncertainties and thereby improve the validity of community epidemiological studies of adult ADHD.

An important opportunity for future epidemiological research on adult ADHD lies in studies of workplace prevalence and indirect costs. The NCS-R findings regarding the workplace costs of ADHD were remarkable: ADHD in the US labor force is associated with 120 million work loss days and an indirect human capital cost of $19.5 billion per year. Such striking results warrant further investigation. Over the past decade, employer interest in the indirect workplace costs of illness has led to a rapid expansion in epidemiological research on the prevalence and adverse workplace consequences of untreated worker health problems, as well as in cost-effective analyses from the employer perspective of targeted workplace health care interventions (Kessler & Stang, 2006). Depression has been the mental disorder of most interest to employers in this regard up to now (Stewart et al. 2003; Wang et al., 2004; Wang, Simon, & Kessler, 2003). However, if the NCS-R results are correct, then ADHD is actually more prevalent among workers than depression at any point in time; in other words, although a higher proportion of workers have depression than ADHD at some time in the year, ADHD is considerably more persistent than depression. Furthermore, the individual-level work impairments associated with ADHD seem to be greater than those associated with depression, especially among blue-collar workers. Given the recent advances in ADHD treatments that have the potential to reduce these work impairments substantially, ADHD in the workplace would seem to be an important target for future epidemiological investigation.

Acknowledgments

This chapter was prepared in conjunction with research on adult ADHD carried out in the US National Comorbidity Survey Replication (NCS-R). The NCS-R is supported by the US National Institute of Mental Health (U01-MH60220) with supplemental support from the US National Institute on Drug Abuse, the Substance Abuse and Mental Health Services Administration, the Robert Wood Johnson Foundation (Grant 044708), and the John W. Alden Trust. The NCS-A ADHD clinical reappraisal study was additionally supported by Eli Lilly and Company. A complete list of NCS publications and the full text of all NCS-R instruments can be found at http://www. hcp.med.harvard.edu/ncs. Send correspondence to ncs@hcp.med.harvard.edu.

The NCS-R is carried out in conjunction with the World Health Organization World Mental Health (WMH) Survey Initiative. We thank the staff of the WMH Data Collection and Data Analysis Coordination Centres for assistance with instrumentation, fieldwork, and consultation on data analysis. These activities were supported by the National Institute of Mental Health (R01 MH070884), the John D. and Catherine T. MacArthur Foundation, the Pfizer Foundation, the US Public Health Service (R13-MH066849, R01-MH069864, and R01 DA016558), the Fogarty International Center (FIRCA R01-TW006481), the Pan American Health Organization, Eli Lilly and Company, Ortho-McNeil Pharmaceutical, Inc., GlaxoSmithKline, and Bristol-Myers Squibb. A complete list of WMH publications can be found at http://www.hcp. med.harvard.edu/wmh.

References

Adler L, Cohen J. (2004). Diagnosis and evaluation of adults with attention-deficit/hyperactivity disorder. *Psychiatr Clin North Am* 27(2):187–201.

Barkley RA, Fischer M, Smallish L, Fletcher K. (2002). The persistence of attention-deficit/hyperactivity disorder into young adulthood as a function of reporting source and definition disorder. *J Abnorm Psychol* 111(2):279–89.

Barkley RA. (1995). ADHD behavior checklist for adults. *ADHD Rep* 3:16.

Barkley RA. (1997). Age dependent decline in ADHD: true recovery or statistical illusion? *ADHD Rep* 5: 1–5.

Biederman J, Mick E, Faraone SV. (2000). Age-dependent decline of symptoms of attention deficit hyperactivity disorder: impact of remission definition and symptom type. *Am J Psychiatry* 157(5):816–8.

Bird HR, Canino G, Rubio-Stipec M, Gould MS, Ribera J, Sesman M, et al. (1988). Estimates of the prevalence of childhood maladjustment in a community survey in Puerto Rico. The use of combined measures. *Arch Gen Psychiatry* 45(12):1120–6.

Cantwell DP. (1985). Hyperactive children have grown up. What have we learned about what happens to them? *Arch Gen Psychiatry* 42(10):1026–8.

Chwastiak LA, Von Korff M. (2003). Disability in depression and back pain: evaluation of the World Health Organization Disability Assessment Schedule (WHO-DAS-II) in a primary care setting. *J Clin Epidemiol* 56(6):507–14.

Cuffe SP, McKeown RE, Jackson KL, Addy CL, Abramson R, Garrison CZ. (2001). Prevalence of attention-deficit/hyperactivity disorder in a community sample of older adolescents. *J Am Acad Child Adolesc Psychiatry* 40(9):1037–44.

Cuffe SP, Moore CG, McKeown RE. (2005). Prevalence and correlates of ADHD symptoms in the national health interview survey. *J Atten Disord* 9(2):392–401.

Demyttenaere K, Bruffaerts R, Posada-Villa J, Gasquet I, Kovess V, Lepine JP, et al. (2004). Prevalence, severity, and unmet need for treatment of mental disorders in the World Health Organization World Mental Health surveys. *JAMA* 291(21):2581–90.

DeQuiros GB, Kinsbourne M. (2001). Adult ADHD: analysis of self-ratings in a behavior questionnaire. *Ann N Y Acad Sci* 931:140–7.

Faraone SV, Biederman J. (2005). What is the prevalence of adult ADHD? Results of a population screen of 966 adults. *J Atten Disord* 9(2):384–91.

Faraone SV, Biederman J, Mick E. (2006). The age-dependent decline of attention deficit hyperactivity disorder: a meta-analysis of follow-up studies. *Psychol Med* 36(2):159–65.

Faraone SV, Sergean J, Gillberg C, Biederman J. (2003). The worldwide prevalence of ADHD: is it an American condition? *World Psychiatry* 2(2):104–13.

Gittelman R, Mannuzza S. (1985). Diagnosing ADD-H in adolescents. *Psychopharmacol Bull* 21(2):237–42.

Heiligenstein E, Conyers LM, Berns AR, Miller MA, Smith MA. (1998). Preliminary normative data on DSM-IV attention deficit hyperactivity disorder in college students. *J Am Coll Health* 46(4):185–8.

Hill JC, Schoener EP. (1996). Age-dependent decline of attention deficit hyperactivity disorder. *Am J Psychiatry* 153(9):1143–6.

Jensen PS, Rubio-Stipec M, Canino G, Bird HR, Dulcan MK, Schwab-Stone ME, et al. (1999). Parent and child contributions to diagnosis of mental disorder: are both informants always necessary? *J Am Acad Child Adolesc Psychiatry* 38(12):1569–79.

Kessler RC, Adler L, Ames M, Barkley RA, Birnbaum HG, Greenberg PE, et al. (2005). The prevalence and effects of adult attention-deficit/hyperactivity disorder on work performance in a nationally representative sample of workers. *J Occup Environ Med* 47(6):565–72.

Kessler RC, Adler L, Ames M, Demler O, Faraone S, Hiripi E, et al. (2005). The World Health Organization Adult ADHD Self-Report Scale (ASRS): a short screening scale for use in the general population. *Psychol Med* 35(2):245–56.

Kessler RC, Adler L, Barkley RA, Biederman J, Connors K, Demler O, et al. (2006). The prevalence and correlates of adult ADHD in the United States: results from the National Comorbidity Survey Replication. *Am J Psychiatry* 163(4):716–23.

Kessler RC, Adler LA, Barkley R, Biederman J, Conners CK, Faraone SV, et al. (2005). Patterns and predictors of attention-deficit/hyperactivity disorder persistence into adulthood: results from the National Comorbidity Survey Replication. *Biol Psychiatry* 57(11):1442–51.

Kessler RC, Ames M, Hymel PA, Loeppke R, McKenas DK, Richling D, et al. (2004). Using the WHO Health and Work Performance Questionnaire (HPQ) to evaluate the indirect workplace costs of illness. *J Occup Environ Med* 46:s23–7.

Kessler RC, Barber C, Beck A, Berglund PA, Cleary PD, McKenas D, et al. (2003). The World Health Organization Health and Work Performance Questionnaire (HPQ). *J Occup Environ Med* 45(2):156–74.

Kessler RC, Merikangas KR. (2004). The National Comorbidity Survey Replication (NCS-R): background and aims. *Int J Methods Psychiatr Res* 13(2):60–8.

Kessler RC, Stang PE, eds. (2006). *Health and Work Productivity: Making the Business Case for Quality Health Care*. Chicago: University of Chicago Press.

Kessler RC, Ustun TB. (2004). The World Mental Health (WMH) Survey Initiative version of the World Health Organization (WHO) Composite International Diagnostic Interview (CIDI). *Int J Methods Psychiatr Res* 13(2):93–121.

Kooij JJ, Buitelaar JK, Van Den Oord EJ, Furer JW, Rijnders CA, Hodiamont PP. (2005). Internal and external validity of attention-deficit hyperactivity disorder in a population-based sample of adults. *Psychol Med* 35(6):817–27.

Mannuzza S, Klein RG, Bessler A, Malloy P, LaPadula M. (1998). Adult psychiatric status of hyperactive boys grown up. *Am J Psychiatry* 155(4):493–8.

Mannuzza S, Klein RG, Klein DF, Bessler A, Shrout P. (2002). Accuracy of adult recall of childhood attention deficit hyperactivity disorder. *American Journal of Psychiatry* 159(11):1882–8.

Mannuzza S, Klein RG, Moulton JL, 3rd. (2003). Persistence of attention-deficit/hyperactivity disorder into adulthood: what have we learned from the prospective follow-up studies? *J Atten Disord* 7(2):93–100.

McBurnett K. (1997). Attention-deficit/hyperactivity disorder: a review of diagnostic issues. In Widiger TA, Francis AJ, Pincus HA, Ross R, First MB, Davis W, eds. *DSM-IV Sourcebook*. Washington, DC: American Psychiatric Association: 111–43.

McGough JJ, Barkley RA. (2004). Diagnostic controversies in adult attention deficit hyperactivity disorder. *Am J Psychiatry* 161(11):1948–56.

Murphy K, Barkley RA. (1996). Attention deficit hyperactivity disorder adults: comorbidities and adaptive impairments. *Compr Psychiatry* 37(6):393–401.

Murphy P, Schachar R. (2000). Use of self-ratings in the assessment of symptoms of attention deficit hyperactivity disorder in adults. *Am J Psychiatry* **157**(7):1156–9.

Pastor PN, Reuben CA. (2005). Racial and ethnic differences in ADHD and LD in young school-age children: parental reports in the National Health Interview Survey. *Public Health Rep* **120**(4):383–92.

Ratey J, Greenberg S, Bemporad. JR, Lindem K. (1992). Unrecognized attention-deficit hyperactivity disorder in adults presenting for outpatient psychotherapy. *J Child Adolesc Psychopharmacol* **4**:267–75.

Resnick RJ. (2005). Attention deficit hyperactivity disorder in teens and adults: they don't all outgrow it. *J Clin Psychol* **61**(5):529–33.

Riccio CA, Wolfe M, Davis B, Romine C, George C, Lee D. (2005). Attention deficit hyperactivity disorder: manifestation in adulthood. *Arch Clin Neuropsychol* **20**(2):249–69.

Robins LN, Helzer JE, Croughan JL, Ratcliff KS. (1981). National Institute of Mental Health Diagnostic Interview Schedule: its history, characteristics and validity. *Arch Gen Psychiatry* **38**(4):381–9.

Robins LN, Wing J, Wittchen H-U, Helzer JE, Babor TF, Burke JD, et al. (1988). The Composite International Diagnostic Interview: an epidemiologic instrument suitable for use in conjunction with different diagnostic systems and in different cultures. *Arch Gen Psychiatry* **45**(12):1069–77.

Rubin DB. (1987). *Multiple Imputation for Nonresponse in Surveys.* New York: Wiley.

Sawilowsky S, Musial JL. (1988). Modeling ADHD exponential decay. *ADHD Rep* **6**(1):10–11.

Seidman LJ, Valera EM, Makris N. (2005). Structural brain imaging of attention-deficit/hyperactivity disorder. *Biol Psychiatry* **57**(11):1263–72.

Shaffer D. (1994). Attention deficit hyperactivity disorder in adults. *Am J Psychiatry* **151**(5):633–8.

Shekim WO, Kashani J, Beck N, Cantwell DP, Martin J, Rosenberg J, et al. (1985). The prevalence of attention deficit disorders in a rural Midwestern community sample of nine-year-old children. *J Am Acad Child Psychiatry* **24**(6):765–70.

Stewart WF, Ricci JA, Chee E, Hahn SR, Morganstein D. (2003). Cost of lost productive work time among US workers with depression. *JAMA* **289**(23):3135–44.

Taylor A. (1986). *The Overactive Child.* London: Spastic Society.

Taylor E, Sandberg S. (1984). Hyperactive behavior in English schoolchildren: a questionnaire survey. *J Abnorm Child Psychol* **12**(1):143–55.

Wang PS, Beck AL, Berglund P, McKenas DK, Pronk NP, Simon GE, et al. (2004). Effects of major depression on moment-in-time work performance. *Am J Psychiatry* **161**(10):1885–91.

Wang PS, Simon G, Kessler RC. (2003). The economic burden of depression and the cost-effectiveness of treatment. *Int J Methods Psychiatr Res* **12**(1):22–33.

Weiss G, Hechtman L, Milroy T, Perlman T. (1985). Psychiatric status of hyperactives as adults: a controlled prospective 15-year follow-up of 63 hyperactive children. *J Am Acad Child Psychiatry* **24**(2):211–20.

Wender PH, Reimherr FW, Wood D, Ward M. (1985). A controlled study of methylphenidate in the treatment of attention deficit disorder, residual type, in adults. *Am J Psychiatry* **142**(5):547–52.

Wender PH, Wolf LE, Wasserstein J. (2001). Adults with ADHD. An overview. *Ann N Y Acad Sci* **931**:1–16.

Wilens TE, Faraone SV, Biederman J. (2004). Attention-deficit/hyperactivity disorder in adults. *JAMA* **292**(5):619–23.

Zucker M, Morris MK, Ingram SM, Morris RD, Bakeman R. (2002). Concordance of self- and informant ratings of adults' current and childhood attention-deficit/ hyperactivity disorder symptoms. *Psychol Assess* **14**(4):379–89.

Chapter 3

Gender differences in ADHD

Patricia Quinn

Introduction

The concept of ADHD – its symptoms, course, and etiology – has evolved over the years. In this process, several long-held assumptions have been set aside. Hyperactivity, once believed to be the essential feature of ADHD, is now understood to present among only a subset of those with the disorder. In addition, ADHD in adults is no longer considered merely a "residual" version of a childhood disorder, but is more accurately recognized as the adult manifestation of a life span disorder. Over the last decade another longstanding assumption has been called into question – that ADHD primarily affects males.

Gender-sensitive profiles of ADHD have been slow to develop, and although we have come a long way in the last decade toward a better understanding of the differences in manifestations of ADHD in men and women, there remains much to learn, with many avenues yet to be explored. This chapter focuses on specific issues related to ADHD in women and includes such topics as the unique presentation and the psychological effects related to late diagnosis, coexisting conditions commonly seen in women with ADHD, and the challenge of providing an appropriate treatment plan for women with ADHD.

Prevalence of ADHD in women

As ADHD in adults became more widely recognized and treated in the mid-1990s, a number of adult ADHD clinics were established. Informal reports emerging from these clinics initially suggested that the percentage of women self-referred to these clinics was much higher than the percentage of females with ADHD previously reported in the literature (Biederman, 1994; Biederman et al., 1994; Stein, 1994).

More recent studies investigating gender ratios of adults with ADHD have found that the difference in prevalence rates for males and females may diminish in adulthood (Faraone et al., 2000; Walker, 1999). Although there are no reliable data on the number of women with ADHD or the true male-to-female ratio of adults with ADHD, all of these reports strongly suggest that women with ADHD represent a more significant proportion of adults with ADHD than has been previously recognized.

Comorbid conditions in women with ADHD

It is estimated that 70–75% of adults presenting for treatment of ADHD have at least one additional psychiatric diagnosis (Shekim, Asarnow, Hess, Zaucha, & Wheeler, 1990; Wilens, Biederman, & Spencer, 2002). Although there is general agreement that gender-related differences exist in comorbid conditions, these differences have been described in clusters: boys have been found to have more "externalizing" disorders, and girls have been described as tending to have more "internalizing" disorders such as anxiety and depression. Although research on adult females with ADHD continues to lag behind that on adult males with ADHD, many clinicians are reporting unique issues and comorbid conditions in women with ADHD within their practices.

Stein and colleagues (1995) using the Wender Utah Rating Scales (WURS), conducted a factor analysis to compare self-reported symptoms of men and women diagnosed with ADHD and found significant gender differences. The responses of women in this study loaded primarily on a "dysphoria" factor, although they also reported problems with attention and organization, conduct problems, and impulsivity. In contrast,

ADHD in Adults: Characterization, Diagnosis and Treatment, ed. Jan Buitelaar, Cornelis Kan and Philip Asherson.
Published by Cambridge University Press. © Cambridge University Press 2011.

men's self-reported symptoms emphasized more conduct and learning problems, stress intolerance, attention difficulties, and poor social skills/awkwardness.

Anxiety and depression

Using self-report and interview data, Rucklidge and Kaplan (1997) found that women in their sample who were diagnosed with ADHD in adulthood were more apt to report depressive symptoms, were more stressed and anxious, had more external locus of control and lower self-esteem, and engaged in more emotion-oriented versus task-oriented coping strategies than women who did not meet diagnostic criteria for ADHD. Similarly in research published by Katz, Goldstein, and Geckle (1998), women diagnosed with ADHD in adulthood were found to have a greater degree of psychological distress than their male counterparts on measures of psychiatric symptoms, but displayed more efficient cognitive strategies on neuropsychological measures.

As previously cited, a study conducted by Stein and colleagues in 1995 found that the ADHD symptoms most frequently reported by women were dysphoria, inattention, organization problems, and impulsive conduct. The largest factor extracted for females was dysphoria, which was described as a reactive moodiness rather than true depression with vegetative signs. A study conducted by Arcia and Conners (1998) also found important differences between male and female responses on self-ratings: adult women had a poorer self-concept and reported fewer assets and more problems than did their males counterparts. In general, females with ADHD report emotional instability characterized by fluctuating anxiety, depression, and sudden mood swings leading to difficulty in self-regulation (J Young, 2002).

Findings recently reported from the preliminary analysis of a comorbidity study involving 3559 individuals with ADHD, ranging in age from 2 to 88 years, also confirmed an increase in mood disorders in females (Turgay et al., 2005). In the adult population only, major depression, anxiety disorders, and dysthymic disorder were the most prevalent comorbid conditions reported. In addition, women were found to have higher rates of major depression, anxiety disorders, and dysthymic disorders than men (54% vs. 36%, 28% vs. 15%, and 16% vs. 13%, respectively).

In another study, investigators highlighted differences between 188 women and 348 men, all self-referred, who participated in a multisite placebo-controlled nonstimulant drug study (Robinson et al., 2005). In comparison with male participants, the women were more likely to have combined-type ADHD and reported more ADHD, depression, and anxiety symptoms. Women also endorsed more emotional dysregulation as measured on the Wender-Reimherr Adult Attention Deficit Disorder Scale.

The gender-specific comorbidity patterns found in the two previous studies diverge from evidence obtained from large clinical studies that lifetime comorbidity rates in ADHD do not vary by gender. Those large studies found that the only gender-related difference in lifetime rates of psychiatric comorbidity were lower rates of conduct disorder and antisocial personality disorder in women than men (Biederman et al., 2004).

Low self-esteem

Research has also highlighted the fact that women with ADHD struggle with a more negative self-image than do men with ADHD (Arcia & Conners, 1998). Societal criticism of impulsive, risk-taking behavior in girls and greater maternal criticism of ADHD behavior in daughters (Barkley, 1994) often become internalized. It is this ingrained low self-regard and lack of faith in one's acceptability, rather than the cognitive challenges of ADHD, that most likely result in the greatest long-term psychological damage seen in women (Rucklidge & Kaplan, 1997).

Social isolation and withdrawal

In her book, *Women with Attention Deficit Disorder* (1995), Solden described women "coming out of the ADHD closet" as they grow in self-acceptance and self-understanding through psychotherapy. Many young girls with ADHD enter this "closet" early in life, spending childhood years anxiously avoiding class participation for fear of embarrassment. Often, these girls isolate themselves socially because of social anxiety and sometimes outright peer rejection. Some research suggests that girls with ADHD experience more peer rejection than boys and that these patterns begin as early as preschool (Berry, Shaywitz, & Shaywitz, 1985). Other studies (Brown, Madan-Swain, & Baldwin, 1991; Hinshaw, 2002) found that peer rejection of girls with ADHD begins early and tends to increase with age.

Because females tend to be more affiliative by nature (Gilligan, 1982; Tannen, 1991), it would be reasonable to speculate that the peer rejection experienced by children with ADHD would have a stronger negative impact on females. Carol Gilligan has written extensively of the lengths to which young women will go to preserve interpersonal relationships, suppressing and disavowing their own feelings. Robin and colleagues (1997) found that adults with ADHD, both men and women, are more introverted and socially withdrawn than adults without ADHD. Although both men and women with ADHD tend to be socially isolated, it seems likely that negative reactions to social isolation would be greater in women as a result of different male–female relational patterns. Many women with ADHD describe painful feelings of "not fitting in," of not finding the social contact and social acceptance that they so strongly desire.

Parenting issues

Women are more likely than men to be the primary parent of their children. In addition, women with ADHD have the strong likelihood of having a child with ADHD. As the abundant literature on children with ADHD attests, raising a child with this disorder is a particularly challenging task, made even more daunting when the mother has ADHD herself. When a marriage ends in divorce, it is the mother who is most likely to have custody of her children. All of these interrelated patterns strongly illustrate the potentially much greater challenge that parenthood poses for women with ADHD than for men.

Yet, although great attention has been paid to the parenting needs of children with ADHD, very little attention has been paid to the needs of mothers with ADHD and the ways that recommended parenting approaches must be adapted to their needs. A study by Weinstein, Apfel, and Weinstein (1998) found that mothers with ADHD are more likely to have relatives with alcoholism and neuropsychiatric disorders, more likely to have neuropsychiatric disorders themselves, and more likely to experience problems with daily living compared to mothers without ADHD.

A recently published study in the *Journal of Abnormal Psychology* provides the first data on how parents with ADHD perform on key parenting tasks (Murray & Johnston, 2006). Results from this study documented the parenting difficulties experienced by mothers with ADHD. Compared to other mothers, mothers with ADHD were less knowledgeable about their child's whereabouts, friends, and activities; were less consistent in their discipline strategies; and generated less effective solutions to child management problems. In most cases, the parenting differences between mothers with and without ADHD were both large and statistically significant, with most effect sizes greater than 1. Despite these difficulties, however, they were no less positive than other mothers in how they related to their child, and they provided their child with similar levels of positive feedback and support.

Emotional instability and interactions with fluctuating hormonal states

Hormonal changes occurring at puberty often affect emotional volatility, leading many girls with ADHD to become emotionally hyperreactive. Ratey, Miller, and Nadeau (1995) were among the first to write about the interaction between changing hormonal states and ADHD in women. It has been proposed that whenever brain estrogen levels "fall below the minimum brain estrogen requirement," for whatever reason and at whatever age, brain dysfunction may result (Arpels, 1996). Low estrogen states could thus be particularly problematic for women with ADHD, who are already experiencing symptoms as a result of neurotransmitter imbalance.

Low estrogen states occur before menstruation, during the postpartum period, and in menopause, although levels begin to decline during perimenopause. Symptoms shared by women in low estrogen states include depression, irritability, sleep disturbance, anxiety, panic, difficulty concentrating, and memory and cognitive dysfunction. Women with ADHD frequently report a worsening of ADHD symptoms during these low estrogen periods. In addition, during the premenstrual period, some women may experience both physical symptoms and mildly depressed mood (premenstrual syndrome; PMS) or a severe mood disturbance that significantly affects their ability to function (premenstrual dysphoric disorder; PMDD).

Eating disorders and ADHD in women

Another recently emerging scientific concept that has unique implications for those diagnosing and treating women with ADHD is the association of eating disorders and ADHD. Eating disorders and ADHD share several key characteristics including impulsivity (lack of impulse control) and low self-esteem. Overlapping clinical characteristics would suggest that eating disorders and ADHD may respond to the same medical treatment. Recently, the potential role of ADHD treatment in the management of bulimia has been described in greater detail (Dukarm, 2005), with several case reports appearing in the medical literature.

In two samples of adults with and without ADHD, significantly greater rates of bulimia nervosa were identified in women with ADHD versus those without ADHD: 12% vs. 3%, $p < 0.05$ for one sample and 11% vs. 1%, $p < 0.05$ for the other sample (Surman, Randall, & Biederman, 2006). Although preliminary and requiring further confirmation, these findings suggest that ADHD may be associated with bulimia nervosa in some women. If confirmed, this association between bulimia nervosa and ADHD could have important clinical and therapeutic implications.

Additionally, two recent studies of adolescent girls previously diagnosed with ADHD also found a significant incidence of eating disorders at follow-up. A large prospective study of adolescent girls with and without ADHD (controls) found that those with ADHD were 3.6 times more likely to develop an eating disorder, defined as either anorexia or bulimia nervosa (Biederman et al., 2007). During the study's 5-year follow-up, 16% of the girls with ADHD (20 girls) and 5% of the controls (5 girls) developed an eating disorder. Compared with the controls, the girls with ADHD were 5.6 times more likely to develop bulimia and 2.7 times more likely to develop anorexia nervosa. They also had significantly higher rates of depression, anxiety disorders, and disruptive behavior.

In a second study, 93 adolescent girls with ADHD-C type, 49 with ADHD-I type, and 88 controls seen at a 5-year follow-up were assessed for eating disorders; it found that baseline impulsivity symptoms best predicted adolescent eating pathology, as did the diagnosis of ADHD-C type. In addition, peer rejection and parent–child relationship patterns also were predictive of eating disorders (Mikami et al., 2008).

The challenge of providing an appropriate treatment plan for women with ADHD

Although diagnostic considerations in females are critical, gender-appropriate treatment issues are equally important. Currently, both diagnostic criteria and treatment protocols are derived from predominantly male populations. Treatment outcome remains dependent on clear and precise diagnosis that addresses unique symptoms, specific functional impairments, and other important variables that will dictate intervention strategies. ADHD is a condition that affects multiple aspects of mood, cognitive abilities, behaviors, and daily life. Therefore, effective treatment for ADHD in adult women may require a multimodal approach that includes medication, cognitive behavioral therapy, stress management, and other support services such as ADHD coaching and professional organizing. Although they have been deemed clinically useful, these last two support services have little to no empirical data to support their usefulness to date. As a result, they are not included in the more in-depth discussion of treatments that follows.

Psychotherapy for women with ADHD

Women fortunate enough to receive an accurate ADHD diagnosis often face a subsequent challenge when they seek appropriate treatment. There are very few clinicians experienced in treating adult ADHD, and even fewer are familiar with the unique issues faced by women with ADHD. As a result, most clinicians use standard psychotherapeutic approaches. Although these approaches can be helpful in gaining insight into emotional and interpersonal issues, they do not help a woman with ADHD learn to better manage her ADHD on a daily basis or learn strategies to lead a more productive and satisfying life.

ADHD-focused cognitive behavioral therapies are currently being developed that focus on a broad range of issues including self-esteem, interpersonal and family issues, daily health habits, daily stress level, and life management skills (Ramsay & Rostain, 2005a, 2005b). In addition, interventions often referred to as "neurocognitive psychotherapies" that combine cognitive behavior therapy with cognitive rehabilitation techniques (Nadeau, 2002; S Young, 2002) are proving quite effective for dealing with the day-to-day challenges faced by women with ADHD. Combining cognitive behavior therapy that focuses on the psychological issues of ADHD (e.g. self-esteem, self-acceptance, self-blame, etc.) with the cognitive rehabilitation approach that focuses on life management skills for improving cognitive functions, learning compensatory strategies, and restructuring the environment has been found to be extremely effective when treating women with ADHD.

Medication in the treatment of women with ADHD

Pharmacotherapy, and more specifically the use of stimulants, continues to be the first line of intervention in the treatment of ADHD for both males and females. Stimulants are highly effective in the treatment of ADHD symptoms in adult patients (Spencer et al., 1996; Weiss & Murray, 2003; Wilens, Spencer, & Biederman, 2000). In fact, many adult patients with uncomplicated cases of ADHD may respond well to pharmacotherapy alone.

However, medication issues for women with ADHD are often more complicated than those for men for several reasons. First, as discussed earlier, women are more likely to suffer from comorbid anxiety and/or depression as well as a range of other conditions (Biederman, 1998; Biederman et al., 1993). Because alcohol and drug use disorders are frequently encountered in women with ADHD and may begin at a young age (Wilens, Spencer, & Biederman, 1995), a careful history of substance use is important. Any effective medication approach for women needs to take into consideration all aspects of the patient's life including the treatment of comorbid conditions as well as ADHD.

Second, the medication picture may be complicated by hormone fluctuations across the menstrual cycle and across the life span (e.g., puberty, perimenopause, and menopause), with an increase in ADHD symptoms whenever estrogen levels fall. In some cases, hormone replacement may need to be integrated into the medication regimen used to treat a woman with ADHD (Quinn, 2002).

Conclusion

For several years now, Barkley has proposed the need to take a fresh look at adult patterns, suggesting that ADHD may be manifested differently in adults. Just as ADHD in adults may be different than, not "less than," ADHD in children, it is also reasonable to propose that ADHD in females may be different from ADHD in males, rather than a "paler" version of male ADHD. However, such differences will not be uncovered if researchers are confined by current diagnostic criteria. In proposing that we take a fresh look at gen-

der differences, it seems most fruitful to look at specific gender differences, rather than in an ill-defined cluster.

We know that comorbid disorders in females with ADHD are often different from those seen in males with ADHD. Higher rates of anxiety, mood, and eating disorders and hormonal fluctuations often complicate the picture of ADHD in women. Clinicians are challenged with disentangling the symptoms of ADHD from symptoms of these comorbid conditions. The interplay of several of these conditions needs to be examined more closely so we can accurately paint the clinical picture of ADHD in women. The coexistence of ADHD and depression, which becomes such an integral part of the disorder in some women, and the role of hormonal fluctuations over the life span need to be explored in particular. Do the depression and anxiety seen in women with ADHD represent fallout from years of ADHD difficulties or are they true comorbid conditions? What is the interaction between estrogen levels and ADHD symptoms levels in women, and does it also play into the depressive picture that frequently emerges? Disordered eating patterns are only now being seen as associated with ADHD because research has focused for too long on male-only populations. What else will emerge as we shine the light of future research on female populations?

Perhaps the most critical next step in the field of ADHD in women is the development of more gender-appropriate diagnostic criteria and tools. Adherence to current diagnostic criteria results in limiting the diagnosis in females to those who most resemble males with ADHD. Without more gender-appropriate diagnostic criteria, females will continue to go undiagnosed or misdiagnosed. Rucklidge and Kaplan's research (1997) has already demonstrated the high cost for women of going undiagnosed. Though their struggles are less overt, the impact of ADHD on women is no less significant. Only with gender-sensitive diagnosis and treatment will the underdiagnosis of ADHD in females be adequately addressed.

References

Arcia E, Conners CK. (1998). Gender differences in ADHD? *J Dev Behav Pediatr* **19**:77–83.

Arnold LE. (1996). Sex differences in ADHD: conference summary. *J Abnorm Child Psychol* **24**:555–69.

Arpels JC. (1996). The female brain hypoestrogenic continuum from the premenstrual syndrome to menopause: a hypothesis and review. *J Reprod Med* **41**:633–9.

Barkley RA. (1994). Personal communication at NIMH Sex Differences Conference, reported in Arnold LE (1996). Sex differences in ADHD: conference summary. *J Abnorm Child Psychol* **24**:555–69.

Berry CA, Shaywitz SE, Shaywitz BA. (1985). Girls with attention deficit disorder: a silent majority? A report on behavioral and cognitive characteristics. *Pediatrics* **76**:801–9.

Biederman J. (1994). Personal communication of preliminary findings at NIMH Sex Differences Conference, reported in Arnold LE (1996). Sex differences in ADHD: conference summary. *J Abnorm Child Psychol* **24**:555–69.

Beiderman J. (1998). Attention-deficit/hyperactivity disorder: a lifespan perspective. *J Clin Psychiatry* **59**:4–16.

Biederman J, Ball SW, Monuteaux MC, Surman CB, Johnson JL, Zeitlin S. (2007). Are girls with ADHD at risk for eating disorders? Results from a controlled, five-year prospective study. *J Dev Behav Pediatr* **28**:302–7.

Biederman J, Faraone SV, Monuteaux MC, Bober M, Cadogen E. (2004). Gender effects on attention-deficit/hyperactivity disorder in adults, revisited. *Biol Psychiatry* **55**:692–700.

Biederman J, Faraone SV, Spencer T, Wilens T, Mick E. (1994). Gender differences in adults with attention deficit hyperactivity disorder. *Psychopharmacol Bull* **30**:65.

Biederman J, Faraone SV, Spencer T, Wilens T, Norman D, Lapey K, et al. (1993). Patterns of psychiatric comorbidity, cognition, and psychosocial functioning in adults with attention deficit hyperactivity disorder. *Am J Psychiatry* **150**:1792–8.

Brown RT, Madan-Swain A, Baldwin K. (1991). Gender differences in a clinic-referred sample of attention deficit disordered children. *Child Psychiatry Hum Dev* **22**:111–28.

Dukarm C. (2005). Bulimia nervosa and ADD: a possible role for stimulant medication. *J Womens Health* **14**:345–50.

Faraone SV, Biederman J, Spencer T, Wilens T, Seidman LJ, Mick E, Doyle AE. (2000). Attention-deficit/hyperactivity disorder in adults: an overview. *Biol Psychiatry* **48**:9–20.

Gilligan C. (1982). *In a Different Voice.* Cambridge, MA: Harvard University Press.

Hinshaw S. (2002). Preadolescent girls with attention-deficit/hyperactivity disorder: I. Background characteristics, comorbidity, cognitive and social functioning, and parenting practices. *J Consult Clin Psychol* **70**:1086–97.

Katz LJ, Goldstein G, Geckle M. (1998). Neuropsychological and personality differences between men and women with ADHD. *J Atten Disord* **2**:239–47.

Mikami AY, Hinshaw SP, Peterson KA, & Lee JC. (2008). Eating pathology among adolescent girls with attention-deficit/hyperactivity disorder. *J Abnorm Psychol* **117**(1):225–35.

Murray C, Johnston C. (2006). Parenting in mothers with and without Attention-Deficit/Hyperactivity Disorder. *J Abnorm Psychol* **115**:52–61.

Nadeau KG. (2002). Neurocognitive psychotherapy for women with ADHD. In: Quinn PO, Nadeau KG, eds. *Gender Issues and ADHD: Research, Diagnosis and Treatment.* Washington DC: Advantage Books: 220–54.

Quinn PO. (2002). Hormonal fluctuations and the influence of estrogen in the treatment of women with ADHD. In: Quinn PO, Nadeau KG, eds. *Gender Issues and ADHD: Research, Diagnosis and Treatment.* Washington DC: Advantage Books: 183–99.

Ramsay JR, Rostain AL. (2005a). Adapting psychotherapy to meet the needs of adults with attention deficit/hyperactivity disorder. *Psychother: Theory, Res, Pract, Training* **42**:72–84.

Ramsay JR, Rostain AL. (2005b). Girl, repeatedly interrupted: the case of a young adult woman with ADHD. *Clin Case Stud* **4**:329–46.

Ratey J, Miller A, Nadeau K. (1995). Special diagnostic and treatment considerations in women with attention deficit disorder. In: Nadeau K, ed. *A Comprehensive Guide to Attention Deficit Disorder in Adults: Research, Diagnosis, and Treatment.* New York: Brunner/Mazel: 260–83.

Robin AL, Tzelepis A, Bedway M, Gilroy G, Sprague D. (1997). The study of ADHD adults: a new beginning. *ADHD Rep* **5**(6):11, 14–15.

Robinson RJ, Reimherr F, Faraone SV, et al. (2005). Gender differences in ADHD adults during clinical trials with atomoxetine. Poster NR 497 presented at: Annual Meeting of the American Psychiatric Association; Atlanta.

Rucklidge JJ, Kaplan BJ. (1997). Psychological functioning in women identified in adulthood with attention-deficit/hyperactivity disorder. *J Atten Disord* **2**:167–76.

Shekim W, Asarnow RF, Hess E, Zaucha K, Wheeler N. (1990). An evaluation of attention deficit disorder-residual type. *Compr Psychiatry* **31**:416–25.

Solden S. (1995). *Women with Attention Deficit Disorder: Embracing Disorganization at Home and in the Workplace.* Grass Valley, CA: Underwood Books.

Spencer T, Biederman J, Wilens T, Harding M, O'Donnell D, Griffin S. (1996). Pharmacotherapy of attention deficit disorder across the life cycle. *J Am Acad Child Adolesc Psychiatry* **35**:409–32.

Stein MA. (1994). Personal communication at the NIMH Sex Differences Conference, reported in Arnold LE (1996). Sex differences in ADHD: conference summary. *J Abnorm Child Psychol* **24**:555–69.

Stein MA, Sandoval R, Szumowski E, Roizen N, Reinecke M, Blondis T, Klein A. (1995). Psychometric characteristics of the Wender Utah Rating Scale (WURS): reliability and factor structure for men and women. *Psychopharmacol Bull* **31**:423–31.

Surman CB, Randall ET, Biederman J. (2006) Association between attention-deficit/hyperactivity disorder and bulimia nervosa: analysis of 4 case-control studies. *J Clin Psychiatry* **67**:351–4.

Tannen D. (1991). *You Just Don't Understand: Women and Men in Conversation*. New York: Ballantine Books.

Turgay A, Ansari R, Schwartz M, et al. (2005). Comorbidity differences in ADHD throughout the life cycle. Paper presented at: Annual Meeting of the American Psychiatric Association; Atlanta.

Walker C. (1999). Gender and genetics in ADHD: genetics matter; gender does not. Paper presented at: ADDA Conference; Chicago.

Weiss M, Murray C. (2003). Assessment and management of attention-deficit hyperactivity disorder in adults. *Can Med Assoc J* **168**:715–22.

Weinstein CS, Apfel RJ, Weinstein SR. (1998). Description of mothers with ADHD with children with ADHD. *Psychiatry* **61**:12–19.

Wilens TE, Biederman J, Spencer TJ. (2002). Attention deficit/hyperactivity disorder across the lifespan. *Annu Rev Med* **53**:113–31.

Wilens TE, Spencer TJ, Biederman J. (1995). Are attention-deficit hyperactivity disorder and the psychoactive substance use disorders really related? *Harv Rev Psychiatry* **3**:260–2.

Wilens TE, Spencer TJ, Biederman J. (2000). Pharmacotherapy of attention-deficit/hyperactivity disorder. In: Brown TE, ed. *Attention Deficit Disorders and Comorbidities in Children, Adolescents, and Adults*. Washington, DC: American Psychiatric Press: 509–35.

Young J. (2002). Depression and anxiety in women with ADHD. In: Quinn PO, Nadeau KG, eds. *Gender Issues and ADHD: Research, Diagnosis and Treatment*. Washington DC: Advantage Books: 270–91.

Young S. (2002). A model of psychotherapy for adults with ADHD. In: Goldstein S, Ellison AT, eds. *Clinician's Guide to Adult ADHD: Assessment and Intervention*. San Diego: Academic Press: 147–63.

Chapter

4

Quantitative and molecular genetic studies of attention-deficit hyperactivity disorder in adults

Philip J. Asherson, Florence Levy, and Steve V. Faraone

Introduction

ADHD is a common, highly heritable neurodevelopmental disorder (Asherson, 2004) affecting around 5% of children (Polanczyk et al., 2007) and 2.5% of adults (Fayyad et al., 2007; Simon et al., 2009). The disorder starts in early childhood and is characterized by pervasive inattention, hyperactivity, and impulsivity that are inappropriate to the developmental stage. The fact that the adult outcome of childhood ADHD is not always benign has been known for a long time. An early review of outcome studies of hyperactive children reported that they experience significant academic, social, and conduct difficulties during adolescence and that social, emotional, and impulse problems persist into young adulthood for the majority (Hechtman & Weiss, 1983). The authors concluded that, although some hyperactive children were found to be functioning normally as adults, a troublesome minority were experiencing severe psychiatric or antisocial problems. Despite some reports that ADHD might be a self-limiting condition (Hill & Schoener, 1996) this view has not been supported by more recent evidence, and we now know that ADHD persists into adult life in the majority of cases either as a full-blown condition (around 15% of cases) or in partial remission (around 50% of cases), with persistence of symptoms associated with significant levels of academic, occupational, or social impairment and high levels of psychiatric comorbidity (Faraone, Biederman, & Mick, 2006).

Although at a descriptive level we know about the developmental trajectory of ADHD into adult life, we know far less about the genetic and environmental contributions to persistence or desistence of the disorder and their influences on the developmental course and outcomes in adult life. Quantitative and molecular genetic studies play a pivotal role in helping us understand the mechanisms involved and the links between ADHD and comorbid disorders in adult life (Asherson, Kuntsi, & Taylor, 2005). Basic research in this area is important because it may help us not only develop novel medical and targeted psychosocial interventions for prevention and treatment but also clarify the nosological distinctions of adult ADHD from other common adult psychiatric disorders. For example, the trait-like characteristics of ADHD symptoms that start during childhood or early adolescence and have a chronic persistent course and the frequency of symptoms such as mood instability that frequently co-occur alongside 'core' ADHD symptoms mean that there is symptom overlap between ADHD, personality disorder, and dysthymia; this overlap leads to considerable confusion about the separate validity of the diagnostic construct of ADHD in adults (Asherson, 2005).

In this chapter we outline family, twin, and adoption studies and recent advances in molecular genetics of ADHD in children and adults. Genetic research on ADHD started with the recognition by Morrison and Stewart (1971) and Cantwell (1972) that hyperactivity aggregates in families. Since then family studies of ADHD have clearly defined a disorder that shows familial clustering both between and across generations. As we shall see, these studies show that ADHD in adults occurs far more frequently among the parents of children with ADHD than the parents of controls and that parents with ADHD have very high rates of ADHD among their offspring. Analyses of extended multigenerational pedigrees have also made an important contribution to the literature, and data from adults with ADHD have been used to map genes for ADHD (Arcos-Burgos, Castellanos, Konecki, et al., 2004; Faraone, Biederman, & Monuteaux, 2000; Palacio et al., 2004; Ribases et al., 2010).

ADHD in Adults: Characterization, Diagnosis and Treatment, ed. Jan Buitelaar, Cornelis Kan and Philip Asherson.
Published by Cambridge University Press. © Cambridge University Press 2011.

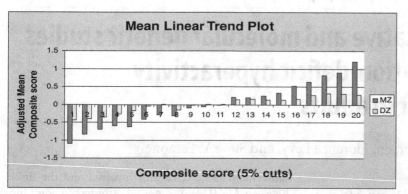

Figure 4.1 ADHD is a quantitative trait. Twin probands are divided into groups based on a composite index of ADHD symptoms scores derived by combining parent and teacher ratings scales for ADHD. The adjusted mean (population mean – co-twin mean) has been plotted for each group. The correlations for MZ (0.78) and DZ (0.28) twin pairs reflect an even distribution of twin-pair similarity, suggesting that genetic liability for ADHD is continuously distributed throughout the population.

Despite these advances we still know little about the balance between genetic and environmental contributions to ADHD in adults and the factors that influence persistence of the disorder into adult life. There are a few genetically sensitive studies of ADHD in adults, consisting of adoption studies of biological and non-biological parents of children with ADHD and in the last year the first twin studies of ADHD symptoms in adults have now been reported. The adoption study data show that parent–offspring associations for ADHD are restricted to biological relatives and therefore are likely to be mediated by genetic factors. Population twin studies are the main method used to estimate the relative influence of genetic and environmental factors on human traits. These find only low heritabilities for ADHD symptoms in adults (Boomsma et al., 2010; Larsson et al., in review), while comparable studies in children and adolescents consistently demonstrate high heritability (Faraone et al., 2005; Thapar et al., 1999) and the stability of genetic influences on ADHD symptoms throughout childhood and adolescence (Kuntsi et al., 2005; Larsson, Larsson, & Lichtenstein, 2004).

Twin studies of ADHD

Studies in children and adolescents

Twin studies compare genetically identical or monozygous (MZ) twins with non-identical or dizygous (DZ) twins who share on average half of their parental genes. For this reason we expect a familial trait that is influenced by genetic factors to show greater similarity or concordance between MZ compared to DZ twins, whereas a trait mediated by shared environmental influences would show the same degree of similarity between the two types of twin pairs. There are two

main ways in which twin data have been used to infer genetic and environmental influences on ADHD. The first approach, referred to as univariate or individual-differences analysis, considers the correlations in trait scores within twin pairs (i.e. twin – co-twin correlations), usually sampled from the general population. There have been numerous studies of this type in children and adolescents, and they all show considerable differences in the size of the correlations for ADHD symptom scores between MZ and DZ twin pairs for both parent and teacher reports of ADHD symptoms and behaviors. Diagnostic checklists for ADHD symptoms consistently correlate around 0.7 to 0.8 for MZ twins compared to 0.35 or lower for DZ twins. The resulting estimate of heritability, the proportion of variance in ADHD symptoms explained by genetic factors, is in the order of 60–90% (Thapar et al., 1999), with an estimated average across studies of 76% (Faraone et al., 2005).

Twin studies suggest that genetic liability for ADHD is continuously distributed throughout the population (Chen et al., 2008). Figure 4.1 illustrates the way that ADHD symptom scores in one twin predict ADHD scores among their co-twins, with no apparent discontinuity in genetic liability from one tail of the distribution to the other. The continuity of ADHD symptoms across the population can be more formally investigated using an alternative approach to twin analysis that links extreme groups, defined as a threshold on a clinical rating scale or using diagnostic criteria, and continuous trait measures among their co-twins. This method, known as DF analysis after the authors De Fries and Fulker (1985), derives an estimate of heritability known as *group heritability*. In DF analysis, twins are identified who fall above a clinical threshold for the disorder and the mean ADHD scores among their co-twins are then compared to the population mean. For disorders that are genetically influenced, the co-twins of affected cases (or those with extreme scores) should regress toward the population mean (while remaining significantly different from the population mean): however, the DZ co-twin mean will be closer to the population mean than the MZ co-twin mean. In contrast, if the disorder stems predominantly from environmental insults such as early traumatic brain injury or obstetric complications, both MZ and DZ co-twin means should regress to the population mean. When the disorder is influenced mainly by shared environmental factors, the familial influences will affect the MZ and DZ co-twins in a similar way, and the mean trait scores for both MZ and DZ co-twins will regress equally to the population mean (while remaining significantly different from the population mean).

Twin studies that have adopted the DF approach for ADHD estimate similar heritabilities to those derived by individual-differences analysis (Gillis et al., 1992; Gjone, Stevenson, & Sundet, 1996; Levy et al., 1997; Price et al., 2001; Stevenson, 1992). For example, a population twin study of 6000 preschool twins found individual-differences heritability ranging from 0.79 to 0.83 and group heritability estimates for the most hyperactive 5%, 10%, and 27% ranging from 0.83 to 0.93 (Price et al., 2005). Subsequent analysis of these data also found that group heritability was similar for the least hyperactive 5%, 10%, and 27%, suggesting that the same genes that confer risk for ADHD influence levels of ADHD symptoms throughout the population. Another study investigated whether the heritability of attention problems increased with their severity (Gjone et al., 1996). This model is useful because one might expect cases at the severe end of the dimension to have a categorical disorder such as ADHD, so that if ADHD accounted for the heritability of attention problems we would expect to see increasing heritability with increasing severity. However, heritability did not change with severity, so the authors concluded that there was in the population a continuously distributed dimension of genetic liability to attention problems.

More recently, we investigated the level of ADHD symptoms among the siblings of ADHD combined type probands aged 6–18 years using the International Multicentre ADHD Genetics (IMAGE) project sample. Using a modified DF approach for sibling data, we found similar estimated correlations between ADHD probands and their siblings to that reported for DZ twins from population twin studies (Chen et al., 2008). Furthermore, we found no evidence for a bimodal distribution of ADHD symptoms scores among the siblings of ADHD probands, thereby confirming the familial association between ADHD in probands and ADHD symptom scores among their siblings.

The perception of ADHD as a quantitative trait is important because it informs us that there is no clear distinction between the clinical disorder and the quantitative trait. Quantitative genetic data therefore support the application of a medical model for ADHD similar to that used to define common forms of anxiety and depression, which emphasizes the links between the number and severity of symptoms and psychiatric morbidity and/or psychosocial impairments. In clinical practice this means that the presence of clinically significant impairments associated with the persistence of ADHD symptoms is a key criterion for the diagnosis of ADHD in adults. The implication for molecular genetic studies is that we should expect that at least some of the genetic variants that increase risk for the clinical disorder will also influence ADHD trait scores in the general population, thus allowing studies of ADHD as a quantitative trait to be adopted alongside more traditional affected–unaffected or case–control designs.

Twin studies in adults

Despite the high heritability reported from child and adolescent twin samples this has not been the case for comparable studies in adults which show heritabilities in the region of 0.30 to 0.40 (Boomsma et al., 2010; Larsson et al., in review). The reasons for this discrepancy are not yet fully understood but may be due, at least in part, to the use of self-rated data in the adult studies rather than informant-rated data used in most child and adolescent studies. This has been shown in the child and adolescent literature where studies that have included self-ratings of ADHD symptoms find far lower heritabilities that those based on parent and teacher reports. One study that investigated this question used parent, teacher, and self-ratings in a sample of 11 to 16 year olds and found no evidence of a heritable phenotype using self-report of ADHD symptoms (Martin. Scourfield, & McGuffin, 2002). In this study, correlations for MZ and DZ pairs were 0.73 and 0.25 for parent ratings and 0.81 and 0.38 for teacher ratings, respectively – giving high estimates of heritability in the region of 0.7–0.8. However, the correlations for self-rated ADHD symptoms among the same 11 to 16 year olds were 0.29 for both MZ and DZ twin pairs, indicating no genetic effects at all and only a moderate familial effect due entirely to environmental factors. Although the self-ratings of ADHD symptoms in this study used a comparatively short scale consisting of only a few broad symptom items, the difference in heritability estimates for self-ratings compared to informant ratings was very striking. In another more detailed study that used interview data with a group of adolescent twins, ADHD symptoms were found to be heritable. However as in the adult self-rated data this was found to be far lower than that found for parent and teacher rated data due to the low correlation for ADHD symptoms among MZ twins of only 0.32 (Ehringer et al., 2006).

At the time of writing one adult population twin study has been published that used self-ratings for current ADHD symptoms and reported a low heritability of around 0.30 (Boosma et al., 2010). Two further published papers using adult twin data report on the heritability of retrospectively rated childhood ADHD symptoms and found this to be in the region of 0.35 to 0.50 (Haberstick et al., 2008; Schultz et al., 2006). Although slightly lower than that reported in childhood twin studies the heritability for retrospectively reported ADHD is around the figure expected given the reliability of retrospective recall compared to data collected at the time. However the estimated heritability of only 0.30 in adults for current self-rated data in the Dutch study from Boomsma and colleagues (2010) is below that expected.

Because there are no other published twin studies for current ADHD symptoms in adults, we report here preliminary data from an unpublished sample of Australian adult twins (Asherson, Hay, Howe-Forbes, unpublished data) and from a larger Swedish twin study (Larsson et al., in review). In the Australian twin study, the data were based on self-ratings for current levels of the 18 *DSM-IV* ADHD items and retrospective childhood ratings for *DSM-IV* items were extracted from the Wender-Utah Rating Scales. There was a moderate phenotypic correlation between current and retrospective ADHD symptom scores of around 0.5 and moderate heritability of around 0.5 for retrospective ratings from childhood which was similar to that reported in the published studies of retrospectively reported childhood ADHD symptoms. However, for current self-rated ADHD symptoms the MZ and DZ correlations

were only 0.15 and 0.05 respectively, giving rise to a much lower heritability estimate of around 0.15. The very low MZ correlation of 0.15 for current self-ratings of ADHD symptoms indicated that in this sample ADHD symptoms in adults were largely non-familial with neither major shared environmental nor genetic influences. The general conclusion of low heritability for self-rated current ADHD symptoms in adults is further supported by a large sample of Swedish adult twins that estimated heritability to be around 0.35 (Larsson et al., in review). This finding is again consistent with that of the adolescent study of self-reported symptoms from Ehringer and colleagues (2006) and the recent adult twin study from Boomsma (2010). In conclusion several published and unpublished studies confirm that heritability for self-rated ADHD in adult population samples is around 30%, with the majority of the phenotypic variance accounted for by unique environmental factors and measurement error.

One explanation for the relatively low heritability could be low test–test reliability of self-reported ratings of ADHD symptoms in adults. When we repeated a set of ADHD rating scales between 1 and 2 years after initial assessment in a group of parents of children with ADHD, we found intraclass correlations to be around 0.8 (Asherson and colleagues, unpublished data) while the study from Boomsma and colleagues reported test-test reliability to be around 0.6–0.7. Poor reliability of the measures used is therefore unlikely to explain the relatively low heritability for self-rated ADHD in adults.

However, we have identified two potential sources of error that might give rise to low heritability estimates in self-ratings of ADHD symptoms in adults and require further exploration. First, as discussed earlier, self-ratings of current ADHD symptoms in adolescence confirm the importance of rater effects because we know there is a major discrepancy in heritability estimates derived from self- and informant ratings during adolescence.

Second, another potentially important factor is age of onset (AOO) of the reported symptoms. We compared the mean scores for ADHD symptoms in adult ADHD probands (*AAP*: n = 233), parents of children with ADHD (*PCA*: n = 512), and parents of control children (*PCC*: n = 456). Surprisingly, the two groups of parents did not differ substantially from each other, with an estimated familial index of only 0.06 (familial index = $[\mu PCA$-$\mu PCC]/[\mu AAP$-$\mu PCC]$). The familial index is an estimation of the familial association in ADHD symptoms between first-degree relatives, because parents of children with ADHD share on average 50% of their genetic variation with their child with ADHD and their mean score for ADHD symptoms is thus expected to be significantly different from controls. In the parent groups, however, AOO for ADHD symptoms showed a bimodal distribution, with the divide around 15 years. By excluding from the analysis parents who reported ADHD symptoms that started after the age of 15, we found greater differences between the parental groups, yielding a revised familial index of 0.25. This figure is comparable with that expected from DZ and sibling pair correlations in childhood ADHD. Our data therefore suggest that AOO might be an important indicator of heterogeneity, with symptoms with AOO younger than 15 years showing familial association to childhood ADHD, whereas those with AOO older than 15 years appearing to be etiologically distinct, perhaps representing epiphenomena of adult-onset disorders.

One firm conclusion is that self-rated ADHD symptoms may not reflect the true extent of the genetic influences on ADHD in adults. Further work is now required to clarify whether more objective measures of ADHD show higher heritability in the same way that informant data appears to show greater heritability than self-report data in children. Self-rating scales should therefore be used with caution in genetic epidemiological studies of ADHD in adults. Studies of ADHD in adults should focus on reporter ratings (spouse, close relative, employer) in addition to self-ratings and on the continuity of symptoms from childhood through to adulthood. However, this issue should not be confused with the positive predictive validity of self-ratings when used within clinical populations with prior evidence for ADHD, which is around 78% (Mannuzza et al., 2002) or more (Kessler et al., 2005).

Adoption studies of adult ADHD

Another important source of information on the genetic influences on adult ADHD is derived from adoption data. Several reports have suggested that the familial risk for ADHD in adults is mediated predominantly by genetic and not environmental influences, based on different rates of ADHD among biological and non-biological (adoptive) parents of children with ADHD. Initial reports from early family studies found that adoptive parents of hyperactive children were less likely than biological parents to have hyperactivity or associated disorders (Cantwell, 1972; Morrison & Stewart, 1971), a finding that was confirmed in three subsequent studies.

The first of these studies compared 176 biological and adoptive parents of hyperactive and normal control children. Biological parents reported more attentional difficulties and slower mean reaction times than the non-biological parents, although they showed similar levels of impulsivity (Alberts-Corush, Firestone, & Goodman, 1986). These findings are in keeping with clinical follow-up studies of children with ADHD that find that inattentive symptoms are more persistent than impulse control problems, which tend to resolve with increasing age (Biederman, Mick, & Faraone, 2000). A second study showed a similar pattern of findings (Sprich et al., 2000). This study investigated the adoptive parents of 25 children with ADHD and compared them to biological parents of 101 ADHD children and 50 control children. The rates of adult ADHD was found to be 18% in the biological parents compared to 6% in the adoptive parents and 3% in the control parents, again suggesting a predominant role for genetic factors. The third study stemmed from the analysis of parents of children taking part in the multimodal treatment study of children with ADHD (Epstein et al., 2000). The pattern of familial aggregation of ADHD symptoms was investigated in the parents of 579 combined-type ADHD probands and of 288 control children without ADHD. Adult ADHD symptoms reported by both self and informant reports were found to be higher among the parents of children with ADHD, with increased levels of inattentiveness and cognitive problems, hyperactivity and restlessness, impulsivity, and emotional lability. The sample contained both biological and non-biological parents, and the informant data showed that among the parents of ADHD children levels of inattention, cognitive problems, impulsivity, and emotional lability were higher for biological parents compared to non-biological parents, although self-ratings were not related to biological status. The informant data but not the self-ratings of ADHD symptoms therefore supported the hypothesis that the familial association of parent ADHD with offspring ADHD is the result of biological factors and therefore likely to be explained by genetic factors shared between parent and offspring.

Another family (but not adoption) study used a combination of objective and self-report data and found that the familial risk was greater for more objective measures of ADHD-related problems compared to self-report measures. The study examined neuropsychological and behavioral function among the parents of 53 preschool children, including a subgroup with ADHD (Curko Kera et al., 2004). In keeping with the known familial inheritance of ADHD, parents of preschool children with ADHD displayed slower reaction times and more commission errors on a continuous performance task than parents of children who did not have ADHD. However, there were no significant differences in behavior using the self-reported Brown Attention-Deficit Disorder Scale for Adults. The lack of evidence for familial effects on self-rated ADHD scores, which is seen in several studies, lends further support to the conclusion that self-ratings of ADHD symptoms are not a good index of genetic liability for ADHD in adults.

Family twin and adoption studies of ADHD and comorbid disorders

Family studies have shown beyond doubt that there is substantial familial clustering of ADHD in both the parents and siblings of child probands with ADHD. Family studies have also focused on increased rates of comorbid traits and disorders in the parents of ADHD offspring. These studies serve to quantify the familial risks associated with ADHD, but cannot differentiate between the effects of shared genes and shared environments in causing familial resemblance. Although some of the early literature highlighted the familial clustering of ADHD with alcohol abuse (e.g. Alterman et al., 1982; Alterman & Tarter, 1983, 1986; Manshadi et al., 1983) more attention has been given to the association between ADHD and antisocial behavioral disorders throughout the life span.

The first carefully controlled family study of ADHD symptoms used a group of unselected and blindly evaluated child and adult relatives of ADHD probands; it found increased rates of both current and retrospectively reported ADHD symptoms, as well as a strong familial association with antisocial behavior among first-degree relatives (Biederman et al., 1990; Faraone et al., 1991). This study used *DSM-III* criteria and was therefore based on probands with a diagnosis of attention deficit disorder (ADD). Its main finding was that both child and adult relatives of child ADD probands were at significantly greater risk for ADD than relatives of both psychiatric and normal controls. Risk for ADD was highest among

relatives of ADD comorbid with conduct disorder probands (ADHD+CD; 38%), moderate among relatives of ADD comorbid with oppositional disorder (ADD+ODD; 17%) and "pure" ADD probands (24%), and lowest among relatives of psychiatric and normal controls (5% for both groups). These data suggested a liability of risk for ADD, or familial loading, that was higher for ADD probands comorbid with conduct disorder than for "pure" ADD probands. By comparison, the risk for antisocial disorders among relatives was highest for ADD+CD (34%) and ADD+ODD (24%) probands, which was significantly greater than the risk to relatives of ADD probands (11%), psychiatric (7%), and normal controls (4%). Finally this study found that both ADD and antisocial disorders co-occurred in the same individuals more often than expected by chance alone. Hence this study came to three main conclusions: ADHD shows familial aggregation both within and between generations, ADHD comorbid with conduct disorder shows greater familial loading for ADHD, and there is familial clustering for comorbidity between ADHD and conduct disorder within families.

The complexity of the links between ADHD and antisocial behavior was described in an adoption study that investigated 283 male adopted-away children of adults displaying antisocial behaviors. Having a biological parent adjudged to be delinquent or to have an adult criminal conviction predicted increased rates of ADHD in their adopted-away sons (Cadoret & Stewart, 1991), suggesting important shared genetic influences between delinquent behavior and ADHD. Among adoptee children ADHD was found to predict aggressive behavior and in turn aggressive behavior predicted increased adult antisocial behavior. Environmental factors were also found to be important: the socioeconomic status and psychiatric problems in adoptive family members correlated significantly with ADHD, aggression, and antisocial measures in the adoptees. The authors concluded that ADHD should be considered a syndrome that has a variety of correlated behaviors, such as aggressive behavior, and that each of these correlated behaviors is influenced by different genetic and environmental factors.

Another study highlighted the extensive range of comorbidities that show familial clustering with ADHD (Chronis et al., 2003). It investigated the level of comorbid syndromes among parents of 98 young children with ADHD and found, as expected, that childhood ADHD was associated with increased rates of maternal and paternal ADHD. Childhood ADHD+ODD/CD were also associated with maternal mood disorders, anxiety disorders, and stimulant/cocaine dependence and with paternal childhood disruptive behavior and adult drinking problems.

Twin studies can clarify the way that genes and environment contribute to the comorbidity and familial clustering of ADHD with conduct disorder (Silberg et al., 1996; Thapar, Harrington, & McGuffin, 2001). Thapar and colleagues using a sample of 2082 twin pairs showed that the overlap between childhood ADHD-related behaviours and conduct problems was explained by common genetic and non-shared environmental influences (Thapar et al., 2001). The genetic contribution to conduct problems was entirely explained by the same genetic factors that influenced ADHD-related behaviors, and the overlap of the two types of behaviour was mainly explained by these genetic influences. Nevertheless, the ADHD-related behaviours and conduct problems appeared to be partly distinct because additional environmental factors influenced conduct problems. In addition the researchers tested the predictions of the liability threshold model for ADHD and ADHD+CD and found that ADHD+CD is best perceived as a quantitatively "more severe" variant of ADHD in the sense that it indexes a higher genetic loading for ADHD. The data fit well with a risk model in which ADHD is an early risk factor for the development of conduct problems and this adverse developmental trajectory is affected by both genetic influences shared with ADHD and familial environmental influences that are specific to the development of conduct problems.

Although twin studies indicate that shared environmental influences play only a limited role in the etiology of ADHD, environmental factors may still be pivotal, acting through mechanisms of gene–environment interaction (Rutter & Silberg, 2002). This is because the heritability component incorporates genetic effects that are mediated by interactions with the familial environment (see Moffitt, Caspi, & Rutter, 2005, for a detailed description of this approach). The impact of exposure to parental ADHD on risk for offspring ADHD therefore requires scientific scrutiny even in the absence of evidence for shared environmental effects. This is an important issue because adults with ADHD are likely to interact with their children in an inconsistent, variable, and irritable way and the lack of consistent parenting may lead to increased rates of ADHD symptoms among their offspring. However, one report has suggested that the impact of exposure to parental ADHD on clinical features and dysfunction in offspring is minimal (Biederman, Faraone, & Monuteaux, 2002). This study reported on 1099 offspring of non-ADHD, remitted ADHD, and persistent ADHD parents. It compared offspring across these three groups on clinical, cognitive, and psychosocial outcomes, adjusting for exposure to other parental psychopathology, offspring ADHD status, and social class. The study found that the risk of ADHD was equally high for the offspring of parents with either remitted ADHD or current (persistent) ADHD compared to the parents who never had ADHD. However, parental ADHD status had an impact on family life since having a parent with persistent adult ADHD predicted higher levels of family conflict and poor family cohesion. This study therefore suggested no direct impact of current parental ADHD on risk for ADHD, although there was a general adverse impact on family life that affected all family members.

Persistence of symptoms and the genetics of ADHD

Two family studies of ADHD in adults (Biederman et al., 1995; Manshadi et al., 1983) found that the risk of ADHD among the offspring of adults with ADHD was much higher than the risk of ADHD among relatives of children with ADHD. For example, the 57% prevalence of ADHD among children of parents with adult ADHD was much higher than the 15% prevalence of ADHD among siblings of children with ADHD (Biederman et al., 1995).

This high familial loading of adult ADHD suggests that genes, or other familial risk factors, may play a greater role in the etiology of persistent ADHD than they do for remitting ADHD. This "persistence" hypothesis was tested in two ways. In a prospective study, 140 ADHD boys and 120 non-ADHD boys were examined at a baseline assessment and completed a 4-year follow-up study. By mid–adolescence, 85% of the ADHD boys continued to have the disorder, whereas 15% showed remission of symptoms. The prevalence of ADHD was significantly higher among the relatives of persistent ADHD probands compared to the relatives of remitted ADHD probands (Biederman et al., 1996). Parents of persistent ADHD probands had a recurrence rate of

ADHD of 16.3% compared to 10.8% for parents of non-persistent ADHD probands, whereas siblings of persistent ADHD probands had a recurrence rate of ADHD of 24.4% compared to 4.6% among siblings of non-persistent ADHD probands (Biederman et al., 1995; Faraone, Biederman, & Friedman, 2000). In a retrospective study, ADHD adolescents having retrospectively reported childhood-onset ADHD were compared with ADHD children. The relatives of adolescent probands had higher rates of ADHD compared with the relatives of child probands (Biederman et al., 1995). Thus, a prospective study of children and a retrospective study of adolescents suggest that, when ADHD persists into adolescence and adulthood, it shows greater familial loading for ADHD than do non-persistent forms of ADHD.

Taken together, these data suggest that, from a familial perspective, not only is the adult ADHD diagnosis valid, but it might actually be more valid than the childhood diagnosis – because the familial transmission of ADHD seems to be greater for adults than children with ADHD. This leads to the straightforward prediction that familial transmission is greater when examining ADHD symptoms in adult relatives than it is when examining symptoms in non adult relatives. To test this prediction, Faraone and colleagues analyzed ADHD symptom data collected by structured interviews from the members of 280 ADHD and 242 non-ADHD families (Faraone, Biederman, Feighner, et al., 2000). For past and current symptoms, ADHD families showed significantly more familial aggregation for adult relatives than for non adult relatives. The pattern of results supporting this hypothesis was seen for both current and past assessments of total ADHD symptoms and for inattentive and hyperactive-impulsive symptoms considered separately. The results also could not be accounted for by gender, psychiatric comorbidity, or ascertainment source because the same pattern of results was found for the subgroups defined by these variables.

Faraone and colleagues also considered the possibility that ADHD in children biases the self-reports of ADHD in their adult relatives (Faraone, Biederman, Feighner, et al., 2000). Because the adult relatives of children with ADHD are usually aware of ADHD symptoms in the ADHD child, that knowledge may bias them to report ADHD symptoms in themselves. If that occurs, then the rates of ADHD among adult relatives of ADHD children would be spuriously high, leading to the incorrect conclusion that adult ADHD

is more familial than child ADHD. However, if ADHD adults are biased to over report symptoms, then the adult relatives of ADHD children should have had a greater number of symptoms than the child relatives. That was not the case. In fact, the adult relatives tended to report fewer symptoms, although the difference was not statistically significant.

This evidence against reporter bias is consistent with a prior report from a different sample (Faraone, Biederman, & Mick, 1997). The study hypothesized the following: if having an ADHD child biased an adult to report ADHD symptoms, then ADHD adults having ADHD children should report more symptoms than ADHD adults who do not have ADHD children. It compared symptom rates between 26 clinically referred ADHD adults who had ADHD children and 49 clinically referred ADHD adults who did not have ADHD children. It rejected the hypothesis by showing that the number of symptoms reported by ADHD adults did not differ between those who did and did not have ADHD children. An additional finding indicated that no individual symptom was more frequent among the ADHD adults who had ADHD children compared with those who did not have ADHD children. This finding was another indication that having an ADHD child did not bias ADHD adults to over report ADHD symptoms.

The literature about persistent ADHD is relatively small, but it suggests that the persistent form of ADHD is familial and shows greater familial loading for ADHD than the non-persistent form. More work from twin and molecular genetic studies is needed to determine if the increased familiality of persistent ADHD reflects the actions of genes or of familial environmental factors.

Gender differences

Levy and colleagues (2005) investigated gender differences in ADHD and comorbidity with oppositional-defiant disorder, conduct disorder, separation anxiety, and measures of reading and language problems in a large sample of child siblings and twins taking part in the Australian Twin ADHD Project (ATAP). The findings indicated that, whereas the pattern of comorbidity differed among three *DSM-IV* subtypes, there were no significant gender differences in comorbidity for externalizing disorders, although girls with the inattentive subtype were more likely to present with symptoms of anxiety. These findings were consistent with those in family studies of few gender differences in externalizing disorders but possible differences in internalizing disorders.

Gender differences in genetic and environmental influences on ADHD have also been investigated in children. Rhee, Waldman, Hay, and Levy (1999) reviewed the twin literature at that time and found that heritability for hyperactivity and inattention did not differ between boys and girls. They also reported on their own study of 1034 MZ twin pairs, 1009 DZ pairs, and 348 sibling pairs aged 3 to 18 years. Overall they found evidence of additive genetic influences (heritability = 0.85 to 0.90) with no influence of shared environmental factors. There were only minor potential differences in the effects of gender, with additive and dominance genetic effects on boys compared to additive effects in girls and some evidence that shared environmental factors might play a small role in girls but not in boys.

The most interesting finding from this paper was support for the polygenic multiple threshold model, which holds that boys are more likely to be affected with ADHD than girls because they have a lower threshold for the liability needed to express itself as the disorder of ADHD. This can be simply understood as the effect of a general factor that shifts the entire distribution of ADHD scores in females downward, with a lower mean score for ADHD symptoms in females compared to males in the general population. Applying the same threshold of clinical severity to both males and females will identify more males as affected. However, in terms of the distribution of liability, female ADHD probands represent a more extreme form of ADHD on the female liability distribution (i.e. representing a more extreme threshold liability) than male probands. This predicts that female ADHD probands would confer a higher familial risk to their siblings than male ADHD probands. We were able to investigate this hypothesis in a large sample of ADHD combined type probands and their siblings from the IMAGE project (Chen et al., 2008) and found that that among 1512 siblings of 1152 male probands there were 239 ADHD cases (15.8%). In contrast, among 226 siblings of 181 female probands there were 57 ADHD cases (25.2%). Hence these data support the liability threshold model as an explanation for the difference in the gender ratio for ADHD in children. Because comparable data are not yet available for adult cohorts we cannot confirm whether these findings will apply equally to ADHD in adults.

Molecular genetic findings

We have already described how international research has established that there is a strong genetically inherited contribution to ADHD. The genetic mechanisms involved are now being sort with considerable success. It is established that certain alleles (sequence variants) of the gene coding for the dopamine D4 receptor (DRD4) occur more frequently in children with ADHD than in healthy controls, and other DNA changes associated with ADHD have been found as well. Several linkage studies that scan the entire human genome (the entire set of human genes) have been completed that indicate suggestive target regions containing one or more risk genes for ADHD.

More recently, enormous expectations have been generated by the development of very high-density genetic marker maps that enable scans of the human genome for association with common genetic variations, using single-nucleotide polymorphism (SNP) arrays that assay hundreds of thousands of markers in one experiment. Genome-wide association strategies have proved to be a powerful method for detecting multiple genetic risk factors of small effect in many complex traits, including blood pressure, obesity, and diabetes (Barrett et al., 2009; Hofker & Wijmenga, 2009; Newton-Cheh et al., 2009). Within psychiatry, genome-wide association studies (GWAS) have clearly identified genetic variants that confer small but significant risks to disorders such as autism and schizophrenia (Barrett et al., 2009; Purcell et al., 2009; Shi et al., 2009; Stefansson et al., 2009).

At the time of writing several GWAS studies have been initiated for ADHD, and initial data have identified several potential genes associated with ADHD that were not the target of previous candidate gene studies (Franke et al., 2009). The strongest of these initial findings is perhaps the association with the Cadherin 13 gene (CDH13). This gene lies within the region of linkage on chromosome 16 identified in the meta-analysis of linkage studies (Zhou, Dempfle, et al., 2008b). SNPs within the CDH13 gene region were reported to be associated with ADHD in a reanalysis of the genome-wide association scan study from the IMAGE sample using a two-stage approach (Lasky-Su et al., 2008) and were within the top 25 findings overall (Neale et al., 2008). Furthermore, the association with ADHD was one of the top findings from a genome-wide association scan using a DNA pooling approach in a German dataset (Lesch et al., 2008) and has also been reported from studies of drug abuse and dependence (Uhl et al., 2009). CDH13 codes for a member of the cell–cell adhesion proteins in addition to playing a role in neural growth regulation. This finding and other hints from GWAS indicate that genes involved in cell division, cell adhesion, neuronal migration and neuronal plasticity may also confer risk for ADHD (Franke et al., 2009).

Yet another approach has been the search for rare mutational events such as copy number variants (CNVs). Initial data are interesting, showing that in cases of ADHD there may be clustering of rare CNVs within genes implicated in other neurodevelopmental disorders, including autism and schizophrenia (Abrahams & Geschwind, 2008; Kirov et al., 2009; Kusenda & Sebat, 2008; Sebat et al., 2007; Stefansson et al., 2008). This finding implies that rare variants that account for ADHD in some cases, are found in genes that also give rise to other neurodevelopmental disorders. For autism around 20% (or more) of all cases may result from rare CNVs (Abrahams & Geschwind, 2008), although we do not yet know whether a similar picture will be found for ADHD.

We should not be surprised by the overlap in genetic risks between ADHD and autism because quantitative genetic studies show overlapping genetic influences, with around 50% of the genetic influences on ADHD symptoms shared with autism symptoms in a population twin sample (Ronald et al., 2006). Therefore, it is of interest that a study in ADHD found clustering of CNVs within genes already implicated in autism (Elia et al., 2010). Furthermore, another study clearly confirmed the association of ADHD with CNVs that have also been implicated in autism and schizophrenia (Williams et al., 2010). We can therefore see that both GWAS and CNV studies are already opening up new avenues of research with the identification of novel genes that had not been previously considered on the basis of prior knowledge of the disorder.

To date nearly all molecular genetic studies have used child ADHD cohorts with a predominance of combined subtype (70–100% in most studies) and inattentive probands (0–30% in most studies). However, this focus will change as large samples of adult ADHD have now been recruited. Only a few genetic studies specifically using adult ADHD samples have been published to date and these have not always yielded the same findings as those seen in children. At this stage there are insufficient data to say whether non-replication in adult samples of some of the findings from childhood ADHD are due to limited sample size and power, measurement error, and the appropriate application of clinical criteria; or whether specific genetic mechanisms are involved in persistence of ADHD into adult life. As we shall see in the case of the dopamine transporter gene, current evidence suggests a different pattern of findings in adults compared to children. However, the fact that adult ADHD is associated with high familial loading for ADHD, has similar effects of stimulant medications on reduction of ADHD symptoms (NICE, 2008), and has similar neurocognitive and functional correlates as in child ADHD suggests that at least some of the same genetic associations will be seen in both children and adults with ADHD. We might therefore expect to see both replications of child findings in adult ADHD samples and genetic differences that relate to the long-term outcomes of ADHD in adults.

Candidate gene association studies

Numerous candidate gene studies have been completed that use genetic association strategies to determine whether genetic variation within genes with an a priori hypothesis for a role in the etiology of ADHD increases the risk for ADHD (Asherson, 2004; Faraone et al., 2005; Galili-Weisstub et al., 2005; Gizer et al., 2009). Much of this work has focused on genes in catecholaminergic systems because the drugs that effectively treat ADHD either increase levels of synaptic dopamine through increased release of dopamine or blockade of reuptake from the synapse (e.g. the stimulants) or serve as norepinephrine reuptake inhibitors (e.g. tricyclic antidepressants, atomoxetine). Compared with genes involved in regulating dopaminergic and noradrenergic systems, gene regulation of serotonergic systems has received relatively little attention in ADHD research. This is because measures of serotonin metabolism are minimally related to the clinical efficacy of the medicines that treat ADHD. Nevertheless, molecular genetic studies have examined serotonergic genes because of the well-known role of serotonin in impulsivity, one of the core symptoms of ADHD (Brunner & Hen, 1997).

One plausible pathway to ADHD was discovered through the study of Coloboma mice, which have a hemizygous deletion of chromosome 2q (Wilson, 2000). The deletion region includes the gene encoding SNAP-25, a neurone-specific protein implicated in the exocytotic release of neurotransmitters from nerve terminals. Coloboma mice show spontaneous hyperactivity, delays in achieving complex neonatal motor abilities, and learning deficiencies. These problems are not seen if the mice are given a functioning SNAP-25 gene through a transgenic procedure. Treatment with amphetamine but not methylphenidate reverses the mouse hyperactivity, which is consistent with the mechanism of action of these medications. Both methylphenidate and amphetamine treat ADHD by blocking the dopamine transporter. However, amphetamine also facilitates the non-vesicular release of dopamine through reverse transport, an activity that would be expected to reverse the deficits in exocytotic neurotransmitter release caused by the Coloboma mutation.

To test genes associated with these biological hypotheses, candidate gene studies have used case-control or family-based designs. Case-control designs compare allele frequencies between patients with ADHD and non-ADHD controls. Alleles that confer risk for ADHD should be more common among ADHD patients compared to controls. The family-based design compares the alleles that parents transmit to their offspring with ADHD to those that they do not transmit. If an allele increases the risk for ADHD, it should be transmitted more commonly from parents to their affected offspring than by chance. From both study designs it is possible to derive an odds ratio (OR) that assesses the magnitude of the association between ADHD and the putative risk alleles (an OR of 1.0 indicates no association, those greater than 1.0 indicate the allele increases risk for ADHD, and those less than 1.0 indicate the allele decreases risk for ADHD).

Faraone et al. (2005) reviewed the ADHD candidate gene literature and examined pooled ORs for candidate risk alleles that had been reported in at least three case-control or family-based association studies. Table 4.1 shows eight findings that provide statistically significant evidence of association with ADHD based on the pooled ORs from three or more studies. These genes encode proteins for the D4 and D5 dopamine receptors (DRD4, DRD5), the dopamine transporter (DAT1), dopamine beta hydroxylase (an enzyme that converts dopamine to noradrenalin), the serotonin transporter, the serotonin 1B receptor, and SNAP-25. Together these genes are thought to contribute around 3–4% to additive genetic variance on ADHD (Kuntsi et al., 2006). Many other genes have been studied but in most cases have yielded either

Table 4.1 Pooled odds ratios for genes examined in three or more studies

Gene	Number of studies	OR	95% CI
FB: DRD4 (VNTR, 7-repeat)	17	1.16	1.03–1.31
CC: DRD4 (VNTR, 7-repeat)	13	1.45	1.27–1.65
FB: DRD5 (CA repeat, 148 bp)	14	1.24	1.12–1.38
FB: SLC6A3 (VNTR, 10-repeat)	14	1.13	1.03–1.24
FB: DBH (TaqI A)n	3	1.33	1.11–1.59
FB: SNAP-25 (T1065G)	5	1.19	1.03–1.38
CC: SLC6A4(5HTTLPR long)	3	1.31	1.09–1.59
FB: HTR1B (G861C)	3	1.44	1.14–1.83

Notes: CC = case control, FB = family-based; OR = odds ratio; Inf. Trans = informative transmissions; CI = confidence interval.
Source: Based on Faraone et al. (2005) and Kuntsi et al. (2006).

negative or uncertain findings either because of discrepancies in the published findings or a lack of further studies to confirm or refute initial observations. These genes include the noradrenergic transporter, catechol-o-methyltransferase and monoamine oxidase (both involved in the breakdown of neurotransmitters such as dopamine), the dopamine D1 and D3 receptors, tyrosine hydroxylase, and other neurotransmitter receptors including noradrenergic, serotonin, acetylcholine, and glutamate 2A receptor subunits.

More recently, several studies have investigated relatively large numbers of candidate genes using multiple markers to capture genetic variation spanning entire gene regions. The first study of this type was completed by the IMAGE project (Brookes, Xu, et al., 2006). Using a sample of 776 *DSM-IV* combined-type probands and their parents for within-family tests of association, they looked for association with 1038 SNPs spanning 51 genes. The genes covered were all involved in the regulation of neurotransmitter pathways, particularly dopamine, norepinephrine, and serotonin pathways, in addition to circadian rhythm genes. Although the study identified nominal significance with one or more SNPs in 18 of the genes investigated, none of the findings withstood correction for multiple testing of markers. However, the study was able to replicate some key findings in the literature (DRD4 and DAT1), as well as potential association in other genes (TPH2, ARRB2, SYP, DAT1, ADRB2, HES1, MAOA, and PNMT). One unusual but interesting finding from the IMAGE sample was the association with a rare SNP in the noradrenergic gene that conferred protection against ADHD. The finding was replicated in a follow-up sample from IMAGE and two independent samples from Dublin and Massachusetts with ORs ranging from 0.26 to 0.54 (Xu et al., 2008).

Another study that adopted a similar approach used both child and adult samples to investigate the association with 19 genes involved in the regulation of serotonergic pathways (Ribases et al., 2007). Using a clinical sample of 451 ADHD patients (188 adults and 263 children) and 400 controls, the study found several significant associations after correcting for multiple testing: the DDC gene was strongly associated with both adulthood ($p = 0.0005$; OR $= 2.2$) and childhood ADHD ($p = 0.0027$; OR $= 1.9$); the MAOB gene was associated in the adult ADHD sample ($p = 0.003$; OR $= 1.9$); and the 5HT2A gene showed evidence of association with the combined ADHD subtype in both adults ($p = 0.004$; OR $= 1.6$) and children ($p = 0.008$; OR $= 1.5$). This study not only identifies serotonergic pathway genes associated with ADHD (subject to further replication and meta-analytic studies) but also is the first to identify associations that replicate between child and adult ADHD samples within the same study.

One of the overall conclusions from the candidate gene studies completed to date is the existence of genetic risk factors for ADHD that each confer only a small amount to the overall genetic risk, with the average ORs for the positive associations ranging from 1.13 to 1.5. These small ORs are consistent with the idea that many genes of small effect mediate the genetic vulnerability to ADHD. Moreover, they indicate that the most common explanation for the frequent failure to replicate initial reports of association is that many individual studies are underpowered to find significant genetic associations (Altshuler & Daly, 2007; Lohmueller et al., 2003).

Such small and often inconsistent effects emphasize the need for future molecular genetic studies to implement strategies that will provide sufficient statistical power. So far, this has been achieved only through meta-analytic studies, although currently very large samples are being made available through consortia projects. Of particular note was a combined analysis of multiple datasets for DRD4, DRD5, and DAT1 resulting in genome-wide levels of significance for DRD4 ($p = 2 \times 1012$) and DRD5 ($p = 8 \times 10^{-8}$) but not for DAT1 (Li et al., 2006).

The dopamine D4 receptor: The most consistent association between ADHD and a common genetic variant is with the dopamine D4 receptor gene (DRD4). As indicated by meta-analysis there is a small but highly significant association with the 7-repeat allele of a variable number tandem repeat (VNTR) marker (Li et al., 2006). Both noradrenaline and dopamine are potent agonists of the dopamine D4 receptor (Lanau et al., 1997), which is prevalent in fronto–subcortical networks implicated in the pathophysiology of ADHD by neuroimaging and neuropsychological studies (Bush, Valera, & Seidman, 2005; Castellanos & Tannock, 2002; Doyle et al., 2005; Seidman, Valera, & Makris, 2005).

The association of ADHD with the 7-repeat allele of a VNTR polymorphism in exon 3 of DRD4 was first described in 1996 in a small sample of 39 children and 39 ethnically matched controls (LaHoste et al., 1996) and followed reports that the 7-repeat allele was associated with adult novelty seeking (Benjamin et al., 1996; Ebstein et al., 1996). The association with novelty seeking is, however, far from conclusive. Meta-analysis of 20 studies that included a total of 3907 individuals concluded that on average there was no effect of this gene on the adult trait of novelty seeking, although 13 studies had found that the 7-repeat allele was more frequent in individuals with higher novelty-seeking scores (Kluger, Siegfried, & Ebstein, 2002). However, there was evidence of *true heterogeneity*, indicating that there were likely to be important moderators that could explain why some studies found evidence for this association and others did not.

Because novelty-seeking traits are known to be associated with adult ADHD (Downey et al., 1997) this raised the possibility that in adults the association between novelty seeking and ADHD is mediated by DRD4. This possibility was investigated in a study that looked at the links among DRD4, ADHD, and novelty-seeking temperament in the parents of children who had taken part in an affected sibling pair linkage study of ADHD (Lynn et al., 2005). These parents were therefore expected to be at high risk for ADHD and to share specific genetic risk factors with their two affected offspring. The lifetime recurrence rate of DSM-IV ADHD among the 171 parents investigated was 33%, and a current ADHD diagnosis was seen in 16%. Among the parents it was found that although novelty seeking predicted a lifetime diagnosis of ADHD and the 7-repeat allele of DRD4 was found to be associated with ADHD (explaining 5% of the variance in adult ADHD symptom scores), there was no association between DRD4 and novelty seeking. The authors concluded that in this unique sample of parents from multiply affected ADHD families, novelty seeking and the 48-bp DRD4 variant were associated with a lifetime history of ADHD; however, the association between novelty seeking and ADHD could not be explained by genetic variation of DRD4.

There have been a few other studies of DRD4 in adult ADHD populations. One used a dataset of adult ADHD probands collected in Toronto by Muglia and colleagues (2000). They tested for the presence of association with DRD4 in two independent samples, one comprising 66 cases and 66 ethnically matched controls and the second made up of nuclear families. Case-control analysis found a significantly higher presence of the 7-repeat allele in the adult ADHD probands ($p = 0.01$), a trend in the dataset of nuclear families, and overall good evidence for the association ($p = .003$).

One other study that found evidence for the DRD4 association used large multiply affected pedigrees from Columbia and incorporated analysis of individuals who were diagnosed with ADHD as adults. Using tests of association that included analysis of co-segregation of the 7-repeat allele with affection status across generations, they found significant evidence for the association with ADHD (Arcos-Burgos, Castellanos, Konecki, et al., 2004). It therefore appears that several studies that have investigated the association between adult ADHD and DRD4 have found evidence for this association.

Finally a recent study from Norway investigated the DRD4 association in a sample of 358 adult ADHD cases (Johansson et al., 2007). They found no evidence of association, but rather a similar frequency of the 7-repeat allele in the ADHD cases and a set of 340 controls.

The dopamine transporter gene: The International Multicentre Persistent ADHD CollaboraTion (IMPACT) group was formed in 2007 from research groups with adult ADHD samples from Germany, Norway, Spain, the Netherlands, the United Kingdom, and the United States. One of their first studies to be completed was the analysis of the two VNTR polymorphisms within the dopamine transporter gene (DAT1) reported to be associated with ADHD in several childhood ADHD samples (Asherson et al., 2007). DAT1 has been one of the most investigated genes in ADHD genetic research, since the initial report of an association with the 10-repeat allele of a VNTR in the 3'untranslated region of the gene (Cook et al., 1995). Despite numerous subsequent studies showing positive evidence of association with the 10-repeat allele

there have also been many negative studies, and the results of meta-analytic studies show little or no effect (Faraone et al., 2005; Li et al., 2006; Maher et al., 2002; Yang et al., 2007). Significant evidence of heterogeneity suggests that the inconsistent findings might relate to identifiable sources of heterogeneity (Li et al., 2006). Potential sources of heterogeneity include association with a specific haplotype (Asherson et al., 2007; Brookes, Mill, et al., 2006), association with ADHD that is not comorbid with conduct disorder (Zhou, Chen, et al., 2008), and interaction with prenatal risk factors (Becker et al., 2008; Kahn et al., 2003; Neuman et al., 2007).

Because some genes may be associated with persistence or desistence of ADHD, another potential source of heterogeneity may be the developmental age of the samples. Although the comparison between persistent and desistent forms of ADHD has yet to be formally evaluated, several groups have examined the 3'UTR polymorphism in adult ADHD samples. Initial results have been inconsistent, with some studies finding evidence for association with the 9-repeat rather than the 10-repeat allele (Barkley et al., 2006b; Bruggemann et al., 2007; Franke et al., 2008; Johansson et al., 2007; Muglia et al., 2002). The IMPACT group has completed a further analysis using a combined dataset that includes a total of 1520 cases and 1854 controls from Germany, Netherlands, Norway, and Spain (Franke et al., 2010). Whereas the 10/10 genotype of the 3'UTR polymorphism was thought to be associated with ADHD in children, this study found that the 9/9 genotype was associated with ADHD in adults ($P = 0.03$), with an average OR of 1.34 (95% CI 1.03–1.76). Although this finding may not be strongly significant it is notable that four of the five samples included in the combined analysis showed the same direction effect. It is therefore feasible that the dopamine transporter gene plays a role in modifying the phenotype rather than causing it, with the 9-repeat associated with persistence of ADHD symptoms into adult life.

Other molecular genetic studies in adult ADHD

Muglia and De Luca previously reported on other genetic associations with adult ADHD, but none have been significant. They conducted studies of the dopamine transporter gene in 152 adult ADHD probands (Muglia, Jain, Inkster, et al., 2002), the dopamine D3 receptor gene in a small sample of only

39 adult ADHD nuclear families (Muglia, Jain, & Kennedy, 2002), and the noradrenergic transporter gene and adrenergic 2C receptor gene in 128 trios (De Luca, Muglia, Jain, et al., 2004; De Luca, Muglia, Vincent, et al., 2004). As reported earlier Ribases and colleagues, using samples collected in Spain, compared child and adult samples directly and were able to find associations in two genes that replicated between the two subsamples (Ribases et al., 2007). Johansson and colleagues from Norway (2007) studied DRD5 and DAT1 in addition to DRD4 and found evidence that the microsatellite allele close to the DRD5 gene associated in the previous studies with child ADHD was also associated in their adult ADHD sample ($p = 0.02$, OR = 1.27).

Genome-wide linkage scans

To date, there have been seven independent ADHD genome-wide linkage scans published. The UCLA (Fisher et al., 2002; Ogdie et al., 2003, 2004) and MGH studies (Faraone et al., 2008) from the United States, the Dutch study (Bakker et al., 2003), the German study (Hedebrand et al., 2006) and a multisite European study (Asherson et al., 2008) used an affected sibling pair (ASP) design; in addition, an extended pedigree study has been completed from a population isolate in Colombia (Arcos-Burgos, Castellanos, Pineda, et al., 2004). All these studies were designed to map genes underpinning the *DSM-IV*-defined categorical ADHD phenotype. Table 4.1 summarizes the linkage signals nominated from the categorical ADHD scans. Using a binary ADHD phenotype, each study identified some genomic regions with significant (LOD > 3.0 or MLS > 3.0) or suggestive (LOD > 2.0 or MLS > 2.0) linkage signals. Three regions – chromosomes 5p, 9p, and 17p – showed suggestive linkage in independent studies. The well-recognized ADHD candidate gene, the dopamine transporter gene (DAT1), is located in the vicinity of the chromosome 5p region and might give rise at least in part to the linkage signal (Friedel et al., 2007). However, none of the linkage regions was consistently detected in all the scans, and the majority were found in only one study.

The linkage study from Arcos-Burgos and colleagues is of interest to adult ADHD because they used 18 extended multigenerational families identified in Colombia (Arcos-Burgos et al., 2002). These families were selected through child probands referred for clinical evaluation for ADHD and subsequent psychiatric

Table 4.2 Summary of nonparametric multipoint LOD scores from published linkage scans

Chromosome region	Bakker 2003	Ogdie 2004	Arcos-Bergos 2004
3q13	1.4	ns	Ns
4p16	1.8	ns	Ns
4q13	ns	ns	2.7
5p13	1.4 *	2.6	Ns
5q33	ns	ns	1.6
6q12	ns	3.3	Ns
6q26	1.2	ns	Ns
7p13	3.0	ns	Ns
8q11	ns	ns	1.9
9q33	2.0	ns	Ns
10cen	1.3	ns	Ns
11q22	ns	ns	4.0
11q25	ns	1.0	Ns
13q33	2.0	0.8	Ns
16p13	ns	3.7	Ns
17p11	ns	3.6	3.0
20q13	ns	1.1	Ns

Note: Score >1.0 is mild evidence, >2.0 moderate evidence, >3.0 strong evidence.
*Broad criteria in study from Bakker et al., 2003.
Sources: Arcos-Burgos et al., 2004; Bakker et al., 2003; Ogdie et al., 2004; Smalley et al., 2002.

interviews were conducted with 433 individuals who were informative for linkage analysis, including 284 adults aged over 17 years. The families were found to contain a very high proportion of individuals affected with ADHD (32.8%); many pedigree members had significant levels of comorbid ADHD with conduct and oppositional-defiant disorders as well as with alcohol and tobacco dependence. The linkage scan used both traditional parametric and nonparametric approaches that took advantage of the affection status for individuals across all generations (Arcos-Burgos, Castellanos, Pineda, et al., 2004). In addition to the overall evidence for linkage shown in Table 4.2, they found that certain families showed strong linkage to different specific genetic loci, with marked co-segregation of certain regions and affection status, suggesting a high level of locus heterogeneity (different genes acting within different pedigrees).

The results of the linkage studies are difficult to interpret for several reasons. First, linkage studies do not have sufficient power to identify most common genetic variation associated with common disorders, which are expected to have small effect sizes far below the resolution of feasible linkage studies (Risch & Merikangas, 1996). Although linkage is a powerful technique for detecting single genes of major effect, it is not as applicable (even for genes of large effect) in cases where there is considerable genetic heterogeneity, with different families segregating different genes. Second, in the analysis of common complex disorders, linkage can only define relatively large chromosomal regions that contain numerous genes, so that considerable additional work is required to move from a positive linkage finding to the identification of a specific gene or functionally significant genetic variant(s).

To gain an overall impression from the ADHD linkage research, a meta-analysis was recently completed that combined data from seven independent studies (Zhou, Dempfle, et al., 2008). In the meta-analysis, genome-wide significant linkage was identified on chromosome 16 between 64 Mb and 83 Mb based on small but consistent findings from this particular location spread across the seven studies. In addition, nine other genomic regions showed nominal or suggestive evidence of linkage. Overall, the linkage results may be informative and could focus the search for novel ADHD susceptibility genes, although specific risk genes that explain the linkage findings have yet to be clearly identified. Of particular interest, however, is the finding from GWAS that a gene called CDH13 may be associated with ADHD; it lies within the chromosome 16 region identified in the meta-analytic study (Zhou, Dempfle, et al., 2008).

One gene that has been specifically identified following an initial linkage strategy is the latrophilin 3 gene (LPHN3) (Arcos-Burgos, Jain, Acosta, et al., 2010; Ribases, Antoni Ramos-Quiroga, Sanchez-Mora, et al., 2010). The original studies used large multi-generational families from the genetically isolated Paisa population in Columbia. A genome linkage study of 16 families found significant linkage on chromosome 4q13 (Arcos-Burgos, Castellanos, Pineda, et al., 2004). Fine-mapping applied to nine of the families narrowed a critical region of around 20,000,000 base pairs. Following studies identified a significant region of association within exons 4 through to 19 of LPHN3 that was replicated in samples from US, German, Spanish and Norwegian samples, with an average odds ratio of around 1.2 (Arcos-Burgos, Jain, Acosta, et al., 2010). Finally, a further study of 334

adults with ADHD and 334 controls from Spain found additional evidence for the association, indicating an association between genetic variants of LPHN3 and ADHD throughout the lifespan (Ribases, Antoni Ramos-Quiroga, Sanchez-Mora, et al., 2010). The role of LPHN3 is not well understood, but it is a G-protein coupled receptor that is thought to be involved in neurotransmission and maintenance of neuronal viability.

Genome-wide association scans of ADHD

Further work is currently underway to generate sufficient GWAS data to identify novel genes associated with ADHD. Although initial data from 958 ADHD proband–parent trios from the IMAGE sample were inconclusive, because none of the genetic markers showed genome-wide levels of significance for the association with ADHD (Neale et al., 2008), further studies are underway to extend the available GWAS data for ADHD and their results will be combined in meta-analytic studies. A recent report combining GWAS datasets from across Europe and the United States failed to detect any further loci that stand out, suggesting that 10,000 or more samples may be needed to clearly identify common risk variants for ADHD in childhood ADHD samples (Neale et al., 2010). The addition of adult samples such as those from the IMPACT group may be important to the search for novel genetic mechanisms in ADHD because of the relatively high familial loading for the adult phenotype. Despite the potential difficulties in accumulating the required sample sizes, the availability of large collaborative datasets means that expectations are high that within 1–2 years novel gene systems that confer increased risk for ADHD will be identified.

Concluding remarks and the authors' perspective

Quantitative genetic studies of ADHD have moved beyond simple estimations of heritability to answer more complex questions about genetic and environmental influences on ADHD course and development. Analysis of ADHD symptoms has found that the stability of ADHD symptoms in childhood is accounted for by shared genetic influences.

In childhood shared genetic factors also explain familial associations between ADHD and comorbid disorders and traits, including conduct disorder, dyslexia, and lower IQ. The recognition of shared genetic influences is conceptually important, suggesting the existence of multiple overlapping (pleiotropic) effects of genes, or risk models (genes → risk for ADHD → risk for comorbid disorder), rather than distinct genetic risk factors for which individual sets of genes map onto individual developmental pathways. Pleiotropic effects are likely because most genes that regulate brain function are expressed in multiple brain regions, and therefore functional genetic variation will have an impact on more than one neuronal pathway/system. Furthermore, individual brain regions may affect multiple brain processes (Kovas & Plomin, 2006). However, shared genetic effects may indicate developmental trajectories by which genes influence disorder A (e.g. ADHD) that in turn increases risk for disorder B (e.g. antisocial behavior). Such developmental trajectories from ADHD to the development of comorbidity will likely be mediated by additional environmental and genetic influences. Finally family and twin studies cannot exclude the possibility that some independent genetic effects act on comorbidities. Identifying the specific genes involved will help clarify the causal relationships between ADHD and co-occurring disorders and traits.

However, genetic investigations of adult ADHD are in their infancy. Twin studies of older adolescents find the same high heritabilities as seen in younger children, and family and adoption studies inform us that the adult disorder is highly familial and may in fact be more valid than child ADHD as an index of risk for ADHD among close family members. Twin studies measuring ADHD symptoms in the adult population suggest that self-rated ADHD symptoms are not a particularly heritable phenotype, and it remains to be clarified whether this finding is due to measurement problems or reflects a true change in the balance of genetic and environmental influences on the adult phenotype. However, adoption studies indicate that the association between offspring and parent ADHD is "biologically driven" and therefore likely to be the result of shared genes and not shared environments.

Molecular genetic studies of childhood ADHD have developed rapidly since the first reports of association with the dopamine D4 receptor and dopamine transporter genes (DAT1). The association with DRD4 has stood the test of time with multiple replications (and nonreplications) and evidence from meta-analyses confirming small but significant effects on

risk for ADHD. Molecular genetic studies of adult ADHD are still relatively few, but there seems to be consistent evidence that the DRD4 association is also seen in the adult ADHD population. This makes sense from an evolutionary perspective because it has been shown that the DRD4 7-repeat allele arose relatively recently as a rare mutation event and has subsequently been positively selected. This means that in some way it has increased the chances of being passed on to subsequent generations (increased fertility), presumably by affecting the behavior of adults who carry one or two copies of this genetic variant (Ding et al., 2002; Wang et al., 2004). Genetic associations with ADHD in children have yet to be fully investigated in adult ADHD.

As discussed earlier, future quantitative and molecular genetic studies of adult ADHD can unravel key questions about the etiological relationship between adult ADHD and comorbid disorders and traits, including mood disorders, personality disorders, antisocial behavior, and drug, alcohol, and tobacco addiction. These studies will be important in clarifying the etiological and nosological distinctions between adult ADHD and comorbid conditions. The status of mood instability is particularly interesting because it commonly co-occurs with ADHD symptoms in adults and is a major cause of diagnostic confusion due to overlapping clinical definitions within current diagnostic systems (Skirrow et al., 2009). One potential pitfall identified from the research so far is the use of self-rating scales for ADHD symptoms in adults. Available data from twin studies find that self-rated ADHD symptoms are far less familial than observer ratings and do not appear to be highly heritable, so the use of reporter accounts and more objective measures will be important. The reason why self-ratings should show such different familial associations is not known; however, on the basis of current data, it may be specific to rating ADHD symptoms in the general population, given that self-ratings of personality traits show greater evidence of genetic effects. Despite these data, family and adoption studies consistently show increased rates of ADHD, related traits, and neuropsychological impairments in the biological parents of children with ADHD.

As in other areas of psychiatry, the "nature–nurture" debate on ADHD has been vociferous over the years. Environmental risks for ADHD were known before genetic influences were established. George Still in 1902 first reported the occurrence of a hyperactive behavior pattern when brain damage was expected, but this finding could not be demonstrated and was hypothesized to include etiological factors such as birth injury or mild anoxia. This laid the foundation for the concept of minimal brain damage/dysfunction, a childhood syndrome that included developmental impairments in control of attention, impulse, and motor function, as well as in perception, conceptualization, language, and memory linked to deviations in the function of the central nervous system. The subsequent finding that genetic factors explain familial aggregation of ADHD suggested a likely role for gene–environment interaction (Rutter & Silberg, 2002).

The role of environmental risks has not been investigated in relation to adult ADHD, but might be involved in persistence of the disorder. To date only a few molecular genetic studies of ADHD incorporate environmental-risk measures. Kahn and colleagues (2003) reported that in preschool children, hyperactivity-impulsivity and oppositional behavior were associated with genetic variation of DAT1, but only in a group exposed to maternal smoking during the pregnancy; this finding was recently replicated by Becker and colleagues (2008). We also reported that the DAT1 association with ADHD might be confined to a group whose mothers were drinking alcohol during pregnancy (Brookes, Mill, et al., 2006). These studies suggest that functional variation of DAT1 might modify the direct effects of tobacco and alcohol on the developing fetal brain and thereby the risk for ADHD. Although this is a plausible neurobiological hypothesis, these data are equally consistent with the effect of damaging parental influences because we know that mothers who smoke during pregnancy are more likely to be antisocial, have children with antisocial men, bring up their children in disadvantaged circumstances, and to be depressed (Maughan et al., 2004). However, new data from the investigation of births following in vitro fertilization have found that maternal use of tobacco during pregnancy is only associated with offspring ADHD when there is a genetic relationship between the mother and offspring, and not where the developing fetus is genetically unrelated to the mother (Thapar et al., 2009). This important finding suggests genetic mediation of the association between offspring ADHD and maternal smoking and raises the possibility that there may be no direct toxic effect of smoking on behavioral outcomes, but rather that there may be a correlation between parental smoking behavior and genetic risks for ADHD.

A major challenge is to identify the neurocognitive processes that mediate genetic influences on ADHD. Although much progress has been made in cognitive experimental research on ADHD, a consensus has yet to emerge on the key underlying processes. One approach to understanding the neurobiology of ADHD is to investigate brain function through performance on cognitive tasks that delineate the underlying cognitive processes. Cognitive studies find widespread impairments in both children and adults with ADHD, with deficits particularly on executive function tasks, especially those measuring response inhibition and sustained attention (Johnson et al., 2009; Willcutt et al., 2005). Among the various cognitive variables investigated, reaction time (RT) variability is one of the most effective in discriminating between ADHD and control samples (Johnson et al., 2009; Klein et al., 2006; Kuntsi et al., 2001), although several other behavioral and cognitive measures are associated with the condition.

In a recent (Kuntsi et al. 2010) study Kuntsi and colleagues used a multivariate (MV) familial factor approach in a large sample of ADHD and control sibling pairs to address the question of whether one or more familial factors underlie the slow and variable reaction times (Andreou et al., 2007; Uebel et al., 2009), impaired response inhibition and sustained attention (Uebel et al., 2009), and choice impulsivity (preference for smaller immediate rewards, incorporating "delay aversion"; Marco et al., 2009) that were previously reported to be associated with ADHD and siblings of ADHD probands, using samples from the IMAGE project. MV methods delineate the architecture of genetic and environmental influences underlying the association between ADHD and task performance, while simultaneously addressing the etiological influences on several separately measured cognitive processes and, further, indicating their relative importance. Results from these analyses indicated the presence of two familial cognitive impairment factors in ADHD. The larger factor, reflecting 70% of the familial variance with ADHD, captured all familial influences on mean RT and RT variability. The smaller factor, reflecting 20% of the familial variance with ADHD, captured all familial influences on omission errors on the go/no-go task and 60% of those on commission errors.

The identification of separate "variability" and "error" factors is predicted by previous cognitive models for ADHD including the arousal-attention model

(Johnson et al., 2007; O'Connell et al., 2008, 2009) and the developmental model from Halperin. Within the developmental framework (Halperin & Schulz, 2006; Halperin et al., 2008), RT variability is proposed to reflect poor state regulation, perceptual sensitivity, and/or weak arousal mechanisms. The model proposes a distinction between two neurocognitive processes: (1) the proposed subcortical dysfunction linked to the etiology of ADHD and (2) prefrontally mediated executive control, linked to persistence or desistence of ADHD during adolescence. As such, one possible interpretation of the two familial factors is that the first factor (RT) represents the core, enduring deficit and the second factor (errors) represents prefrontally mediated executive control. The model predicts that the extent to which executive control functions, which develop throughout childhood and adolescence, can compensate for the more primary and enduring subcortical deficits, can determine the degree of recovery from ADHD symptoms. Future research could apply the current model of two familial factors within a longitudinal design to test the predictions emerging from the developmental model (Kuntsi et al., 2010).

In conclusion, the new genetics heralded by the near completion of the human genome sequence has been followed by a rapid increase in the number of identified genetic variants. It has shifted the goal of behavioral genetic research from gene discovery toward gene functionality (McGuffin & Plomin, 2004). Quantitative genetic findings have shifted perception of ADHD toward that of a quantitative trait sharing etiological influences with other developmental, behavioral, and cognitive traits. Molecular genetics has confirmed a priori hypotheses of dopamine system dysregulation and promises to identify additional genes and gene systems in the coming decade. Combining genetic, environmental, and neurobiological research has the potential to delineate causal links between ADHD and the developmental course of the disorder, including persistence of ADHD symptoms into adulthood and comorbidity with adult psychiatric disorders and traits. At a time when the role of developmental or "life span" disorders is increasingly being recognized within adult as well as child psychiatry, the knowledge generated by the use of quantitative and molecular genetic holds promise for increased understanding of the influences in persistence/desistence of ADHD, the links between ADHD and comorbid disorders, and the development of improved clinical approaches to the treatment and diagnosis of ADHD in the adult population.

References

Abrahams BS, Geschwind DH. (2008). Advances in autism genetics: on the threshold of a new neurobiology. *Nat Rev Genet* 9:341–55.

Alberts-Corush J, Firestone P, Goodman JT. (1986). Attention and impulsivity characteristics of the biological and adoptive parents of hyperactive and normal control children. *Am J Orthopsychiatry* 56:413–23.

Alterman AI, Petrarulo E, Tarter R, McGowan JR. (1982). Hyperactivity and alcoholism: familial and behavioral correlates. *Addict Behav* 7:413–21.

Alterman AI, Tarter RE. (1983). The transmission of psychological vulnerability. Implications for alcoholism etiology. *J Nerv Ment Dis* 171:147–54.

Alterman AI, Tarter RE. (1986). An examination of selected typologies. Hyperactivity, familial, and antisocial alcoholism. *Recent Dev Alcohol* 4:169–89.

Altshuler D, Daly M. (2007). Guilt beyond a reasonable doubt. *Nat Genet* 39:813–15.

Andreou P, Neale BM, Chen W, Christiansen H, Gabriels I, Heise A, et al. (2007). Reaction time performance in ADHD: improvement under fast-incentive condition and familial effects. *Psychol Med* 37:1703–15.

Arcos-Burgos M, Castellanos FX, Konecki D, Lopera F, Pineda D, Palacio JD, et al. (2004). Pedigree disequilibrium test (PDT) replicates association and linkage between DRD4 and ADHD in multigenerational and extended pedigrees from a genetic isolate. *Mol Psychiatry* 9:252–9.

Arcos-Burgos M, Castellanos FX, Lopera F, Pineda D, Palacio JD, Garcia M, et al. (2002). Attention-deficit/hyperactivity disorder (ADHD): feasibility of linkage analysis in a genetic isolate using extended and multigenerational pedigrees. *Clin Genet* 61:335–43.

Arcos-Burgos M, Castellanos FX, Pineda D, Lopera F, Palacio JD, Palacio LG, et al. (2004). Attention-deficit/hyperactivity disorder in a population isolate: linkage to loci at 4q13.2, 5q33.3, 11q22, and 17p11. *Am J Hum Genet* 75:998–1014.

Arcos-Burgos M, Jain M, Acosta MT, et al. (2010). A common variant of the latrophilin 3 gene, LPHN3, confers susceptibility to ADHD and predicts effectiveness of stimulant medication. *Mol Psychiatry*.

Asherson P. (2004). Attention-Deficit Hyperactivity Disorder in the post-genomic era. *Eur Child Adolesc Psychiatry* 13(suppl 1):I50–70.

Asherson P. (2005). Clinical assessment and treatment of attention deficit hyperactivity disorder in adults. *Expert Rev Neurother* 5:525–39.

Asherson P, Brookes K, Franke B, Chen W, Gill M, Ebstein RP, et al. (2007). Confirmation that a specific haplotype of the dopamine transporter gene is associated with combined-type ADHD. *Am J Psychiatry* 164:674–7.

Asherson P, Kuntsi J, Taylor E. (2005). Unravelling the complexity of attention-deficit hyperactivity disorder: a behavioural genomic approach. *Br J Psychiatry* 187:103–5.

Asherson P, Zhou K, Anney RJ, Franke B, Buitelaar J, Ebstein R, et al. (2008). A high-density SNP linkage scan with 142 combined subtype ADHD sib pairs identifies linkage regions on chromosomes 9 and 16. *Mol Psychiatry* 13(5):514–21.

Bakker SC, Van Der Meulen EM, Buitelaar JK, Sandkuijl LA, Pauls DL, Monsuur AJ, et al. (2003). A whole-genome scan in 164 Dutch sib pairs with attention-deficit/hyperactivity disorder: suggestive evidence for linkage on chromosomes 7p and 15q. *Am J Hum Genet* 72:1251–60.

Barkley RA, Smith KM, Fischer M, Navia B. (2006). An examination of the behavioral and neuropsychological correlates of three ADHD candidate gene polymorphisms (DRD4 7+, DBH TaqI A2, and DAT1 40 bp VNTR) in hyperactive and normal children followed to adulthood. *Am J Med Genet B Neuropsychiatr Genet* 141B(5):487–98.

Barrett JC, Clayton DG, Concannon P, Akolkar B, Cooper JD, Erlich HA, et al. (2009). Genome-wide association study and meta-analysis find that over 40 loci affect risk of type 1 diabetes. *Nat Genet* 41:703–7.

Becker K, El-Faddagh M, Schmidt MH, Esser G, Laucht M. (2008). Interaction of dopamine transporter genotype with prenatal smoke exposure on ADHD symptoms. *J Pediatr* 152:263–9.

Benjamin J, Li L, Patterson C, Greenberg BD, Murphy DL, Hamer DH. (1996). Population and familial association between the D4 dopamine receptor gene and measures of Novelty Seeking. *Nat Genet* 12:81–4.

Biederman J, Faraone SV, Keenan K, Knee D, Tsuang MT. (1990). Family-genetic and psychosocial risk factors in DSM-III attention deficit disorder. *J Am Acad Child Adolesc Psychiatry* 29:526–33.

Biederman J, Faraone SV, Mick E, Spencer T, Wilens T, Kiely K, et al. (1995). High risk for attention deficit hyperactivity disorder among children of parents with childhood onset of the disorder: a pilot study. *Am J Psychiatry* 152:431–5.

Biederman J, Faraone S, Milberger S, Curtis S, Chen L, Marrs A, et al. (1996). Predictors of persistence and remission of ADHD into adolescence: results from a four-year prospective follow-up study. *J Am Acad Child Adolesc Psychiatry* 35:343–51.

Biederman J, Faraone SV, Monuteaux MC. (2002). Differential effect of environmental adversity by gender: Rutter's index of adversity in a group of boys and girls with and without ADHD. *Am J Psychiatry* 159:1556–62.

Biederman J, Mick E, Faraone SV. (2000). Age-dependent decline of symptoms of attention deficit hyperactivity disorder: impact of remission definition and symptom type. *Am J Psychiatry* 157:816–18.

Brookes KJ, Mill J, Guindalini C, Curran S, Xu X, Knight J, et al. (2006). A common haplotype of the dopamine transporter gene associated with attention-deficit/hyperactivity disorder and interacting with maternal use of alcohol during pregnancy. *Arch Gen Psychiatry* 63:74–81.

Brookes K, Xu X, Chen W, Zhou K, Neale B, Lowe N, et al. (2006). The analysis of 51 genes in DSM-IV combined type attention deficit hyperactivity disorder: association signals in DRD4, DAT1 and 16 other genes. *Mol Psychiatry* 11:934–53.

Bruggemann D, Sobanski E, Alm B, Schubert T, Schmalzried H, Philipsen A, et al. (2007). No association between a common haplotype of the 6 and 10-repeat alleles in intron 8 and the 3'UTR of the DAT1 gene and adult attention deficit hyperactivity disorder. *Psychiatr Genet* 17(2):121.

Brunner D, Hen R. (1997). Insights into the neurobiology of impulsive behavior from serotonin receptor knockout mice. *Ann N Y Acad Sci* 836:81–105.

Bush G, Valera EM, Seidman LJ. (2005). Functional neuroimaging of attention-deficit/hyperactivity disorder: a review and suggested future directions. *Biol Psychiatry* 57:1273–84.

Cadoret RJ, Stewart MA. (1991). An adoption study of attention deficit/hyperactivity/aggression and their relationship to adult antisocial personality. *Compr Psychiatry* 32:73–82.

Cantwell DP. (1972). Psychiatric illness in the families of hyperactive children. *Arch Gen Psychiatry* 27:414–7.

Castellanos FX, Tannock R. (2002). Neuroscience of attention-deficit/hyperactivity disorder: the search for endophenotypes. *Nat Rev Neurosci* 3:617–28.

Chen W, Zhou K, Sham P, Franke B, Kuntsi J, Campbell D, et al. (2008). DSM-IV combined type ADHD shows familial association with sibling trait scores: A sampling strategy for QTL linkage. *Am J Med Genet B Neuropsychiatr Genet* 147B(8):1450–60.

Chronis AM, Lahey BB, Pelham WE, Jr., Kipp HL, Baumann BL, Lee SS. (2003). Psychopathology and substance abuse in parents of young children with attention-deficit/hyperactivity disorder. *J Am Acad Child Adolesc Psychiatry* 42:1424–32.

Cook EH, Jr., Stein MA, Krasowski MD, Cox NJ, Olkon DM, Kieffer JE, Leventhal BL. (1995). Association of attention-deficit disorder and the dopamine transporter gene. *Am J Hum Genet* **56**:993–8.

Curko Kera EA, Marks DJ, Berwid OG, Santra A, Halperin JM. (2004). Self-report and objective measures of ADHD-related behaviors in parents of preschool children at risk for ADHD. *CNS Spectr* **9**:639–47.

Curran S, Rijsdijk F, Martin N, Marusic K, Asherson P, Taylor E, Sham P. (2003). CHIP: Defining a dimension of the vulnerability to attention deficit hyperactivity disorder (ADHD) using sibling and individual data of children in a community-based sample. *Am J Med Genet B Neuropsychiatr Genet* **119**(1):86–97.

De Luca V, Muglia P, Jain U, Kennedy JL. (2004). No evidence of linkage or association between the norepinephrine transporter (NET) gene MnlI polymorphism and adult ADHD. *Am J Med Genet B Neuropsychiatr Genet* **124B**:38–40.

De Luca V, Muglia P, Vincent JB, Lanktree M, Jain U, Kennedy JL. (2004). Adrenergic alpha 2C receptor genomic organization: association study in adult ADHD. *Am J Med Genet B Neuropsychiatr Genet* **127B**: 65–7.

DeFries JC, Fulker DW. (1985). Multiple regression analysis of twin data. *Behav Genet* **15**:467–73.

Ding YC, Chi HC, Grady DL, Morishima A, Kidd JR, Kidd KK, et al. (2002). Evidence of positive selection acting at the human dopamine receptor D4 gene locus. *Proc Natl Acad Sci USA* **99**:309–14.

Downey KK, Stelson FW, Pomerleau OF, Giordani B. (1997). Adult attention deficit hyperactivity disorder: psychological test profiles in a clinical population. *J Nerv Ment Dis* **185**:32–8.

Doyle AE, Willcutt EG, Seidman LJ, Biederman J, Chouinard VA, Silva J, Faraone SV. (2005). Attention-deficit/hyperactivity disorder endophenotypes. *Biol Psychiatry* **57**:1324–35.

Ebstein RP, Novick O, Umansky R, Priel B, Osher Y, Blaine D, et al. (1996). Dopamine D4 receptor (D4DR) exon III polymorphism associated with the human personality trait of Novelty Seeking. *Nat Genet* **12**: 78–80.

Ehringer MA, Rhee SH, Young S, Corley R, Hewitt JK. (2006). Genetic and environmental contributions to common psychopathologies of childhood and adolescence: a study of twins and their siblings. *J Abnorm Child Psychol* **34**:1–17.

Elia J, Gai X, Xie HM, Perin JC, Geiger E, Glessner JT, et al. (2010). Rare structural variants found in attention-deficit hyperactivity disorder are preferentially associated with neurodevelopmental genes. *Mol Psychiatry* **15**(6):637–46.

Epstein JN, Conners CK, Erhardt D, Arnold LE, Hechtman L, Hinshaw SP, et al. (2000). Familial aggregation of ADHD characteristics. *J Abnorm Child Psychol* **28**:585–94.

Faraone SV, Biederman J, Feighner JA, Monuteaux MC. (2000). Assessing symptoms of attention deficit hyperactivity disorder in children and adults: which is more valid? *J Consult Clin Psychol* **68**:830–42.

Faraone SV, Biederman J, Friedman D. (2000). Validity of DSM-IV subtypes of attention-deficit/hyperactivity disorder: a family study perspective. *J Am Acad Child Adolesc Psychiatry* **39**:300–7.

Faraone SV, Biederman J, Keenan K, Tsuang MT. (1991). Separation of DSM-III attention deficit disorder and conduct disorder: evidence from a family-genetic study of American child psychiatric patients. *Psychol Med* **21**:109–21.

Faraone SV, Biederman J, Mick E. (1997). Symptom reports by adults with attention deficit hyperactivity disorder: are they influenced by attention deficit hyperactivity disorder in their children? *J Nerv Ment Dis* **185**:583–4.

Faraone SV, Biederman J, Mick E. (2006). The age-dependent decline of attention deficit hyperactivity disorder: a meta-analysis of follow-up studies. *Psychol Med* **36**:159–65.

Faraone SV, Biederman J, Monuteaux MC. (2000). Attention-deficit disorder and conduct disorder in girls: evidence for a familial subtype. *Biol Psychiatry* **48**: 21–9.

Faraone SV, Doyle AE, Lasky-Su J, Sklar PB, D'Angelo E, Gonzalez-Heydrich J, et al. (2008). Linkage analysis of attention deficit hyperactivity disorder. *Am J Med Genet B Neuropsychiatr Genet* **147B**:1387–91.

Faraone SV, Perlis RH, Doyle AE, Smoller JW, Goralnick JJ, Holmgren MA, Sklar P. (2005). Molecular genetics of attention-deficit/hyperactivity disorder. *Biol Psychiatry* **57**:1313–23.

Fayyad J, De Graaf R, Kessler R, Alonso J, Angermeyer M, Demyttenaere K, et al. (2007). Cross-national prevalence and correlates of adult attention-deficit hyperactivity disorder. *Br J Psychiatry* **190**:402–9.

Fisher SE, Francks C, McCracken JT, McGough JJ, Marlow AJ, MacPhie IL, et al. (2002). A genomewide scan for loci involved in attention-deficit/hyperactivity disorder. *Am J Hum Genet* **70**:1183–96.

Franke B, Hoogman M, Arias Vasquez A, Heister JG, Savelkoul PJ, Naber M, et al. (2008). Association of the dopamine transporter (SLC6A3/DAT1) gene 9–6 haplotype with adult ADHD. *Am J Med Genet B Neuropsychiatr Genet* **147B**:1576–9.

Franke B, Neale BM, Faraone SV. (2009). Genome-wide association studies in ADHD. *Hum Genet* **126**:13–50.

Franke B, Vasquez AA, Johansson S, Hoogman M, Romanos J, Boreatti-Hummer A, et al. (2010). Multicenter analysis of the SLC6A3/DAT1 VNTR haplotype in persistent ADHD suggests differential involvement of the gene in childhood and persistent ADHD. *Neuropsychopharmacology* 35(3): 656–64.

Friedel S, Saar K, Sauer S, Dempfle A, Walitza S, Renner T, et al. (2007). Association and linkage of allelic variants of the dopamine transporter gene in ADHD. *Mol Psychiatry* 12:923–33.

Galili-Weisstub E, Levy S, Frisch A, Gross-Tsur V, Michaelovsky E, Kosov A, et al. (2005). Dopamine transporter haplotype and attention-deficit hyperactivity disorder. *Mol Psychiatry* 10:617–8.

Gillis JJ, Gilger JW, Pennington BF, DeFries JC. (1992). Attention deficit disorder in reading-disabled twins: evidence for a genetic etiology. *J Abnorm Child Psychol* 20:303–15.

Gizer IR, Ficks C, Waldman ID. (2009). Candidate gene studies of ADHD: a meta-analytic review. *Hum Genet* 126:51–90.

Gjone H, Stevenson J, Sundet JM. (1996). Genetic influence on parent-reported attention-related problems in a Norwegian general population twin sample. *J Am Acad Child Adolesc Psychiatry* 35:588–96; discussion 596–8.

Haberstick BC, Timberlake D, Hopfer CJ, Lessem JM, Ehringer MA, Hewitt JK. (2008). Genetic and environmental contributions to retrospectively reported DSM-IV childhood attention deficit hyperactivity disorder. *Psychol Med* 38:1057–66.

Halperin JM, Schulz KP. (2006). Revisiting the role of the prefrontal cortex in the pathophysiology of attention-deficit/hyperactivity disorder. *Psychol Bull* 132:560–81.

Halperin JM, Trampush JW, Miller CJ, Marks DJ, Newcorn JH. (2008). Neuropsychological outcome in adolescents/young adults with childhood ADHD: profiles of persisters, remitters and controls. *J Child Psychol Psychiatry* 49:958–66.

Hebebrand J, Dempfle A, Saar K, Thiele H, Herpertz-Dahlmann B, Linder M. (2006). A genome-wide scan for attention-deficit/hyperactivity disorder in 155 German sib-pairs. *Mol Psychiatry* 11(2):196–205.

Hechtman L, Weiss G. (1983). Long-term outcome of hyperactive children. *Am J Orthopsychiatry* 53:532–41.

Hill JC, Schoener EP. (1996). Age-dependent decline of attention deficit hyperactivity disorder. *Am J Psychiatry* 153:1143–6.

Hofker M, Wijmenga C. (2009). A supersized list of obesity genes. *Nat Genet* 41:139–40.

Johansson S, Halleland H, Halmoy A, Jacobsen KK, Landaas ET, Dramsdahl M, et al. (2007). Genetic analyses of dopamine related genes in adult ADHD patients suggest an association with the DRD5-microsatellite repeat, but not with DRD4 or SLC6A3 VNTRs. *Am J Med Genet B Neuropsychiatr Genet* 47B(8):1470–5.

Johnson KA, Kelly SP, Bellgrove MA, Barry E, Cox M, Gill M, Robertson IH. (2007). Response variability in attention deficit hyperactivity disorder: evidence for neuropsychological heterogeneity. *Neuropsychologia* 45:630–8.

Johnson KA, Wiersema JR, Kuntsi J. (2009). What would Karl Popper say? Are current psychological theories of ADHD falsifiable? *Behav Brain Funct* 5:15.

Kahn RS, Khoury J, Nichols WC, Lanphear BP. (2003). Role of dopamine transporter genotype and maternal prenatal smoking in childhood hyperactive-impulsive, inattentive, and oppositional behaviors. *J Pediatr* 143:104–10.

Kessler RC, Adler L, Ames M, Demler O, Faraone S, Hiripi E, et al. (2005). The World Health Organization Adult ADHD Self-Report Scale (ASRS): a short screening scale for use in the general population. *Psychol Med* 35(2):245–56.

Kirley A, Lowe N, Mullins C, McCarron M, Daly G, Waldman I, et al. (2004). Phenotype studies of the DRD4 gene polymorphisms in ADHD: association with oppositional defiant disorder and positive family history. *Am J Med Genet B Neuropsychiatr Genet* 131B: 38–42.

Kirov G, Grozeva D, Norton N, Ivanov D, Mantripragada KK, Holmans P, et al. (2009). Support for the involvement of large copy number variants in the pathogenesis of schizophrenia. *Hum Mol Genet* 18:1497–503.

Klein C, Wendling K, Huettner P, Ruder H, Peper M. (2006). Intra-subject variability in attention-deficit hyperactivity disorder. *Biol Psychiatry* 60: 1088–97.

Kluger AN, Siegfried Z, Ebstein RP. (2002). A meta-analysis of the association between DRD4 polymorphism and novelty seeking. *Mol Psychiatry* 7:712–7.

Kovas Y, Plomin R. (2006). Generalist genes: implications for the cognitive sciences. *Trends Cogn Sci* 10: 198–203.

Kuntsi J, Neale BM, Chen W, Faraone SV, Asherson P. (2006). The IMAGE project: methodological issues for the molecular genetic analysis of ADHD. *Behav Brain Funct* 2:27.

Kuntsi J, Oosterlaan J, Stevenson J. (2001). Psychological mechanisms in hyperactivity: I. Response inhibition deficit, working memory impairment, delay aversion, or something else? *J Child Psychol Psychiatry* 42:199–210.

Kuntsi J, Rijsdijk F, Ronald A, Asherson P, Plomin R. (2005). Genetic influences on the stability of attention-deficit/hyperactivity disorder symptoms from early to middle childhood. *Biol Psychiatry* 57:647–54.

Kusenda M, Sebat J. (2008). The role of rare structural variants in the genetics of autism spectrum disorders. *Cytogenet Genome Res* 123:36–43.

LaHoste GJ, Swanson JM, Wigal SB, Glabe C, Wigal T, King N, Kennedy JL. (1996). Dopamine D4 receptor gene polymorphism is associated with attention deficit hyperactivity disorder. *Mol Psychiatry* 1:121–4.

Lanau F, Brockhaus M, Pink JR, Franchet C, Wildt-Perinic D, Goepfert C, et al. (1997). Development and characterization of antibodies against the N terminus of the human dopamine D4 receptor. *J Neurochem* 69:2169–78.

Larsson JO, Larsson H, Lichtenstein P. (2004). Genetic and environmental contributions to stability and change of ADHD symptoms between 8 and 13 years of age: a longitudinal twin study. *J Am Acad Child Adolesc Psychiatry* 43:1267–75.

Lasky-Su J, Neale BM, Franke B, Anney RJ, Zhou K, Maller JB, et al. (2008). Genome-wide association scan of quantitative traits for attention deficit hyperactivity disorder identifies novel associations and confirms candidate gene associations. *Am J Med Genet B Neuropsychiatr Genet* 147B:1345–54.

Lesch KP, Timmesfeld N, Renner TJ, Halperin R, Roser C, Nguyen TT, et al. (2008). Molecular genetics of adult ADHD: converging evidence from genome-wide association and extended pedigree linkage studies. *J Neural Transm* 115:1573–85.

Levy F, Hay DA, Bennett KS, McStephen M. (2005). Gender differences in ADHD subtype comorbidity. *J Am Acad Child Adolesc Psychiatry* 44:368–76.

Levy F, Hay DA, McStephen M, Wood C, Waldman I. (1997). Attention-deficit hyperactivity disorder: a category or a continuum? Genetic analysis of a large-scale twin study. *J Am Acad Child Adolesc Psychiatry* 36:737–44.

Li D, Sham PC, Owen MJ, He L. (2006). Meta-analysis shows significant association between dopamine system genes and attention deficit hyperactivity disorder (ADHD). *Hum Mol Genet* 15:2276–84.

Lohmueller KE, Pearce CL, Pike M, Lander ES, Hirschhorn JN. (2003). Meta-analysis of genetic association studies supports a contribution of common variants to susceptibility to common disease. *Nat Genet* 33:177–82.

Lynn DE, Lubke G, Yang M, McCracken JT, McGough JJ, Ishii J, et al. (2005). Temperament and character profiles

and the dopamine D4 receptor gene in ADHD. *Am J Psychiatry* 162:906–13.

Maher BS, Marazita ML, Ferrell RE, et al. (2002). Dopamine system genes and attention deficit hyperactivity disorder: a meta-analysis. *Psychiatr Genet* 12:207–15.

Mannuzza S, Klein RG, Klein DF, Bessler A, Shrout P. (2002). Accuracy of adult recall of childhood attention deficit hyperactivity disorder. *Am J Psychiatry* 159:1882–8.

Manshadi M, Lippmann S, O'Daniel RG, Blackman A. (1983). Alcohol abuse and attention deficit disorder. *J Clin Psychiatry* 44:379–80.

Marco R, Miranda A, Schlotz W, Melia A, Mulligan A, Muller U, et al. (2009). Delay and reward choice in ADHD: an experimental test of the role of delay aversion. *Neuropsychology* 23:367–80.

Martin N, Scourfield J, McGuffin P. (2002). Observer effects and heritability of childhood attention-deficit hyperactivity disorder symptoms. *Br J Psychiatry* 180:260–5.

Maughan B, Taylor A, Caspi A, Moffitt TE. (2004). Prenatal smoking and early childhood conduct problems: testing genetic and environmental explanations of the association. *Arch Gen Psychiatry* 61:836–43.

McGuffin P, Plomin R. (2004). A decade of the Social, Genetic and Developmental Psychiatry Centre at the Institute of Psychiatry. *Br J Psychiatry* 185:280–2.

Moffitt TE, Caspi A, Rutter M. (2005). Strategy for investigating interactions between measured genes and measured environments. *Arch Gen Psychiatry* 62:473–81.

Morrison JR, Stewart MA. (1971). A family study of the hyperactive child syndrome. *Biol Psychiatry* 3: 189–95.

Muglia P, Jain U, Inkster B, Kennedy JL. (2002). A quantitative trait locus analysis of the dopamine transporter gene in adults with ADHD. *Neuropsychopharmacology* 27:655–62.

Muglia P, Jain U, Kennedy JL. (2002). A transmission disequilibrium test of the Ser9/Gly dopamine D3 receptor gene polymorphism in adult attention-deficit hyperactivity disorder. *Behav Brain Res* 130:91–5.

Muglia P, Jain U, Macciardi F, Kennedy JL. (2000). Adult attention deficit hyperactivity disorder and the dopamine D4 receptor gene. *Am J Med Genet* 96:273–7.

Neale BM, Lasky-Su J, Anney R, Franke B, Zhou K, Maller JB, et al. (2008). Genome-wide association scan of attention deficit hyperactivity disorder. *Am J Med Genet B Neuropsychiatr Genet* 147B:1337–44.

Neale BM, Medland SE, Ripke S, et al. (2010). Meta-analysis of genome-wide association studies of attention-deficit/hyperactivity disorder. *J Am Acad Child Adolesc Psychiatry* **49**:884–97.

Neuman RJ, Lobos E, Reich W, Henderson CA, Sun LW, Todd RD. (2007). Prenatal smoking exposure and dopaminergic genotypes interact to cause a severe ADHD subtype. *Biol Psychiatry* **61**:1320–8.

Newton-Cheh C, Johnson T, Gateva V, Tobin MD, Bochud M, Coin L, et al. (2009). Genome-wide association study identifies eight loci associated with blood pressure. *Nat Genet* **41**:666–76.

NICE. (2008). *Attention Deficit Hyperactivity Disorder: Diagnosis and Management of ADHD in Children, Young People and Adolescents.* London: Royal College of Psychiatry.

O'Connell RG, Bellgrove MA, Dockree PM, Lau A, Fitzgerald M, Robertson IH. (2008). Self-Alert Training: volitional modulation of autonomic arousal improves sustained attention. *Neuropsychologia* **46**:1379–90.

O'Connell RG, Bellgrove MA, Dockree PM, Lau A, Hester R, Garavan H, et al. (2009). The neural correlates of deficient error awareness in attention-deficit hyperactivity disorder (ADHD). *Neuropsychologia* **47**:1149–59.

Ogdie MN, Fisher SE, Yang M, Ishii J, Francks C, Loo SK, et al. (2004). Attention deficit hyperactivity disorder: fine mapping supports linkage to 5p13, 6q12, 16p13, and 17p11. *Am J Hum Genet* **75**:661–8.

Ogdie MN, MacPhie IL, Minassian SL, Yang M, Fisher SE, Francks C, et al. (2003). A genomewide scan for attention-deficit/hyperactivity disorder in an extended sample: suggestive linkage on 17p11. *Am J Hum Genet.* **72**:1268–79.

Palacio JD, Castellanos FX, Pineda DA, Lopera F, Arcos-Burgos M, Quiroz YT, et al. (2004). Attention-deficit/hyperactivity disorder and comorbidities in 18 Paisa Colombian multigenerational families. *J Am Acad Child Adolesc Psychiatry* **43**:1506–15.

Polanczyk G, de Lima MS, Horta BL, Biederman J, Rohde LA. (2007). The worldwide prevalence of ADHD: a systematic review and metaregression analysis. *Am J Psychiatry* **164**:942–8.

Price TS, Simonoff E, Asherson P, Curran S, Kuntsi J, Waldman I, Plomin R. (2005). Continuity and change in preschool ADHD symptoms: longitudinal genetic analysis with contrast effects. *Behav Genet* **35**:121–32.

Price TS, Simonoff E, Waldman I, Asherson P, Plomin R. (2001). Hyperactivity in preschool children is highly heritable. *J Am Acad Child Adolesc Psychiatry* **40**:1362–4.

Purcell SM, Wray NR, Stone JL, Visscher PM, O'Donovan MC, Sullivan PF, et al. (2009). Common polygenic variation contributes to risk of schizophrenia and bipolar disorder. *Nature* **460**:748–52.

Purper-Ouakil D, Wohl M, Mouren MC, et al. (2005). Meta-analysis of family-based association studies between the dopamine transporter gene and attention deficit hyperactivity disorder. *Psychiatr Genet* **15**:53–9.

Rhee SH, Waldman ID, Hay DA, Levy F. (1999). Sex differences in genetic and environmental influences on DSM-III-R attention-deficit/hyperactivity disorder. *J Abnorm Psychol* **108**:24–41.

Ribases M, Antoni Ramos-Quiroga J, Sanchez-Mora C, et al. (2010). Contribution of Latrophilin 3 (LPHN3) to the genetic susceptibility to ADHD in adulthood: a replication study. *Genes Brain Behav.*

Ribases M, Ramos-Quiroga JA, Hervas A, Bosch R, Bielsa A, Gastaminza X, et al. (2007). Exploration of 19 serotoninergic candidate genes in adults and children with attention-deficit/hyperactivity disorder identifies association for 5HT2A, DDC and MAOB. *Mol Psychiatry* **14**:71–85.

Risch N, Merikangas K. (1996). The future of genetic studies of complex human diseases. *Science* **273**:1516–7.

Ronald A, Happe F, Bolton P, Butcher LM, Price TS, Wheelwright S, et al. (2006). Genetic heterogeneity between the three components of the autism spectrum: a twin study. *J Am Acad Child Adolesc Psychiatry* **45**:691–9.

Rutter M, Silberg J. (2002). Gene-environment interplay in relation to emotional and behavioral disturbance. *Annu Rev Psychol* **53**:463–90.

Schultz MR, Rabi K, Faraone SV, Kremen W, Lyons MJ. (2006). Efficacy of retrospective recall of attention-deficit hyperactivity disorder symptoms: a twin study. *Twin Res Hum Genet* **9**:220–32.

Sebat J, Lakshmi B, Malhotra D, Troge J, Lese-Martin C, Walsh T, et al. (2007). Strong association of de novo copy number mutations with autism. *Science* **316**: 445–9.

Seidman LJ, Valera EM, Makris N. (2005). Structural brain imaging of attention-deficit/hyperactivity disorder. *Biol Psychiatry* **57**:1263–72.

Shi J, Levinson DF, Duan J, Sanders AR, Zheng Y, Pe'er I, et al. (2009). Common variants on chromosome 6p22.1 are associated with schizophrenia. *Nature* **460**:753–7.

Silberg J, Rutter M, Meyer J, Maes H, Hewitt J, Simonoff E, et al. (1996). Genetic and environmental influences on the covariation between hyperactivity and conduct disturbance in juvenile twins. *J Child Psychol Psychiatry* **37**:803–16.

Simon V, Czobor P, Bálint S, et al. (2009). Prevalence and correlates of adult attention-deficit hyperactivity disorder: Meta-analysis. *British Journal of Psychiatry* **194**:204–11.

Skirrow C, McLoughlin G, Kuntsi J, Asherson P. (2009). Behavioral, neurocognitive and treatment overlap between attention-deficit/hyperactivity disorder and mood instability. *Expert Rev Neurother* 9: 489–503.

Sprich S, Biederman J, Crawford MH, Mundy E, Faraone SV. (2000). Adoptive and biological families of children and adolescents with ADHD. *J Am Acad Child Adolesc Psychiatry* 39:1432–7.

Stefansson H, Ophoff RA, Steinberg S, Andreassen OA, Cichon S, Rujescu D, et al. (2009). Common variants conferring risk of schizophrenia. *Nature* 460: 744–7.

Stefansson H, Rujescu D, Cichon S, Pietilainen OP, Ingason A, Steinberg S, et al. (2008). Large recurrent microdeletions associated with schizophrenia. *Nature* 455:232–6.

Stevenson J. (1992). Evidence for a genetic etiology in hyperactivity in children. *Behav Genet* 22:337–44.

Thapar A, Harrington R, McGuffin P. (2001). Examining the comorbidity of ADHD-related behaviours and conduct problems using a twin study design. *Br J Psychiatry* 179:224–9.

Thapar A, Holmes J, Poulton K, Harrington R. (1999). Genetic basis of attention deficit and hyperactivity. *Br J Psychiatry* 174:105–11.

Thapar A, Rice F, Hay D, Boivin J, Langley K, Van Den Bree M, et al. (2009). Prenatal smoking might not cause attention-deficit/hyperactivity disorder: evidence from a novel design. *Biol Psychiatry* 66(8):722–7.

Uebel H, Albrecht B, Asherson P, Borger NA, Butler L, Chen W, et al. (2010). Performance variability, impulsivity errors and the impact of incentives as gender-independent endophenotypes for ADHD. *J Child Psychol Psychiatry* 51(2):210–18.

Uhl GR, Drgon T, Johnson C, Liu QR. (2009). Addiction genetics and pleiotropic effects of common haplotypes that make polygenic contributions to vulnerability to substance dependence. *J Neurogenet* 23(3):272–82.

Wang E, Ding YC, Flodman P, Kidd JR, Kidd KK, Grady DL, et al. (2004). The genetic architecture of selection at the human dopamine receptor D4 (DRD4) gene locus. *Am J Hum Genet* 74:931–44.

Willcutt EG, Doyle AE, Nigg JT, Faraone SV, Pennington BF. (2005). Validity of the executive function theory of attention-deficit/hyperactivity disorder: a meta-analytic review. *Biol Psychiatry* 57:1336–46.

Wilson MC. (2000). Coloboma mouse mutant as an animal model of hyperkinesis and attention deficit hyperactivity disorder. *Neurosci Biobehav Rev* 24:51–7.

Xu X, Hawi Z, Brookes KJ, Anney R, Bellgrove M, Franke B, et al. (2008). Replication of a rare protective allele in the noradrenaline transporter gene and ADHD. *Am J Med Genet B Neuropsychiatr Genet* 147B:1564–7.

Yang B, Chan RC, Jing J, et al. (2007). A meta-analysis of association studies between the 10-repeat allele of a VNTR polymorphism in the 3′-UTR of dopamine transporter gene and attention deficit hyperactivity disorder. *Am J Med Genet B Neuropsychiatr Genet* 144B:541–50.

Zhou K, Chen W, Buitelaar J, Banaschewski T, Oades RD, Franke B, et al. (2008). Genetic heterogeneity in ADHD: DAT1 gene only affects probands without CD. *Am J Med Genet B Neuropsychiatr Genet* 147B:1481–7.

Zhou K, Dempfle A, Arcos-Burgos M, Bakker SC, Banaschewski T, Biederman J, et al. (2008). Meta-analysis of genome-wide linkage scans of attention deficit hyperactivity disorder. *Am J Med Genet B Neuropsychiatr Genet* 147B:1392–8.

Chapter

Structural and functional magnetic resonance imaging findings in adults with ADHD

Yannis Paloyelis and Philip J. Asherson

Introduction

The purpose of this chapter is to provide an overview of findings from structural and functional magnetic resonance imaging (MRI) research focusing on adults with ADHD. According to current diagnostic criteria, which require symptom onset in childhood, adult ADHD is conceptualized as the long-term negative outcome of a condition that began early in life. Therefore, by definition, adults with ADHD present a "worse outcome" group. It is only relatively recently that adult ADHD has been the focus of neuroimaging research, reflecting a relative reluctance in the recognition of the adult syndrome as a valid diagnostic category (Asherton et al., 2007).

Neuroimaging research with adults with ADHD has the potential to address a range of issues. It can examine if there are deficits characteristic of the adolescent ADHD brain that tend to remain relatively stable and whether abnormalities observed in adulthood are the outcome of long-term neurodevelopmental processes associated with a negative clinical outcome. The adult ADHD brain may also present unique characteristics, which could be the outcome of long-term adaptation to dysfunctional activation during childhood (Hesslinger et al., 2002) or be due to chronic treatment effects. Moreover, differences could also be attributed to the use of compensatory mechanisms or be related to symptoms that are associated more closely with the adult manifestation of the disorder.

It is evident that neuroanatomic and functional alterations in adult ADHD cannot be discussed without reference to data from childhood. In the following sections we summarize existing knowledge from structural and functional neuroimaging research in ADHD (including studies published by March 2009). We briefly discuss findings from studies with children

and adolescents, but we focus more on developmental studies and studies using adult samples. We conclude by critically discussing the hypothesis that ADHD may be the outcome of delayed brain maturation; recent neuroimaging data have provided new support for this hypothesis.

Neuroanatomic deficits in the ADHD brain

Children and adolescents with ADHD

Cross-sectional findings

ADHD has been associated with global and regional brain volume reductions. Two recent meta-analyses summarized evidence from a large number of studies and identified the brain regions showing the most robust deficits (Ellison-Wright, Ellison-Wright, & Bulmore, 2008; Valera et al., 2007). The first meta-analytic review aggregated data from region-of-interest studies published before January 2005 (Valera et al., 2007). Among regions studied more frequently, total and right cerebral volumes, areas in the cerebellum, the splenium of the corpus callosum, and the right caudate showed the largest and most robust neuroanatomic deficits. Among less frequently studied areas, regions in the frontal lobes showed large deficits (Valera et al., 2007). In a meta-analysis of six voxel-based morphometry studies including a total of 114 ADHD cases and 143 controls, a region of decreased gray matter was identified in the right putamen/globus pallidus of the ADHD group (Ellison-Wright et al., 2007). This area is neuroanatomically associated with the right caudate identified in the region-of-interest review, forming the right striatum. Region-of-interest studies have also shown reductions in the putamen (Aylward et al., 1996; Castellanos et al., 1996), but

ADHD in Adults: Characterization, Diagnosis and Treatment, ed. Jan Buitelaar, Cornelis Kan and Philip Asherson.
Published by Cambridge University Press. © Cambridge University Press 2011.

Box 5.1 Overview of neuroanatomic deficits in children and adolescents with ADHD.

Overall cortical volume/thickness

Reductions in global measures of cortical volume (Wolosin et al., 2009; Yang et al., 2008) and thickness (Shaw et al., 2006) have been reported, although they have not always reached significance (Durston et al., 2004; Filipek et al., 1997; McAlonan et al., 2007). Wolosin et al. (2009) found that a cortical volume reduction of about 8% in the ADHD group was due to a decrease in cortical folding rather than cortical thickness.

Frontal lobes

Reductions in bilateral frontal gray and white matter volumes are commonly reported and have provided the largest effect sizes (Carmona et al., 2005; Li et al., 2007; McAlonan et al., 2007; Plessen et al., 2006; Valera et al., 2007; Wang et al., 2007; but see Garrett et al., 2008, for an exception). Reductions in the dorsolateral prefrontal cortex are reported more consistently (Seidman et al., 2005). Decreased cortical thickness in medial, superior frontal, and precentral regions has also been reported in a study with a very large sample size (Shaw et al., 2006).

Orbitofrontal cortex – limbic brain

Neuroanatomic deficits in the orbitofrontal cortex (Carmona et al., 2005; Plessen et al., 2006; Shaw, Gornick, et al., 2007) and limbic areas (i.e. the amygdala and the hippocampus; Lopez-Larson et al., 2009; Plessen et al., 2006) have also been reported. Interregional connectivity between the amygdala and the orbitofrontal cortex in ADHD may be disturbed (Plessen et al., 2006). The orbitofrontal cortex and the limbic brain provide the neural substrate for learning stimulus–outcome associations, reward processing, the regulation of behavior in accordance with context and expected outcomes, and the regulation of emotional processes (Moghaddam & Homayoun, 2008); a dysfunction in this system may contribute to behavioral disinhibition, impulsivity, and emotional lability, which are characteristic of ADHD.

Cingulate cortex

Despite the frequent implication of the cingulate cortex in functional neuroimaging studies (Paloyelis et al., 2007) and the theoretical importance of the anterior cingulate cortex in the neurobiology of ADHD, given its role in error detection, response selection, and other aspects of cognitive and emotional processing (Bush et al., 1999), the cingulate cortex has been the focus of relatively few studies. Some earlier reports failed to find a deficit in the anterior cingulate cortex (Kates et al., 2002; Mostofsky et al., 2002), yet improvements in spatial resolution and bigger sample sizes revealed deficits in the anterior (Carmona et al., 2005; Pliszka et al., 2006; Shaw et al., 2006) and posterior cingulate cortices (Carmona et al., 2005; Overmeyer et al., 2001). Inconsistencies could result from sample differences in medication history, as one study found anterior cingulate cortex deficits in treatment-naive children compared to healthy controls, but not in chronically treated children (Pliszka et al., 2006).

Corpus callosum

ADHD is associated with a highly localized deficit in the splenium of the corpus callosum, which connects homologous temporal and parietal areas (Seidman et al., 2005; Valera et al., 2007). Three-dimensional surface-based modeling of the corpus callosum, affording high spatial resolution, confirmed the presence of neuroanatomic deficits particularly in a posterior region (the isthmus), after excluding cases with comorbid oppositional-defiant disorder (Luders et al., 2009). Such deficits could indicate differences in the degree of myelination or deficits in tissue structure (e.g. number of neurons) and organization in homologous temporal/parietal regions (Luders et al., 2009; Seidman et al., 2005).

Basal ganglia

Robust evidence exists for decreased gray matter volume in the right striatum (caudate, putamen; Ellison-Wright et al., 2008; Valera et al., 2007), whereas evidence for deficits in the globus pallidus has been equivocal (Qiu et al., 2009; Valera et al., 2007). Recent studies not included in the meta-analyses reviewed in this chapter have shown reduced volumes in the left (Qiu et al., 2009), right (Tremols et al., 2008), and bilateral caudate (Pliszka et al., 2006; Yang et al., 2008) or the lack of significant volume differences (Lopez-Larson et al., 2009). It is unclear whether volume decreases exist only in boys (Qiu et al., 2009) or both genders (Yang et al., 2008), and there were no differences between youths with the combined or inattentive ADHD subtypes (Qiu et al., 2009). The developmental trajectories of the caudate in ADHD and healthy control groups have been shown to converge by late adolescence, due to an increased rate of caudate volume reduction in healthy controls (Castellanos et al., 2002). Studies using older adolescent samples have found increased caudate volumes in ADHD (Garrett et al., 2008; Mataro et al., 1997), which could be consistent with this trend. New evidence on the putamen has been equivocal, showing either volume reductions (Qui et al., 2009) or no differences (Wellington et al., 2006). Volume reductions in ADHD seem to be unaffected by stimulant medication (Castellanos et al., 2002; Pliszka et al., 2006). Asymmetry abnormalities in the caudate (Tremols et al., 2008; Uhlikova et al., 2007) and the putamen (Wellington et al., 2006) have also been reported.

Cerebellum
Volume reductions in the cerebellum, particularly the cerebellar vermis, are among the most consistent findings (McAlonan et al., 2007; Seidman et al., 2005; Valera et al., 2007; Yang et al., 2008). Some evidence points to deficits in the inferior vermis (Valera et al., 2007) and the superior vermis (Bledsoe et al., 2009; Mackie et al., 2007).

Other areas
Volume reductions have also been observed in temporal, parietal, and occipital gray and white mater areas (Carmona et al., 2005; Mackie et al., 2007; McAlonan et al., 2007; Wang et al., 2007). Using very large sample sizes, Shaw et al. (2006; Shaw, Gornick, et al., 2007) found reduced cortical thickness in the right anterior temporal (consistent with Sowell et al., 2003), right medial temporal, and the right posterior parietal cortices.

White matter microstructure
Diffusion-tensor imaging (DTI) allows the assessment of the integrity, organization, and development of white matter tracts (Ashtari et al., 2005). It has shown localized deficits in white matter microstructure in ADHD that would be undetectable by conventional MRI (Anjari et al., 2007). Lower fractional anisotropy (FA) values express a lesser degree of myelination, density, and organization of white matter fibers, which have been reported in motor and attentional circuits and frontostriatal tracts in samples with ADHD (Ashtari et al., 2005; Hamilton et al., 2008; Skranes et al., 2007). Increased FA values, reflecting increased diffusion along the primary tract direction but decreased diffusion along secondary and tertiary tract directions, have also been reported in the center of major motor and attention pathways, which are thought to reflect abnormal branching and crossing of fibers in children with ADHD (Silk et al., 2009). FA values have been shown to correlate with inattention scores (Ashtari et al., 2005) and to be associated with performance on perceptual, cognitive, and motor tasks (Skranes et al., 2007), as well as with behavioral performance and blood-oxygen-level-dependent activation in frontostriatal regions during a cognitive control task (Casey et al., 2007).

they were not significant probably because of a lack of power due to the small total sample size.

Box 5.1 provides a qualitative overview of regions presenting neuroanatomic deficits in children and adolescents with ADHD. We summarize evidence from recent structural neuroimaging studies, whereas information on findings from studies published before 2005 is mainly based on previous reviews (Seidman, Valera, & Makris, 2005; Valera et al., 2007).

Longitudinal evidence
Longitudinal studies conducted at the US National Institutes for Health (Castellanos et al., 2002; Shaw, Eckstrand, et al., 2007; Shaw, Gornick, et al., 2007; Shaw et al., 2006) of two large cohorts of youths with ADHD (mostly combined subtype) and healthy controls provide unique insight into the developmental trajectories of healthy and ADHD brains. Gray/white matter volume growth followed parallel trajectories in both groups, except for the caudate, as discussed in Box 5.1 (Casetellanos et al., 2002). The use of methods offering high spatial resolution showed that, despite similarities in the temporal sequence of cortical devel-

opment, in the brains of the ADHD group there was a delay of 2 to 5 years in the median age by which peak cortical thickness was achieved in the superior and middle frontal gyri (areas showing the longest delay), medial prefrontal cortex, and the posterior superior and middle temporal gyri (extending to the middle occipital gyrus; Shaw, Eckstrand, et al., 2007). An exception was found in the primary motor cortex, where the ADHD group reached peak cortical thickness 5 months earlier than the comparison group. In the rest of the brain either a model that allowed for the detection of peaks (quadratic model) did not fit either group, or the extrapolated age of peak thickness was beyond the age range of the sample. However, this *maturational lag* in cortical development was not followed by an eventual "normalization" of absolute differences in cortical thickness, as earlier evidence of highly regional cortical thinning in ADHD (Shaw et al., 2006) still held in this somewhat expanded sample (Philip Shaw, personal communication).

Cortical thickness growth was not found to differ as a function of clinical outcome, with the exception of a region in the right parietal cortex where developmental trajectories converged in late adolescence; this convergence was driven largely by the different developmental course of a better outcome group, as assessed by scores on the Children's Global Assessment Scale (CGAS; Shaw et al., 2006). In the cerebellum, volumes in the left anterior cerebellar lobe tended to converge by late adolescence, yet this convergence was not statistically significant for the worse outcome group (Mackie et al., 2007). Conversely, the developmental trajectories of total cerebellar volumes (particularly in the posterior-inferior vermis) for the worse outcome group progressively diverged from those of healthy controls from mid-adolescence onward (Mackie et al., 2007).

Cortical thickness growth was associated with a variable number tandem repeat polymorphism of the dopamine receptor 4 (DRD4) gene at exon 3 (Shaw, Gornick, et al., 2007). ADHD carriers of the DRD4 7-repeat allele showed the least cortical thickness and a reduced rate of cortical thinning at the right supramarginal/angular gyri and the right inferior frontal/lateral orbitofrontal cortex, so that by age 17 cortical thickness differences among all groups had diminished.

Effects of long-term stimulant medication

Adults with ADHD are likely to have a history of long-term stimulant treatment. Therefore, it is important to consider the possible effects of chronic stimulant treatment on brain development before discussing evidence from adult studies. Overall, evidence from cross-sectional and prospective studies suggests that chronic stimulant treatment may be associated with a protective effect on brain development, diminishing differences from healthy control groups. Treatment-naive youths with ADHD, compared to medicated or healthy control children, have shown smaller white matter volumes (Castellanos et al., 2002), posterior-inferior cerebellar vermis area (Bledsoe, Semrud-Clikeman, & Pliszka, 2009) and right anterior cingulate cortex volumes (Pliszka et al., 2006). They have also shown smaller cerebellums, temporal gray matter, and total cerebral volumes compared to healthy controls, as well as trends for decreased frontal and parietal gray matter volumes (Castellanos et al., 2002). In a prospective study, Shaw et al. (2009) found that when ADHD youths who interrupted treatment in early adolescence were rescanned about 4 years later, they showed evidence for an increased rate of cortical thinning in the left inferior/middle frontal gyrus,

the right medial and inferolateral precentral gyri, and the right parieto-occipital region, compared to both adolescents with ADHD who continued treatment and healthy controls. The latter groups did not differ from each other, and the rate of cortical thinning was not associated with clinical outcome. Shaw et al. (2009) suggested that the localization of differences in rates of cortical thinning at regions that show sensitivity to methylphenidate treatment (Mehta et al., 2000) and the tendency of stimulant medication to enhance performance and normalize functional activation might be examples of "activity-dependent neuroplasticity."

Neuroanatomic deficits in adults with ADHD

So far, seven studies (Biederman et al., 2008; Hesslinger et al., 2002; Makris et al., 2007, 2008; Monuteaux et al., 2008; Perlov et al., 2008; Seidman et al., 2006) have examined neuroanatomic deficits in adults with ADHD (see Table 5.1). Two other studies used a sample of women with comorbid ADHD and borderline personality disorder (Rusch, Luders, et al., 2007; Rusch, Weber, et al., 2007).

In a series of reports using fully or partially overlapping samples and a range of neuroimaging techniques, investigators have reported neuroanatomic abnormalities in frontostriatal and right parietal neural circuits underlying executive functions and attentional processes in adults with ADHD. Seidman et al. (2006) showed cortical volume reductions in bilateral frontal lobes, particularly the left superior frontal gyrus (13.1% decrease) and the right anterior cingulate cortex (13.2% decrease), whereas a later study with a slightly larger sample added a significant decrease in right cerebellar gray matter (Biederman et al., 2008). Using a segmentation method that allowed a more refined localization of differences, Makris et al. (2007) found reduced cortical thickness in the a priori defined attention and executive function brain circuits (bilateral middle and superior frontal gyri, cingulate cortex, and right angular and supramarginal gyri) as well as in the orbitofrontal cortex.

Abnormalities in the microstructure of white matter tracts underpinning attention and executive function networks, namely the right cingulum and the right superior lateral fascicle II, have also been reported in adults with current or childhood ADHD (Makris et al., 2008). The superior lateral fascicle II provides bidirectional connections between prefrontal and posterior parietal areas, possibly mediating the

Study	N	Age mean (SD)	Age range	% Males	Clinic/ community sample	Early onset	Current DSM-IV criteria	Medication history (N)	IQ	Comorbidity	Method	ROIs	Findings
Biederman 2008*	ADHD: 26 Control: 23 BD: 18 ADHD+BD: 31	ADHD: 36.9 (11.1) Controls: 34.0 (9.6) BD: 39.9 (6.5) ADHD+BD: 35.7 (12.0)	18–59	ADHD: 50%; Control: 57%; BD: 44%; ADHD+BD: 61%;	Both	Yes	Yes	ADHD: 1 Control: 1 BD: 11 ADHD+BD: 13	>74	ADHD: 4 MAD, 13 SUD; Control: 7 SUD; BD: 2 MAD, 9 SUD; ADHD+BD: 4 MAD, 7 SUD.	Morphometric (volumes); Semi-automatic segmentation and ROI definition	ROIs: FC, SFG, MFG, Non-DLPFC, OFC, ACC, A, TH; TCGM; CRB GM. Exploratory: TC/PC/OC, Caud, Nacc, Put, GP.	ADHD<Control (independent of BD); FC, non-DLPFC, left SFG, right ACC, Right CRB GM. BD<Control (independent of ADHD): left OFC; BD>Control (independent of ADHD): right TH; No differences in Caud, Put, GB, Nacc, TC/PC/OC.
Makris 2008	ADHD: 12 Controls: 17	ADHD: 41.3(2.1) Controls: 40.5(2.1)	37–46	ADHD: 58.3%; Controls: 47.1%	Community	Yes	5/12 participants	ADHD:1	>74	None reported	White matter FA.	CB, SLF II; Fornix (control region); Exploratory: forebrain WM	Right CB & SLF II FA: ADHD<Control (sig. after controlling for forebrain WM); Fornix & forebrain WM: no difference. Both groups had higher FA in left CB; ADHD>Controls. Selective abnormalities over WM ROIs implicated in attentional & EF systems.
Monuteaux 2008*	ADHD (7R): 24 (6) Control (7R): 20 (6) ADHD+BD (7R): 19(7)	32.5–38.4 (8.9–15.9)	18–59	ADHD: 50% Control: 65% ADHD+BD: 68%	Both	Yes	Yes	Not stated	>74	ADHD: 1 MDD, 12 SUD; Control: 5 SUD; ADHD+BD: 7 MDD, 3 MAD, 15 SUD	Morphometric analyses (volumes); Genetic imaging.	SFG, MFG, ACC, CRB GM	7R carriers had smaller volumes in SFG (D=.68) & CRB GM (D=0.56) only in the ADHD group.
Perlov 2008	ADHD: 27 Control: 27	ADHD:32.4(10.6) Control: 30.7(7.8)	ADHD: 19–55 Control: 22–46	ADHD: 63% Control: 56%	Clinic	Not specified	Yes	MPH Naïve: 26; Medication-free for 6 months; Other medication history not reported	–	No Axis I/II comorbidity	Manual volumetry	Hippocampus, amygdala	No sig. group differences with respect to hippocampus/amygdala or TBV (age/sex corrected).

(cont.)

Table 5.1 (cont.)

Study	N	Age mean (SD)	Age range	% Males	Clinic/ community sample	Early onset	Current DSM-IV criteria	Medication history	IQ	Comorbidity	Method	ROIs	Findings
Makris 2007*	As In Seidman 2006	As In Seidman 2006	As In Seidman 2006	As In Seidman 2006	Both	Yes	Yes; ADHD subtypes: 12 CT, 9 IN, 2 HI.	As In Seidman 2006	>79	As In Seidman 2006	Cortical thickness.	SFG, MFG, OFC, anterior & posterior CG, AG, anterior & posterior SG, PO; Exploratory: vertices outside ROIs	ADHD<Controls: SFG, MFG, OFC, ACC, PCC, right AG, ASG, right PSG. After covarying mean cortical thickness: ADHD<Controls: right MFG, bilateral ACC, right AG & left PCC. ADHD>Controls: right PCC exploratory: ADHD<Control: right occipital pole (BA17)
Seidman 2006*	ADHD: 24 Control: 18	ADHD: 38 (2.2); Control: 34.8 (2.5)	18–59.	ADHD: 50% Control: 50%	Both	Yes	Yes; ADHD subtypes: 12 CT, 9 IN, 2 HI.	ADHD: 7 CONTROL: 4	>79	ADHD: 4 Mood; 4 GAD; 12 SUD. Control: 4 Mood; 6 SUD.	Morphometric (volumes)/3D isosurface differences (for ACC); Semi-automatic segmentation and ROI definition	ROIs: TCV, total GM, PFC (esp. DLPFC), ACC, CRB GM, Caud; Exploratory: Nacc, all other parcelated areas.	ADHD<Controls: Cortical GM. Specifically: bilateral FL (D=0.59–0.61); left SFG, D=0.67), right medial paralimbic areas (D=0.58; E.G. right ACC, D=0.53, particularly subgenual and dorsal regions); ADHD>Controls: cortical WM, Nacc (trends); Ns: TCV, WBV, Caud, Put, GP, A, Hip, Th, CRB, brain stem, ventricles.
Hesslinger 2002	ADHD: 8 Controls: 17	ADHD: 31.2 (4.4); Controls: 30.2 (7.9)	19–40	100%	Clinic	Yes (onset <7)	Yes; Plus emotional instability symptoms	None	–	Excluded: MDD, BD, Schiz, SUD	Manual volumetry	OFC	Left OFC: ADHD<Controls; Right OFC>Controls; Ns: TBV: Ns

Note: *Same or partially overlapping samples. Abbreviations: A: amygdala; ACC: anterior cingulate cortex; AG: angular gyrus; BD: bipolar disorder; Caud: caudate; CB: cingulum bundle; CG: cingulate gyrus; CRB: cerebellum; CT: combined subtype; DLPFC: dorsolateral prefrontal cortex; FA: fractional anisotropy; FC: frontal cortex; FL: frontal lobes; GAD: generalised anxiety disorder; GM: gray matter; GP: globus pallidus; HI: hyperactive/impulsive subtype; Hip: hippocampus; IN: inattentive subtype; MAD: multiple anxiety disorder; MDD: major depressive disorder; MFG: middle frontal gyrus; MPH: methylphenidate; Nacc: nucleus accumbens; OC: occipital cortex; OFC: orbitofrontal cortex; PC: parietal cortex; PCG: posterior cingulate gyrus; PO: parietal operculum; Put: putamen; ROI: region of interest; SFG: superior frontal gyrus; SG: supramarginal gyrus; SLF: superior longitudinal fascicle; SUD: substance use disorder; SZ: schizophrenia; TBV: total brain volume; TC: temporal cortex; TCGM: total cerebral gray matter; TCV: total cerebral volume; TH: thalamus; WBV: whole brain volume; WM: white matter.

regulation of spatial attention processes, whereas the cingulum provides connections between the anterior cingulate cortex and prefrontal, parietal, thalamic, and limbic areas, contributing to the integration of motivational/affective processes with attention and executive functions (Makris et al., 2008).

Seidman et al. (2006) failed to find any differences in the basal ganglia. Initially, a trend for increased volumes in the nucleus accumbens was reported, but it was not replicated with a larger sample (Biederman et al., 2008). No differences were observed in other limbic areas (amygdala, hippocampus; Biederman et al., 2008; Perlov et al., 2008; Seidman et al., 2006) or the thalamus (Biederman et al., 2008; Seidman et al., 2006).

Interestingly, adults with ADHD did not show a reduction in total brain volume compared to controls in any of the three independent samples where differences in brain volume were examined (Biederman et al., 2008; Hesslinger et al., 2002; Monuteaux et al., 2008; Perlov et al., 2008; Seidman et al., 2006). This is striking, given that a global reduction in total cerebral volume is a consistent finding in children/adolescents with ADHD (Valera et al., 2007). The failure to find such a volume reduction could be due to the effects of chronic treatment with stimulant medication (Castellanos et al., 2002). It could also reflect abnormalities in the balance between gray and white matter development; Seidman et al. (2006) found that cortical gray matter volume reduction was compensated for by an equivalent increase in white matter volume.

Frequent but short-lived mood swings, irritability, and emotional overreaction to stressors are other characteristics that are frequently observed in adults and youths with ADHD (Asherson et al., 2007; Skirrow et al., 2009; Wender, Wolf, & Wasserstein, 2001). Such symptoms of emotional dysregulation and lability have led to the hypothesis that adults with ADHD would show structural abnormalities in the orbitofrontal cortex (Hesslinger et al., 2002), an area that plays a key role in the regulation of behavior and emotional processes (Mega & Cummings, 1994; Tekin & Cummings, 2002). Indeed, adults with ADHD have shown decreased volumes and cortical thickness in this region (Hesslinger et al., 2002; Makris et al., 2007). Using a female adult sample with comorbid ADHD and borderline personality disorder, Rusch, Weber, et al. (2007) reported abnormalities in the structural integrity of white matter in the inferior frontal lobes, which correlated with affective dysregulation.

The symptomatic overlap and shared characteristics between ADHD and other mood and personality disorders, such as bipolar disorder and borderline personality disorder, and their substantial comorbidity (Biederman et al., 2008; Rusch, Luders, et al., 2007; Rusch, Weber, et al., 2007) present problems in their differential classification. Magnetic resonance imaging could provide a means to disentangle such disorders by assessing similarities and differences in morphometric abnormalities among samples with "pure" and comorbid forms of the disorders. Using this approach, Biederman et al. (2008) found that each syndrome was associated with relatively selective regional deficits in the cerebral cortex (but not subcortical structures). ADHD (independently of bipolar disorder status) was associated with volume reductions in regions associated with executive function/attention networks (left superior frontal gyrus, right anterior cingulate cortex, right cerebellar gray matter), confirming previous reports (Seidman et al., 2006). Bipolar disorder (independent of ADHD status) was associated with neuroanatomic differences in limbic-prefrontal regions involved in emotional regulation (i.e. with a volume reduction in the left orbitofrontal cortex and a volume increase in the right thalamus). Volumetric abnormalities in the comorbid cases involved deficits in regions associated with each disorder separately. This evidence supports the idea that, in adults, ADHD and bipolar disorder represent truly comorbid disorders and that their co-occurrence is not simply a case of misdiagnosis (Biederman et al., 2008). Recent genetic evidence adds further complexity to this issue though: the DRD4 7-repeat allele was associated with decreased gray matter volumes in the superior frontal gyrus and the cerebellum in adults with "pure ADHD" but not in those with comorbid bipolar disorder (Monuteaux et al., 2008). If replicated, this finding could be suggestive of a distinct familial ADHD and bipolar disorder subtype (which has received support by familial evidence; Faraone et al., 2001), without excluding other possibilities such as interactions among genes in the comorbid cases (Monuteaux et al., 2008).

The case of early-onset bipolar disorder, which differs in its clinical presentation from adult bipolar disorder (Lopez-Larson et al., 2009), and ADHD might be different. Lopez-Larson et al. (2009) found that, although youths with comorbid early-onset bipolar disorder and ADHD did not show any neuroanatomic differences in subcortical structures from youths with pure bipolar disorder, they did show distinct neuroanatomic abnormalities from youths with pure ADHD; these abnormalities were localized in limbic brain structures. Early-onset bipolar disorder was associated with smaller hippocampi and larger nucleus accumbens volumes, whereas ADHD was associated with volume reductions in the striatum and the amygdala. These findings would support the notion that comorbid bipolar disorder and ADHD in youths is a subtype or a more severe form of early-onset bipolar disorder (Lopez-Larson et al., 2009). Differentiating between bipolar disorder and ADHD and understanding the causes of their comorbidity may have important implications for treatment (Biederman et al., 2008; Marks, Newcorn, & Halperin, 2001; Monuteaux et al., 2008).

Evaluation of neuroanatomic deficits in adults with ADHD

Only three studies have examined neuroanatomic deficits over a relatively wider range of brain regions, using different methods on the same or overlapping samples. They have produced findings that are consistent with what we would expect on the basis of cross-sectional and longitudinal evidence from children and adolescents (Biederman et al., 2008; Makris et al., 2007; Seidman et al., 2006). Adults with ADHD showed volume/thickness reductions over a network of frontal and parietal regions involved in attention/executive functions, the orbitofrontal cortex, and the cerebellum. They also showed deficits in associated white matter tracts (Makris et al., 2008). The lack of volume differences in the caudate and other basal ganglia (Biederman et al., 2008; Hesslinger et al., 2002; Makris et al., 2007; Seidman et al., 2006) was expected (Castellanos et al., 2002), although the lack of volumetric differences in the amygdala and the hippocampus was inconsistent with limited evidence from children/adolescents with ADHD. Finally, the lack of differences in total brain volume could be due to chronic effects of medication or abnormal white matter development.

Functional MRI studies in ADHD

Task-dependent functional deficits in children and adolescents with ADHD

The majority of fMRI studies in ADHD have focused on the neural mechanisms underpinning executive function deficits. It is beyond the scope of this chapter to provide a comprehensive review of this area. Here we provide a brief overview of existing research based both on an earlier systematic review of fMRI research in ADHD (Paloyelis et al., 2007) and an examination of some more recent work in this area.

Most of the studies used a narrow range of tasks that examined inhibitory control and attention processes and consistently reported atypical brain activation in frontal and striatal areas. However, there were inconsistencies in the direction of the difference in the frontal lobes (some studies showing hypoactivation and others hyperactivation), as well as in the laterality of the findings and the exact regions involved. A decrease in striatal activation was perhaps the most consistent finding, reported in all but one study, which found significant group differences. Studies that examined other cognitive functions – tapping attention processes, motor function, working memory, or temporal processing – consistently showed reduced brain activation in ADHD in more widespread regions, including areas in the temporal and parietal cortices (Rubia et al., 2007; Smith et al., 2008; Stevens, Pearlson, & Kiehl, 2007; Vance et al., 2007). Meta-analytic evidence confirmed hypoactivation in frontal, parietal, and striatal areas, whereas hyperactivation was also observed in certain regions (Dickstein et al., 2006). Recent studies have provided further evidence for hypoactivation in a wide network of brain regions, including the cerebellum, in ADHD (e.g. Durston et al., 2007; Suskauer et al., 2007; Vance et al., 2007), whereas Sheridan, Hinshaw, and D'Esposito (2007) suggested that increased activation during a working memory task may be indicative of less efficient neural processing in ADHD.

Task-dependent functional deficits in adults with ADHD

Studies have shown both regional and network-wide deficits during the performance of working memory tasks by adults with ADHD. Decreased activation, compared to healthy controls, has been found in the left inferior frontal gyrus, the occipital gyrus, and the cerebellum (Valera et al., 2005; Wolf et al., 2009) as well as the right insula and the medial frontal gyrus (Wolf et al., 2009), whereas increased activation at the right cerebellum was associated with lower ADHD symptoms. Adults with ADHD have also shown abnormal functional connectivity patterns in nodes of working memory/executive function and attention networks, such as the inferior and superior frontal gyri, the anterior cingulate cortex, and the superior parietal lobule (Wolf et al., 2009). Enhanced functional connectivity of the right inferior frontal gyrus was associated with improved task performance in the high load condition in the ADHD group (Wolf et al., 2009).

An interesting study has suggested that the commonly observed executive function deficits in ADHD may be partly caused by deficits in more fundamental processes (Hale et al., 2007). Adults with ADHD showed atypical brain activation in task-related networks while performing both variations of a task that differed in their load on executive functions. *Digit span backward* is considered to be an executive function/ working memory task, whereas *digit span forward* involves a single component process requiring the simple repetition of a series of numbers. The authors suggested that deficits in higher mental processes, such as executive functions, may stem from dysfunction in more fundamental neural systems engaged in "access to, or generation of, phonologically represented information" (Hale et al., 2007). Thus ADHD may be associated with a dysfunction in fundamental neural systems that may lead to a deficit in higher order executive functions such as inhibitory control. For example, a deficit in a verbal representation system may have an impact on subvocal articulation, which constitutes an important component process of inhibitory control according to some authors (Barkley, 1997).

Another interesting finding that came from this study was that the systematic training of participants to use a single mental strategy resulted in no differences in the frontal lobes in the digit span backward condition. This finding could suggest that the often reported frontal lobe abnormalities associated with executive functions in ADHD might be due, to some extent at least, to the use of different strategies (Hale et al., 2007).

Adults with ADHD have also shown atypical brain activation while responding/inhibiting responses to stimuli and during performance-related feedback presentation in a go/no-go task (Dibbets et al., 2009). Successful performance in response inhibition trials was associated with increased activation in the ADHD group, compared to controls, in the left inferior frontal gyrus and the right putamen, whereas increased activation in the inferior frontal gyrus was associated with an increased error rate. Increased activation in the left inferior and the right middle frontal gyri in the ADHD group was also observed during simple stimulus response trials (Dibbets et al., 2009). Despite the lack of behavioral evidence for differential sensitivity to negative feedback in the ADHD group, the ADHD group showed increased activation in the left inferior frontal gyrus when activation associated with positive feedback was subtracted from activation associated with negative feedback. Positive feedback presentation was accompanied by lower activation in the inferior/middle frontal gyri and orbitofrontal cortex, as well as the caudate, in the ADHD group compared to controls, whereas negative feedback was associated with lower activation in the hippocampus/ nucleus accumbens area. This study suggests that adult ADHD is associated with alterations in neural mechanisms underlying executive functions and reward/motivational processes (Dibbets et al., 2009).

Deficits associated with reward/motivational processes and reward-related decision making

Recently, studies have started to investigate the function of the mesolimbic dopaminergic reward/ motivation circuitry in ADHD, deficits in which have been linked with the disorder (Paloyelis et al., submitted; Scheres et al., 2007; Strohle et al., 2008; Volkow et al., 2010). Individual differences in the function of the dopaminergic reward circuitry have been associated with individual differences in reward-related impulsivity (Hanh et al., 2009; Hariri et al., 2006). Therefore, understanding the pathophysiology of this system in ADHD is important, given that youths with ADHD have consistently shown higher levels of reward-related impulsivity than controls (Paloyelis, Asherson, & Kuntsi, 2009; Paloyelis et al., 2010, Scheres et al., 2010), and that dysfunctions in this system may lead to the development of ADHD symptom according to influential neurobiological models of the disorder (Sagvolden et al., 2005; Sonuga-Barke, 2005; Tripp & Wickens, 2008).

Currently, few studies have investigated this area, especially in adults. Using a cued-reaction time task, initial evidence from adolescents and adults with ADHD reported decreased ventral striatal activation (compared to controls) in response to anticipated cue-signaled monetary gains (Scheres et al., 2007; Strohle et al., 2008) (but not monetary losses; Scheres et al., 2007), while the adult study also reported that the ADHD group showed increased activation in prefrontal regions and the caudate nucleus following reward delivery (Strohle et al. 2008). A recent study with a much larger and more homogeneous sample of male adolescents with ADHD-combined subtype, and typically developing controls has confirmed the latter observation from the adult group (Paloyelis et al., submitted), while it failed to support previous evidence for reduced responsivity to cue-signaled rewards in the ventral striatum (Scheres et al., 2007; Strohle et al., 2008). Paloyelis et al. (submitted) further reported evidence for increased striatal responsivity to anticipated rewards in the ADHD group (compared to controls) if genetic variation in the gene for the dopamine transporter (*DAT1/SLC6A3*) is taken into account. The area of altered reward/motivation processes in ADHD is developing fast, and future studies will need to illuminate how the pathophysiology of this circuitry relates to ADHD-typical behavior, such as impulsivity and the development of ADHD symptoms.

Atypical brain activation in the fronto-striatal circuitry involved in reward processing has also been observed with a simple decision-making task (Plichta et al., 2009). When faced with choices between monetary sums available at different delays, adults with ADHD showed patterns of brain activation that differed from controls in a manner that varied as a function of the available options and caudate nucleus subregion. They showed lower activation in the ventral striatum (compared to controls) when an immediate option was present, whereas they showed higher activation in dorsal areas of the caudate when the decision was between two delayed amounts (Plichta et al., 2009). Making a choice between two delayed amounts was further accompanied by amygdala hyperresponsiveness compared to controls (and the reverse when an immediate option was present), which could be explained by a more aversive emotional reaction to the implied presence of delay, in line with delay aversion theory (Sonuga-Barke, 2005).

Studies using dyads of parents and children with ADHD

Variations among scanning protocols and behavioral paradigms, as well as sample heterogeneity, may be sources of inconsistencies when comparing different studies, particularly when the studies use cross-sectional samples at different developmental stages. In this section we review a series of studies using a clever design in which researchers employed dyads of adolescents with a family history of ADHD and their affected

parents (Casey et al., 2007; Epstein et al., 2007; Garrett et al., 2008). A family history of ADHD may increase sample homogeneity and biological risk, as well as the probability that observed similarities may be biologically based given the high heritability of ADHD. Overall, these studies link deficient frontostriatal gray and white matter development with response inhibition deficits and suggest that neuroanatomical deficits are heritable in ADHD (Casey et al., 2007).

Using a response inhibition (go/no-go) task, Epstein et al. (2007) found decreased activation in the right inferior frontal gyrus and the left caudate during successful inhibition in both adolescents and parents, suggesting that frontostriatal dysfunction may be a developmentally stable characteristic of ADHD. Increased activation in these regions was associated with a greater sensitivity to target detection. Adolescents showed decreased activation in a wider network of regions extending to the middle frontal gyrus, inferior parietal lobule, and anterior cingulate cortex, whereas adults with ADHD showed increased activation in the left inferior parietal cortex and the anterior cingulate cortex.

In two other studies, Casey et al. (2007) and Garrett et al. (2008) linked neuroanatomic deficits to behavioral performance and functional activation in frontostriatal regions. Abnormalities in the microstructure of frontostriatal white matter tracts were associated with impaired performance and decreased activation in the caudate and the inferior frontal gyrus during a response inhibition task in parents and adolescents with ADHD. There was also a positive correlation between fractional anisotropy values in adolescents with ADHD and their parents in frontostriatal white matter tracts.

Garrett et al. (2008) found that caudate volumes correlated negatively with functional activation in the left caudate and the right inferior frontal gyrus during successful inhibition trials. The ADHD group showed increased caudate and inferior frontal gyrus volumes compared to controls, which could be due to the older age range of the participants (see also Mataro et al., 1997). As Castellanos et al. (2002) have shown, caudate differences tend to disappear by late adolescence. However, increased volumes were still associated with activation deficits, and as in an earlier study, increased caudate volumes were associated with impaired performance in an attention test and with the presence of more ADHD symptoms. Therefore, this study shows that an apparent lack of the expected volumetric deficits does not necessarily imply "normalization" but may result from aberrant maturational processes (e.g. reduced pruning).

Acute stimulant effects in adults with ADHD

Stimulant medication generally tends to "normalize" atypical brain activity in both adults and youths with ADHD, decreasing or increasing activation in frontal regions, the basal ganglia, and the cerebellum accordingly (Anderson et al., 2002; Epstein et al., 2007; O'Gorman et al., 2008; Shafritz et al., 2004; Telcher et al., 2000; Vaidya et al., 1998; but not in Kobel et al. (2009)).

In a randomized, placebo-controlled study (Bush et al., 2008), methylphenidate hydrochloride osmotic-release oral system (OROS) was found to increase activation in the dorsal anterior cingulate cortex and other areas of a distributed cingulate-fronto-parietal cognitive/attention network, as well as the thalamus, caudate, and cerebellum, during a cognitive interference control task. Increases in functional activation were related to treatment response. In an earlier study using a similar cognitive interference control task (Bush et al., 1999), adults with ADHD showed decreased dorsal anterior cingulate cortex activation compared to healthy controls.

In a parent–child dyad study described earlier, administration of methylphenidate increased brain activation at prefrontal regions, the caudate, the inferior parietal lobe, and the anterior cingulate in adolescents with ADHD who had showed decreased activation in these regions while off medication. Similarly, acute administration of methylphenidate increased activation in the left caudate in their parents, but it also altered brain activation in other regions that had not shown differences in activation compared to controls at baseline (Epstein et al., 2007).

O'Gorman et al. (2008) used continuous arterial spin labeling (CASL) MRI to assess quantitative group differences in blood perfusion between a group of adults who were off their normal stimulant medication for a week and a group of healthy controls, as well as the effects of reinstating their usual treatment regime on blood perfusion. Adults with ADHD off medication showed increased blood perfusion in the caudate and frontal and parietal regions, compared to healthy controls. The reinstatement of treatment "normalized" blood perfusion in the caudate and frontal and parietal

regions and decreased it further in some other regions (e.g. parahippocampal gyrus).

Spontaneous brain activity

The investigation of spontaneous brain activity while participants are resting is an emerging and fascinating subfield in fMRI research. New methodologies are being developed to address a wide range of questions regarding the functional integrity of specific regions, whole networks, or network nodes, and in applications such as discriminating between groups (Zhu et al., 2008) or inferring resting-state brain activity (Tian et al., 2008). Evidence from studies examining spontaneous brain activity in youths (e.g. Cao et al., 2006; Tian et al., 2006; Zang et al., 2007) and adults (Castellanos et al., 2008; Uddin et al., 2008) with ADHD is consistent with a dysfunction in more general processes, rather than deficits pertaining to narrowly defined cognitive processes (e.g. executive functions).

Some methods examine the temporal coherence between the time-series of a particular voxel and its nearest neighbors, assessing regional integrity (Cao et al., 2006), or between a seed region and other regions, mapping networks of potentially functionally related areas (functional connectivity; Castellanos et al., 2008). Such methods are sensitive to the initial selection of seed voxel/region, and this sensitivity may lead to inconsistent results in different studies. Network homogeneity analysis provides an unbiased method to examine coherence within a network and identify regions that may show reduced connectivity (Uddin et al., 2008).

There is evidence to suggest the existence of a "default mode network" comprising medial prefrontal and parietal and lateral parietal regions, which is active during the resting state and which shows task-induced deactivations during attentional/cognitive tasks and negative correlations with activation in task-related regions (Raichle et al., 2001, 2007). One role of this network may involve the suppression of mental processes that are not related to current behavior. Weissman et al. (2006) have shown that momentary lapses in attention – represented by slower response times on a trial by trial basis and contributing to increased intrasubject variability, a common behavioral finding in ADHD (Castellanos et al., 2005; Klein et al., 2006) – were preceded by decreased activity in frontal attention-control regions (i.e. the right inferior and middle frontal gyri and the dorsal anterior cingulate cortex) before the presentation of task-related stimuli and were associated with reduced task-induced deactivation of a default mode neural network.

Adults with ADHD have shown decreased functional connectivity between default mode components (particularly the precuneus and ventromedial prefrontal cortex; Castellanos et al., 2008); the deficient connectivity of the precuneus was confirmed in the same sample using network homogeneity analysis (Uddin et al., 2008). The strength of the functional connectivity between default mode network components has been positively associated with performance in working memory tasks (Hampson et al., 2006), on which participants with ADHD show deficits (Marinussen et al., 2005; Willcutt et al., 2005). Furthermore, ADHD participants showed abnormal anti-correlations between the dorsal anterior cingulate cortex and posterior regions of the default mode network (precuneus/posterior cingulate cortex) relative to healthy controls (Castellanos et al., 2008). This pattern may represent the decreased efficiency of the dorsal anterior cingulate cortex in regulating task-induced deactivation of the default mode network in ADHD, thereby resulting in an increase in attentional lapses during goal-directed activity (and perhaps increased intrasubject variability in response times). The degree of the anti-correlations was also negatively associated with ADHD symptoms (Castellanos et al., 2008).

The maturational delay hypothesis

Recent evidence from longitudinal studies showing a delay in the age by which peak cortical thickness is reached in the ADHD brain (Shaw, Eckstrand, et al., 2007) has led some authors to suggest that ADHD may be the outcome of a *"maturational lag that eventually normalizes in a considerable proportion of children"* (Rubia, 2007). Although a maturational lag may indeed be contributing to ADHD, the idea of eventual "normalization" is more problematic.

To begin with, despite the similarity in the temporal sequence of cortical development between children with ADHD and healthy controls (Shaw, Eckstrand, et al., 2007), robust neuroanatomic deficits in cortical volumes and thickness remain (Castellanos et al., 2002; Shaw et al., 2006), at least in adults who continue to show the full syndrome. Persistence of ADHD in adulthood, either as the full-blown syndrome or in partial remission with significant impair-

ment, is common and affects 65% of those diagnosed with childhood ADHD (Faraone, Biederman, & Mick, 2006). Therefore, whether normalization of neuroanatomic deficits and associated cognitive and behavioral deficits occurs is an empirical question, and in any case it could only concern the portion of children with ADHD who show full recovery in adulthood.

A second problem with the idea of an eventual normalization concerns the existence of appropriate criteria that could be used to assess it. The apparent lack of volumetric/thickness differences is probably an inadequate and invalid criterion, as *both* the maturational lag and the apparent maturational recovery (see for example the developmental trajectories of caudate volumes in children with ADHD and healthy controls; Castellanos et al., 2002) may reflect deficient maturational processes. We saw earlier that study participants with ADHD in their late adolescence have shown increased caudate volumes compared to healthy controls (Garrett et al., 2008; Mataro et al., 1997), contrary to the robust observation of decreased caudate volumes in children with ADHD (e.g., Valera et al., 2007). However, in both cases increased caudate volumes were associated with impaired performance, activation deficits, and more ADHD symptoms (Garrett et al., 2008; Mataro et al., 1997).

The precise association among region-specific structural changes, underlying neural processes, and functional development is largely unknown; thus, different developmental trajectories, followed by apparent diminution of volumetric or other structural differences with age, may not necessarily imply normalization. Although the idea of a maturational lag underlying ADHD remains a very interesting one, a maturational "catching-up" and consequent symptom improvement do not necessarily follow. The role of compensatory mechanisms in mediating behavioral/cognitive improvements is also largely unappreciated. Further longitudinal research is required, following up children with ADHD into adulthood and including participants with the full range of possible outcomes, as well as the use of multimodal imaging methods, before this question can begin to be addressed.

Final remarks

There is still a lack of sufficient functional and structural neuroimaging data from adults with ADHD, which prevents us from drawing any firm conclusions.

Existing evidence is largely consistent with functional and structural data from children and adolescents with ADHD, suggesting the presence of persistent deficits. Although the ADHD brain may show a maturational lag, its development may prove to be more sophisticated than implied by a model in which it is simply "limping behind" (Rubia, 2007) the normal brain. Crucially, future studies must carefully take into consideration the impact of medication history and comorbidity. Chronic treatment with stimulant medication and possibly other psychotropic drugs to target comorbid disorders can affect brain development, and the presence of comorbid disorders, such as a history and/or current substance abuse in 50% or more of the sample, may introduce important confounds.

References

Anderson CM, Polcari A, Lowen SB, Renshaw PF, Teicher MH. (2002). Effects of methylphenidate on functional magnetic resonance relaxometry of the cerebellar vermis in boys with ADHD. *Am J Psychiatry* 159(8): 1322–8.

Anjari M, Srinivasan L, Allsop JM, Hajnal JV, Rutherford MA, Edwards AD, et al. (2007). Diffusion tensor imaging with tract-based spatial statistics reveals local white matter abnormalities in preterm infants. *Neuroimage* 35(3):1021–7.

Asherson P, Chen W, Craddock B, Taylor E. (2007). Adult attention-deficit hyperactivity disorder: recognition and treatment in general adult psychiatry. *Br J Psychiatry* 190:4–5.

Ashtari M, Kumra S, Bhaskar SL, Clarke T, Thaden E, Cervellione KL, et al. (2007). Attention-deficit/hyperactivity disorder: a preliminary diffusion tensor imaging study. *Biol Psychiatry* 57(5):448–55.

Aylward EH, Reiss AL, Reader MJ, Singer HS, Brown JE, Denckla MB. (1996). Basal ganglia volumes in children with attention-deficit/hyperactivity disorder. *J Child Neurol* 11(2):112–15.

Barkley RA. (1997). Behavioral inhibition, sustained attention, and executive functions: constructing a unifying theory of ADHD. *Psychol Bull* 121(1):65–94.

Biederman J, Makris N, Valera EM, Monuteaux MC, Goldstein JM, Buka S, et al. (2008). Towards further understanding of the co-morbidity between attention deficit hyperactivity disorder and bipolar disorder: a MRI study of brain volumes. *Psychol Med* 38(7):1045–56.

Bledsoe J, Semrud-Clikeman M, Pliszka SR. (2009). A magnetic resonance imaging study of the cerebellar vermis in chronically treated and treatment-naive children with attention-deficit/hyperactivity disorder combined type. *Biol Psychiatry* 7:620–4.

Bush G, Frazier JA, Rauch SL, Seidman LJ, Whalen PJ, Jenike MA, et al. (1999). Anterior cingulate cortex dysfunction in attention-deficit/hyperactivity disorder revealed by fMRI and the Counting Stroop. *Biol Psychiatry* 45(12):1542–52.

Bush G, Spencer TJ, Holmes J, Shin LM, Valera EM, Seidman LJ, et al. (2008). Functional magnetic resonance imaging of methylphenidate and placebo in attention-deficit/hyperactivity disorder during the multi-source interference task. *Arch Gen Psychiatry* 65(1):102–14.

Cao Q, Zang Y, Sun L, Sui M, Long X, Zou Q, et al. (2006). Abnormal neural activity in children with attention deficit hyperactivity disorder: a resting-state functional magnetic resonance imaging study. *Neuroreport* 17(10):1033–6.

Carmona S, Vilarroya O, Bielsa A, Tremols V, Soliva JC, Rovira M, et al. (2005). Global and regional gray matter reductions in ADHD: a voxel-based morphometric study. *Neurosci Lett* 389(2):88–93.

Casey BJ, Epstein JN, Buhle J, Liston C, Davidson MC, Tonev ST, et al. (2007). Frontostriatal connectivity and its role in cognitive control in parent-child dyads with ADHD. *Am J Psychiatry* 164(11):1729–36.

Castellanos FX, Giedd JN, Marsh WL, Hamburger SD, Vaituzis AC, Dickstein DP, et al. (1996). Quantitative brain magnetic resonance imaging in attention-deficit hyperactivity disorder. *Arch Gen Psychiatry* 53(7):607–16.

Castellanos FX, Lee PP, Sharp W, Jeffries NO, Greenstein DK, Clasen LS, et al. (2002). Developmental trajectories of brain volume abnormalities in children and adolescents with attention-deficit/hyperactivity disorder. *JAMA* 288(14):1740–8.

Castellanos FX, Margulies DS, Kelly C, Uddin LQ, Ghaffari M, Kirsch A, et al. (2008). Cingulate-precuneus interactions: a new locus of dysfunction in adult attention-deficit/hyperactivity disorder. *Biol Psychiatry* 63(3):332–7.

Castellanos FX, Sonuga-Barke EJ, Scheres A, Di Martino A, Hyde C, Walters JR. (2005). Varieties of attention-deficit/hyperactivity disorder-related intra-individual variability. *Biol Psychiatry* 57(11):1416–23.

Dibbets P, Evers L, Hurks P, Marchetta N, Jolles J. (2009). Differences in feedback- and inhibition-related neural activity in adult ADHD. *Brain Cogn* 70(1):73–83.

Dickstein SG, Bannon K, Castellanos FX, Milham MP. (2006). The neural correlates of attention deficit hyperactivity disorder: an ALE meta-analysis. *J Child Psychol Psychiatry* 47(10):1051–62.

Durston S, Davidson MC, Mulder MJ, Spicer JA, Galvan A, Tottenham N, et al. (2007). Neural and behavioral correlates of expectancy violations in attention-deficit hyperactivity disorder. *J Child Psychol Psychiatry* **48**(9):881–9.

Durston S, Hulshoff Pol HE, Schnack HG, Buitelaar JK, Steenhuis MP, Minderaa RB, et al. (2004). Magnetic resonance imaging of boys with attention-deficit/hyperactivity disorder and their unaffected siblings. *J Am Acad Child Adolesc Psychiatry* **43**(3): 332–40.

Ellison-Wright I, Ellison-Wright Z, Bullmore E. (2008). Structural brain change in Attention Deficit Hyperactivity Disorder identified by meta-analysis. *BMC Psychiatry* **8**:51.

Epstein JN, Casey BJ, Tonev ST, Davidson MC, Reiss AL, Garrett A, et al. (2007). ADHD- and medication-related brain activation effects in concordantly affected parent-child dyads with ADHD. *J Child Psychol Psychiatry* **48**(9):899–913.

Faraone SV, Biederman J, Mick E. (2006). The age-dependent decline of attention deficit hyperactivity disorder: a meta-analysis of follow-up studies. *Psychol Med* **36**(2):159–65.

Faraone SV, Biederman J, Monuteaux MC. (2001). Attention deficit hyperactivity disorder with bipolar disorder in girls: Further evidence for a familial subtype? *J Affect Disord* **64**(1):19–26.

Filipek PA, Semrud-Clikeman M, Steingard RJ, Renshaw PF, Kennedy DN, Biederman J. (1997). Volumetric MRI analysis comparing subjects having attention-deficit hyperactivity disorder with normal controls. *Neurology* **48**(3):589–601.

Garrett A, Penniman L, Epstein JN, Casey BJ, Hinshaw SP, Glover G, et al. (2008). Neuroanatomical abnormalities in adolescents with attention-deficit/hyperactivity disorder. *J Am Acad Child Adolesc Psychiatry* **47**(11):1321–8.

Hahn, T, Dresler, T, Ehlis, A-C, Plichta, MM, Heinzel, S, Polak, T, et al. (2009). Neural response to reward anticipation is modulated by Gray's impulsivity. *NeuroImage* **46**:1148–53.

Hale TS, Bookheimer S, McGough JJ, Phillips JM, McCracken JT. (2007). Atypical brain activation during simple & complex levels of processing in adult ADHD: an fMRI study. *J Atten Disord* **11**(2):125–40.

Hamilton LS, Levitt JG, O'Neill J, Alger JR, Luders E, Phillips OR, et al. (2008). Reduced white matter integrity in attention-deficit hyperactivity disorder. *Neuroreport* **19**(17):1705–8.

Hampson M, Driesen NR, Skudlarski P, Gore JC, Constable RT. (2006). Brain connectivity related to working memory performance. *J Neurosci* **26**:13338–43.

Hariri, AR, Brown, SM, Williamson, DE, Flory, JD, de Wit, H, & Manuck, SB. (2006). Preference for

immediate over delayed rewards is associated with magnitude of ventral striatal activity. *Journal of Neuroscience* **26**(51):13213–17.

Hesslinger B, Tebartz van Elst L, Thiel T, Haegele K, Hennig J, Ebert D. (2002). Frontoorbital volume reductions in adult patients with attention deficit hyperactivity disorder. *Neurosci Lett* **328**(3):319–21.

Kates WR, Frederikse M, Mostofsky SH, Folley BS, Cooper K, Mazur-Hopkins P, et al. (2002). MRI parcellation of the frontal lobe in boys with attention deficit hyperactivity disorder or Tourette syndrome. *Psychiatry Res* **116**(1–2):63–81.

Klein C, Wendling K, Huettner P, Ruder H, Peper M. (2006). Intra-subject variability in attention-deficit hyperactivity disorder. *Biol Psychiatry* **60**(10):1088–97.

Kobel M, Bechtel N, Weber P, Specht K, Klarhofer M, Scheffler K, et al. (2009). Effects of methylphenidate on working memory functioning in children with attention deficit/hyperactivity disorder. *Eur J Paediatr Neurol* **13**(6):516–23.

Li X, Jiang J, Zhu W, Yu C, Sui M, Wang Y, et al. (2007). Asymmetry of prefrontal cortical convolution complexity in males with attention-deficit/hyperactivity disorder using fractal information dimension. *Brain Dev* **29**(10):649–55.

Lopez-Larson M, Michael ES, Terry JE, Breeze JL, Hodge SM, Tang L, et al. (2009). Subcortical differences among youths with attention-deficit/hyperactivity disorder compared to those with bipolar disorder with and without attention-deficit/hyperactivity disorder. *J Child Adolesc Psychopharmacol* **19**(1):31–9.

Luders E, Narr KL, Hamilton LS, Phillips OR, Thompson PM, Valle JS, et al. (2009). Decreased callosal thickness in attention-deficit/hyperactivity disorder. *Biol Psychiatry* **65**(1):84–8.

Mackie S, Shaw P, Lenroot R, Pierson R, Greenstein DK, Nugent TF, 3rd, et al. (2007). Cerebellar development and clinical outcome in attention deficit hyperactivity disorder. *Am J Psychiatry* **164**(4): 647–55.

Makris N, Biederman J, Valera EM, Bush G, Kaiser J, Kennedy DN, et al. (2007). Cortical thinning of the attention and executive function networks in adults with attention-deficit/hyperactivity disorder. *Cereb Cortex* **17**(6):1364–75.

Makris N, Buka SL, Biederman J, Papadimitriou GM, Hodge SM, Valera EM, et al. (2008). Attention and executive systems abnormalities in adults with childhood ADHD: A DT-MRI study of connections. *Cereb Corte* **18**(5):1210–20.

Marks DJ, Newcorn JH, Halperin JM. (200). Comorbidity in adults with attention-deficit/hyperactivity disorder. *Ann NY Acad Sci* **931**:216–38.

Martinussen R, Hayden J, Hogg-Johnson S, Tannock R. (2005). A meta-analysis of working memory impairments in children with attention-deficit/ hyperactivity disorder. *J Am Acad Child Adolesc Psychiatry* **44**(4):377–84.

Mataro M, Garcia-Sanchez C, Junque C, Estevez-Gonzalez A, Pujol J. (1997). Magnetic resonance imaging measurement of the caudate nucleus in adolescents with attention-deficit hyperactivity disorder and its relationship with neuropsychological and behavioral measures. *Arch Neurol* **54**(8): 963–8.

McAlonan GM, Cheung V, Cheung C, Chua SE, Murphy DG, Suckling J, et al. (2007). Mapping brain structure in attention deficit-hyperactivity disorder: a voxel-based MRI study of regional grey and white matter volume. *Psychiatry Res* **154**(2):171–80.

Mega MS, Cummings JL. (1994). Frontal-subcortical circuits and neuropsychiatric disorders. *J Neuropsychiatry Clin Neurosci* **6**(4):358–70.

Mehta MA, Owen AM, Sahakian BJ, Mavaddat N, Pickard JD, Robbins TW. (2000). Methylphenidate enhances working memory by modulating discrete frontal and parietal lobe regions in the human brain. *J Neurosci* **20**(6):RC65.

Moghaddam B, Homayoun H. (2008). Divergent plasticity of prefrontal cortex networks. *Neuropsychopharmacology* **33**(1):42–55.

Monuteaux MC, Seidman LJ, Faraone SV, Makris N, Spencer T, Valera E, et al. (2008). A preliminary study of dopamine D4 receptor genotype and structural brain alterations in adults with ADHD. *Am J Med Genet B Neuropsychiatr Genet* **147B**(8):1436–41.

Mostofsky SH, Cooper KL, Kates WR, Denckla MB, Kaufmann WE. (2002). Smaller prefrontal and premotor volumes in boys with attention-deficit/hyperactivity disorder. *Biol Psychiatry* **52**(8):785–94.

O'Gorman RL, Mehta MA, Asherson P, Zelaya FO, Brookes KJ, Toone BK, et al. (2008). Increased cerebral perfusion in adult attention deficit hyperactivity disorder is normalised by stimulant treatment: a non-invasive MRI pilot study. *Neuroimage* **42**(1): 36–41.

Overmeyer S, Bullmore ET, Suckling J, Simmons A, Williams SC, Santosh PJ, et al. (2001). Distributed grey and white matter deficits in hyperkinetic disorder: MRI evidence for anatomical abnormality in an attentional network. *Psychol Med* **31**(8):1425–35.

Paloyelis Y, Asherson P, Kuntsi J. (2009). Are ADHD symptoms associated with delay aversion or choice impulsivity? A general population study. *J Am Acad Child Adolesc Psychiatry* **48**(8):837–36.

Paloyelis, Y, Asherson, P, Mehta, MA, Faraone, SV, & Kuntsi, J. (2010). DAT1 and COMT Effects on Delay Discounting and Trait Impulsivity in Male Adolescents with Attention Deficit/Hyperactivity Disorder and Healthy Controls. *Neuropsychopharmacology* **35**:2414–26.

Paloyelis, Y, Mehta, MA, Faraone, SV, Asherson, P, & Kuntsi, J. (submitted). Is attention deficit/hyperactivity disorder characterized by neural *hypo-* or *hyper*-sensitivity to rewards? The role of *DAT1*.

Paloyelis Y, Mehta MA, Kuntsi J, Asherson P. (2007). Functional MRI in ADHD: a systematic literature review. *Expert Rev Neurother* **7**(10):1337–56.

Perlov E, Philipsen A, Tebartz van Elst L, Ebert D, Henning J, Maier S, et al. (2008). Hippocampus and amygdala morphology in adults with attention-deficit hyperactivity disorder. *J Psychiatry Neurosci* **33**(6):509–15.

Plessen KJ, Bansal R, Zhu H, Whiteman R, Amat J, Quackenbush GA, et al. (2006). Hippocampus and amygdala morphology in attention-deficit/hyperactivity disorder. *Arch Gen Psychiatry* **63**(7):795–807.

Plichta MM, Vasic N, Wolf RC, Lesch KP, Brummer D, Jacob C, et al. (2009). Neural hyporesponsiveness and hyperresponsiveness during immediate and delayed reward processing in adult attention-deficit/ hyperactivity disorder. *Biol Psychiatry* **65**(1): 7–14.

Pliszka SR, Lancaster J, Liotti M, Semrud-Clikeman M. (2006). Volumetric MRI differences in treatment-naive vs chronically treated children with ADHD. *Neurology* **67**(6):1023–7.

Qiu A, Crocetti D, Adler M, Mahone EM, Denckla MB, Miller MI, et al. (2000). Basal ganglia volume and shape in children with attention deficit hyperactivity disorder. *Am J Psychiatry* **166**(1):74–82.

Raichle ME, MacLeod AM, Snyder AZ, Powers WJ, Gusnard DA, Shulman GL. (2001). A default mode of brain function. *Proc Natl Acad Sci USA* **98**(2):676–82.

Raichle ME, Snyder AZ. A default mode of brain function: a brief history of an evolving idea. (2007). *Neuroimage* **37**(4):1083–90; discussion 97–9.

Rubia K, Smith AB, Brammer MJ, Taylor E. (2007). Temporal lobe dysfunction in medication-naive boys with attention-deficit/hyperactivity disorder during attention allocation and its relation to response variability. *Biol Psychiatry* **62**(9):999–1006.

Rubia K. (2002). The dynamic approach to neurodevelopmental psychiatric disorders: use of fMRI combined with neuropsychology to elucidate the dynamics of psychiatric disorders, exemplified in ADHD and schizophrenia. *Behav Brain Res* **130**(1–2):47–56.

Rubia K. Neuro-anatomic evidence for the maturational delay hypothesis of ADHD. (2007). *Proc Natl Acad Sci USA* **104**(50):19663–4.

Rusch N, Luders E, Lieb K, Zahn R, Ebert D, Thompson PM, et al. (2007). Corpus callosum abnormalities in women with borderline personality disorder and comorbid attention-deficit hyperactivity disorder. *J Psychiatry Neurosci* **32**(6):417–22.

Rusch N, Weber M, Il'yasov KA, Lieb K, Ebert D, Hennig J, et al. (2007). Inferior frontal white matter microstructure and patterns of psychopathology in women with borderline personality disorder and comorbid attention-deficit hyperactivity disorder. *Neuroimage* **35**(2):738–47.

Sagvolden, T, Johansen, EB, Aase, H, & Russell, VA. (2005). A dynamic developmental theory of attention-deficit/hyperactivity disorder (ADHD) predominantly hyperactive/impulsive and combined subtypes. *Behavioral and Brain Sciences* **28**(3):397–419.

Scheres A, Milham MP, Knutson B, Castellanos FX. (2007). Ventral striatal hyporesponsiveness during reward anticipation in attention-deficit/hyperactivity disorder. *Biol Psychiatry* **61**(5):720–4.

Scheres, A, Tontsch, C, Thoeny, AL, & Kaczkurkin, A. (2010). Temporal Reward Discounting in Attention-Deficit/Hyperactivity Disorder: The Contribution of Symptom Domains, Reward Magnitude, and Session Length. *Biological psychiatry* **67**(7): 641–48.

Seidman LJ, Valera EM, Makris N. (2005). Structural brain imaging of attention-deficit/hyperactivity disorder. *Biol Psychiatry* **57**(11):1263–72.

Seidman LJ, Valera EM, Makris N, Monuteaux MC, Boriel DL, Kelkar K, et al. (2006). Dorsolateral prefrontal and anterior cingulate cortex volumetric abnormalities in adults with attention-deficit/hyperactivity disorder identified by magnetic resonance imaging. *Biol Psychiatry* **60**(10):1071–80.

Shafritz KM, Marchione KE, Gore JC, Shaywitz SE, Shaywitz BA. (2004). The effects of methylphenidate on neural systems of attention in attention deficit hyperactivity disorder. *Am J Psychiatry* **161**(11): 1990–7.

Shaw P, Eckstrand K, Sharp W, Blumenthal J, Lerch JP, Greenstein D, et al. (2007). Attention-deficit/ hyperactivity disorder is characterized by a delay in cortical maturation. *Proc Natl Acad Sci USA* **104**(49):19649–54.

Shaw P, Gornick M, Lerch J, Addington A, Seal J, Greenstein D, et al. (2007). Polymorphisms of the dopamine D4 receptor, clinical outcome, and cortical structure in attention-deficit/hyperactivity disorder. *Arch Gen Psychiatry* **64**(8):921–31.

Shaw P, Lerch J, Greenstein D, Sharp W, Clasen L, Evans A, et al. (2006). Longitudinal mapping of cortical thickness and clinical outcome in children and adolescents with attention-deficit/hyperactivity disorder. *Arch Gen Psychiatry* **63**(5):540–9.

Shaw P, Sharp WS, Morrison M, Eckstrand K, Greenstein DK, Clasen LS, et al. (2009). Psychostimulant treatment and the developing cortex in attention deficit hyperactivity disorder. *Am J Psychiatry* **166**(1): 58–63.

Sheridan MA, Hinshaw S, D'Esposito M. (2007). Efficiency of the prefrontal cortex during working memory in attention-deficit/hyperactivity disorder. *J Am Acad Child Adolesc Psychiatry* **46**(10):1357–66.

Silk TJ, Vance A, Rinehart N, Bradshaw JL, Cunnington R. (2009). White-matter abnormalities in attention deficit hyperactivity disorder: A diffusion tensor imaging study. *Hum Brain Mapp* **30**(9):2757–65.

Skirrow C, McLoughlin G, Kuntsi J, Asherson P. (2009). Behavioural, neurocognitive and treatment overlap between Attention Deficit Hyperactivity Disorder and mood instability. *Expert Rev Neurother* **9**(4): 489–503.

Skranes J, Vangberg TR, Kulseng S, Indredavik MS, Evensen KA, Martinussen M, et al. (2007). Clinical findings and white matter abnormalities seen on diffusion tensor imaging in adolescents with very low birth weight. *Brain* **130**(Pt 3):654–66.

Smith AB, Taylor E, Brammer M, Halari R, Rubia K. (2008). Reduced activation in right lateral prefrontal cortex and anterior cingulate gyrus in medication-naive adolescents with attention deficit hyperactivity disorder during time discrimination. *J Child Psychol Psychiatry* **49**(9):977–85.

Sonuga-Barke EJS. (2005). Causal models of attention-deficit/hyperactivity disorder: From common simple deficits to multiple developmental pathways. *Biol Psychiatry* **57**(11):1231–8.

Sowell ER, Thompson PM, Welcome SE, Henkenius AL, Toga AW, Peterson BS. (2003). Cortical abnormalities in children and adolescents with attention-deficit hyperactivity disorder. *Lancet* **362**(9397): 1699–707.

Stevens MC, Pearlson GD, Kiehl KA. (2007). An FMRI auditory oddball study of combined-subtype attention deficit hyperactivity disorder. *Am J Psychiatry* **164**(11):1737–49.

Strohle A, Stoy M, Wrase J, Schwarzer S, Schlagenhauf F, Huss M, et al. (2008). Reward anticipation and outcomes in adult males with attention-deficit/hyperactivity disorder. *Neuroimage* **39**(3):966–72.

Suskauer SJ, Simmonds DJ, Fotedar S, Blankner JG, Pekar JJ, Denckla MB, et al. (2008). Functional magnetic resonance imaging evidence for abnormalities in response selection in attention deficit hyperactivity disorder: differences in activation associated with response inhibition but not habitual motor response. *J Cogn Neurosci* **20**(3):478–93.

Teicher MH, Anderson CM, Polcari A, Glod CA, Maas LC, Renshaw PF. (2000). Functional deficits in basal ganglia of children with attention-deficit/hyperactivity disorder shown with functional magnetic resonance imaging relaxometry. *Nat Med* **6**(4):470–3.

Tekin S, Cummings JL. (2002). Frontal-subcortical neuronal circuits and clinical neuropsychiatry: an update. *J Psychosom Res* **53**(2):647–54.

Tian L, Jiang T, Liang M, Zang Y, He Y, Sui M, et al. (2008). Enhanced resting-state brain activities in ADHD patients: a fMRI study. *Brain Dev* **30**(5): 342–8.

Tian L, Jiang T, Wang Y, Zang Y, He Y, Liang M, et al. (2006). Altered resting-state functional connectivity patterns of anterior cingulate cortex in adolescents with attention deficit hyperactivity disorder. *Neurosci Lett* **400**(1–2):39–43.

Tremols V, Bielsa A, Soliva J-C, Raheb C, Carmona S, Tomas J, et al. (2008). Differential abnormalities of the head and body of the caudate nucleus in attention deficit-hyperactivity disorder. *Psychiatry Research: Neuroimaging* **163**(3):270–8.

Tripp, G, & Wickens, JR. (2008). Research review: dopamine transfer deficit: a neurobiological theory of altered reinforcement mechanisms in ADHD. *Journal of Child Psychology and Psychiatry and Allied Disciplines* **49**(7):691–704.

Uddin LQ, Kelly AM, Biswal BB, Margulies DS, Shehzad Z, Shaw D, et al. (2008). Network homogeneity reveals decreased integrity of default-mode network in ADHD. *J Neurosci Methods* **169**(1):249–54.

Uhlikova P, Paclt I, Vaneckova M, Morcinek T, Seidel Z, Krasensky J, et al. (2007). Asymmetry of basal ganglia in children with attention deficit hyperactivity disorder. *Neuro Endocrinol Lett* **28**(5):604–9.

Vaidya CJ, Austin G, Kirkorian G, Ridlehuber HW, Desmond JE, Glover GH, et al. (1998). Selective effects of methylphenidate in attention deficit hyperactivity disorder: a functional magnetic resonance study. *Proc Natl Acad Sci USA* **95**(24):14494–9.

Valera EM, Faraone SV, Biederman J, Poldrack RA, Seidman LJ. (2005). Functional neuroanatomy of working memory in adults with attention-deficit/ hyperactivity disorder. *Biol Psychiatry* **57**(5):439–47.

Valera EM, Faraone SV, Murray KE, Seidman LJ. (2007). Meta-analysis of structural imaging findings in attention-deficit/hyperactivity disorder. *Biol Psychiatry* **61**(12):1361–9.

Vance A, Silk TJ, Casey M, Rinehart NJ, Bradshaw JL, Bellgrove MA, et al. (2007). Right parietal dysfunction in children with attention deficit hyperactivity disorder, combined type: a functional MRI study. *Mol Psychiatry* **12**(9):826–32, 793.

Volkow, ND, Wang, G-J, Newcorn, JH, Kollins, SH, Wigal, TL, Telang, F, et al. (2010). Motivation deficit in ADHD is associated with dysfunction of the dopamine reward pathway. *Molecular psychiatry* 1–8.

Wang J, Jiang T, Cao Q, Wang Y. (2007). Characterizing anatomic differences in boys with attention-deficit/ hyperactivity disorder with the use of deformation-based morphometry. *Am J Neuroradiol* **28**(3):543–7.

Weissman DH, Roberts KC, Visscher KM, Woldorff MG. (2006). The neural bases of momentary lapses in attention. *Nat Neurosci* **9**(7):971–8.

Wellington TM, Semrud-Clikeman M, Gregory AL, Murphy JM, Lancaster JL. (2006). Magnetic resonance imaging volumetric analysis of the putamen in children with ADHD: combined type versus control. *J Atten Disord* **10**(2):171–80.

Wender PH, Wolf LE, Wasserstein J. (2001). Adults with ADHD. An overview. *Ann NY Acad Sci* **931**:1–16.

Willcutt EG, Doyle AE, Nigg JT, Faraone SV, Pennington BF. (2005). Validity of the executive function theory of attention-deficit/hyperactivity disorder: a meta-analytic review. *Biol Psychiatry* **57**(11):1336–46.

Wolf RC, Plichta MM, Sambataro F, Fallgatter AJ, Jacob C, Lesch KP, et al. (2009). Regional brain activation changes and abnormal functional connectivity of the ventrolateral prefrontal cortex during working memory processing in adults with attention-deficit/hyperactivity disorder. *Hum Brain Mapp* **30**(7):2252–66.

Wolosin SM, Richardson ME, Hennessey JG, Denckla MB, Mostofsky SH. (2009). Abnormal cerebral cortex structure in children with ADHD. *Hum Brain Mapp* **30**(1):175–84.

Yang P, Wang PN, Chuang KH, Jong YJ, Chao TC, Wu MT. (2008). Absence of gender effect on children with attention-deficit/hyperactivity disorder as assessed by optimized voxel-based morphometry. *Psychiatry Res* **164**(3):245–53.

Zang YF, He Y, Zhu CZ, Cao QJ, Sui MQ, Liang M, et al. (2007). Altered baseline brain activity in children with ADHD revealed by resting-state functional MRI. *Brain Dev* **29**(2):83–91.

Zhu CZ, Zang YF, Cao QJ, Yan CG, He Y, Jiang TZ, et al. (2008). Fisher discriminative analysis of resting-state brain function for attention-deficit/hyperactivity disorder. *Neuroimage* **40**(1):110–20.

Chapter

Electrophysiological studies of adult ADHD

Gráinne McLoughlin, Jonna Kuntsi, and Philip J. Asherson

Longitudinal outcome studies indicate that the cardinal symptoms of ADHD – inattentiveness, hyperactivity, and impulsiveness – persist into adulthood in the majority of cases (Faraone & Biederman, 2005). As some symptoms of ADHD decline in severity throughout development, many individuals who fulfilled symptom criteria for ADHD as children may no longer reach full criteria for ADHD as adults, even though in many cases persistence of some symptoms continues to cause significant clinical impairments (Asherson et al., 2007). Although currently there are no specific criteria for ADHD in adults and research on adult ADHD is as yet limited, adult ADHD is increasingly being recognized as a reliable and valid diagnostic entity that shares many features with ADHD in children (Asherson, 2005). Convergent data from cognitive-experimental, neuropsychological (Boonstra et al., 2005; Hervey, Epstein, & Curry, 2004; Woods, Lovejoy, & Bush, 2002), neuroimaging, and neurochemical studies (Hesslinger et al., 2002; Seidman, Valera, & Bush, 2004; Seidman et al., 2006; Volkow et al., 2007) suggest that metabolic and structural differences associated with ADHD persist into adulthood. Similarly, investigations of adult ADHD, which use electrophysiological techniques (electroencephalography [EEG] and event-related potential [ERPs]), have indicated persistence of neurophysiological abnormalities in ADHD.

The aim of this chapter is to provide an overview of the electrophysiological findings, to date, in adult ADHD. To provide a lifespan perspective of the electrophysiology of ADHD, these findings in adults are discussed in relation to those in children. This discussion highlights where there is developmental stability in the neurophysiology and, conversely, where there is evidence of maturational changes. Electro-

physiological methods have specific advantages over both brain imaging and cognitive methodologies, and we outline them here. We also review findings from both quantitative EEG research and functional studies using ERPs in adult ADHD. Additionally, in considering another advantage of electrophysiological techniques, we discuss their usefulness in combination with genetic methodologies.

Advantages of electrophysiological techniques

Electrophysiology measures neural activation with millisecond resolution, which allows precise tracking of differential steps in information processing. This constitutes a significant advantage of these methods over behavioral and brain imaging techniques (e.g. PET, fMRI), which have a temporal resolution in the order of seconds. However, electrophysiological methods are more limited than neuroimaging techniques for localizing brain processes. This is due to the inverse problem, which means that several distinct source distributions can give rise to an observed scalp distribution recorded from the cortex. In addition, the scalp, skull, and other tissues in between the neural circuitry and the measuring electrode diffuse even localized electrical brain activity over most of the scalp. Therefore the observed activity does not always bear a direct relationship to any specific underlying brain structure. To localize the source of activity it is necessary to model and separate these sources, which is becoming increasingly accurate with high-density electrode source-modeling algorithms (Makeig et al., 1997). These advances mean that the spatial resolution in electrophysiology is less than an order of magnitude worse than in fMRI (approximately 1 cm). In addition, distributed source modeling and statistics are now

ADHD in Adults: Characterization, Diagnosis and Treatment, ed. Jan Buitelaar, Cornelis Kan and Philip Asherson.
Published by Cambridge University Press. © Cambridge University Press 2011.

available (Strik et al., 1998), and realistic models of the head for the source modeling are constructed from MRI images (e.g. Statistical Parametrical Mapping, Wellcome Department, UK), greatly enhancing the spatial localization.

Electrophysiological measures also have specific advantages over cognitive methodologies. Mental processes are not directly observable; rather, their existence and function must be inferred from the manner in which task performance changes in different contexts, involving different levels of experimental variables. Because underlying processes can be measured only indirectly, conclusions based on performance data alone may lead to the incorrect characterization of deficits. Electrophysiological parameters are ideal for the study of higher level cognitive processes, such as attention, response selection, and decision making. Sensory-cognitive information processing occurs very rapidly in the brain, so the determination of the sequence of activity in real time allows for the identification of covert information processing even in the absence of performance differences; it can also detect processes that cannot be inferred directly from performance measures alone.

Quantitative EEG studies

EEG measures brain function by analyzing the electrical activity at the scalp as generated by underlying brain structures. In quantitative EEG, multielectrode recordings are quantified in the frequency range of interest, which usually extends from about 1–70 Hz. This frequency range has traditionally been separated into five wide frequency bands, typically defined as delta (1.5–3.5 Hz), theta (3.5–7.5 Hz), alpha (7.5–12.5 Hz), beta (12.5–30 Hz), and gamma (30–70 Hz). This procedure has the advantage of being able to accurately index neural activity in the brain, both when it is engaged and when it is at rest.

The most consistent finding from EEG studies in ADHD is that children, adolescents, and adults with the disorder exhibit increased theta activity when compared with controls, particularly relative to other frequencies during the eyes-closed resting condition (Bresnahan, Anderson, & Barry, 1999; Chabot & Serfontein, 1996; Clarke et al. 2001a, 2001b, 2002a, 2002b, 2008b; Janzen et al., 1995; Koehler et al., 2009; Lazzaro et al., 1998; Mann et al., 1992; Matsuura et al., 1993). This slow-wave activity occurs in the frequency band of 3.5–7.5 cycles per second (Hz) range and is

associated with drowsiness and cortical underarousal. Decreased high-frequency beta activity (12.5–30 Hz) has also been reported in EEG studies of children, adolescents, and adults (Bresnahan et al., 1999; Bresnahan & Barry, 2002; Clarke et al. 1998, 2001b; Lazzaro et al., 1998). However, there does seem to be a shift toward normalization of beta activity in adult ADHD, in that the difference in beta power between the ADHD and control groups appears to diminish with age (Bresnahan et al., 1999, 2006; Bresnahan & Barry, 2002; Hermens et al., 2004; Koehler et al., 2009), particularly in frontal and central sites (Bresnahan et al., 1999). This normalization was tentatively suggested to be related to the reduction in hyperactive symptoms reported in adults with ADHD (Biederman, Mick, & Faraone, 2000), but this hypothesis has not been tested directly (Bresnahan et al., 1999).

A number of studies suggest increased alpha activity in adults with ADHD (Bresnahan et al., 1999; Koehler et al., 2009; Noland White, Hutchens, & Lubar, 2005), both during eyes-closed resting and task conditions, although there has been some inconsistency in this finding (Clarke et al., 2008b). An increase in alpha activity may represent a developmental effect, as findings in children indicate normal or decreased alpha activity (Barry, Clarke, & Johnstone, 2003; Callaway, Halliday, & Naylor, 1983; Clarke et al., 2001a; Dykman et al., 1982). There is inconsistency in the findings related to delta activity in adult ADHD, with two studies reporting increased activity (Bresnahan et al., 2006; Hermens et al., 2004), one reporting a reduction in activity (Clarke et al., 2008b), and another reporting no differences in delta activity between cases and controls (Koehler et al., 2009).

As the frequencies of the EEG act in concert, it has been suggested that examining frequency ratios is a better way of capturing the degree of cortical involvement (Monastra, Lubar, & Linden, 2001; Noland White et al., 2005). Because of the higher level of theta power in ADHD, the ratio of theta activity to the faster beta activity is higher in ADHD than in control groups throughout the lifespan (Bresnahan & Barry, 2002; El Sayed et al., 2002; Monastra et al., 2001). As the theta/beta ratio decreases with normal development, the higher ratio in ADHD was suggested to indicate a delay in the maturation of the central nervous system (Mann et al., 1992). Yet the persistence of the increased theta/beta ratio in adults with ADHD (Bresnahan et al., 1999; Bresnahan & Barry, 2002) suggests persistent neuronal inefficiency and cortical underarousal, rather than a maturational delay. A study investigating the theta/beta ratio in relation to performance on neuropsychological tests reported that in adults with ADHD there was an association between poorer performance on attention tasks and increased theta/beta ratios (Noland White et al., 2005). The theta/beta ratio yields sensitivity rates of 0.8–0.9 and specificity rates of 0.7–0.9 in children, adolescents, and adults with ADHD (Mann et al., 1992; Snyder & Hall, 2006); it also distinguishes adults who have ADHD from those who display some ADHD symptoms but fail to meet diagnostic criteria (Bresnahan & Barry, 2002).

Studies investigating the effects of stimulant medication in children and adolescents have found that medication decreases the slow-wave (theta) activity and increases the faster beta activity (Clarke et al., 2002a. 2002b; Loo et al., 2004). These medication-related increases in cortical activation have also been associated with improvements in behavior and cognitive function (Loo et al., 2004), although in one study there was no clear change in the EEG patterns despite an improvement in task performance (Lubar et al., 1999). An investigation of medication effects in adults found that, post medication, the EEG profiles of adults with ADHD approached those of healthy controls (Bresnahan et al., 2006). In this study, theta power failed to completely normalize, but this is similar to the findings in children with ADHD (Bresnahan et al., 2006; Clarke et al., 2002a, 2002b).

ERP studies

A useful electrophysiological technique for the investigation of brain function is the study of ERPs. ERPs are small voltage fluctuations resulting from evoked brain activity – a response evoked by a stimulus. These electrical charges represent the averaged electrical response of the brain over many trials (typically 25–100 trials) and are time-locked to repeated occurrences of sensory, cognitive, or motor events. Averaging removes the spontaneous background EEG fluctuations, which are random relative to when the event occurred. These electrical signals contain a characteristic sequence of maps, which coincide with a number of characteristic peaks and troughs and reflect only that activity that is consistently associated with event processing in a time-locked way. The ERP component thus reflects, with high-temporal resolution, the patterns of neuronal activity evoked by a stimulus.

Determination of the functional significance of the component requires simultaneous consideration of its eliciting conditions; scalp distribution (topography), which includes polarity at selected channels (P=positive and N=negative); and mean latency in milliseconds after stimulus presentation (e.g. parietal P360, P550, and so on) or order of occurrence (occipital P1, N1, P2, N2, and so on; see Fig. 6.1). The high-temporal resolution of ERP measures allows the brain activity in ADHD to be sequenced in real time.

Several theories postulate deficits in ADHD that have effects across many executive functions or on more narrowly defined aspects of executive functioning, such as response inhibition, attention, or working memory. A recent meta-analysis confirmed that children with ADHD often perform more poorly than control children on tasks measuring inhibition, vigilance, working memory, and planning (Willcutt et al., 2005). Yet, there are many possible explanations for the observed performance deficits (reviewed in Kuntsi, McLoughlin, & Asherson, 2006). In contrast to performance measures, such as speed and accuracy, which provide indirect indices of underlying processes, ERPs provide a direct, precise temporal measure of covert brain activity. This is especially true for neuronal processes occurring in the absence of overt behavior, such as preparatory and inhibitory processes. Hence ERPs can distinguish among different covert processes and elucidate whether behavioral impairments are preceded or caused by certain neuronal deficits.

One of the prominent theories of ADHD proposes that a core deficit of response inhibition processing underlies the development of broader deficits in executive function, which in turn cause the wide range of dysfunctional behaviors in ADHD (Barkley & Murphy, 2005). ERP studies have indicated that there is abnormal inhibitory processing in child and adult ADHD (Banaschewski et al., 2003, 2004; Brandeis et al., 1998; Dumaishuber & Rothenberger, 1992; Fallgatter et al., 2005; McLoughlin, Albrecht, Banaschewski, Rothenberger, et al., 2009; Perchet et al., 2001; Pliszka, Liotti, & Woldorff, 2000; van Leeuwen et al., 1998; Wiersema et al., 2006). Although a recent study failed to find any inhibitory processing problems in adult ADHD (Prox et al., 2007), this finding could be due to the small sample size of this study. When there are deficits in inhibitory processing in both adults and children, they are typically

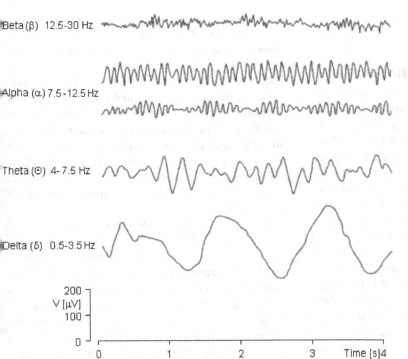

Figure 6.1 Frequency bands that have been investigated in ADHD (adapted from Malmivuo & Plonsey, 1995).

accompanied by early processing abnormalities, prior to any inhibitory processing, which suggests that ADHD is not caused by an inhibition deficit (Banaschewski et al., 2003, 2004; Brandeis et al., 1998; van Leeuwen et al., 1998).

The stop-signal task is often used in the investigation of inhibitory processing in ADHD. In this task, participants are instructed to respond to a given signal, but to inhibit their response if a stop signal, usually a tone, is presented. This requires the suppression of a response that is already in the process of being executed, and the less time that participants are given to stop the response, the harder the process becomes. An ERP study using the stop task to investigate adult ADHD reported that the auditory N1 to the stop signal, which reflects attentional orienting and occurs before response inhibition processing, was altered in adults with ADHD (Bekker, Kenemans, & Verbaten, 2004). Similarly, in the cued continuous performance task, the most consistent deficit in childhood ADHD is deficient covert attentional orienting to the cue, as indexed by the P3 (Banaschewski et al., 2003; Bekker et al., 2004; van Leeuwen et al., 1998); recently this has also been found to be abnormal in adult ADHD (McLoughlin, Albrecht, Banaschewski,

Brandeis, et al., 2009). Reduced amplitudes of the contingent negative variation (CNV) component indicate further deficits related to cognitive preparation in children and adults with ADHD (Banaschewski et al., 2004; McLoughlin, Albrecht, Banaschewski, Rothenberger, et al., 2009; Perchet et al., 2001). These abnormal preparatory states in ADHD have been interpreted as relating to posterior attentional systems (van Leeuwen et al., 1998) and suboptimal state regulation (Banaschewski et al., 2004).

The process of performance monitoring is an essential prerequisite for adaptively altering behavior and decision making and comprises error detection and conflict monitoring. Recent studies indicate that ERP correlates of performance monitoring – N2 and error negativity (Ne) – are abnormal in both childhood and adulthood ADHD, particularly in tasks that have a high level of conflict monitoring and induce a large number of errors (Albrecht et al., 2008; McLoughlin, Albrecht, Banaschewski, Brandeis, et al., 2009).

A study investigating medication effects on the P3 and the N2 in a go/no-go task did not find any differences between medicated and unmedicated ADHD adults (Ohlmeier et al., 2007). This is in contrast to previous findings in children with ADHD (Seifert et al.,

2003) and to medication-related changes seen in the EEGs of adults with ADHD (Bresnahan et al., 2006).

Inter- and intrahemispheric transfer

The coherence of EEG activity between two sites is conceptualized as the correlation in the frequency domain between two EEG time points measured simultaneously at different scalp locations (Shaw, 1981) and provides information about the consistency in brain activity between two sites. EEG coherence can be regarded as an index for both structural and functional brain characteristics; in other words, how different parts of the brain relate during different tasks (French & Beaumont, 1984). An early study of hyperkinetic disorder found that interhemispheric coherences were slightly reduced in hyperkinetic children, whereas intrahemispheric coherences were slightly elevated (Montagu, 1975). More recent studies have indicated that both intra- and interhemispheric coherence are elevated in ADHD but predominantly in the frontal areas of the brain (Barry et al., 2002; Chabot et al., 1999) and, in particular, relates to slow-wave (delta and theta) activity (Barry et al., 2002). As such, ADHD in children appears to be associated with reduced cortical differentiation and specialization, particularly in circuits involving slow-wave activity.

A recent study that investigated interhemispheric coherences in adult with ADHD suggested that the abnormalities in theta coherence normalize with development, with the main differences related to alpha activity (Clarke et al., 2008a). This finding is reflected in the childhood literature (Barry et al., 2002). Another study, which investigated interhemispheric transfer using ERPs in adults, found that participants diagnosed with combined-type ADHD exhibited faster transfer from left to right, whereas those who had inattentive subtype demonstrated slower right-to-left hemisphere transfer (Rolfe, Kirk, & Waldie, 2007). This preliminary finding suggests that abnormal interhemispheric transfer is a core abnormality of ADHD throughout the life span and that discrepancies between the findings may be due to differences between the ADHD subtypes.

Electrophysiological parameters as endophenotypes

Given its high heritability (60–90%; Faraone et al., 2005), ADHD has been the focus of numerous molecu-

lar genetic investigations, and several candidate genes have been linked to ADHD (Thapar et al., 2007). However, the identification of candidate genes has been impeded by ADHD's etiological complexity (Asherson, 2004), because the causal pathway is likely to involve the incremental contribution of many genes of small effect size, which may interact and correlate with the environment in complex ways. In consideration of these complexities, there has been much recent interest, in genetic research on psychiatric disorders, in heritable intermediate phenotypes between genetic risk factors and measurable behavior/diagnosis known as "endophenotypes."

Electrophysiological indices are ideal for endophenotype research for several reasons. As outlined in this chapter, they elicit striking group differences, which are developmentally stable and reliable (Fallgatter et al., 2001, 2002). In addition, the collection of these data is cost efficient, enabling the recruitment of larger numbers of participants, which is essential for adequate power to detect genes of small effect size. A third important advantage is that these indices are highly heritable. Heritability estimates for EEG power in all frequency bands range from 79–89% (van Beijsterveldt et al., 1996; Zietsch et al., 2007) and for interhemispheric transfer of EEG activity are approximately 50% for frontal sites (Chorlian et al., 2007). Further, adult twin studies showed that approximately 50% of the variance in components associated with inhibition and error monitoring – the N2, P3, and Ne, which are developmentally stable deficits in ADHD (McLoughlin, Albrecht, Banaschewski, Brandeis, et al., 2009; McLoughlin, Albrecht, Banaschewski, Rothenberger, et al., 2009) – can be attributed to genetic factors, suggesting that these parameters may potentially serve as endophenotypes (Anokhin, Golosheykin, & Heath, 2008; Anokhin, Heath, & Myers, 2004). Further, a recent study indicated that the Ne shares familial effects with ADHD (McLoughlin, Albrecht, Banaschewski, Brandeis, et al., 2009). These promising findings warrant further study, including investigation of possible associations of electrophysiological parameters with genes implicated in ADHD.

Conclusions

Collectively, the EEG and ERP findings in children, adolescents, and adults with ADHD suggest that electrophysiological indices represent underlying processes that are developmentally stable. In particular, there is evidence for persistence of increased theta activity across frontal regions and for an increased ratio of this slow-wave activity compared to the faster beta activity throughout the lifespan. Electrophysiological assessments enable measurement of covert processes, and the superior temporal resolution enables precise tracking of different steps in information processing, which is critical for ADHD theory. The functional ERP findings indicate that patterns of abnormal processing, firmly established in childhood ADHD, persist in adult ADHD, particularly preparatory and inhibitory processes. These findings provide external validation of the ADHD diagnosis in adults, which is becoming increasingly recognized as a common psychiatric disorder in adulthood (Asherson, 2005; Nutt et al., 2007). Given these findings that indicate electrophysiological parameters as developmentally stable and heritable indices of brain function, they may be particularly useful in studies that aim to further our understanding of the processes that mediate genetic influences on the behaviors associated with ADHD.

Acknowledgments

The authors thank Tobias Banaschewski and Daniel Brandeis for their earlier expert advice on ERP research in ADHD, which has also benefited this review.

References

Albrecht B, Brandeis D, Uebel H, Heinrich H, Mueller UC, Hasselhorn M, et al. (2008). Action monitoring in boys with attention-deficit/hyperactivity disorder, their nonaffected siblings, and normal control subjects: evidence for an endophenotype. *Biol Psychiatry* 64(7):615–25.

Anokhin AP, Golosheykin S, Heath AC. (2008). Heritability of frontal brain function related to action monitoring. *Psychophysiology* 45:524–34.

Anokhin AP, Heath AC, Myers E. (2004). Genetics, prefrontal cortex, and cognitive control: a twin study of event-related brain potentials in a response inhibition task. *Neurosci Lett* 368:314–8.

Asherson P. (2004). Attention-Deficit Hyperactivity Disorder in the post-genomic era. *Eur Child Adolesc Psychiatry* 13(suppl 1):I50–70.

Asherson P. (2005). Clinical assessment and treatment of attention deficit hyperactivity disorder in adults. *Expert Rev Neurother* 5:525–39.

Asherson P, Chen W, Craddock B, Taylor E. (2007). Adult attention-deficit hyperactivity disorder: recognition and treatment in general adult psychiatry. *Br J Psychiatry* 190:4–5.

Banaschewski T, Brandeis D, Heinrich H, Albrecht B, Brunner E, Rothenberger A. (2003). Association of ADHD and conduct disorder–brain electrical evidence for the existence of a distinct subtype. *J Child Psychol Psychiatry* 44:356–76.

Banaschewski T, Brandeis D, Heinrich H, Albrecht B, Brunner E, Rothenberger A. (2004). Questioning inhibitory control as the specific deficit of ADHD–evidence from brain electrical activity. *J Neural Transm* 111:841–64.

Barkley R, Murphy KR. (2005). *Attention-Deficit Hyperactivity Disorder: A Clinical Workbook*. New York: Guilford.

Barry RJ, Clarke AR, Johnstone SJ. (2003). A review of electrophysiology in attention-deficit/hyperactivity disorder: I. Qualitative and quantitative electroencephalography. *Clin Neurophysiol* 114: 171–83.

Barry RJ, Clarke AR, McCarthy R, Selikowitz M. (2002). EEG coherence in attention-deficit/hyperactivity disorder: a comparative study of two DSM-IV types. *Clin Neurophysiol* 113:579–85.

Bekker EM, Kenemans JL, Verbaten MN. (2004). Electrophysiological correlates of attention, inhibition, sensitivity and bias in a continuous performance task. *Clin. Neurophysiol* 115:2001–13.

Biederman J, Mick E, Faraone SV. (2000). Age-dependent decline of symptoms of attention deficit hyperactivity disorder: impact of remission definition and symptom type. *Am J Psychiatry* 157:816–18.

Boonstra AM, Oosterlaan J, Sergeant JA, Buitelaar JK. (2005). Executive functioning in adult ADHD: a meta-analytic review. *Psychol Med* 35:1097–1108.

Brandeis D, van Leeuwen TH, Rubia K, Vitacco D, Steger J, Pascual-Marqui RD, Steinhausen HC. (1998). Neuroelectric mapping reveals precursor of stop failures in children with attention deficits. *Behav Brain Res* 94:111–25.

Bresnahan SM, Anderson JW, Barry RJ. (1999). Age-related changes in quantitative EEG in attention-deficit/hyperactivity disorder. *Biol Psychiatry* 46:1690–7.

Bresnahan SM, Barry RJ. (2002). Specificity of quantitative EEG analysis in adults with attention deficit hyperactivity disorder. *Psychiatry Res* 112:133–44.

Bresnahan SM, Barry RJ, Clarke AR, Johnstone SJ. (2006). Quantitative EEG analysis in dexamphetamine-responsive adults with attention-deficit/hyperactivity disorder. *Psychiatry Res* 141:151–9.

Callaway E, Halliday R, Naylor H. (1983). Hyperactive children's event-related potentials fail to support underarousal and maturational-lag theories. *Arch Gen Psychiatry* 40:1243–8.

Chabot RJ, Orgill AA, Crawford G, Harris MJ, Serfontein G. (1999). Behavioral and electrophysiologic predictors of treatment response to stimulants in children with attention disorders. *J Child Neurol* 14:343–51.

Chabot RJ, Serfontein G. (1996). Quantitative electroencephalographic profiles of children with attention deficit disorder. *Biol Psychiatry* 40:951–63.

Chorlian DB, Tang, Y, Rangaswamy M, O'Connor S, Rohrbaugh J, Taylor R, Porjesz B. (2007). Heritability of EEG coherence in a large sib-pair population. *Biol Psychol* 75:260–6.

Clarke AR, Barry RJ, Bond D, McCarthy R, Selikowitz M. (2002a). Effects of stimulant medications on the EEG of children with attention-deficit/hyperactivity disorder. *Psychopharmacology (Berl)* 164:277–84.

Clarke AR, Barry RJ, Bond D, McCarthy R, Selikowitz M. (2002b). EEG analysis of children with attention-deficit/hyperactivity disorder and comorbid reading disabilities. *J Learn Disabil* 35:276–85.

Clarke AR, Barry RJ, Heaven PC, McCarthy R, Selikowitz M, Byrne MK. (2008a). EEG coherence in adults with attention-deficit/hyperactivity disorder. *Int J Psychophysiol* 67:35–40.

Clarke AR, Barry RJ, Heaven PC, McCarthy R, Selikowitz M, Byrne MK. (2008b). EEG in adults with attention-deficit/hyperactivity disorder. *Int J Psychophysiol* 70:176–83.

Clarke AR, Barry RJ, McCarthy R, Selikowitz M. (1998). EEG analysis in Attention-Deficit/Hyperactivity Disorder: a comparative study of two subtypes. *Psychiatry Res* 81:19–29.

Clarke AR, Barry RJ, McCarthy R, Selikowitz M. (2001a). EEG-defined subtypes of children with attention-deficit/hyperactivity disorder. *Clin Neurophysiol* 112:2098–105.

Clarke AR, Barry RJ, McCarthy R, Selikowitz M. (2001b). Electroencephalogram differences in two subtypes of attention-deficit/hyperactivity disorder. *Psychophysiology* 38:212–21.

Dumaishuber C, Rothenberger A. (1992). Psychophysiological correlates of orienting, anticipation and contingency changes in children with psychiatric-disorders. *J Psychophysiol*, 225–39.

Dykman RA, Holcomb PJ, Oglesby DM, Ackerman PT. (1982). Electrocortical frequencies in hyperactive, learning-disabled, mixed, and normal children. *Biol Psychiatry* 17:675–85.

El Sayed E, Larsson JO, Persson HE, Rydelius PA. (2002). Altered cortical activity in children with attention-deficit/hyperactivity disorder during attentional load task. *J. Am Acad Child Adolesc Psychiatry* 41:811–19.

Fallgatter AJ, Aranda DR, Bartsch AJ, Herrmann MJ. (2002). Long-term reliability of electrophysiologic response control parameters. *J Clin Neurophysiol* 19:61–6.

Fallgatter AJ, Bartsch AJ, Strik WK, Mueller TJ, Eisenack SS, Neuhauser B, et al. (2001). Test-retest reliability of electrophysiological parameters related to cognitive motor control. *Clin Neurophysiol* 112:198–204.

Fallgatter AJ, Ehlis AC, Rosler M, Strik WK, Blocher D, Herrmann MJ. (2005). Diminished prefrontal brain function in adults with psychopathology in childhood related to attention deficit hyperactivity disorder. *Psychiatry Res* 138:157–69.

Faraone SV, Biederman J. (2005). What is the prevalence of adult ADHD? Results of a population screen of 966 adults. *J Atten Disord* 9:384–91.

Faraone SV, Perlis RH, Doyle AE, Smoller JW, Goralnick JJ, Holmgren MA, Sklar P. (2005). Molecular genetics of attention-deficit/hyperactivity disorder. *Biol Psychiatry* 57:1313–23.

French CC, Beaumont JG. (1984). A critical review of EEG coherence studies of hemisphere function. *Int J Psychophysiol* 1:241–54.

Hermens DF, Williams LM, Lazzaro I, Whitmont S, Melkonian D, Gordon E. (2004). Sex differences in adult ADHD: a double dissociation in brain activity and autonomic arousal. *Biol Psychol* 66:221–33.

Hervey AS, Epstein JN, Curry JF. (2004). Neuropsychology of adults with attention-deficit/hyperactivity disorder: a meta-analytic review. *Neuropsychology* 18:485–503.

Hesslinger B, Tebartz VE, Thiel T, Haegele K, Hennig J, Ebert D. (2002). Frontoorbital volume reductions in adult patients with attention deficit hyperactivity disorder. *Neurosci Lett* 328:319–21.

Janzen T, Graap K, Stephanson S, Marshall W, Fitzsimmons G. (1995). Differences in baseline EEG measures for ADD and normally achieving preadolescent males. *Biofeedback Self Regul* 20:65–82.

Koehler S, Lauer P, Schreppel T, Jacob C, Heine M, Boreatti-Hummer A, et al. (2009). Increased EEG power density in alpha and theta bands in adult ADHD patients. *J Neural Transm* 116:97–104.

Kuntsi J, McLoughlin G, Asherson P. (2006). Attention deficit hyperactivity disorder. *Neuromolecular Med* 8:461–84.

Lazzaro I, Gordon E, Whitmont S, Plahn M, Li W, Clarke S, et al. (1998). Quantified EEG activity in adolescent attention deficit hyperactivity disorder. *Clin Electroencephalogr* 29:37–42.

Loo SK, Hopfer C, Teale PD, Reite ML. (2004). EEG correlates of methylphenidate response in ADHD: association with cognitive and behavioral measures. *J Clin Neurophysiol* 21:457–64.

Lubar JF, White JN, Jr, Swartwood MO, Swartwood JN. (1999). Methylphenidate effects on global and complex measures of EEG. *Pediatr Neurol* 21:633–7.

Makeig S, Jung TP, Bell AJ, Ghahremani D, Sejnowski TJ. (1997). Blind separation of auditory event-related brain responses into independent components. *Proc Natl Acad Sci USA* 94:10979–84.

Malmivuo, J, Plonsey R. (1995). *Bioelectromagnetism*. New York: Oxford University Press.

Mann CA, Lubar JF, Zimmerman AW, Miller CA, Muenchen RA. (1992). Quantitative analysis of EEG in boys with attention-deficit-hyperactivity disorder: controlled study with clinical implications. *Pediatr Neurol* 8:30–6.

Matsuura M, Okubo Y, Toru M, Kojima T, He Y, Hou Y, et al. (1993). A cross-national EEG study of children with emotional and behavioral problems: a WHO collaborative study in the Western Pacific Region. *Biol Psychiatry* 34:59–65.

McLoughlin G, Albrecht B, Banaschewski T, Brandeis D, Kuntsi J, Asherson P. (2009). Error processing and conflict monitoring show evidence of familiality in adult ADHD. *Neuropsychologia* 47(14):3134–42.

McLoughlin G, Albrecht B, Banaschewski T, Rothenberger A, Brandeis D, Kuntsi J. (under review). Electrophysiological evidence for abnormal preparatory states and inhibitory processing in adult ADHD. *Behavioral and Brain Functions.*

Monastra VJ, Lubar JF, Linden M. (2001). The development of a quantitative electroencephalographic scanning process for attention deficit-hyperactivity disorder: reliability and validity studies. *Neuropsychology* 15:136–44.

Montagu JD. (1975). Hyperkinetic child – behavioral, electrodermal and EEG investigation. *Dev Med Child Neurol* 17:299–305.

Noland White J, Hutchens TA, Lubar JF. (2005). Quantitative EEG assessment during neuropsychological task performance in adults with attention deficit hyperactivity disorder. *J Adult Dev* 12:113–21.

Nutt DJ, Fone K, Asherson P, Bramble D, Hill P, Matthews K, et al. (2007). Evidence-based guidelines for management of attention-deficit/hyperactivity disorder in adolescents in transition to adult services and in adults: recommendations from the British Association for Psychopharmacology. *J Psychopharmacol* 21: 10–41.

Ohlmeier MD, Prox V, Zhang Y, Zedler M, Ziegenbein M, Emrich HM, Dietrich DE. (2007). Effects of methylphenidate in ADHD adults on target evaluation processing reflected by event-related potentials. *Neurosci Lett* 424:149–54.

Perchet C, Revol O, Fourneret P, Mauguiere F, Garcia-Larrea L. (2001). Attention shifts and anticipatory mechanisms in hyperactive children: an ERP study using the Posner paradigm. *Biol Psychiatry* 50(1):44–57.

Pliszka SR, Liotti M, Woldorff MG. (2000). Inhibitory control in children with attention-deficit/hyperactivity disorder: event-related potentials identify the processing component and timing of an impaired right-frontal response-inhibition mechanism. *Biol. Psychiatry* 48:238–46.

Prox V, Dietrich DE, Zhang Y, Emrich HM, Ohlmeier MD. (2007). Attentional processing in adults with ADHD as reflected by event-related potentials. *Neurosci Lett* 419:236–41.

Rolfe MH, Kirk IJ, Waldie KE. (2007). Interhemispheric callosal transfer in adults with attention-deficit/hyperactivity disorder: an event-related potential study. *Neuroreport* 18:255–59.

Seidman LJ, Valera EM, Bush G. (2004). Brain function and structure in adults with attention-deficit/hyperactivity disorder. *Psychiatr Clin North Am* 27:323–47.

Seidman LJ, Valera EM, Makris N, Monuteaux MC, Boriel DL, Kelkar K, et al. (2006). Dorsolateral prefrontal and anterior cingulate cortex volumetric abnormalities in adults with attention-deficit/hyperactivity disorder identified by magnetic resonance imaging. *Biol Psychiatry* 60:1071–80.

Seifert J, Scheuerpflug P, Zillessen KE, Fallgatter A, Warnke A. (2003). Electrophysiological investigation of the effectiveness of methylphenidate in children with and without ADHD. *J Neural Transm* 110:821–9.

Shaw JC. (1981). An introduction to the coherence function and its use in EEG signal analysis. *J Med Eng Technol* 5:279–88.

Snyder SM, Hall JR. (2006). A meta-analysis of quantitative EEG power associated with attention-deficit hyperactivity disorder. *J Clin Neurophysiol* 23: 440–55.

Strik WK, Fallgatter AJ, Brandeis D, Pascual-Marqui RD. (1998). Three-dimensional tomography of event-related potentials during response inhibition: evidence for phasic frontal lobe activation. *Electroencephalogr Clin Neurophysiol* 108:406–13.

Thapar A, Langley K, Owen MJ, O'Donovan MC. (2007). Advances in genetic findings on attention deficit hyperactivity disorder. *Psychol Med* 37:1681–92.

van Beijsterveldt CE, Molenaar PC, de Geus EJ, Boomsma DI. (1996). Heritability of human brain functioning as assessed by electroencephalography. *Am J Hum Genet* 58:562–73.

van Leeuwen TH, Steinhausen HC, Overtoom CC, Pascual-Marqui RD, van't Klooster B, Rothenberger A, et al. (1998). The continuous performance test revisited with neuroelectric mapping: impaired orienting in children with attention deficits. *Behav Brain Res* 94:97–110.

Volkow ND, Wang GJ, Newcorn J, Telang F, Solanto MV, Fowler JS, et al. (2007). Depressed dopamine activity in caudate and preliminary evidence of limbic involvement in adults with attention-deficit/hyperactivity disorder. *Arch Gen Psychiatry* 64:932–40.

Wiersema R, Van Der MJ, Antrop I, Roeyers H. (2006). State regulation in adult ADHD: an event-related potential study. *J Clin Exp Neuropsychol* 28:1113–26.

Willcutt EG, Doyle AE, Nigg JT, Faraone SV, Pennington BF. (2005). Validity of the executive function theory of attention-deficit/hyperactivity disorder: a meta-analytic review. *Biol Psychiatry* 57:1336–46.

Woods SP, Lovejoy DW, Ball JD. (2002). Neuropsychological characteristics of adults with ADHD: a comprehensive review of initial studies. *Clin Neuropsychol* 16:12–34.

Zietsch BP, Hansen JL, Hansell NK, Geffen GM, Martin NG, Wright MJ. (2007). Common and specific genetic influences on EEG power bands delta, theta, alpha, and beta. *Biol Psychol* 75:154–64.

Chapter

7

Emission tomography in adult ADHD

Mitul A. Mehta and Johanna Krause

The primary pharmacological treatments for ADHD in both children and adults are thought to exert their efficacy by increasing the levels of catecholamines in the brain. This mode of action suggests a pathophysiological substrate within the dopaminergic or noradrenergic systems or an abnormality in brain regions that can be ameliorated via altered catecholaminergic transmission. The undoubted success of the psychomotor stimulant drugs has driven a vast literature on the pharmacological treatment of ADHD. However, the presence of a primary abnormality within the catecholamine system in patients with ADHD is far from confirmed, with studies to date providing, at best, an incomplete picture of possible neuroreceptor differences. In addition, the relatively recent introduction of novel pharmacological treatments such as modafinil for which the mechanism of action is not understood leaves open the possibility of a final common pathway for treatment efficacy, while simultaneously broadening targets for novel treatments and unexplored pathophysiology.

Neuroimaging allows the study in vivo of neurotransmitter receptor densities, endogenous neurotransmitter release, and drug occupancy of particular receptor targets. The two techniques that have been used are single photon emission computed tomography (SPECT) and positron emission tomography (PET). These techniques provide exquisite sensitivity to delineate different aspects of brain neurophysiology, but are also limited. The principal limitation in the use of emission tomography is the need for radioisotopes, which restricts the number of investigations per individual. It is nonetheless more acceptable to use these techniques in adults than in children and adolescents.

The general consensus that ADHD symptomatology and the associated diagnosis sometimes persist into adulthood opens up the study of the neurobiology

of ADHD through emission tomography. This chapter reviews emission tomography studies in ADHD that address the neurobiology of this disorder and treatment effects; it also examines the potential for these imaging techniques to help undercover possible mechanisms underlying the behavioral and cognitive changes that follow treatment (a summary of the studies in adults is provided in Table 7.1).

Single photon emission computed tomography

SPECT has been used to measure brain perfusion (regional cerebral blood flow) and receptor densities in ADHD. It uses single photon (gamma) emitters "attached" to biological molecules and relies on measuring the line of response for each registered event. The measurement of direction is partially forced by using lead collimators, which results in a reduction in sensitivity because of a reduction in the number of photons detected. The main advantages of SPECT are the availability of cameras and radionuclides, which can even be bought commercially due to their long half-lives. The need to use labels that are uncommon in human tissue such as Technetium-99 (Tc-99m) can be seen as a disadvantage of SPECT because they have potential differences in metabolism compared to the native molecule, and these differences may have an impact on interpretation. The use of carbon-11 ligands allows the theoretical possibility of radiolabeling any biological molecule. Such radioligands are suitable for positron emission tomography.

Positron emission tomography

PET has been used to measure perfusion and dopaminergic markers in ADHD. Like SPECT, PET is

ADHD in Adults: Characterization, Diagnosis and Treatment, ed. Jan Buitelaar, Cornelis Kan and Philip Asherson.
Published by Cambridge University Press. © Cambridge University Press 2011.

Table 7.1 ADHD

Study/category	Design	Age	Method and radiotracer	Result	Comments
Cerebral glucose metabolism					
Zametkin et al. 1990	25 ADHD, 18m 50 Cont, 28m Auditory CPT	ADHD: 37.4 Cont: 36.3	FDG-PET	↓ global metabolism ↓ regional metabolism (after correction for global changes) in 4/60 regions	
Ernst et al. 1998	39 ADHD, 24m 56 Cont, 26m Auditory CPT	ADHD: 35.2 Cont: 28.6	FDG-PET	↓ global metabolism in ADHD females	Controls younger than ADHD
Blood flow					
Schweitzer et al. 2000	6 ADHD, m 6 Cont, m Working memory addition task	ADHD: 28.5 Cont: 25.7	H2O-PET	ADHD: Activation of precuneus, inferior parietal lobe Cont: Activation of superior temporal gyrus and lateral frontal gyrus	No direct comparison between groups
Schweitzer et al. 2003	10 ADHD, m Resting state scans at baseline and after 3 weeks optimization of methylphenidate dose.	ADHD: 31.5	H2O-PET	↑ cerebellum ↓ precentral gyrus, left caudate nucleus Highest symptom scores, smallest reductions in rCBF in midbrain and cerebellum	
Ernst et al. 2003	10 ADHD, m 12 Cont, 6m Decision-making task	ADHD: 28.8 Cont: 29.9	H2O-PET	ADHD: ↑ activation in anterior cingulate, post central gyrus, and superior temporal gyrus and ↓ insula, hippocampus, inferior temporal, and fusiform gyri	
Schweitzer et al. 2004	10 ADHD, m 11 Cont, m Auditory addition task at baseline and after methylphenidate (patients only)	ADHD: 31.5 Cont: 29.2	H2O-PET	Unmedicated patients: ↓ activation in several cortical regions and ↑ activation in largely subcortical regions. Methylphenidate: ↓ activation in medial and middle frontal gyrus and ↑ activation in thalamus and precentral gyrus	Same patients as (25)
O'Gorman et al.	9 ADHD, m 11 Cont, m Resting state perfusion on and off medication (patients only)	ADHD: 30 Cont: 30	ASL-MRI*	Unmedicated patients: ↑ perfusion in left caudate, frontal and parietal gray and white matter Medication: ↓ (normalized) perfusion in left caudate. ↓ perfusion in parahippocampal gyrus and regions of inferior frontal and parietal gray matter	
Dopamine synthesis					
Ernst et al. 1998	17 ADHD, 8m 23 Cont, 13m	ADHD: 39.3 Cont: 33.7	[18F]DOPA PET	↓ FDOPA uptake in medial and left prefrontal cortex (50%); lower uptake in left prefrontal cortex related to higher scores on retrospective rating scale for childhood ADHD	

Table 7.1 (*cont.*)

Study/category	Design	Age	Method and radiotracer	Result	Comments
Ludolph et al. (2008)	20 ADHD, m 18 Cont, m 8 patients never treated	ADHD untreated: 21.3 ADHD treated: 19.9 Cont: 22.2	[^{18}F]DOPA PET	↓ FDOPA uptake in putamen, amygdala, and dorsal midbrain in both groups of patients and brainstem in treated ↑ FDOPA uptake in anterior cingulate in both groups and insula/amygdala in untreated ↓ Anterior cingulate, putamen, amygdala, and insula in treated vs. untreated	
Dopamine transporter					
Dougherty et al. 1999	6 ADHD, 2m 30 Cont (database)	ADHD: 41.33 Cont: 21–60	[^{123}I]altropane SPECT	↑ Striatal DAT 70% in ADHD	
Dresel et al. 2000	17 ADHD, 7m 14 Cont, 8m	ADHD: 38 Cont: 37	[^{99m}Tc]TRODAT SPECT	↑ Striatal DAT 17%	
Krause et al. 2000	10 ADHD, 3m 10 Cont, 3m	ADHD: 21–63 Cont: 22–63	[^{99m}Tc]TRODAT SPECT	↑ Striatal DAT 16%	
Krause et al. 2002	11 ADHD smokers, 8m 11 ADHD, nonsmokers, 8m All patients unmedicated	ADHD: 32.6 Cont: 34.5	[^{99m}Tc]TRODAT SPECT	↑ Striatal DAT in nonsmokers	
Van Dyck et al. 2002	9 ADHD, 6m 9 Cont, 6m	ADHD: 41 Cont: 41	[^{123}I]β-CIT SPECT	↔ Striatal DAT	
Larisch et al. 2006 (70)	20 ADHD, 11m 20 Cont, 9m	ADHD: 35 Cont: 32	[^{123}I]FP-CIT SPECT	↑ Striatal DAT 5%	
Hesse et al. 2006	17 ADHD, 7m 14 Cont, 5m	ADHD: 31 Cont: 32	[^{123}I]FP-CIT SPECT	↓ Striatal DAT 23%	Partial analysis of Hesse et al. 2009
La Fougere et al. 2006	16 ADHD treatment responders: 7m 6 ADHD treatment nonresponders: 4m	ADHD responders: 37.8 ADHD nonresponders: 44.2	[^{99m}Tc]TRODAT SPECT	17/22 ADHD ↑ Striatal DAT 24% 16 of these were responders 5/22 ADHD ↓ Striatal DAT 14% All of these were nonresponders	
Spencer et al. 2007	21 ADHD, 14m 26 Cont, 11m	ADHD: 34.4 Cont: 27.4	[^{123}I]altropane SPECT	↔ Striatal DAT uncorrected for age ↑ Right caudate DAT 15% after age correction	Controls younger than ADHD
Volkow et al. 2007	20 ADHD, 10m 25 Cont, 19m All patients unmedicated	ADHD: 32 Cont: 31	[^{11}C]cocaine PET	↓ Left caudate DAT 13% ↓ Left accumbens DAT 60% Putamen DAT positively correlated with attention scores for both groups	
Hesse et al. 2009	17 ADHD, 8m 14 Cont, 8m All patients treatment naive	ADHD: 32 Cont: 32	[^{123}I]FP-CIT SPECT	↓ Striatal DAT ~19% right, ~18% left	

(*cont.*)

Table 7.1 (cont.)

Study/category	Design	Age	Method and radiotracer	Result	Comments
Volkow et al. 2009	53 ADHD, 27m 44 Cont, 30m All patients unmedicated	ADHD: 32 Cont: 31	[^{11}C]cocaine	↓ Caudate DAT 20% ↓ Accumbens DAT 11% ↓ Midbrain DAT 44% Midbrain DAT correlated with attention scores for both groups combined	Includes sample from Volkow et al. 2007
Dopamine receptors and release					
Volkow et al. 2007	19 ADHD, 9m 24 Cont, 18m All patients unmedicated Scanned after placebo and methylphenidate injection	ADHD: 32 Cont: 30	[^{11}C]raclopride PET	↓ Left caudate D2 8.5% ↓ dopamine release in ADHD in left and right caudate Exploratory analysis showed reduced extent of dopamine release in hippocampus and amygdala in ADHD Lower dopamine release in ADHD predicted by lower baseline attention scores	
Volkow et al. 2009	53 ADHD, 27m 44 Cont, 30m All patients unmedicated	ADHD: 32 Cont: 31	[^{11}C]raclopride	↓ Caudate D2 12% ↓ Accumbens D2 6% ↓ Midbrain D2 36% ↓ Hypothalamic D2 67% Left regions correlated with attention scores for both groups combined	

↓ ↔ ↑ Decreased, unchanged, or increased compared to comparison group.
* The novel technique of ASL-MRI has the potential to replace SPECT and PET perfusion, allowing for completely noninvasive investigations.

an imaging tool that uses noninvasive measurements of radioactive decay to index aspects of regional tissue function in vivo. PET is based on the annihilation of positrons (together with an electron), which results in the simultaneous release of two gamma rays in opposite directions. An array of gamma cameras use coincidence detection to define a series of lines of response that are used to reconstruct the PET image. The ability to label molecules with carbon-11, nitrogen-13, oxygen-15, and fluorine-18 (which can be used as a hydrogen substitute) affords PET a degree of flexibility that allows the measurement of various neurobiological parameters such as perfusion, blood volume, glucose metabolism, receptor density, neurotransmitter release, and drug uptake and occupancy.

Perfusion and metabolism in ADHD

The dominant neuroimaging techniques currently in use for understanding functional dysregulation in ADHD are functional magnetic resonance imaging (fMRI; see Chapter 5) and electroencephalography (EEG; see Chapter 6). Cognitive activation paradigms can be defined to a higher degree of temporal resolution with both these methods compared to PET and SPECT, although at the time of the earliest studies of *regional* changes in blood flow and metabolism, fMRI was not yet developed.

Cerebral metabolism as measured using fluorodeoxyglucose-positron emission tomography (FDG-PET) was initially used in adults with ADHD (Zametkin et al., 1990). This early study found a reduction in global cerebral metabolism of about 8% in a group of 25 patients with a mean age of 37. After correction for global metabolism, reductions remained in four regions, with no differences observed between the 18 males and 7 females. During the scans the patients and 50 controls performed a continuous performance task. In a series of follow-up investigations, reductions in global cerebral glucose metabolism were predominantly found in adolescent girls or women with ADHD, with some regional differences (Ernst, Liebenauer, et al., 1994; Ernst, Zametkin, Phillips, et al., 1998; Zametkin et al., 1993).

These already complex results from FDG-PET studies are further complicated by the effects of treatment with methylphenidate or amphetamine. No changes in global metabolism were observed after acute or chronic treatment in three studies of adults with ADHD, approximately two-thirds of whom were male (Ernst, Zametkin, et al., 1994; Matochik et al., 1993, 1994). After chronic treatment (6–15 weeks, fixed-order design) amphetamine produced no regional changes in glucose metabolism (i.e. after correction for global metabolism), whereas methylphenidate was associated with reduced regional metabolism in the right anterior putamen and increases in posterior frontal areas. For the two single-dose studies different sets of local increases and decreases were observed. As with the studies comparing controls to patients, continuous performance tasks were performed during the scanning sessions.

The standardization of a cognitive-behavioral state rather than an unspecified "resting" state (Raichle, 2006) can produce a large reduction in within- and between-subject variability (60–70%) as compared to scans acquired in the resting state (Deutsch et al., 1997; Duara et al., 1987). As such, the choice of the continuous performance tasks, although potentially improving the sensitivity of steady-state studies using FDG-PET or perfusion imaging (see later), may also influence the findings, because such tasks produce small but significant changes in regional cerebral perfusion (e.g. Coull, 1998). For studies in which only one measurement is taken the use of a task state may be advantageous, but the degree to which the findings would differ if a different state such as a resting state or a different task was used is not known.

Perfusion imaging measures regional cerebral blood flow, which correlates with metabolic measurements, even in the presence of dopaminergic agonists (McCullogh, Kelly, & Ford, 1982). The first, landmark studies of Lou and colleagues (1984, 1989, 1990, 1998) used Xenon-133 SPECT and acquired perfusion information from a single 17-mm slice that included the basal ganglia in overlapping groups of children aged 6–15. The cognitive state of patients and controls ranged from rest to passive listening and object naming/detection. The analyses ranged from qualitative descriptions to formal statistical testing (uncorrected for multiple comparison testing across the brain regions). The most consistent finding from these studies was reduced perfusion in the striatum, which was increased by methylphenidate in a sub-

group of children scanned on and off treatment. Subsequent studies using I-123, 99 Tc-ethylcysteinate, and 99 Tc-HMPAO SPECT, all in children and adolescents, showed reduced perfusion in frontal and temporal regions (Amen, 1997; Kaya et al., 2002; Kim et al., 2002; Lorberboym et al., 2004; Sieg et al., 1995). Increases in perfusion were also seen in posterior parietal lobe regions (Kim et al., 2002; Oner et al., 2005), the dorsal anterior cingulate, and motor and premotor cortices (Langleben et al., 2002).

Many of these SPECT studies have been criticized for including a heterogeneous mix of patients with comorbidities, having poor control groups (e.g. including patients with epilepsy) or no control groups, and using qualitative or semi-quantitative analysis techniques (Castellanos, 2002). The requirement to administer radiolabeled tracers explains some of the difficulties in obtaining adequate control groups of children in these studies. The comparison of groups of patients differing in treatment (Schweitzer et al., 2003; Szobot et al., 2003) or genotype (Szobot et al., 2005) obviates some of these difficulties, although studies in adults will allow greater flexibility here.

The effects of treatment with methylphenidate were tested in three studies in addition to those from Lou and colleagues. These studies demonstrated (1) increased perfusion in the frontal cortex, caudate nucleus, thalamus, and temporal lobe (Kim et al., 2001) in a group of 32 male patients aged 7–14 tested before and after treatment; (2) reduced perfusion in the left posterior parietal lobe in a group of 19 patients (age 11.5) on treatment compared to 17 patients matched for age on placebo (Szobot et al., 2003); and (3) decreased perfusion in the precentral gyrus and left caudate nucleus and cerebellar increases in perfusion (Schweitzer et al., 2003). This last study is one of only three reports in adults with ADHD that used PET blood flow imaging with patients in the resting state.

In the study of regional cerebral blood flow in adults with ADHD just mentioned (Schweitzer et al., 2003), 10 patients were scanned twice: once at baseline and once at their optimal treatment dose (selected from 0.5, 0.75, or 1.0 mg/kg/day over a number of weeks). One hour after ingestion of methylphenidate, two $H_2{}^{15}O$ scans were performed 60 minutes apart. Each scan lasted 90 seconds. With the exception of one patient all methylphenidate scans were performed after a baseline scan, and patients were not blind to treatment (no placebo arm is reported). The decreases

79

and increases in blood flow reported in the pre-central gyrus, caudate nucleus, and cerebellum may reflect the influence of methylphenidate on motor and executive/attention networks and would be consistent with neurobiological theories of ADHD and treatment effects (Castellanos & Tannock, 2002; Swanson et al., 2007). It is interesting to note that where these changes overlap with findings in children with ADHD (i.e. caudate nucleus) the direction of the effect was the opposite; that is, perfusion increased in children, but decreased in adults. Within the 10 patients there was also a suggestion that baseline symptom levels scored using the questionnaire of Murphy and Barkley (1996) were predictive of changes in regional cerebral blood flow in the midbrain, cerebellum, and middle frontal gyrus, with those scoring the highest having the small-est changes in these regions.

Because there were no relationships between treat-ment effects at the brain and behavioral level, it is unclear what these results signify in terms of under-lying mechanisms of treatment response, and there-fore larger studies are needed to address such an issue. This small study also does not address whether methylphenidate has different effects in patients com-pared to healthy adults without ADHD beyond baseline-dependent differences as seen in children using fMRI during a response inhibition task (Vaidya et al., 1998). However, the increase in cerebellar blood flow has also been observed previously in healthy vol-unteers given methylphenidate (Mehta et al., 2000) and matches its effects on cerebral glucose metabolism (Volkow et al., 1997). The low density of dopamine transporters (DATs) in the cerebellum suggests a com-mon substrate of effects mediated via noradrener-gic mechanisms, although direct evidence for this is lacking.

Task-dependent changes in regional cerebral blood flow were also measured in the same patients (Schweitzer et al., 2003) and formed the basis of a later publication (Schweitzer et al., 2004). This work extended an earlier report of working memory task activations in ADHD that only qualitatively compared patients with controls and is not discussed here, although it is included in Table 7.1 (Schweitzer et al., 2000). In a fast-paced serial addition task and a number-generating control condition, control participants activated a brain network encompassing the middle temporal gyri, right prefrontal cortex, ventral anterior cingulate cortex, precuneus, fusiform gyrus, and hippocampus. Unmedicated patients with ADHD had reduced activation in cortical regions – inferior frontal, superior temporal, and ventral anterior cingulate gyri – and increased activation in largely subcortical regions – the midbrain, pons, right caudate nucleus – and the cerebellar vermis and middle frontal gyrus. Methylphenidate was associated with reduced activation in the middle and medial frontal gyrus and increased activation in the thalamus and precentral gyrus. The decreased baseline (or resting) signal in the precentral gyrus may underlie the task-related increase in regional cerebral blood flow, but their potential relationship was not explored. Nonetheless the differences between patients and controls observed during the serial addition task were considerably more widespread than the changes observed using fMRI in a group of 20 adults with ADHD performing a sustained attention task with a working memory component (n-back), during which only cerebellar activation was altered (Valera et al., 2005). However, in contrast to Schweitzer et al. (2004), a reduction in activation was seen in the study of Valera et al. (2005).

Because aberrant motivation in ADHD may affect decision making, decision-making networks in adults with ADHD were investigated in a group of 10 patients compared to 12 controls (Ernst et al., 2003). The task was a computerized gambling game based on the task of Bechara and colleagues (2000). This complex task involves selecting cards from four decks that have different reward and punishment values. Although performance did not differ between groups, brain acti-vation patterns showed that controls recruited the insula, hippocampus, and temporal and fusiform gyri more than patients, whereas patients showed greater activation in the anterior cingulate gyrus and post cen-tral and superior temporal gyri compared to controls. The complex nature of the task, involving learning, working memory, and other component functions of decision making (Dunn, Dalgliesh, & Lawrence, 2006), makes interpretation of this study difficult. Functional magnetic imaging studies that are able to delineate dif-ferent trial types and anticipation from feedback will be important in determining the precise abnormali-ties in motivational decision making in adult ADHD, as have already been successfully applied to younger groups (Scheres et al., 2007).

In summary, SPECT and PET studies of regional cerebral blood flow in adults with ADHD are severely limited, with no published studies using SPECT and the two sets of data using PET suggesting abnormal brain physiology or neural activation patterns in widespread cortical and subcortical regions. The sensitivity of these methods to psychomotor stimulant treatment is clear, although the changes observed in adults with ADHD and children may differ in direction, an observation confirmed by one of the authors using MRI-based perfusion imaging (O'Gorman et al., 2008).

Neurotransmitter receptors and release

The mechanism of action of the largely successful psychomotor stimulant medications has fueled catecholamine hypotheses of ADHD. The effects on dopamine (Levy & Swanson, 2001), noradrenaline (Arnsten & Dudley, 2005; Pliszka, 2007), and serotonin (Gainetdinov et al., 1999) are all thought to be important in explaining the therapeutic efficacy of stimulant medication. Whereas serotonergic markers are available for use in human neuroimaging, noradrenergic markers are currently under development (Ding et al., 2006; Schou et al., 2007). Because only dopaminergic markers have been tested in vivo in ADHD, the focus here is on this system.

Ligands have been used in ADHD to index dopamine synthesis (uptake of the precursor for a non-rate-limiting enzyme in the manufacture of dopamine), dopamine transporter density, dopamine transporter occupancy by medication, dopamine D2 receptor density, and dopamine release. Such measurement of components of the dopaminergic system allows direct testing of hypotheses regarding dopaminergic dysfunction in ADHD, including dopamine deficit (Levy & Swanson, 2001) and dopamine excess theories (Solanto, 1998).

Dopamine synthesis

Using the PET ligand [fluorine-18]fluorodopa ([18F]DOPA) the integrity of the presynaptic dopaminergic system was initially found to be compromised in adults with ADHD (n=17) compared to 23 healthy controls (Ernst, Zametkin, Matochik, et al., 1998). [18F]DOPA uptake was reduced by 50% in medial and left prefrontal cortical areas, with opposite gender effects in patients (m < f) compared to controls (f < m). This prefrontal dopaminergic abnormality was hypothesized to be secondary to increased midbrain [18F]DOPA uptake found in a

group of 10 medication-free adolescents with ADHD (Ernst et al., 1999), a finding that was not present in the adults. [^{11}C]DOPA PET has more recently been used in a group of eight medication-free adolescent males with ADHD compared to six controls (Forssberg et al., 2006). Two analysis methods were applied to the data, first describing [^{11}C]DOPA uptake across 28 predefined brain regions and then using a partial least squares regression discriminant analysis to examine different patterns of uptake across the regions. In the first analysis most regions showed reduced uptake, although only the midbrain region reached statistical significance. The 25% reduction in uptake was in the opposite direction to that described previously in adolescents (Ernst et al., 1999). The multivariate analysis was able to discriminate ADHD patients from controls with a pattern of general decreases in subcortical dopamine synthesis with little change in cortical values. For the eight patients there was also a relationship between attention scores (obtained using *DSM-IV* criteria) and regional [^{11}C]DOPA uptake values, which was negative in subcortical regions (e.g. the caudate, midbrain, nucleus accumbens) and positive in fronto-cortical regions (e.g. dorso- and ventrolateral and orbitofrontal cortex). Thus, low subcortical dopamine synthesis measurements were accompanied by ADHD with more severe attention symptoms, with the opposite for the frontal cortex.

The general reduction in DOPA uptake was confirmed in a group of young adult males diagnosed with ADHD, including 8 treatment-naive patients, 12 previously treated patients, and 18 controls (Ludolph et al., 2008). The frontal cortical effects demonstrated in the initial study of presynaptic dopamine function in ADHD were not confirmed, with the predominant effect being a reduction in [^{18}F]DOPA uptake in subcortical and brainstem regions. In a voxel-wise analysis there was also a suggestion of increased uptake in the anterior cingulate cortex in ADHD, an area that also differentiated between treated and untreated patients. In addition, uptake in the putamen, amygdala, and insula also differed, with it being lower in the treated group.

In summary, the four studies of presynaptic dopamine function conducted to date produced different results, with the two studies in adolescents presenting opposite findings within the midbrain and the studies in adults suggesting a reduction in tracer uptake in prefrontal regions (the first study) and in subcortical and cingulate regions (the second study).

The use of different tracers and populations (e.g. age and gender) may be proffered as possible explanations for the differences observed, but it is clear that larger scale studies, although difficult, are necessary to resolve these inconsistencies.

Dopamine transporter

Dopamine transport was first described more than 30 years ago (Iversen, 1971), whereas the dopamine transporter (DAT) itself was identified many years later (Giros et al., 1992). The human DAT gene is localized on chromosome 5p15.3 (Donovan et al., 1995; Giros et al., 1992; Vandenbergh et al., 1992), and genetic polymorphisms of the DAT gene have been reliably associated with ADHD (see Chapter 4). DATs are expressed in a small number of neurons in the brain, mainly in striatum and the nucleus accumbens, but also in the globus pallidus, cingulate cortex, olfactory tubercle, amygdala, and the midbrain (Ciliax et al., 1995).

[^{123}I] Altropane was used in the first study of DAT availability in patients with ADHD (Dougherty et al., 1999). This ligand binds to the human striatal DAT with high affinity, enters the brain rapidly, and accumulates in the striatum within 30 minutes (Fischman et al., 1998; Madras et al., 1998). In six unmedicated adult patients with ADHD, age-corrected DAT levels were approximately 70% higher than in controls drawn from a database (Dougherty et al., 1999). Subsequent studies using [^{99m}Tc]TRODAT-1 found much smaller increases in DAT density in ADHD (Dresel et al., 2000; Krause et al., 2000). Although the specificity for DAT is lower than for altropane, ^{99m}Tc has numerous advantages: 99mTc is the radionuclide of choice for nuclear medicine because it is readily available and relatively inexpensive and gives lower radiation exposure than ^{123}I, so that [^{99m}Tc]TRODAT-1 may be easily used in most nuclear medicine facilities. Ten never-medicated adults with ADHD presented with a 16% increase in striatal specific binding compared to controls matched for age and sex (Krause et al., 2000). The same group reported a 17% increase in striatal specific binding in 17 adults with ADHD.

Although these changes are considerably smaller than the original report by Dougherty et al. (1999), a follow-up study using [^{11}C]altropane in 26 unmedicated, nonsmoking adult patients and 21 well-characterized but younger controls reported a 15% increase in caudate DAT binding (Spencer et al., 2007),

although this result only emerged after age correction of DAT binding. The effects of smoking on DAT binding were initially highlighted by Krause et al. (2002) in a study in which 11 unmedicated nonsmokers with ADHD showed higher DAT density than 11 smoking patients, despite higher ADHD scores for the smokers. It is not clear in which way nicotine alters the measurement of DAT, but this finding suggests that one possibility is that nicotine decreases striatal DAT in a similar way to methylphenidate (either via down-regulation or occupancy of transporters by endogenous dopamine). Self-medication hypotheses of smoking behavior in ADHD would predict cognitive improvements in nonsmokers with ADHD who were administered nicotine, which do occur for response inhibition measured with the stop-signal task (Potter & Newhouse, 2008).

These early studies and a recent review (Spencer et al., 2005) suggest that striatal DAT densities are increased in ADHD, although the most recent studies have questioned this conclusion. Using [^{123}I]β-CIT SPECT imaging in nine adults with ADHD, no changes in striatal binding were seen compared to controls (van Dyck et al., 2002). This tracer has poor selectivity for the dopamine transporter (approx 1:1 sensitivity with the serotonin transporter), although a similar result was reported in a group of 12 adolescents with ADHD using the more selective PET ligand [^{11}C]PE21 (Jucaite et al., 2005). The latter study did report decreased DAT binding in the midbrain. It is important to note that in this study of adolescents with ADHD the controls were 10 adults; the precise effect on the results of using adults as controls is unknown. In two independent SPECT studies using [^{123}I]FP-CIT, a small increase (5%) in striatal DAT binding in 20 adults with ADHD (Larisch et al., 2006) and an 18–19% decrease in a group of 17 adults (Hesse et al., 2009) were reported respectively. The only studies conducted in children with ADHD initially reported an increase in striatal DAT binding of 28% using [^{123}I]IPT (Cheon et al., 2003), but subsequently showed a dramatic reduction of approximately 60% in four children with the 9/10 DAT allele and a smaller increase of about 14% in seven children with the 10/10 DAT allele (Cheon et al., 2005).

The most recent studies using PET imaging with [^{11}C]cocaine (Volkow, Wang, Newcorn, Fowler, et al., 2007; Volkow et al., 2009) also showed a reduction of 20% DAT binding in the caudate nucleus, 11% in the region of the nucleus accumbens, and 44% in the midbrain, with no change in the putamen, a finding that remained after the removal of smokers (Volkow, Wang, Newcorn, Fowler, et al., 2007). In the first of these studies putamen DAT binding, although not different between the adults with ADHD and controls, did correlate with the attention subscale of a questionnaire (Conners, 1998). Those with poorer attention had higher DAT binding, and this was the case for the controls as well as the patients. As expected the patients' scores were higher than the controls, but DAT binding in the putamen was not lower. In the second of these studies with a larger sample size, DAT binding in the midbrain was correlated to attention symptoms, such that those with lower binding had more problems, although this relationship may have been confounded by the group differences in both DAT binding and attention scores; the correlation was not reported for the ADHD group or controls alone (Volkow et al., 2009). In a group of 22 nonsmoking, never-treated adults with ADHD, general improvement after treatment (assessed using the Clinical Global Improvement Scale) was found in 16 of 17 patients whose DAT binding was elevated compared to a control sample, whereas the remaining 5 patients did not improve and all had lower DAT binding compared to controls (La Fougere et al., 2006).

DAT binding is unlikely to be a stable, trait biological marker because DAT levels are known to vary as a function of dopamine levels, with six children with ADHD demonstrating down-regulation after 3 months of treatment with methylphenidate (Vles et al., 2003). However, medication status or history does not seem a likely reason for the discrepancies among the numerous studies of DAT levels in ADHD (see Table 7.1) because most of the patients were unmedicated and different studies using never-medicated patients have shown opposite results (Krause et al., 2000; Volkow, Wang, Newcorn, Fowler, et al., 2007). The effect of the DAT genotype is also a candidate for explaining differences among the studies, but the effects were inconsistent and the group sizes generally small (e.g. Cheon et al., 2005; Krause et al., 2006). Other potential candidates are methodological, such as the use of different imaging methodologies and ligands. Studies with [^{11}C]altropane and [^{11}C]cocaine suggest that the use of different ligands is an unlikely cause of differences because the detected occupancies of oral methylphenidate using these two ligands are similar (Spencer et al., 2006; Volkow, Wang, et al., 1998).

Therefore, the issue of altered DAT binding in ADHD is currently unresolved, with increases, decreases, and no change being reported to date. Although factors such as symptom levels, genotype, and smoking may indeed alter DAT densities, none of these factors can sufficiently account for the current discrepancies in the literature. A notable observation is that, with the exception of the most recent study in which only the age-corrected analysis revealed differences (Spencer et al., 2007), the elevation in DAT binding in ADHD is chronologically reduced. The first study noted a 70% increase in DAT binding and one of the latest a 20% reduction in DAT binding. Diagnostic variation and ADHD subtypes therefore must be considered as plausible candidates for the observed differences across studies, although the numbers of patients typically included have not allowed for a systematic analysis of these issues. Ultimately meta-analyses and meta-regression are required to accurately summarize this literature. Nonetheless, despite the recent results that have questioned the developing story of increased DAT levels in ADHD, dopaminergic deficits remain important candidates for neurobiological abnormality in ADHD, possibly indexed by other receptors (dopamine receptors are classified as D1–D5) or evoked dopamine release.

Dopamine D2 receptors and dopamine release

Several ligands are now available for imaging dopamine receptors. The dopamine system has five distinct subtypes, although they are classically grouped into two superfamilies (Neve & Neve, 1997): D1-like (D1 and D5) and D2-like (D2, D3, and D4). Currently only receptors associated with each superfamily have been indexed with PET and SPECT, although newer ligands may have increased sensitivity to receptors within each superfamily. [^{11}C]raclopride and [^{123}I]IBZM, which are ligands for D2-like receptors, have been used in ADHD; they are best suited to index dopamine D2 and D3 receptor availability within the striatum (D4 receptors predominate within the neocortex). Both ligands are also sensitive to changes in endogenous dopamine levels and therefore can also be used to index dopamine release.

Initially, in a study of nine children with ADHD scanned with [^{123}I]IBZM SPECT, baseline dopamine D2 receptor availability was higher compared to average values in young healthy adults. Three months after methylphenidate treatment, dopamine D2 receptor availability was reduced across the striatum. Baseline dopamine D2 receptor binding was predictive of the percentage reduction in hyperactivity scores and teacher ratings after the three months (Ilgin et al., 2001). A control group was absent in a study of six adolescents who were born preterm (who have higher risk of ADHD), in which methylphenidate (0.3 mg/kg oral) induced reduction of [^{11}C]raclopride binding consonant with the expected increase in extracellular dopamine; the reduction in binding potential was associated with increased commission errors on tests of impulsivity and inattention (Rosa Neto et al., 2002). That is, those who had greater dopamine release after methylphenidate performed worse on tests sensitive to ADHD.

Subsequently a group of nine adolescents who met criteria for ADHD showed the same relationship between larger methylphenidate-induced change in [^{11}C]raclopride binding and poor performance on the test of variables of attention (TOVA; Greenberg & Waldman, 1993). If poor attentional task performance reflects an underlying impairment in dopamine function in ADHD, then these results can be seen as consistent with elevated or reduced levels of basal dopamine. Elevated levels of basal dopamine release could theoretically be enhanced with methylphenidate, which acts to block reuptake rather than release dopamine. In addition, lower basal dopamine levels could theoretically lead to reduced feedback inhibition effects on synthesis and release, thereby allowing for a greater effect of methylphenidate. Even so, these studies provided a proof of the principle that markers of dopamine release can be related to cognitive and behavioral indices of ADHD.

More recently the early suggestion of elevated [^{11}C]raclopride binding (Ilgin et al., 2001) was not replicated in a group of 12 adolescents with ADHD (Lou et al., 2004), although as with Ilgin et al. (2001) a young adult control group was used for comparison. This finding may be important because there are developmental changes in the dopamine system from childhood/adolescence into adulthood (Tseng et al., 2007). Nonetheless, measured motor activity was positively related to [^{11}C]raclopride binding in the right caudate nucleus within the ADHD group, suggesting that dopamine transmission within this structure may underlie some of the features of ADHD. Indeed smaller caudate nucleus volume in ADHD is one of the

few volumetric features that seem to diminish in adulthood (Castellanos et al., 2002).

Using appropriately matched controls, Volkow and colleagues (Volkow, Wang, Newcorn, Telang, et al., 2007; Volkow et al., 2009) have recently demonstrated *reduced* dopamine D2 receptor availability in adults with ADHD. In the first of two studies, dopamine D2 receptor availability was measured in 19 patients and 24 healthy controls with [^{11}C]raclopride, once after injection of saline placebo and once after intravenous methylphenidate (0.5 mg/kg). Although the route of administration in clinical treatment of ADHD is oral, this study allowed examination of the endogenous neurochemical responsiveness in the presence of clear blockade of DAT. On placebo, caudate [^{11}C]raclopride binding was lower in ADHD, achieving statistical significance in the left hemisphere, a finding subsequently replicated in a group of 53 patients and extended to the accumbens, midbrain, and hypothalamic region (Volkow et al., 2009). The larger sample sizes and carefully matched control groups in this study question the earlier suggestion of raised [^{11}C]raclopride binding in ADHD observed in adolescents (but compared to young adults). Given that radioligand binding measurements (binding potential) represent a ratio of receptor density and affinity, lower binding in ADHD could reflect lower receptor density or increased endogenous dopamine levels. It was argued that the former was more likely based on the reduced dopamine release in ADHD after methylphenidate compared to controls. Across both groups intravenous methylphenidate reduced [^{11}C]raclopride binding across the striatum (caudate and putamen) with a significantly smaller change in ADHD within the caudate nucleus. The level of dopamine release was negatively correlated with symptom scores (based on *DSM-IV*) of inattention and memory problems, such that those with reduced dopamine release experienced higher symptom scores.

These correlations parallel the recent findings with [^{11}C]DOPA in adolescents with ADHD described earlier (Forssberg et al., 2006), in which lower dopamine synthesis (structural and/or functional presynaptic dopamine function) was associated with poorer attention scores based on *DSM-IV*. Taken together the studies suggest that ADHD may be associated with reduced presynaptic dopamine function, resulting in reduced evoked dopamine release, and that these deficits may underlie some of the attentional, but not hyperactive symptoms. This is the opposite of the subcortical dopamine dysfunction in schizophrenia, in which DOPA uptake and dopamine release are both increased (Laruelle et al., 2003). In an exploratory analysis, dopamine release in adults with ADHD given intravenous methylphenidate also showed reduced dopamine release in the amygdala and hippocampus, but in terms of the number of voxels passing a predefined statistical threshold (spatial extent) rather than the difference at a voxel level (amplitude of response).

In summary, studies of dopamine receptor density and release in ADHD have suggested increased or no change in dopamine D2 receptor density in adolescents compared to adult controls (Ilgin et al., 2001; Lou et al., 2004) and clear decreased caudate D2 receptor density in recent, well-controlled studies of adults with ADHD (Volkow, Wang, Newcorn, Telang, et al., 2007; Volkow et al., 2009). The same adults also had blunted dopamine release after the administration of methylphenidate, suggesting lower endogenous spontaneous release of dopamine. A primary deficit in dopamine cells is supported by a recent observation of reduced [^{11}C]DOPA uptake in ADHD, although a similar result was not observed in earlier studies of adolescents (Ernst et al., 1999) and adults (Ernst, Zametkin, Matochik et al., 1998). Alternatively, as with the developing theories of schizophrenia (Laruelle et al., 2003), abnormal regulation of subcortical dopamine systems by the prefrontal cortex (via the glutamatergic projections from the prefrontal cortex to striatum) may also be responsible for attenuated dopamine release. Although such a model is consistent with functional and structural neuroimaging findings in adults with ADHD (see Chapter 5), it does not account for the differences between prefrontal cortical dysfunction in schizophrenia and ADHD, leading to apparently opposite changes in subcortical control of dopamine release.

Conclusions

Overall, SPECT and PET studies of cerebral perfusion and dopamine synthesis, release, and receptors have shown clear sensitivity to ADHD, with differential measurements across all modalities. The initial findings of abnormal striatal perfusion are still relevant. Striatal markers of perfusion and functional activation in adults are proving important in understanding functional deficits in ADHD (see Chapter 5). In addition, striatal dopamine markers potentially relevant in mediating differences in cognition (Reeves et al., 2005; Volkow, Gur, et al., 1998) and personality (Farde, Gustavsson, & Jonsson, 1997; Reeves et al., 2007; Tomer et al., 2008) differ in both children and adults with ADHD. However, in the neurochemical literature in ADHD there are considerable differences and inconsistencies across studies. The multiple replications of elevated DAT density in ADHD (Spencer et al., 2005) have not only been questioned, but the most recent results suggest the opposite finding of reduced DAT density in adults with ADHD (Hesse et al., 2009; Volkow, Wang, Newcorn, Fowler, et al., 2007; Volkow et al., 2009). The most recent studies have also suggested reduced dopamine release in ADHD, a conclusion more consistent with the dopamine excess hypothesis put forward by Seeman and Madras (1998, 2002) than a simple dopamine deficit hypothesis. In this model increased dopamine tone leads to greater feedback inhibition and decreased impulse-triggered dopamine release. The use of cognitive tasks known to evoke dopamine release and the influence of methylphenidate on such release (Volkow et al., 2004) will be important in fully testing such hypotheses. The incorporation of genetic variations for the DAT in these studies is also important, as is the transition from differential markers to functional abnormalities (Dreher et al., 2009). It is also widely acknowledged that abnormal dopamine function is unlikely to account for all the deficits and variability in behavior in ADHD; therefore the differences within other neurotransmitter systems such as the noradrenergic system will be an important topic in the coming years, particularly with recent computational models making specific predictions regarding the differential role of dopamine and noradrenaline in cognitive deficits in ADHD (Frank et al., 2007).

Despite these advances, clarification of the inconsistencies in the neurotransmitter studies of ADHD in childhood and adult will require mapping of the developmental trajectory of supposed dopamine dysfunction while controlling for the influence of medication status, comorbidities, and substance use history. Doing so will require longitudinal studies, although carefully controlled cross-sectional designs in medication-naive and treated populations as well as healthy volunteers will go some way in addressing some of the apparent inconsistencies in the literature to date. The most recent studies have confirmed that dopaminergic markers are indeed valuable targets for understanding the neurobiology of ADHD, while suggesting that the dynamic responsiveness of the system to treatment needs to be taken into account in fully interpreting studies.

References

Amen DG, Carmichael BD. (1997). High-resolution brain SPECT imaging in ADHD. *Ann Clin Psychiatry* **9**(2):81–6.

Arnsten AF, Dudley AG. (2005). Methylphenidate improves prefrontal cortical cognitive function through alpha2 adrenoceptor and dopamine D1 receptor actions: relevance to therapeutic effects in Attention Deficit Hyperactivity Disorder. *Behav Brain Funct* **1**(1):2.

Bechara A, Damasio H, Damasio AR. (2000). Emotion, decision making and the orbitofrontal cortex. *Cereb Cortex* **10**(3):295–307.

Castellanos FX, Lee PP, Sharp W, Jeffries NO, Greenstein DK, Clasen LS, et al. (2002). Developmental trajectories of brain volume abnormalities in children and adolescents with attention-deficit/hyperactivity disorder. *JAMA* **288**(14):1740–8.

Castellanos FX. (2002). Proceed, with caution: SPECT cerebral blood flow studies of children and adolescents with attention deficit hyperactivity disorder. *J Nucl Med* **43**(12):1630–3.

Castellanos FX, Tannock R. (2002). Neuroscience of attention-deficit/hyperactivity disorder: the search for endophenotypes. *Nat Rev Neurosci* **3**(8): 617–28.

Cheon KA, Ryu YH, Kim JW, Cho DY. (2005). The homozygosity for 10-repeat allele at dopamine transporter gene and dopamine transporter density in Korean children with attention deficit hyperactivity disorder: relating to treatment response to methylphenidate. *Eur Neuropsychopharmacol* **15**(1):95–101.

Cheon KA, Ryu YH, Kim YK, Namkoong K, Kim CH, Lee JD. (2003). Dopamine transporter density in the basal ganglia assessed with [123I]IPT SPET in children with attention deficit hyperactivity disorder. *Eur J Nucl Med Mol Imaging* **30**(2):306–11.

Ciliax BJ, Heilman C, Demchyshyn LL, Pristupa ZB, Ince E, Hersch SM, et al. (1995). The dopamine transporter: immunochemical characterization and localization in brain. *J Neurosci* **15**(3 Pt 1):1714–23.

Conners CK. (1998). Rating scales in attention-deficit/ hyperactivity disorder: use in assessment and treatment monitoring. *J Clin Psychiatry* **59**(suppl 7): 24–30.

Coull JT. (1998). Neural correlates of attention and arousal: insights from electrophysiology, functional neuroimaging and psychopharmacology. *Prog Neurobiol* **55**(4):343–61.

Deutsch G, Mountz JM, Katholi CR, Liu HG, Harrell LE. (1997). Regional stability of cerebral blood flow measured by repeated technetium-99m-HMPAO SPECT: implications for the study of state-dependent change. *J Nucl Med* **38**(1):6–13.

Ding YS, Lin KS, Logan J. (2006). PET imaging of norepinephrine transporters. *Curr Pharm Des* **12**(30):3831–45.

Donovan DM, Vandenbergh DJ, Perry MP, Bird GS, Ingersoll R, Nanthakumar E, et al. (1995). Human and mouse dopamine transporter genes: conservation of 5'-flanking sequence elements and gene structures. *Brain Res Mol Brain Res* **30**(2):327–35.

Dougherty DD, Bonab AA, Spencer TJ, Rauch SL, Madras BK, Fischman AJ. (1999). Dopamine transporter density in patients with attention deficit hyperactivity disorder. *Lancet* **354**(9196):2132–3.

Dreher JC, Kohn P, Kolachana B, Weinberger DR, Berman KF. (2009). Variation in dopamine genes influences responsivity of the human reward system. *Proc Nat Acad Sci USA* **106**(2):617–22.

Dresel S, Krause J, Krause KH, La Fougere C, Brinkbaumer K, Kung HF, et al. (2000). Attention deficit hyperactivity disorder: binding of [99mTc]TRODAT-1 to the dopamine transporter before and after methylphenidate treatment. *Eur J Nucl Med* **27**(10):1518–24.

Duara R, Gross-Glenn K, Barker WW, Chang JY, Apicella A, Loewenstein D, et al. (1987). Behavioral activation and the variability of cerebral glucose metabolic measurements. *J Cereb Blood Flow Metab* **7**(3):266–71.

Dunn BD, Dalgleish T, Lawrence AD. (2006). The somatic marker hypothesis: a critical evaluation. *Neurosci Biobehav Rev* **30**(2):239–71.

Ernst M, Kimes AS, London ED, Matochik JA, Eldreth D, Tata S, et al. (2003). Neural substrates of decision making in adults with attention deficit hyperactivity disorder. *Am J Psychiatry* **160**(6):1061–70.

Ernst M, Liebenauer LL, King AC, Fitzgerald GA, Cohen RM, Zametkin AJ. (1994). Reduced brain metabolism in hyperactive girls. *J Am Acad Child Adolesc Psychiatry* **33**(6):858–68.

Ernst M, Zametkin AJ, Matochik JA, Jons PH, Cohen RM. (1998). DOPA decarboxylase activity in attention deficit hyperactivity disorder adults. A [fluorine-18]fluorodopa positron emission tomographic study. *J Neurosci* **18**(15):5901–7.

Ernst M, Zametkin AJ, Matochik JA, Liebenauer L, Fitzgerald GA, Cohen RM. (1994). Effects of intravenous dextroamphetamine on brain metabolism in adults with attention-deficit hyperactivity disorder (ADHD). Preliminary findings. *Psychopharmacol Bull* **30**(2):219–25.

Ernst M, Zametkin AJ, Matochik JA, Pascualvaca D, Jons PH, Cohen RM. (1999). High midbrain [18F]DOPA accumulation in children with attention deficit hyperactivity disorder. *Am J Psychiatry* **156**(8): 1209–15.

Ernst M, Zametkin AJ, Phillips RL, Cohen RM. (1998). Age-related changes in brain glucose metabolism in adults with attention-deficit/hyperactivity disorder and control subjects. *J Neuropsychiatry Clin Neurosci* **110**(2):168–77.

Farde L, Gustavsson JP, Jonsson E. (1997). D2 dopamine receptors and personality traits. *Nature* **385**(6617):590.

Fischman AJ, Bonab AA, Babich JW, Palmer EP, Alpert NM, Elmaleh DR, et al. (1998). Rapid detection of Parkinson's disease by SPECT with altropane: a selective ligand for dopamine transporters. *Synapse* **29**(2): 128–41.

Forssberg H, Fernell E, Waters S, Waters N, Tedroff J. (2006). Altered pattern of brain dopamine synthesis in male adolescents with attention deficit hyperactivity disorder. *Behav Brain Funct* **2**:40.

Frank MJ, Santamaria A, O'Reilly RC, Willcutt E. (2007). Testing computational models of dopamine and noradrenaline dysfunction in attention deficit/hyperactivity disorder. *Neuropsychopharmacology* **32**(7):1583–99.

Gainetdinov RR, Wetsel WC, Jones SR, Levin ED, Jaber M, Caron MG. (1999). Role of serotonin in the paradoxical calming effect of psychostimulants on hyperactivity. *Science* **283**(5400):397–401.

Giros B, el Mestikawy S, Godinot N, Zheng K, Han H, Yang-Feng T, et al. (1992). Cloning, pharmacological characterization, and chromosome assignment of the human dopamine transporter. *Mol Pharmacol* **42**(3):383–90.

Greenberg LM, Waldman ID. (1993). Developmental normative data on the test of variables of attention (T.O.V.A.). *J Child Psychol Psychiatry* **34**:1019–30.

Hesse S, Ballaschke O, Barthel H, Sabri O. (2009). Dopamine transporter imaging in adult patients with attention-deficit/hyperactivity disorder. *Psychiatry Res* **171**(2):120–8.

Hesse S, Ballaschke O, Barthel H, von Cramon DY, Sabri O. (2006). The striatal dopamine transporter availability is reduced in adults with attention-deficit/hyperactivity disorder. *J Nucl Med* **47**(suppl 1):142.

Ilgin N, Senol S, Gucuyener K, Gokcora N, Sener S. (2001). Is increased D2 receptor availability associated with response to stimulant medication in ADHD? *Dev Med Child Neurol* **43**(11):755–60.

Iversen LL. (1971). Role of transmitter uptake mechanisms in synaptic neurotransmission. *Br J Pharmacol* **41**(4):571–91.

Jucaite A, Fernell E, Halldin C, Forssberg H, Farde L. (2005). Reduced midbrain dopamine transporter binding in male adolescents with attention-deficit/hyperactivity disorder: association between striatal dopamine markers and motor hyperactivity. *Biol Psychiatry* **57**(3):229–38.

Kaya GC, Pekcanlar A, Bekis R, Ada E, Miral S, Emiroglu N, et al. (2002). Technetium-99m HMPAO brain SPECT in children with attention deficit hyperactivity disorder. *Ann Nucl Med* **16**(8):527–31.

Kim BN, Lee JS, Cho SC, Lee DS. (2001). Methylphenidate increased regional cerebral blood flow in subjects with attention deficit/hyperactivity disorder. *Yonsei Med J* **42**(1):19–29.

Kim BN, Lee JS, Shin MS, Cho SC, Lee DS. (2002). Regional cerebral perfusion abnormalities in attention deficit/hyperactivity disorder. Statistical parametric mapping analysis. *Eur Arch Psychiatry Clin Neurosci* **252**(5):219–25.

Krause KH, Dresel SH, Krause J, Kung HF, Tatsch K. (2000). Increased striatal dopamine transporter in adult patients with attention deficit hyperactivity disorder: effects of methylphenidate as measured by single photon emission computed tomography. *Neurosci Lett* **285**(2):107–10.

Krause KH, Dresel SH, Krause J, Kung HF, Tatsch K, Ackenheil M. (2002). Stimulant-like action of nicotine on striatal dopamine transporter in the brain of adults with attention deficit hyperactivity disorder. *Int J Neuropsychopharmacol* **5**(2):111–3.

Krause J, Dresel SH, Krause KH, La Fougere C, Zill P, Ackenheil M. (2006). Striatal dopamine transporter availability and DAT-1 gene in adults with ADHD: no higher DAT availability in patients with homozygosity for the 10-repeat allele. *World J Biol Psychiatry* **7**(3):152–7.

La Fougere C, Krause J, Krause KH, Josef Gildehaus F, Hacker M, Koch W, et al. (2006). Value of 99mTc-TRODAT-1 SPECT to predict clinical response to methylphenidate treatment in adults with attention deficit hyperactivity disorder. *Nucl Med Commun* **27**(9):733–7.

Langleben DD, Acton PD, Austin G, Elman I, Krikorian G, Monterosso JR, et al. (2002). Effects of methylphenidate discontinuation on cerebral blood flow in prepubescent boys with attention deficit hyperactivity disorder. *J Nucl Med* **43**(12):1624–9.

Larisch R, Sitte W, Antke C, Nikolaus S, Franz M, Tress W, et al. (2006). Striatal dopamine transporter density in drug naive patients with attention-deficit/hyperactivity disorder. *Nucl Med Commun* **27**(3):267–70.

Laruelle M, Kegeles LS, Abi-Dargham A. (2003). Glutamate, dopamine, and schizophrenia: from pathophysiology to treatment. *Ann N Y Acad Sci* **1003**:138–58.

Levy F, Swanson JM. (2001). Timing, space and ADHD: the dopamine theory revisited. *Aust N Z J Psychiatry* **35**(4):504–11.

Lorberboym M, Watemberg N, Nissenkorn A, Nir B, Lerman-Sagie T. (2004). Technetium 99m ethylcysteinate dimer single-photon emission computed tomography (SPECT) during intellectual stress test in children and adolescents with pure versus comorbid attention-deficit hyperactivity disorder (ADHD). *J Child Neurol* **19**(2):91–6.

Lou HC, Andresen J, Steinberg B, McLaughlin T, Friberg L. (1998). The striatum in a putative cerebral network activated by verbal awareness in normals and in ADHD children. *Eur J Neurol* **5**(1):67–74.

Lou HC, Henriksen L, Bruhn P. (1984). Focal cerebral hypoperfusion in children with dysphasia and/or attention deficit disorder. *Arch Neurol* **41**(8):825–9.

Lou HC, Henriksen L, Bruhn P. (1990). Focal cerebral dysfunction in developmental learning disabilities. *Lancet* **335**(8680):8–11.

Lou HC, Henriksen L, Bruhn P, Borner H, Nielsen JB. (1989). Striatal dysfunction in attention deficit and hyperkinetic disorder. *Arch Neurol* **46**(1):48–52.

Lou HC, Rosa P, Pryds O, Karrebaek H, Lunding J, Cumming P, et al. (2004). ADHD: increased dopamine receptor availability linked to attention deficit and low neonatal cerebral blood flow. *Dev Med Child Neurol* **46**(3):179–83.

Ludolph AG, Kassubek J, Schmeck K, Glaser C, Wunderlich A, Buck AK, et al. (2008). Dopaminergic dysfunction in attention deficit hyperactivity disorder (ADHD), differences between pharmacologically treated and never treated young adults: a 3,4-dihdroxy-6-[18F]fluorophenyl-l-alanine PET study. *Neuroimage* **41**(3):718–27.

Madras BK, Meltzer PC, Liang AY, Elmaleh DR, Babich J, Fischman AJ. (1998). Altropane, a SPECT or PET imaging probe for dopamine neurons: I. Dopamine transporter binding in primate brain. *Synapse* **29**(2):93–104.

Matochik JA, Liebenauer LL, King AC, Szymanski HV, Cohen RM, Zametkin AJ. (1994). Cerebral glucose metabolism in adults with attention deficit hyperactivity disorder after chronic stimulant treatment. *Am J Psychiatry* **151**(5):658–64.

Matochik JA, Nordahl TE, Gross M, Semple WE, King AC, Cohen RM, et al. (1993). Effects of acute stimulant medication on cerebral metabolism in adults with hyperactivity. *Neuropsychopharmacology* **8**(4):377–86.

McCulloch J, Kelly PAT, Ford I. (1982). Effect of apomorphine on the relationship between local cerebral glucose utilization and local berebral blood flow (with an appendix on its statistical analysis). *J Cereb Blood Flow Metab* **2**:487–99.

Mehta MA, Owen AM, Sahakian BJ, Mavaddat N, Pickard JD, Robbins TW. (2000). Methylphenidate enhances working memory by modulating discrete frontal and parietal lobe regions in the human brain. *J Neurosci* **20**(6):RC65.

Murphy K, Barkley RA. (1996). Prevalence of DSM-IV ADHD symptoms in an adult community sample of licensed drivers. *J Atten Disord* **1**:147–61.

Neve KA, Neve RL. (1997). *The Dopamine Receptors*. Totowa, NJ: Humana.

O'Gorman RL, Mehta MA, Asherson P, Zelaya FO, Brookes KJ, Toone BK, et al. (2008). Increased cerebral perfusion in adult attention deficit hyperactivity disorder is normalised by stimulant treatment: a non-invasive MRI pilot study. *Neuroimage* **42**(1): 36–41.

Oner O, Oner P, Aysev A, Kucuk O, Ibis E. (2005). Regional cerebral blood flow in children with ADHD: changes with age. *Brain Dev* **27**:279–85.

Pliszka SR. (2007). Pharmacologic treatment of attention-deficit/hyperactivity disorder: efficacy, safety and mechanisms of action. *Neuropsychol Rev* **17**(1):61–72.

Potter AS, Newhouse PA. (2008). Acute nicotine improves cognitive deficits in young adults with attention-deficit/hyperactivity disorder. *Pharmacol Biochem Behav* **88**(4):407–17.

Raichle ME. (2006). Neuroscience. The brain's dark energy. *Science* **314**(5803):1249–50.

Reeves SJ, Grasby PM, Howard RJ, Bantick RA, Asselin MC, Mehta MA. (2005). A positron emission tomography (PET) investigation of the role of striatal dopamine (D2) receptor availability in spatial cognition. *Neuroimage* **28**(1):216–26.

Reeves SJ, Mehta MA, Montgomery AJ, Amiras D, Egerton A, Howard RJ, et al. (2007). Striatal dopamine (D2) receptor availability predicts socially desirable responding. *Neuroimage* **34**(4):1782–9.

Rosa Neto P, Lou H, Cumming P, Pryds O, Gjedde A. (2002). Methylphenidate-evoked potentiation of extracellular dopamine in the brain of adolescents with premature birth: correlation with attentional deficit. *Ann N Y Acad Sci* **965**:434–9.

Scheres A, Milham MP, Knutson B, Castellanos FX. (2007). Ventral striatal hyporesponsiveness during reward anticipation in attention-deficit/hyperactivity disorder. *Biol Psychiatry* **61**(5):720–4.

Schou M, Pike VW, Halldin C. (2007). Development of radioligands for imaging of brain norepinephrine transporters in vivo with positron emission tomography. *Curr Top Med Chem* 7(18):1806–16.

Schweitzer JB, Faber TL, Grafton ST, Tune LE, Hoffman JM, Kilts CD. (2000). Alterations in the functional anatomy of working memory in adult attention deficit hyperactivity disorder. *Am J Psychiatry* 157(2): 278–80.

Schweitzer JB, Lee DO, Hanford RB, Tagamets MA, Hoffman JM, Grafton ST, et al. (2003). A positron emission tomography study of methylphenidate in adults with ADHD: alterations in resting blood flow and predicting treatment response. *Neuropsychopharmacology* 28(5):967–73.

Schweitzer JB, Lee DO, Hanford RB, Zink CF, Ely TD, Tagamets MA, et al. (2004). Effect of methylphenidate on executive functioning in adults with attention-deficit/hyperactivity disorder: normalization of behavior but not related brain activity. *Biol Psychiatry* 56(8): 597–606.

Seeman P, Madras BK. (1998). Anti-hyperactivity medication: methylphenidate and amphetamine. *Mol Psychiatry* 3(5):386–96.

Seeman P, Madras B. (2002). Methylphenidate elevates resting dopamine which lowers the impulse-triggered release of dopamine: a hypothesis. *Behav Brain Res* 130(1–2):79–83.

Sieg KG, Gaffney GR, Preston DF, Hellings JA. (1995). SPECT brain imaging abnormalities in attention deficit hyperactivity disorder. *Clin Nucl Med* 20(1):55–60.

Solanto MV. (1998). Neuropsychopharmacological mechanisms of stimulant drug action in attention-deficit hyperactivity disorder: a review and integration. *Behav Brain Res* 94(1):127–52.

Spencer TJ, Biederman J, Ciccone PE, Madras BK, Dougherty DD, Bonab AA, et al. (2006). PET study examining pharmacokinetics, detection and lieability, and dopamine transporter occupancy of short- and long-acting oral methylphenidate. *Am J Psychiatry* 163:387–95.

Spencer TJ, Biederman J, Madras BK, Dougherty DD, Bonab AA, Livni E, et al. (2007). Further evidence of dopamine transporter dysregulation in ADHD: a controlled PET imaging study using altropane. *Biol Psychiatry* 62(9):1059–61.

Spencer TJ, Biederman J, Madras BK, Faraone SV, Dougherty DD, Bonab AA, et al. (2005). In vivo neuroreceptor imaging in attention-deficit/hyperactivity disorder: a focus on the dopamine transporter. *Biol Psychiatry* 57(11):1293–300.

Swanson JM, Kinsbourne M, Nigg J, Lanphear B, Stefanatos GA, Volkow N, et al. (2007). Etiologic subtypes of attention-deficit/hyperactivity disorder: brain imaging, molecular genetic and environmental

factors and the dopamine hypothesis. *Neuropsychol Rev* 17(1):39–59.

Szobot CM, Ketzer C, Cunha RD, Parente MA, Langleben DD, Acton PD, et al. (2003). The acute effect of methylphenidate on cerebral blood flow in boys with attention-deficit/hyperactivity disorder. *Eur J Nucl Med Mol Imaging* 30(3):423–6.

Szobot C, Roman T, Cunha R, Acton P, Hutz M, Rohde LA. (2005). Brain perfusion and dopaminergic genes in boys with attention-deficit/hyperactivity disorder. *Am J Med Genet B Neuropsychiatr Genet* 132(1):53–8.

Tomer R, Goldstein RZ, Wang GJ, Wong C, Volkow ND. (2008). Incentive motivation is associated with striatal dopamine asymmetry. *Biol Psychiatry* 77(1): 98–101.

Tseng KY, O'Donnell P. (2007). Dopamine modulation of prefrontal cortical interneurons changes during adolescence. *Cereb Cortex* 17:1235–40.

Vaidya CJ, Austin G, Kirkorian G, Ridlehuber HW, Desmond JE, Glover GH, et al. (1998). Selective effects of methylphenidate in attention deficit hyperactivity disorder: a functional magnetic resonance study. *Proc Nat Acad Science USA* 95(24):14494–9.

Valera EM, Faraone SV, Biederman J, Poldrack RA, Seidman LJ. (2005). Functional neuroanatomy of working memory in adults with attention-deficit/hyperactivity disorder. *Biol Psychiatry* 57(5): 439–47.

Vandenbergh DJ, Persico AM, Hawkins AL, Griffin CA, Li X, Jabs EW, et al. (1992). Human dopamine transporter gene (DAT1) maps to chromosome 5p15.3 and displays a VNTR. *Genomics* 14(4):1104–6.

van Dyck CH, Quinlan DM, Cretella LM, Staley JK, Malison RT, Baldwin RM, et al. (2002). Unaltered dopamine transporter availability in adult attention deficit hyperactivity disorder. *Am J Psychiatry* 159(2):309–12.

Vles JS, Feron FJ, Hendriksen JG, Jolles J, van Kroonenburgh MJ, Weber WE. (2003). Methylphenidate down-regulates the dopamine receptor and transporter system in children with attention deficit hyperkinetic disorder (ADHD). *Neuropediatrics* 34(2):77–80.

Volkow ND, Gur RC, Wang GJ, Fowler JS, Moberg PJ, Ding YS, et al. (1998). Association between decline in brain dopamine activity with age and cognitive and motor impairment in healthy individuals. *Am J Psychiatry* 155(3):344–9.

Volkow ND, Wang GJ, Fowler JS, Gatley SJ, Logan J, Ding YS, et al. (1998). Dopamine transporter occupancies in the human brain induced by therapeutic doses of oral methylphenidate. *Am J Psychiatry* 155(10): 1325–31.

Volkow ND, Wang GJ, Fowler JS, Logan J, Angrist B, Hitzemann R, et al. (1997). Effects of methylphenidate on regional brain glucose metabolism in humans: relationship to dopamine D2 receptors. *Am J Psychiatry* **154**(1):50–5.

Volkow ND, Wang GJ, Fowler JS, Telang F, Maynard L, Logan J, et al. (2004). Evidence that methylphenidate enhances the saliency of a mathematical task by increasing dopamine in the human brain. *Am J Psychiatry* **161**(7):1173–80.

Volkow ND, Wang GJ, Kollins SH, Wigal TL, Newcorn JH, Telang F, et al. (2009). Evaluating dopamine reward pathway in ADHD: clinical implications. *JAMA* **302**(10):1084–91.

Volkow ND, Wang GJ, Newcorn J, Fowler JS, Telang F, Solanto MV, et al. (2007). Brain dopamine transporter levels in treatment and drug naive adults with ADHD. *Neuroimage* **34**(3):1182–90.

Volkow ND, Wang GJ, Newcorn J, Telang F, Solanto MV, Fowler JS, et al. (2007). Depressed dopamine activity in caudate and preliminary evidence of limbic involvement in adults with attention-deficit/hyperactivity disorder. *Arch Gen Psychiatry* **64**(8):932–40.

Zametkin AJ, Liebenauer LL, Fitzgerald GA, King AC, Minkunas DV, Herscovitch P, et al. (1993). Brain metabolism in teenagers with attention-deficit hyperactivity disorder. *Arch Gen Psychiatry* **50**(5):333–40.

Zametkin AJ, Nordahl TE, Gross M, King AC, Semple WE, Rumsey J, et al. (1990). Cerebral glucose metabolism in adults with hyperactivity of childhood onset. *N Engl J Med* **323**(20):1361–6.

Chapter

8

Diagnosing ADHD in adults

Leonard A. Adler and David Shaw

Introduction

Attention-deficit hyperactivity disorder (ADHD) is one of the most common mental health disorders in children, with estimates showing that it affects 6–9% of children worldwide (Kessler, Adler, Ames, et al., 2005; Kessler, Adler, Barkley, et al., 2005). ADHD in children was first recognized in the early 1900s, but recognition of the disorder's persistence into adulthood did not occur until the 1970s (Adler & Chua, 2002). Recent longitudinal follow-up studies have shown that clinically significant symptoms of the disorder persist for 60% of children into adulthood, equaling approximately 4% of adults worldwide who are affected by the disorder (Kessler, Adler, Ames, et al., 2005; Kessler, Adler, Barkley, et al., 2005). In the United States, it is believed that as many as 8 million adults have ADHD (Barkley, 2006; Weiss & Murray, 2003), making it one of the most common mental health disorders (Kessler, Adler, Barkley et al., 2005).

Partly as a result of this time lag in recognition, childhood ADHD is fixed firmly in the public consciousness, while adult ADHD is still gaining awareness. Because of its relatively recent emergence as a diagnosis, ADHD remains underrecognized and undertreated in adults (Biederman & Faraone, 2005). More than 40% of adults diagnosed with ADHD in the United States in the 2004 National Comorbidity Survey (NCS) reported seeing a health care professional in the previous year and yet remained undiagnosed. Results from a recent survey of 400 primary care physicians (PCPs) in the United States about their level of familiarity with diagnosing and treating ADHD in adults found that many believe they receive substantially less training in adult ADHD as compared with anxiety and depressive disorders, and they were three times less comfortable diagnosing adult ADHD than diagnosing these disorders (Adler, 2004a). Neverthe-less, much is known about the persistence of the disorder into adulthood, the common presenting problems of adults with ADHD, and the manifestations of the disorder that are unique to adults.

Diagnosing ADHD in adults: an historical perspective

The *Diagnostic and Statistical Manual of Mental Disorders* (DSM) has been relatively slow to acknowledge the disorder's persistence into adulthood, a hesitancy that is consistent with the mental health community's understanding of adult ADHD (Adler, 2004a; Adler & Cohen, 2004; American Psychiatric Association, 1968, 1984, 1994). The first definition of the disorder in the *DSM* appeared in its second edition (*DSM-II*). *DSM-II* defined the disorder as "hyperkinetic syndrome," solely emphasizing motoric overactivity (American Psychiatric Association, 1968; Biederman, Mick, & Faraone, 2000; Mick, Faraone, & Biederman, 2004). In 1980, the third edition (*DSM-III*) provided the first equal emphasis on inattentive symptoms by classifying the disorder as attention deficit disorder, with and without hyperactivity (American Psychiatric Association, 1980). However, *DSM-III* provides only a brief mention of the possibility for ADHD to persist into adolescence or adulthood and no description of adult symptoms. Yet, it was the first diagnostic tool to provide the criteria for an individual to be diagnosed primarily based on the impairment from inattentive symptoms without evidence of hyperactive/impulsive symptoms.

The *Diagnostic and Statistical Manual of Mental Disorders*, third edition, revised (*DSM-III-R*) expanded on the definition, stating that "approximately one third of children with ADHD continue to show some signs of the disorder in adulthood"

(American Psychiatric Association, 1984). Though this edition still did not code adult ADHD as a separate category, it was the first one that went so far as to recognize the possibility of ADHD in adults by listing diagnostic criteria for residual ADHD in adults. In *DSM-III-R*, as in the later editions, adults who showed signs of ADHD were considered to have the disorder, provided that they had experienced those symptoms since early childhood. Other revisions in *DSM-III-R* included changing the name of the disorder to attention-deficit/hyperactivity disorder and placing more emphasis on overactivity than did *DSM-III*.

The acknowledgment that full-fledged ADHD can persist into adulthood was included in the fourth edition (*DSM-IV*), which stated, "In most individuals, symptoms attenuate during late adolescence and adulthood, although a minority of individuals experience the full complement of symptoms of Attention-Deficit/Hyperactivity Disorder into mid-adulthood" (American Psychiatric Association, 2000). By *DSM-IV*'s definition, ADHD must begin in childhood, and evidence of the condition must be demonstrated by age 7. Although this edition recognizes the common continued presentation of ADHD into adulthood, adult-onset ADHD is not considered a valid diagnosis and most likely represents another condition. Another change in the fourth edition is the placement of impulsive and hyperactive symptoms in the same list but keeping them separately identified. It also draws a distinction between the inattentive symptoms and other symptom clusters.

Symptoms of adult ADHD chronicled by the *DSM-IV-TR*

According to the *Diagnostic and Statistical Manual of Mental Disorders,* 4th edition, text revision (*DSM-IV-TR*), individuals must meet all criteria in sections B through E and must have a minimum of six symptoms listed in sections A1 (inattention) or A2 (hyperactivity and impulsivity) for a diagnosis of ADHD. These symptoms must have persisted for at least 6 months, and they must also be manifested "to a degree that [they are] maladaptive and inconsistent with developmental level."

For inattention, those symptoms are:

a) Often fails to give close attention to details or makes careless mistakes in schoolwork, work, or other activities;

b) Often has difficulty sustaining attention in tasks or play activities;

c) Often does not seem to listen when spoken to directly;

d) Often does not follow through on instructions and fails to finish schoolwork, chores, or duties in the workplace (not due to oppositional behavior or failure to understand instructions);

e) Often has difficulty organizing tasks and activities;

f) Often avoids, dislikes, or is reluctant to engage in tasks that require sustained mental effort (such as schoolwork or homework);

g) Often loses things necessary for tasks or activities (e.g. toys, school assignments, pencils, books, or tools);

h) Is often easily distracted by extraneous stimuli;

i) Is often forgetful in daily activities.

For hyperactivity, those symptoms are:

a) Often fidgets with hands or feet or squirms in seat;

b) Often leaves seat in classroom or in other situations in which remaining seated is expected;

c) Often runs about or climbs excessively in situations in which it is inappropriate (in adolescents or adults, may be limited to subjective feelings of restlessness);

d) Often has difficulty playing or engaging in leisure activities quietly;

e) Is often "on the go" or acts as if "driven by a motor";

f) Often talks excessively.

For impulsivity, those symptoms are:

a) Often blurts out answers before questions have been completed;

b) Often has difficulty awaiting one's turn;

c) Often interrupts or intrudes on others (e.g. butts into conversations or games).

Individuals must also meet all of the final four criteria:

1. Some hyperactive-impulsive or inattentive symptoms that caused impairment were present before age 7 years;

2. Some impairment from the symptoms is present in two settings (e.g. school, work, home);

3. There must be clear evidence of clinically significant impairment in social, academic, or occupational functioning;

4. The symptoms do not happen only during the course of a pervasive developmental disorder, schizophrenia, or other psychotic disorder. The symptoms are not better accounted for by another mental disorder (e.g. mood disorder, anxiety disorder, dissociative disorder, or a personality disorder (Adler, 2004; American Psychiatric Association, 2000).

As *DSM-IV-TR* criteria now stand, individuals who present at least six of the nine clinically significant inattentive symptoms would be diagnosed with the inattentive subtype. Those who present at least six of the nine clinically significant hyperactive/impulsive symptoms would be diagnosed with the hyperactive/impulsive subtype. Finally, those with at least six clinically significant symptoms in each category would be diagnosed with the combined subtype.

A recent trial of atomoxetine in 536 patients with ADHD showed that 31% of the study participants were classified with the inattentive subtype, 3% were classified predominantly with hyperactive subtype, and 66% were classified with the combined subtype (Michelson et al., 2003). However, in another clinical trial, an equal number of participants were classified with the inattentive subtype as with the combined subtype (Spencer et al., 2001). Longitudinal studies of youths with ADHD have shown that symptoms of hyperactivity and impulsivity tend to wane, whereas inattention tends to persist into adulthood (Mick et al., 2004). Other studies have found clinically significant levels of hyperactivity and impulsivity in approximately half of ADHD-diagnosed adults and prominent inattention symptoms in up to 90%.

Manifestations and impairments of ADHD in adults

Adults may have not been diagnosed as children partly because the firm structure and relatively minimal demands of childhood limited potential impairment from their symptoms. Some research suggests that these individuals experience greater impairment later in life partly because adult settings tend to be more complex and provide less structure than traditional youth settings (Adler, 2004a; Millstein et al., 1997; Murphy & Adler, 2004). It is therefore important when considering a diagnosis of ADHD to recognize specific impairments experienced by adults.

Executive dysfunction: Occupational challenges

Adults with significant and impairing inattentive symptoms often experience specific executive function deficits, including difficulties with manipulating and organizing information (Achenbach et al., 1998; Barkley, 1997; Millstein et al., 1997; Wilens, Faraone, & Biederman, 2004). Problems related to executive functioning often persist in the professional world, and many patients with ADHD present with complaints of problems in their work setting, either related to completing tasks or to interacting with coworkers. Although the high-energy, "driven by a motor" feeling can be an advantage in some instances, more often than not these types of symptoms lead to poor occupational outcomes (Barkley et al., 2004; Barkley & Murphy, 1998). The Milwaukee Young Adult Outcome Study – a long-term sample of children with ADHD and a comorbid conduct disorder – found that employees with ADHD are more likely to be fired, to display more behavioral or attitude problems on the job, and to garner lower work performance ratings (as rated by current supervisors; Barkley et al., 2004; Barkley & Murphy, 1998). Adults with ADHD also often have a low frustration tolerance, which can lead to issues such as high job turnover rates and explosive or irritable episodes. They frequently present with occupational problems, such as difficulty finding and keeping jobs, underperforming or underachieving at work, or an inability to perform up to their intellectual level in school or training (Wolf & Wasserstein, 2001). Moreover, adults with ADHD are more likely to be of a lower social class and to be self-employed: 35% are self-employed by their 30s (Barkley & Murphy, 1998).

To determine the level of occupational impairment that patients are experiencing, it is useful to ask specific questions about their history of work-related difficulties. These questions, which are often interpersonal rather than cognitive, include, "How often have you changed jobs? What was the reason for the job change? Has it been hard to get along with bosses?" (Wender, 1995). Many adults with ADHD do not regulate themselves well and do not self-correct when problems arise, in part because of a lack of self-monitoring. Poor time management and difficulty completing and changing tasks are common manifestations of inattention. Where possible, adults often attempt to compensate for limited organizational skills by enlisting organizational assistance from a life skills coach, an executive assistant or other support staff at work, or a significant other at home (Murphy & Adler, 2004; Weiss, Hechtman, & Weiss, 1999; Wolf & Wasserstein, 2001). Such overt forms of compensation, as well as more subtle ones, provide further evidence toward an ADHD diagnosis when impairment seems less obvious.

Executive dysfunction: Educational challenges

Achieving educational success is another challenge for adults with ADHD, and many present to clinicians with problems related to higher education or vocational training. According to evidence from self-reports and high school transcripts in the Milwaukee Young Adult Outcome Study (Barkley, 1998; Barkley et al., 2004), students with ADHD experience significantly more grade retention, and more students with ADHD are suspended or expelled. The dropout rate is higher, and on average, students with ADHD have lower class rankings and lower grade point averages. Fewer high school students with ADHD enter college than non-ADHD students. For those who do go to college, students with ADHD have a much lower graduation rate than their non-ADHD peers (Barkley, 2002; Barkley et al., 2004; Barkley & Murphy, 1998). It is important for clinicians to note when adults are performing below expectations during educational or vocational training as this can assist in diagnosing ADHD, particularly if the educational difficulties have persisted since early childhood (Barkley, 2002, 2006; Wender, 1995).

Barkley and other authors have suggested that many of the problems experienced by adults with ADHD originate from poor control over executive functioning, which is linked to deficits in the frontal regions of the brain (Barkley, 1998). According to Barkley, when the behavioral inhibition system is functioning properly, it provides a setting that allows one to perform four key executive functions – non-verbal working memory, internalization of speech (verbal working memory), the self-regulation of affect/motivation/arousal, and reconstitution. When problems arise in one or more of the three areas of behavioral inhibition (e.g. inhibiting an initial response to an event, stopping a response once it has started, and protecting a response from interference and distracters), executive functioning difficulties may

occur. This description helps conceptualize how symptoms of both inattention and hyperactivity/impulsivity could arise from similar deficits.

Mood dysregulation

Adults with ADHD often present with mood lability at home or at work and may report lower self-esteem (Wolf & Wasserstein, 2001). One of the pioneers of adult ADHD research, Paul Wender (1995), has suggested that certain key features of a patient's history and functioning are harbingers of difficulty regulating mood. However, he has cautioned that, when depressive ideation is a component of mood volatility, a distinction needs to be made between depressive symptoms resulting from living with undiagnosed ADHD and a comorbid (or primary) diagnosis of depression (dysthymia or major depression). According to Wender (1995), if ADHD is the primary diagnosis, then it is more likely that the depression is secondary to mood lability, and the depressive ideation will be more transient and context-based, as compared with the more consistent dysphoria of major depression or dysthymia.

Mood lability can also make it difficult to distinguish ADHD from the persistent and more pervasive mood changes in bipolar disorder. Querying the patient regarding the longitudinal nature of symptoms, whether they are driven situationally and whether they antedate the attentional symptoms, may be of some help in establishing the differential diagnosis. It should be noted that the longitudinal differential diagnosis with bipolar disorder is further complicated in that several researchers have found that nearly all patients with childhood-onset bipolar disorder also have ADHD (Faraone et al., 1997; Wozniak et al., 1995). Conversely, other research supports the notion that high rates of mood symptoms in patients with adult ADHD may be related to comorbid disorders rather than being a core element of ADHD (Wilens et al., 2004).

Sexuality, family life, and romantic relationships

Research has shown that adults with ADHD may face increased sexual reproductive risks compared with non-ADHD adults. The Milwaukee Young Adult Outcome Study found that, on average, adolescents with ADHD begin sexual activity earlier, at age 15 as opposed to age 16, and tend to have more sexual partners (18.6 vs. 6.5). In addition, adolescents with ADHD are less likely to use contraception, face a greater risk of teen pregnancy (38% vs. 4%), and are at higher risk for STDs (16% vs. 4%) than their non-ADHD peers. Finally, individuals with ADHD report spending less time with each romantic partner (Barkley, 2002; Barkley et al., 2004; Barkley & Murphy, 1998).

Domestically, adults with ADHD tend to report more familial discord within their immediate families than adults without ADHD. Research has shown that adults with ADHD reported having more difficulty with fulfilling parental responsibilities such as helping get their children ready for school, preparing meals, and helping their children with homework than adults without ADHD (Adler, 2002; Adler & Chua, 2002). Some research has shown that adults with ADHD who have significant hyperactive/impulsive symptoms create tensions with other family members because of their tendency toward constant activity (Weiss et al., 1999). Other research has shown that households containing both a parent and a child with ADHD experience more difficulties surrounding organization, setting and keeping routines, day-to-day supervision, stress tolerance, mood stability, compliance with ADHD treatment plans, and increased familial discord than those in which only the parent has the disorder (Faraone et al., 2000; Wolf & Wasserstein, 2001).

Finally, adults with ADHD may often have difficulty managing or sustaining intimate relationships. Adler and Chua (2002) found that adults with ADHD have higher rates of divorce or separation compared to non-ADHD controls. Furthermore, adults with ADHD are more likely to have been to marital therapy or may be experiencing relationship strife (Wender, 1995). Just making the diagnosis of ADHD can help considerably, and effective treatment for a partner's or spouse's ADHD may lessen or eliminate problems that a couple is experiencing (Wender, 1995). Discord in a couple's relationship may indicate a diagnosis of ADHD when such problems arise due to complaints about one partner's frequent interruptions, being inattentive when his or her partner or spouse is speaking, or having a disorganized or inattentive approach to household responsibilities (Wender, 1995).

Gender and cultural considerations

In reviewing extant literature on childhood ADHD, clinicians may be inclined to expect that the majority of adult ADHD patients will be men. There has been a longstanding gender gap in clinical samples of childhood ADHD, with boys outnumbering girls 10 to 1 (Gaub & Carlson, 1997). However, Biederman (2004) and colleagues have suggested that this gender ratio may be misleading because of a difference in behavioral comorbidity between boys and girls with ADHD (Gaub & Carlson, 1997). Girls have lower rates of conduct and oppositional disorder than boys and are less likely to have disruptive behavior be the primary reason for an initial referral, thus leading to an underidentification of girls with ADHD (Biederman, 2004). In epidemiological samples of adults, the ratio of ADHD in men to women is closer to 3 to 2 (Biederman et al., 1994).

Moreover, in a recent study examining gender differences among adults with and without ADHD, Biederman and colleagues (2004) found no evidence that gender was related to current or lifetime comorbid psychiatric disorders, the expression of ADHD symptoms, or patterns of cognitive and psychosocial functioning. Overall, Biederman et al. (2004) reported nearly equal impairments in psychiatric and cognitive functioning from ADHD across genders. However, they did report that women in their study were more likely than men to exhibit the "talks excessively" symptom of ADHD but that men were significantly more likely to have had at least one comorbid psychiatric disorder in their lifetime and were more at risk for all substance use disorders and antisocial personality disorder.

Although the prevalence of ADHD is similar across cultures, cultural differences can be a major factor in determining whether ADHD symptoms are seen by individuals as problematic and, if they are, whether a person seeks care and remains compliant with treatment (Goldman et al., 1998). Cultural differences in familial, educational, and social expectations can affect whether people seek treatment, as do attitudes and beliefs about illness, choice of care, access to care, degree of trust toward majority institutions and authority figures, religious beliefs, and tolerance for certain behaviors (Livingston, 1999). Clinicians should be aware of such differences because they may obscure a proper diagnosis of adult ADHD.

Driving with ADHD

Another significant area of impairment for adults with ADHD is the operation of motor vehicles. The driving skills and habits of adults with ADHD have been examined by a multitude of measures such as self-reports, driving records, lab testing, and driving simulators. Results from driving histories and in driving simulators have shown that adults with ADHD have poorer steering and motor control, more scrapes and crashes, more false braking, and slower reaction times than non-ADHD adults (Barkley & Murphy, 1998; Barkley et al., 2002). Drivers with ADHD also tend to have fewer safe driving habits, are more likely to drive before obtaining the proper permit to operate a motor vehicle, and have more accidents, including more at-fault accidents, than non-ADHD drivers (Barkley & Murphy, 1998; Barkley et al., 2002): 26% percent of drivers with ADHD have three or more vehicular crashes versus 9% of non-ADHD drivers (Barkley et al., 2002). ADHD drivers also experience more severe accidents than non-ADHD drivers as they tend to have higher damage costs and a greater likelihood of receiving injuries from a crash (Barkley & Murphy, 1998; Barkley et al., 2002). In addition, one study found drivers with ADHD to have a lifetime average of 3.9 ± 5.2 SD speeding citations, which was significantly higher than the lifetime average of 2.4 ± 1.5 SD citations for non-ADHD drivers (Barkley et al., 2002). Finally, drivers with ADHD report having significantly more license suspensions or license revocations (mean 0.5 ± 1.26 SD) than those with ADHD (0.1 ± .21 SD; Barkley et al., 2002). In all, motor vehicle operation is a significant area of impairment for adults with ADHD and should be investigated during a clinical evaluation.

Comorbidity and ADHD

In addition to learning disabilities, particularly processing problems such as dyslexia and auditory processing deficits, for which the comorbidity rate is 20% (Barkley & Murphy, 1998), psychiatric disorders often co-present with ADHD. The presence of at least one psychiatric comorbidity in adult ADHD patients is very common, with estimates ranging as high as 77% (Barkley & Murphy, 1998; Biederman et al., 1993; Kessler et al., 2006). It should also be noted that high rates of comorbidity have been documented in epidemiological samples (Kessler, Adler, Barkley, et al., 2005; Willoughby et al., 2000) and are not caused by

Berkson's bias in clinic samples. Thus, assessing the absence or presence of symptoms of other disorders versus ADHD is a key part of an ADHD diagnosis.

Numerous studies have been conducted to assess the prevalence of these comorbidities. Mood disorders as a group have been found to be present in as many as 59% of adults with ADHD (Roy-Byrne et al., 1997): major depressive disorders in 10–50% (Biederman, 2004; Biederman et al., 1998; Murphy & Barkley, 1996; Shekim et al., 1990; Roy-Byrne et al., 1997); bipolar disorder in 9–19% (Biederman, 2004; Roy-Byrne et al., 1997); and dysthymic disorder in 25–32% (Murphy & Barkley, 1996; Shekim et al., 1990; Roy-Byrne et al., 1997). According to the National Comorbidity Survey Replication (NCS-R) – a nationally representative survey conducted in the United States of approximately 10 000 English-speaking household residents aged 18 years and older interviewed between 2001 and 2003 (Kessler et al., 2006; Kessler & Merikangas, 2004) – the mood disorders as a group have a lifetime comorbidity rate with ADHD of 45%: major depressive episode, 41%; bipolar disorder, 18%; and dysthymia, 13% (Kessler et al., 2006). Dysthymia is particularly significant because, in some cases, it may be present as a result of living for years with undiagnosed, untreated ADHD. In other cases, the dysthymia may be co-occurring but not connected.

The lifetime comorbidity rate for adult antisocial behavior may be as high as 28%, and antisocial personality disorder has been diagnosed in 12–19% of adults with ADHD (Barkley & Murphy, 1998; Biederman, 2004; Biederman et al., 1998). Generalized anxiety disorder has been diagnosed in as many as 53% of adults with ADHD (Biederman et al., 1993; Murphy & Barkley, 1996; Shekim et al., 1990). The NCS-R found lifetime comorbidity rates of 9% for antisocial personality disorder, 59% for any anxiety disorder, 70% for impulse disorders, and 21% for intermittent explosive disorder (Kessler et al., 2006). These rates give an overall picture of an ADHD population in which ADHD is rarely the sole psychiatric disorder.

When discussing comorbidity and impairment, it is necessary to consider substance use disorders. Comorbid substance use disorders often accompany ADHD (Kessler et al., 2006). Previous studies have shown that 20–55% of adults with ADHD report a lifetime history of a substance use disorder – two to four times that of non-ADHD controls – with up to 44% of adults with ADHD abusing and/or becoming dependent on alcohol at some point during their lifetime (Biederman et al., 1993, 1997, 1998; Biederman, Wilens, et al., 1995). The NCS-R found a lifetime rate of comorbidity for any substance use disorder at nearly 36%. This rate encompasses a lifetime rate of alcohol abuse at 31% and other drug abuse – including marijuana and cocaine – at 27%. Although rates of self-medication with nicotine and excessive doses of caffeine were not included in the NCS-R, they can also signal the presence of the disorder. Studies have shown that cigarette smoking and nicotine dependence are more common in adults with ADHD than in non-ADHD controls (Sullivan & Rudnik-Levin, 2001) and that adolescents with ADHD are more likely to smoke and to smoke at an earlier age than controls without the disorder (Milberger et al., 1997; Tercyak, Lerman & Audrain, 2002). However, in a comparison of adolescents with ADHD treated with stimulants versus an untreated cohort, Wilens and colleagues found that pharmacotherapy substantially reduced the risk of such abuse (Wilens et al., 2004). Other research has also shown that pharmacotherapy for ADHD, particularly stimulant therapy in childhood, decreases the risk for subsequent substance use disorders to a level similar to that of the general population (Biederman, 2003; Wilens et al., 2003). This supports the concept that a portion of the initial substance use in adolescents and adults with ADHD may be secondary to self-medication.

Given that patients presenting with other mental health disorders also commonly have adult ADHD, it is important to distinguish a comorbid psychiatric disorder from ADHD because it may be the case that ADHD-like symptoms are simply the product of another psychiatric disorder, such as a mood or anxiety disorder (Alpert et al., 1996; Fones et al., 2000; Nierenberg et al., 2005; Wilens, 2004). This will certainly be the case if the symptoms first developed in adulthood without any related or precursory childhood symptoms. By combining the use of ADHD diagnostic and symptom rating scales with a structured interview assessment tool such as the Structured Clinical Interview for DSM-IV Axis I Disorders (SCID), ADHD is diagnosable and discernible from comorbidities (Adler, 2004a; Dowson et al., 2004). This is because most common ADHD comorbidities have reliably different symptoms from ADHD across a set of characteristics, despite the fact that some overlap. Although comorbidities often add layers of complexity to the making of a diagnosis of ADHD in adults, between the structured clinical interview, the use of self-reporting rating scales, collaboration with informants, and the occasional use of other testing mechanisms such as neuropsychological tests, ADHD can be reliably diagnosed and distinguished from comorbidities that have common symptoms. It is important to note that diagnostic tools are essential to this diagnosis process, and currently available diagnostic tools are discussed later in this chapter.

Recognizing ADHD

Presenting signs and symptoms

As discussed, patients with ADHD often present with varied and diverse symptoms. It is warranted to screen a patient presenting with difficulties with concentration, organization, or establishing and maintaining a routine. A patient presenting with a sense of poor self-discipline or low self-esteem is also a candidate for screening, as is a patient presenting with symptoms related to forgetfulness, poor memory, confusion, or trouble thinking clearly (Wolf & Wasserstein, 2001). Adults with ADHD may also cite concerns about procrastination, lack of motivation, and mood lability (Weiss & Murray, 2003; Wolf & Wasserstein, 2001). Furthermore, adults with ADHD often present with chronic conflicts with authority and difficulties in spouse and peer relationships, particularly leading to frequent job changes or poor academic performance despite average (or above-average) intelligence (Elliott, 2002). Comorbidities such as substance abuse and mood disorders may drive patient presentation; if such comorbidities have been unresponsive to treatment, ADHD may be a driving factor in their persistence. Identifying ADHD as an explanatory force for such a presentation or ruling it out can greatly assist the selection of treatment regimens. Finally, because of the high genetic load associated with ADHD, it is highly probable that a child with the condition will have a parent or close family member who also has the disorder (Biederman et al., 1995; Faraone et al., 2005; Frick et al., 1991; Schachar & Wachsmuth, 1990).

It is important to note that, although no single one of the impairments discussed so far indicates that a patient necessarily has ADHD, a patient who exhibits a number of these characteristics is a likely candidate for ADHD and should be screened appropriately. It is also important for clinicians to recognize that they should not treat adults simply as grown-up children. Although symptoms of adult ADHD can be quite similar to those experienced in childhood, they often reflect the changes in activities and responsibilities that come with age. An adult who experienced aimless restlessness in childhood may experience purposeful restlessness in adulthood: the sense of internal restlessness in many adults with ADHD, sometimes manifested as a feeling of ambition and a desire to accomplish, can lead to a compulsive tendency to overwork or to a choice of occupation in which getting up and down and being energetic are essential components of the job, such as sales and marketing. Other childhood hyperactive symptoms such as difficulty remaining seated, running and climbing excessively, squirming and fidgeting, difficulty playing quietly, and talking excessively are commonly manifested in adults with adaptive behaviors, such as working two jobs, working long hours, or choosing a very active job (Weiss et al., 1999). Deficits stemming from inattentive symptoms in particular tend to be more prominent in adults than children, a phenomenon that some research suggests is due in part to adult settings tending to be more complex and providing less structure than traditional youth settings (Adler, 2004a; Millstein et al., 1997; Murphy & Adler, 2004).

Recognizing ADHD during the clinical interview

Diagnosing adults with ADHD is an inherently complex task. The symptoms of ADHD include characteristics seen to varying degrees in all people with and without the disorder, and there is no blood or neurological test on which to rely. However, as we have noted, ADHD can be consistently diagnosed in adults who are experiencing current symptoms of the disorder and who can give a history of their symptoms dating back to early childhood. An accurate diagnosis can be established by a clinical interview as long as the interview establishes the four main diagnostic criteria: (1) an early childhood onset of the disorder, (2) at least six of nine significant symptoms of inattention or hyperactivity, (3) meaningful impairment in at least two settings, and (4) symptoms that are best explained by ADHD and not another psychiatric disorder (Adler, 2004a; American Psychiatric Association, 2000). Research shows that clinical interviews, such as the Adult ADHD Rating Scale (ADHD-RS), Adult ADHD Investigator Symptom Rating Scale (AISRS), and the Conners rating scale, which incorpo-

rate the *DSM-IV* criteria for ADHD, are highly valid and reliable instruments.

Clinical assessments based on adult self-report of childhood symptoms may have certain limitations. Diagnoses in childhood (nonretrospective) are made based on informant reports (i.e. teachers, parents, guardians), as children tend to be unaware of their own symptoms (Jensen et al., 1999). When adults who are being diagnosed with ADHD for the first time are asked to retrospectively describe childhood symptoms, they may have trouble accurately reporting those symptoms, either because of poor memory or a lack of awareness at the time. However, given the frequent unavailability of retrospective informant reports, physicians must rely on retrospective self-assessments (Wender, Wolf, & Wasserstein, 2001). Another, though far less common, limitation is that a patient self-report cannot fully correct for potential malingering – defined as the conscious fabrication or exaggeration of physical or psychological symptoms, including misrepresentations of symptoms, distortions of self-reports, or dishonesty (Quinn, 2003).

In light of these complications, it is clear that a comprehensive clinical interview is essential for diagnosing adult ADHD. Key questions based on the following should focus the interview. Are inattention, hyperactivity, and impulsivity clearly present? Is there hard evidence that symptoms cause impairment in school, work, and social environments and in daily functioning? Have symptoms been observed since childhood? If not, is there an explanation for how symptoms could have gone unnoticed? Is there evidence that symptoms are not due to a lack of dedication or situational or environmental circumstances? Would symptoms be better explained by another medical or psychiatric diagnosis? Finally, do psychiatric comorbidities exist (Murphy & Adler, 2004)? Covering these diagnostic bases during an in-depth, interpersonal interview, combined with the use of certain diagnostic and assessment tools as secondary evaluative instruments, is the most reliable means of diagnosing ADHD in adults (Murphy & Adler, 2004).

Coping strategies

Adults with ADHD have dealt with their symptoms for years, and most have developed compensatory strategies to mitigate the impact of symptoms. To properly diagnose adult ADHD and to accurately assess the impact of the disorder's symptomatology, it is imperative to account for such coping strategies. Clinicians must be aware that elaborate coping strategies make impairment seem less severe, but the coping strategy may be impairing in and of itself and this impairment should be taken into account when rating symptom severity. Because of the adult's use of coping strategies, impairment may also seem limited to a few symptoms, but even infrequent problems can be serious. For example, a clinician might have a patient who controls the impulse to interrupt people most of the time, but if the interruptions happen at critical junctures, such as with his or her boss or in a courtroom, the behavior could have serious consequences (Murphy & Adler, 2004). Similarly, even occasional inattentiveness can have major consequences for a person driving a vehicle or operating heavy machinery (Expert Roundtable, 2004). Some individuals arrange their life to help cope with difficulties stemming from their ADHD symptoms by selecting occupations below their potential or choosing a spouse who provides organizational assistance. The diagnosis sometimes is missed, because clinical interviews tend to focus on cross-sectional questioning, sometimes neglecting the sorts of developmental questions that highlight difficulties with inattention, hyperactivity, and impulsivity that may have persisted for decades (Wender, 1995). As a result, it is essential to develop a comprehensive picture of the life of an adult with ADHD so as not to miss a diagnosis due to the presence of elaborate coping mechanisms that abate impairment.

Current diagnostic and assessment tools

Rating scales are generally cost effective and valuable as they enable clinicians to obtain a large amount of data quickly, including information on the presence and severity of symptoms. They not only aid diagnosis but also measure response to treatment. Rating scales can also assist clinicians who have limited experience in working with adult ADHD as they provide structure and can include prompts to help probe patients further. However, rating scales are limited because they require reliable familiarity with the patient's behavior, they do not account for distorted self-perception due to psychopathology, and some self-report scales may have questionable reliability (Murphy & Adler, 2004). Self-report rating scales in particular, although often used as symptom assessment mech-

anisms, should be combined with clinical interviews and corroborated by data from other sources such as parents, employers, and significant others and from documents such as report cards and work performance assessment records (Murphy & Adler, 2004). Still, Murphy and Adler (2004) asserted, "If designed well and administered properly, ADHD rating scales can accurately reflect the frequency and severity of ADHD symptoms."

It is important for rating scales to assess the 18 core symptoms of the disorder as outlined in the *DSM-IV-TR*, as these symptoms have been established as valid and reliable for diagnosing ADHD and determining disease severity. Furthermore, individuals with these core symptoms often have other objective characteristics, such as the impairments, comorbidities, cognitive deficits, genetic associations and candidate genes, and structural and functional neuroimaging abnormalities that characterize ADHD. Scales that use these core symptoms can detect drug–placebo differences in anti-ADHD medication. Several diagnostic systems and rating scales assess domains outside of the traditional *DSM-IV-TR* core symptoms. Social and occupational deficits are important features of ADHD, but these deficits are not specific to ADHD and have often been observed in individuals without ADHD who suffer from other disorders (Adler & Cohen, 2004). Although this information may prove useful, the relationship of these additional domains to ADHD remains unclear without further study.

Diagnostic scales

A number of available scales can be used to assist in the diagnosis of adult ADHD. The Conners Adult ADHD Diagnostic Interview for *DSM-IV* is a clinician-administered interview designed to assess the presence of the 18 symptoms for ADHD as defined by *DSM-IV*. Each question is accompanied by specific prompts and examples of symptoms, and the interview screens for impairment in school/work, home, and social settings present in childhood and adulthood. The interview begins by asking patients, "What is going on in your life that leads you to believe you have attention-deficit/hyperactivity disorder or ADHD?" The interviewer then asks the patient about his or her childhood history, including gestation, delivery, and temperament and developmental, environmental, and medical history risk factors. Childhood academic history and adult educational, occupational, and social/interpersonal histories are also examined, as are health history and psychiatric history. Finally, the patient is screened briefly for comorbidities. The completed interview can then be used to determine the presence or absence of ADHD and, if present, the subtype (Adler & Cohen, 2004).

Barkley's Current Symptoms Scale–Self-Report Form is a self-report scale of 18 items that correspond to the symptoms listed in the *DSM-IV* diagnostic criteria. The items alternate between assessing inattentive symptoms (odd-numbered questions) and hyperactive/impulsive symptoms (even-numbered questions) on a Likert-type frequency scale ranging from 0 (never or rarely) to 3 (very often). Over the course of the 18 questions, patients are asked how often these symptoms interfere with school, relationships, work, and home life and at what age symptoms began. This form then concludes with eight questions about symptoms of comorbid oppositional-defiant disorder (ODD). Barkley also has developed several supplemental scales, including the Childhood Symptoms Scale–Self-Report Form; the Developmental Employment, Health, and Social History Form; and the Work Performance Rating Scale–Self-Report Form. These supplemental scales can be sent to patients to complete before their first clinic visit and so produce a thorough diagnostic picture. In addition, the Barkley scales can capture second-person observations through the use of Other Report Forms. Ideally, the patient's parent (if available) should complete the Childhood Symptoms Scale – Other Report Form and the Childhood School Performance Scale – Other Report Form, whereas the Current Symptoms Scale – Other Report Form should be completed by someone who regularly sees the patient on a day-to-day basis, such as a spouse or significant other. Together, these scales form a comprehensive picture of the patient's past and present symptoms and functioning (Adler & Cohen, 2004).

The Brown ADD Scales Diagnostic Form is a clinician-administered measure that begins with questions about clinical history, including the impact of symptoms on work, school, leisure, peer interactions, self-image, and early schooling. The clinician asks about the patient's family history, physical health, drug use, and sleep habits. The clinician also obtains collateral data from an observer or significant other and screens for comorbidity. A Wechsler Adult Intelligence Scale can be used to set a baseline for use in comparing the patient's concentration level with verbal and spatial capabilities. All of these data are looked at in conjunction with the patient's score on the 40-item ADD Scale (which can be either clinician- or patient-administered) to establish a diagnosis (Adler & Cohen, 2004).

The Kiddie-SADS (K-SADS) Diagnostic Interview section on ADHD includes extensive prompts that clinicians can use to assess for ADHD according to the *DSM-IV* criteria. However, its use with adults is limited as the questions are clearly designed for pediatric patients. For example, prompts for the item "Difficulty Remaining Seated" include "Was there ever a time when you got out of your seat a lot at school? Did you get into trouble for this? Was it hard to stay in your seat at school? What about at dinnertime?" (Adler & Cohen, 2004).

The Adult ADHD Clinician Diagnostic Scale (ACDS v1.2) is a semi-structured interview that documents current adult symptomatology. Adapted from the *DSM-IV* domains and K-SADS, the ACDS v1.2 includes suggested prompts for the clinician, which are intended to probe for the impact and severity of these symptoms on patient functioning. This scale includes a retrospective childhood history evaluation and an evaluation of current symptom status (Adler, 2004b). The ACDS v1.2 establishes the cornerstone criteria of a *DSM-IV* diagnosis of adult ADHD, including (1) assessment of severity of childhood symptoms and age of onset, (2) severity of adult ADHD symptoms, (3) documentation of duration of symptoms, and (4) assessment of impairment.

The adult ADHD prompts included in the ACDS v1.2 create a semi-structured interview instrument. The prompts can also be inserted into the Attention-Deficit/Hyperactivity Disorder Rating Scale (ADHD-RS, discussed in the next section), which is a current-symptom assessment instrument, to create a semi-structured measurement. These prompts have been validated in the reexamination of the prevalence of adult ADHD in the National Comorbidity Survey-Replication (Kessler, Adler, Ames, et al., 2005) and a variety of treatment trials (Spencer et al., 1995, 2001, 2005).

Current-symptom surveys and rating scales

Current-symptom surveys can be divided into clinician-administered and self-report forms. A number of the scales are normed and can provide population comparisons. Self-report scales are an effective way to capture the symptoms of adults with ADHD, as symptoms such as internalized restlessness, feeling disorganized, and distraction may be more readily apparent to the patient than to observers (O'Donnell, McCann, & Pluth, 2001). Semi-structured scales are also useful when assessing new patients who may be less aware about their symptoms as they allow the use of an extensive list of example prompts to establish a comprehensive baseline for impairment. Some scales adhere more strictly to the *DSM-IV-TR* symptom domains, whereas others expand the adult ADHD symptomatology to include assessment of mood regulation and executive function (Adler & Cohen, 2004).

The ADHD-RS is an 18-item rating scale that measures symptoms using a 4-point Likert-based severity scale (0 = none, 1 = mild, 2 = moderate, and 3 = severe). This scale is based on the *DSM-IV-TR* criteria for ADHD, with nine items assessing inattentive symptoms and nine items assessing hyperactive and impulsive symptoms. The ADHS-RS has been developed and standardized for use in children, but clinicians can be trained to use it with adult patients (Adler & Cohen, 2004; DuPaul et al., 1998). A recent advance has been the use of the ADHD-RS paired with the prompts contained in the ACDS v1.2, as was discussed earlier (Murphy & Adler, 2004).

The Brown ADD Scale is a frequency scale with 40 items. Patients respond in terms of frequency (0 = never, 1 = once a week or less, 2 = twice a week, or 3 = almost daily), based on symptom descriptions such as "misunderstands directions for assignments, completion of forms, etc." and "starts tasks (e.g. paperwork, chores) but doesn't complete them." This assessment has normed, standardized, and validated clinician-rated and self-report versions (Adler & Cohen, 2004).

The Wender-Reimherr Adult Attention Deficit Disorder Scale (WRAADS) uses the Utah Criteria in adults with ADHD to measure the severity of symptoms in seven categories: attention difficulties, hyperactivity/restlessness, temper, affective lability, emotional overreactivity, disorganization, and impulsivity. The scale rates the individual items from 0 (not present) to 2 (clearly present) and summarizes each of the seven categories on a scale of 0 (none) to 4 (very much). The WRAADS may be particularly useful for assessing mood lability symptoms of ADHD. A recent study found the WRAADS to be an effective tool for measuring improvement of mood dysregulation during a large, controlled trial of the norepinephrine reuptake inhibitor atomoxetine (Reimherr et al., 2003).

The screening version of the Conners' Adult ADHD Rating Scale (CAARS) is a 30-item frequency scale with items like "has difficulty organizing tasks and activities" and "is 'on the go' or acts as if 'driven by a motor.'" Symptoms are assessed on a combination of frequency and severity. Patients respond on a 4-point Likert-type scale (0 = not at all, never; 1 = just a little, once in a while; 2 = pretty much, often; and 3 = very much, very frequently). All 18 items from the *DSM-IV* can be extrapolated from the CAARS. There are also observer and self-report versions of the CAARS. Both the clinician-administered and self-rated versions of this scale have been validated and normed (Adler & Cohen, 2004).

The Adult ADHD Self-Report Scales (ASRS) consist of a 6-item screening tool for general use and an 18-item symptom checklist for patients who might be at risk. These scales were developed by the workgroup on adult ADHD and are copyrighted by the World Health Organization. The ASRS symptom checklist asks patients about the 18 symptom domains identified in the *DSM-IV*, modified to reflect the adult presentation of ADHD symptoms, with a context basis of symptoms provided. Symptoms are rated on a frequency basis, ranging from 0 (none) to 4 (very often). The 6-item screening version, the ASRS v1.1 screener (extracted from the full 18-item symptom assessment scale), is available for assessing patients in the community to establish whether they are at increased risk for ADHD and is designed to be used before the symptom checklist. The six items in the ASRS screener were selected based on psychometric factor analyses of the diagnostic interviews of patients with and without ADHD in the NCS-R (Adler, 2004b).

Neither the 6-item ASRS v1.1 screener nor the full ASRS 18-item symptom assessment version is meant to be a stand-alone diagnostic tool. The diagnosis of ADHD remains predicated on assessment of current symptoms, impairment, and childhood onset of symptoms. The ASRS symptom checklist and other symptom assessment tools are designed to assess the breadth of ADHD symptoms in fulfilling the first criteria. Of note, the ASRS v1.1 screener has been shown to have a 94.3% predictive value and is useful in identifying adults at risk for ADHD (Adler, 2004b).

Finally, the Adult ADHD Quality of Life (AAQoL) scale is a current-symptom psychometric scale that identifies and assesses five ADHD-related quality-of-life domains: daily activities, work, psychological well-being, physical well-being, and relationships (Brod et al., 2004). The AAQoL consists of 23 self-rated items encompassing these five domains. Respondents rate each item on a 5-point scale, from "not at all" to "extremely." The AAQoL assists clinicians in determining the impact of ADHD symptomatology and of treatment on quality of life (Brod et al., 2004).

Summary

Although some areas of understanding of adult ADHD remain limited, there is a strong sense of how to proceed with diagnosis, using current *DSM-IV-TR* criteria as a guide. A thorough clinical interview, aided by the use of rating scales for current symptoms, collateral information about childhood from parents or siblings, and the use of a clinical evaluation to determine comorbidity, forms the backbone of the diagnostic assessment. The poor psychosocial outcomes of patients with ADHD, often a consequence of unrecognized, untreated disorder manifestation, can also serve as a diagnostic indicator. Accordingly, adult ADHD remains a valid clinical diagnosis, and the clinician-administered interview that adheres to the cardinal *DSM-IV-TR* criteria for making the diagnosis remains the cornerstone of the diagnostic evaluation.

References

Achenbach TM, Howell CT, McConaughy SH, Stanger C. (1998). Six-year predictors of problems in a national sample: IV. Young adult signs of disturbance. *J Am Acad Child Adolesc Psychiatry* 37(7):718–27.

Adler LA. (2002). Issues in the diagnosis and treatment of the adult patient with ADHD. *Johns Hopkins Advanced Stud Med* 2:902–5.

Adler LA. (2004a). Adult ADHD: current understanding. Abstract presented at: 51st Annual Meeting of the American Academy of Child & Adolescent Psychiatry; Washington, DC.

Adler LA. (2004b). Adult ADHD diagnostic and self-report symptom scales: development and validation in the National Comorbidity Survey Replication (NCS-R) cohort. Symposium presented at: 157th Annual Meeting of the American Psychiatric Association; New York.

Adler LA, Chua HC. (2002). Management of ADHD in adults. *J Clin Psychiatry* 63(suppl 12):29–35.

Adler LA, Cohen J. (2004). Diagnosis and evaluation of adults with attention-deficit/hyperactivity disorder. *Psychiatr Clin North Am* 27(2):187–201.

Alpert JE, Maddocks A, Nierenberg AA, et al. (1996). Attention deficit hyperactivity disorder in childhood among adults with major depression. *Psychiatry Res* 62(3):213–9.

American Psychiatric Association. (1968). *Diagnostic and Statistical Manual of Mental Disorders*. 2nd ed. Washington, DC: American Psychiatric Association.

American Psychiatric Association. (1980). *Diagnostic and Statistical Manual of Mental Disorders*. 3rd ed. Washington, DC: American Psychiatric Association.

American Psychiatric Association. (1984). *Diagnostic and Statistical Manual of Mental Disorders*. 3rd ed. rev. Washington, DC: American Psychiatric Association.

American Psychiatric Association. (1994). *Diagnostic and Statistical Manual of Mental Disorders*. 4th ed. Washington, DC: American Psychiatric Association.

American Psychiatric Association. (2000). *Diagnostic and Statistical Manual of Mental Disorders*. 4th ed, text revision. Washington, DC: American Psychiatric Association.

Barkley RA. (1997). Behavioral inhibition, sustained attention, and executive functions: constructing a unifying theory of ADHD. *Psychol Bull* 121(1):65–94.

Barkley RA. (1998). *Attention-Deficit Hyperactivity Disorder: A Handbook for Diagnosis and Treatment*. 2nd ed. New York: Guilford Press.

Barkley RA. (2002). Major life activity and health outcomes associated with attention-deficit/hyperactivity disorder. *J Clin Psychiatry* 63(suppl 12):10–15.

Barkley RA. (2006). Primary symptoms, diagnostic criteria, prevalence, and gender differences. In Barkley RA, ed. *Attention Deficit Hyperactivity Disorder: A Handbook for Diagnosis and Treatment*. 3rd ed. New York: Guilford Press: 76–121.

Barkley RA, Fischer M, Smallish L, Fletcher K. (2004). Young adult follow-up of hyperactive children: antisocial activities and drug use. *J Child Psychol Psychiatry* 45(2):195–211.

Barkley RA, Murphy KR. *Attention-Deficit Hyperactivity Disorder: A Clinical Workbook*. 2nd ed. New York: Guilford Press.

Barkley RA, Murphy KR, Dupaul GI, Bush T. (2002). Driving in young adults with attention deficit hyperactivity disorder: knowledge, performance, adverse outcomes, and the role of executive functioning. *J Int Neuropsychol Soc* 8(5):655–72.

Biederman J. (2003). Pharmacotherapy for attention-deficit/hyperactivity disorder (ADHD) decreases the risk for substance abuse: findings from a longitudinal follow-up of youths with and without ADHD. *J Clin Psychiatry* 64(suppl 11):3–8.

Biederman J. (2004). Impact of comorbidity in adults with attention-deficit/hyperactivity disorder. *J Clin Psychiatry* 65(suppl 3):3–7.

Biederman J, Faraone SV. (2005). Attention-deficit hyperactivity disorder. *Lancet* **366**(9481):237–48.

Biederman J, Faraone SV, Mick E, et al. (1995). High risk for attention deficit hyperactivity disorder among children of parents with childhood onset of the disorder: a pilot study. *Am J Psychiatry* **152**(3):431–5.

Biederman J, Faraone SV, Monuteaux MC, Bober M, Cadogen E. (2004). Gender effects on attention-deficit/hyperactivity disorder in adults, revisited. *Biol Psychiatry* **55**(7):692–700.

Biederman J, Faraone SV, Spencer T, Wilens T, Mick E, Lapey KA. (1994). Gender differences in a sample of adults with attention deficit hyperactivity disorder. *Psychiatry Res* **53**(1):13–29.

Biederman J, Faraone SV, Spencer T, Wilens T, Norman D, Lapey KA, et al. (1993). Patterns of psychiatric comorbidity, cognition, and psychosocial functioning in adults with attention deficit hyperactivity disorder. *Am J Psychiatry* **150**(12):1792–8.

Biederman J, Mick E, Faraone SV. (2000). Age-dependent decline of symptoms of attention deficit hyperactivity disorder: impact of remission definition and symptom type. *Am J Psychiatry* **157**(5):816–8.

Biederman J, Wilens TE, Mick E, Faraone SV, Spencer T. (1998). Does attention-deficit hyperactivity disorder impact the developmental course of drug and alcohol abuse and dependence? *Biol Psychiatry* **44**(4):269–73.

Biederman J, Wilens T, Mick E, Faraone SV, Weber W, Curtis S, et al. (1997). Is ADHD a risk factor for psychoactive substance use disorders? Findings from a four-year prospective follow-up study. *J Am Acad Child Adolesc Psychiatry* **36**(1):21–9.

Biederman J, Wilens T, Mick E, Milberger S, Spencer TJ, Faraone SV. (1995). Psychoactive substance use disorders in adults with attention deficit hyperactivity disorder (ADHD): effects of ADHD and psychiatric comorbidity. *Am J Psychiatry* **152**(11):1652–8.

Brod M, Johnston J, Able S, Swindle R. (2004). Adult ADHD quality of life (AAQoL): a new measure. Abstract presented at the 51st Annual Meeting of the American Academy of Child & Adolescent Psychiatry, Washington, DC.

Dowson JH, McLean A, Bazanis E, et al. (2004). The specificity of clinical characteristics in adults with attention-deficit/hyperactivity disorder: a comparison with patients with borderline personality disorder. *Eur Psychiatry* **19**(2):72–8.

DuPaul GJ, Power TJ, Anastopoulos AD, et al. (1998). *ADHD Rating Scale–IV: Checklists, Norms, and Clinical Interpretation.* New York: Guilford Press.

Elliott H. (2002). Attention deficit hyperactivity disorder in adults: a guide for the primary care physician. *South Med J* **95**(7):736–42.

Expert roundtable highlights: stimulants and atomoxetine in the treatment of attention-deficit/hyperactivity disorder. (2004). *J Clin Psychiatry* **19**:1–23.

Faraone SV, Biederman J, Friedman D. (2000). Validity of DSM-IV subtypes of attention-deficit/hyperactivity disorder: a family study perspective. *J Am Acad Child Adolesc Psychiatry* **39**(3):300–7.

Faraone SV, Biederman J, Mennin D, Wozniak J, Spencer T. (1997). Attention-deficit hyperactivity disorder with bipolar disorder: a familial subtype? *J Am Acad Child Adolesc Psychiatry* **36**(10):1378–87.

Faraone SV, Perlis RH, Doyle AE, et al. (2005). Molecular genetics of attention-deficit/hyperactivity disorder. *Biol Psychiatry* **57**(11):1313–23.

Fones CS, Pollack MH, Susswein L, Otto M. (2000). History of childhood attention deficit hyperactivity disorder (ADHD) features among adults with panic disorder. *J Affect Disord* **58**(2):99–106.

French MT, Zarkin GA, Hartwell TD, Bray JW. (1995). Prevalence and consequences of smoking, alcohol use, and illicit drug use at five worksites. *Public Health Rep* **110**(5):593–9.

Frick PJ, Lahey BB, Christ MG, Loeber R, Green S. (1991). History of childhood behavior problems in biological relatives of boys with attention-deficit hyperactivity disorder and conduct disorder. *J Clin Child Psychol* **20**(4):445–51.

Gaub M, Carlson CL. (1997). Gender differences in ADHD: a meta-analysis and critical review. *J Am Acad Child Adolesc Psychiatry* **36**(8):1036–45.

Goldman LS, Genel M, Bezman RJ, Slanetz PJ, for the Council on Scientific Affairs AMA. (1998). Diagnosis and treatment of attention-deficit/hyperactivity disorder in children and adolescents. *JAMA* **279**(14): 1100–7.

Greene RW, Biederman J, Faraone SV, Wilens TE, Mick E, Blier HK. (1999). Further validation of social impairment as a predictor of substance use disorders: findings from a sample of siblings of boys with and without ADHD. *J Clin Child Psychol* **28**(3):349–54.

Jensen PS, Rubio-Stipec M, Canino G, et al. (1999). Parent and child contributions to diagnosis of mental disorder: are both informants always necessary? *J Am Acad Child Adolesc Psychiatry* **38**(12):1569–79.

Kessler RC, Adler L, Ames M, et al. (2005). The World Health Organization Adult ADHD Self-Report Scale (ASRS): a short screening scale for use in the general population. *Psychol Med* **35**(2):245–56.

Kessler RC, Adler L, Barkley RA, Biederman J, Conners CK, Demler O, et al. (2006). The prevalence and correlates of adult ADHD in the United States: Results from the National Comorbidity Survey Replication. *Am J Psychiatry* **163**(4):716–23.

Kessler RC, Adler LA, Barkley R, Biederman J, Conners CK, Faraone SV, et al. (2005). Patterns and predictors of attention-deficit/hyperactivity disorder persistence into adulthood: results from the national comorbidity survey replication. *Biol Psychiatry* **57**(11):1442–51.

Kessler RC, Merikangas KR. (2004). The National Comorbidity Survey Replication (NCS-R): background and aims. *Int J Methods Psychiatr Res* **13**(2):60–8.

Livingston R. (1999). Cultural issues in diagnosis and treatment of ADHD. *J Am Acad Child Adolesc Psychiatry* **38**(12):1591–4.

Michelson D, Adler L, Spencer T, et al. (2003). Atomoxetine in adults with ADHD: two randomized, placebo-controlled studies. *Biol Psychiatry* **53**(2): 112–20.

Mick E, Faraone SV, Biederman J. (2004). Age-dependent expression of attention-deficit/hyperactivity disorder symptoms. *Psychiatr Clin North Am*; **27**(2):215–24.

Milberger S, Biederman J, Faraone SV, Chen L, Jones J. (1997). ADHD is associated with early initiation of cigarette smoking in children and adolescents. *J Am Acad Child Adolesc Psychiatry* **36**(1):37–44.

Millstein RB, Wilens T, Biederman J, Spencer J. (1997). Presenting ADHD symptoms and subtypes in clinically referred adults with ADHD. *J Attent Disord* **2**(3): 159–66.

Murphy KR, Adler LA. (2004). Assessing attention-deficit/hyperactivity disorder in adults: focus on rating scales. *J Clin Psychiatry* **65**(suppl 3):12–17.

Murphy K, Barkley RA. (1996). Attention deficit hyperactivity disorder adults: comorbidities and adaptive impairments. *Compr Psychiatry* **37**(6):393–401.

Nierenberg AA, Miyahara S, Spencer T, Wisniewski SR, Otto MW, Simon N, et al. (2005) Clinical and diagnostic implications of lifetime attention-deficit/hyperactivity disorder comorbidity in adults with bipolar disorder: data from the first 1000 STEP-BD participants. *Biol Psychiatry* **57**(11):1467–73.

O'Donnell JP, McCann KK, Pluth S. (2001). Assessing adult ADHD using a self-report symptom checklist. *Psychol Rep* **88**(3 pt 1):871–81.

Quinn CA. (2003). Detection of malingering in assessment of adult ADHD. *Arch Clin Neuropsychol* **18**(4):379–95.

Reimherr F, Strong RE, Hedges DW, et al. (2003). Emotional dysregulation in ADHD and response to atomoxetine. Abstract presented at: 156th Annual Meeting of the American Psychiatric Association; San Francisco.

Roy-Byrne P, Scheele L, Brinkley J, et al. (1997). Adult attention-deficit hyperactivity disorder: assessment guidelines based on clinical presentation to a specialty clinic. *Compr Psychiatry* **38**(3):133–40.

Schachar R, Wachsmuth R. (1990). Hyperactivity and parental psychopathology. *J Child Psychol Psychiatry* **31**(3):381–92.

Shekim WO, Asarnow RF, Hess E, Zaucha K, Wheeler N. (1990). A clinical and demographic profile of a sample of adults with attention deficit hyperactivity disorder, residual state. *Compr Psychiatry* **31**(5):416–25.

Spencer T, Biederman J, Wilens T, Doyle R, Surman C., Prince J, et al. (2005). A large, double-blind, randomized clinical trial of methylphenidate in the treatment of adults with attention-deficit/hyperactivity disorder. *Biol Psychiatry* **57**(5):456–63.

Spencer T, Biederman J, Wilens T, Faraone S, Prince J, Gerard K, et al. (2001). Efficacy of a mixed amphetamine salts compound in adults with attention-deficit/hyperactivity disorder. *Arch Gen Psychiatry* **58**(8):775–82.

Spencer T, Wilens T, Biederman J, Faraone SV, Ablon JS, Lapey K. (1995). A double-blind, crossover comparison of methylphenidate and placebo in adults with childhood-onset attention-deficit hyperactivity disorder. *Arch Gen Psychiatry* **52**(6):434–43.

Sullivan MA, Rudnik-Levin F. (2001). Attention deficit/hyperactivity disorder and substance abuse. Diagnostic and therapeutic considerations. *Ann N Y Acad Sci* **931**:251–70.

Tercyak KP, Lerman C, Audrain J. (2002). Association of attention-deficit/hyperactivity disorder symptoms with levels of cigarette smoking in a community sample of adolescents. *J Am Acad Child Adolesc Psychiatry* **41**(7):799–805.

Weiss MA, Hechtman LT, Weiss G. (1999). *ADHD in Adulthood: A Guide to Current Theory, Diagnosis, and Treatment.* Baltimore: Johns Hopkins University Press.

Weiss MA, Murray C. (2003). Assessment and management of attention-deficit hyperactivity disorder in adults. *Can Med Assoc J* **168**(6):715–22.

Wender PH. (1995). *Attention-Deficit/Hyperactivity Disorder in Adults.* New York: Oxford University Press.

Wender PH, Wolf LE, Wasserstein J. (2001). Adults with ADHD. An overview. *Ann N Y Acad Sci* **931**: 1–16.

Wilens TE. (2004). Attention-deficit/hyperactivity disorder and the substance use disorders: the nature of the relationship, subtypes at risk, and treatment issues. *Psychiatr Clin North Am* **27**(2):283–301.

Wilens TE, Dodson W. (2004). A clinical perspective of attention-deficit/hyperactivity disorder into adulthood. *J Clin Psychiatry* **65**(10):1301–13.

Wilens TE, Faraone SV, Biederman J. (2004). Attention-deficit/hyperactivity disorder in adults. *JAMA* **292**(5):619–23.

Wilens TE, Faraone SV, Biederman J, Gunawardene S. (2003). Does stimulant therapy of attention-deficit/hyperactivity disorder beget later substance abuse? A meta-analytic review of the literature. *Pediatrics* **111**(1):179–85.

Willoughby MT, Curran PJ, Costello EJ, Angold A. (2000). Implications of early versus late onset of attention-deficit/hyperactivity disorder symptoms.

J Am Acad Child Adolesc Psychiatry **39**(12): 1512–9.

Wolf LE, Wasserstein J. (2001). Adult ADHD: concluding thoughts. *Ann N Y Acad Sci* **931**:396–408.

Wozniak J, Biederman J, Kiely K, et al. (1995). Mania-like symptoms suggestive of childhood-onset bipolar disorder in clinically referred children. *J Am Acad Child Adolesc Psychiatry* **34**(7):867–76.

Chapter

9

Neurocognitive characteristics of adults with attention-deficit hyperactivity disorder

Jonathan H. Dowson and Andrew D. Blackwell

Introduction

ADHD, as defined by *DSM-IV* (American Psychiatric Association, 1994), is one of the most common disorders of childhood and involves inattention, overactivity, and impulsivity. Most prevalence estimates have ranged between 3–7% (American Psychiatric Association, 1994; Barbaresi et al., 2002; Biederman, Mick, & Faraone, 2000; Sachdev, 1999; Wender, Wolf, & Wasserstein, 2001), and prospective studies have shown that clinically significant features of ADHD can persist into adulthood in at least one-third (and perhaps up to two-thirds) of those with a diagnosis in childhood (Wender et al., 2001). An estimate of the prevalence of adult ADHD in a U.S. sample aged between 18–44 in 2006 was 4.4% (Kessler et al., 2006). However, in general, there is a decline in severity in adolescence, in particular for overactivity (Biederman et al., 2000).

A diagnosis of ADHD encompasses heterogeneous presentations in relation to the combinations and severity of the syndrome's characteristics, and because these presentations vary throughout the whole population (Levy et al., 1999), a naturally occurring diagnostic threshold does not exist. Moreover, diagnosis can be confounded by comorbid psychopathology (Sachdev, 1999). Therefore, the level of dysfunction required for a diagnosis is arbitrary and, in part, usually reflects a clinician's judgment. Although for most subjects the etiology of ADHD is "strongly genetic in nature" (Wender et al., 2001), involving variable combinations of the effects of many genes (Sachdev, 1999), genetic factors interact with other environmental causal factors (Banerjee, Middleton, & Faraone, 2007). A recent meta-analysis of molecular genetic studies on variants in the dopamine D4 gene and D5 receptor gene has shown that these variants have been repeatedly asso-

ciated with ADHD (Thapar et al., 2007). It is possible that, in a minority of subjects, examples of the syndrome, as currently defined, may be due to nongenetic factors alone.

Heterogeneity of the behavioral abnormalities in ADHD has motivated the search for "endophenotypes," which are those characteristics of a disorder that are linked relatively closely to its neurobiological substrates (Doyle et al., 2005). Neurocognitive measures are potential candidates (Castellanos & Tannock, 2002; Kuntsi, Oosterlaan, & Stevenson, 2001; Sanuga-Barke & Castellanos, 2005; Swanson et al., 1998). The identification of endophenotypes could lead to more etiologically homogeneous samples, which would be expected to benefit further research, help overcome problems of reliability in relation to current assessment methods, and enable more accurate prediction of treatment response.

Various neurocognitive domains have been proposed as possible candidate endophenotypes for ADHD. Indeed, attempts have been made to identify a single neurocognitive deficit that could be used as a diagnostic test; for example, in relation to various executive functions (EFs) that "maintain an appropriate problem-solving set to attain a later goal" (Willcutt et al., 2005). However, groups of ADHD subjects show considerable heterogeneity in relation to any single neurocognitive deficit (Nigg, 2005). For example, on one measure of EF – the stop-signal reaction time – only about half of three samples of children with ADHD showed a deficit (Nigg, 2005). Whereas it has been reported that nearly 80% of children with ADHD have a deficit on at least one measure of EF, this can also be said of around half of control subjects (Pennington, 2005). A meta-analysis of 83 studies involving EFs found consistently identified deficits on group

---

ADHD in Adults: Characterization, Diagnosis and Treatment, ed. Jan Buitelaar, Cornelis Kan and Philip Asherson.
Published by Cambridge University Press. © Cambridge University Press 2011.

measures of response inhibition, vigilance, working memory, and planning, but noted moderate effect sizes and lack of universality (Willcutt et al., 2005).

Thus, single-domain neurocognitive endophenotypes in ADHD are likely to have limited validity. Adequate neurocognitive assessment in ADHD is likely to require a battery of tests measuring several neurocognitive domains. A profile of neurocognitive impairments has been proposed as the basis for multiple-deficit models for new definitions of ADHD subtypes (Pennington, 2005).

The aim of this chapter is to provide an overview of the neurocognitive impairments that have been reported in groups of adults with ADHD and to highlight the challenges faced by researchers in attempting to measure the neurocognitive characteristics associated with ADHD. The chapter concludes by examining the effects of pharmacological treatments for ADHD on neurocognitive performance and by considering the role of neurocognitive assessment in current and future clinical practice.

Neurocognitive deficits associated with adult ADHD

Neurocognitive deficits, particularly involving attention and EFs, have been reported in numerous studies of children (Barkley, Grodzinsky, & DuPaul, 1992; Barnett et al., 2001; Burden & Mitchell, 2005; Grodzinsky & Diamond, 1992; Kempton et al., 1999; Osterlaan, Scheres, & Sergeant, 2005; Pennington & Ozonoff, 1996; Rhodes, Coghill, & Matthews, 2005; Seidman et al., 1997; Tannoch, Ickowicz, & Schachar, 1995; Williams et al., 2000) and adults (Bekker et al., 2005; Boonstra et al., 2005; Gallagher & Blader, 2001; Johnson et al., 2001; Kovner et al., 1998; Lijffijt et al., 2005; Tsal, Shalev, & Mevorach, 2005; Woods, Lovejoy, & Ball, 2002) with ADHD. These studies have implicated a range of neurocognitive domains and intrasubject performance variability (Castellanos et al., 2005; Toplak & Tannock, 2005) involving sustained attention (Gallagher & Blader, 2001; Lijffijt et al., 2005), verbal fluency (Boonstra et al., 2005), set shifting (Boonstra et al., 2005; Gallagher & Blader, 2001), word reading (Boonstra et al., 2005), color naming (Boonstra et al., 2005), working memory (Castellanos & Tannock, 2002), response inhibition (Boonstra et al., 2005; Lijffijt et al., 2005), delay aversion, temporal information processing (Castellanos & Tannock, 2002; Nigg, 2005; Yang et al., 2007), speed of information

processing, arithmetic skills, motivational dysfunction (involving frontostriatal reward circuits and impaired signaling of delayed reward; Castellanos & Tannock, 2002; Sonuga-Barke, 2005), and "cognitive-energetic" dysfunction (with impaired regulation of activation and effort needed for ongoing information processing; Sergeant, 2005). The last dysfunction is consistent with slower performance and greater intrasubject variability in ADHD subjects (Pennington, 2005).

Several theories have proposed "core" or primary neurocognitive deficits; for example, response inhibition deficit (Bekker et al., 2005), working memory dysfunction, and delay aversion (Kuntsi et al., 2001) have been suggested as possible candidates underlying hyperactivity. As noted earlier, consistent candidates for a core deficit have been one or more EFs, but although specific examples of EFs, such as response inhibition, have been shown to be impaired in both children and adults (Bekker et al., 2005). accumulating evidence has indicated that both children and adults with ADHD can show a wider range of cognitive impairments (Kuntsi, McLouglin, & Asherson, 2006; McLean et al., 2004).

At least some of the diverse manifestations of cognitive impairment may share a common neuropathological substrate involving dysregulation of frontostriatal networks. Indeed, converging evidence from neuroimaging studies offers support for the hypothesis of frontostriatal brain dysfunction in ADHD (Himelstein, Newcorn, & Halperin, 2000). Studies employing magnetic resonance imaging (MRI) have indicated abnormalities in the size and shape of the caudate and pallidum (Castellanos et al., 1994, 1996; Hynd, Semrud-Clikeman, et al., 1991: Hynd et al., 1993) and reductions in right frontal cortex volume (Castellanos et al., 1996; Hynd et al., 1990). Investigation of cerebral blood flow using single photon emission computer tomography (SPECT) has revealed frontal and striatal hypoperfusion in ADHD children, effects that were ameliorated by the administration of stimulant medication (Lou, Henriksen, & Bruhn, 1984; Lou et al., 1989). More recently, functional MRI has demonstrated atypical frontostriatal function in ADHD children when performing two response inhibition tasks. In addition, methylphenidate was shown to differentially modulate striatal activation in the ADHD group relative to the control group (Vaidya et al., 1998).

In a 2001 review of brain imaging studies of ADHD, it was concluded that frontostriatal and cerebellar dysfunction are consistently implicated in subjects with ADHD (Giedd, Blumenthal, Molloy, & Castellanos, 2001). Although most neuroimaging investigations have focused on ADHD in childhood or adolescence, there is now an emerging literature suggesting that abnormalities in the same brain regions underlie the syndrome in adults (Faraone et al., 2000; Makris et al., 2007). The observation that the most commonly observed cognitive deficits in adult ADHD tend to be shown on tests with known sensitivity to frontal lobe dysfunction, coupled with the emerging neuropathological literature demonstrating abnormality in frontostriatal systems, suggests that frontostriatal dysregulation and associated cognitive impairments may be an important factor in the cognitive-behavioral phenotype of adult ADHD. A recent review of brain imaging studies of ADHD has noted that changes are related to extrafrontal regions as well as frontostriatal circuits (Kelly, Margulies, & Castellanos, 2007), and differential right hemisphere dysfunction has been claimed (Geeraerts et al., 2007).

A review of neurocognitive performance in 2001 concluded that adult ADHD is associated with impaired performance in tasks involving sustained attention, set shifting, and working memory and that the last domain "may be particularly impaired" (i.e. in relation to other psychiatric disorders that have been associated with neurocognitive deficits; Gallagher & Blader, 2001). This conclusion is consistent with the findings of a study of 19 unmedicated adults with ADHD and 19 healthy volunteers, matched for age, gender, and verbal IQ (McLean et al., 2004). Although this chapter summarizes the wide range and variability of neurocognitive impairments associated with ADHD, details of this study – which used a computer-administered neurocognition test battery (CANTAB; see www.cantab.com, validated in more than 500 publications involving a wide range of neuropsychiatric disorders) – are provided as examples of EF measurements.

Relative to controls, the adults with ADHD exhibited a range of neurocognitive impairments including marked deficits on a test of self-ordered spatial working memory (CANTAB-SWM; see Fig. 9.1A; McLean et al., 2004). This task measures the ability to retain spatial information and to manipulate remembered items in working memory. During this task, a number of colored boxes are shown on a touch-sensitive computer screen. By touching (and therefore opening) the boxes and using a process of elimination, the partici-

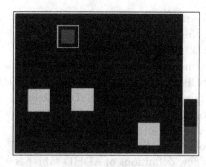

Figure 9.1A
CANTAB spatial working memory.

pant must find the one blue "token" per trial and use them to fill up an empty column on the right-hand side of the screen (only one box contains the hidden blue "token" in each of a succession of trials). The number of boxes is gradually increased, until it is necessary to search a total of eight boxes. The critical instruction is that, in each trial, the participant must not return to a box where a token has previously been found. Therefore the participant must search through the boxes while retaining a spatial map of previously opened boxes. This task also enables evaluation of strategy use by quantifying how systematic the participant is in searching through boxes.

Performance on this spatial working memory (SWM) task has been shown to be impaired by damage to the prefrontal cortex, especially the dorsolateral prefrontal cortex (Manes et al., 2002; Owen et al., 1990). In neuroimaging studies in healthy volunteers, SWM performance has been shown to be associated with activations in the dorsolateral and mid ventrolateral prefrontal cortex (Owen, Evans, & Petrides, 1996). As can be seen in Figure 9.1B, at both easy and more difficult stages of the task, individuals with ADHD made significantly more errors than controls. These errors were shown by a tendency to return to a box where a token had previously been found and by a failure to use a systematic strategy in searching the boxes.

In the study of McLean and colleagues (2004), frontal-type cognitive deficits were not restricted to working memory. For example, the ADHD patients also showed deficits in the performance of a test of planning that has been demonstrated to be sensitive to frontal lobe damage (Owen et al., 1990); in addition, functional brain imaging studies have shown that performance on this task activates a neural network that includes the dorsolateral prefrontal cortex (Baker et al., 1996). In this task the subject is presented with two separate arrays of three colored balls hanging in pockets (see Fig. 9.2A; McLean et al., 2004). The displays are presented in such a way that they can

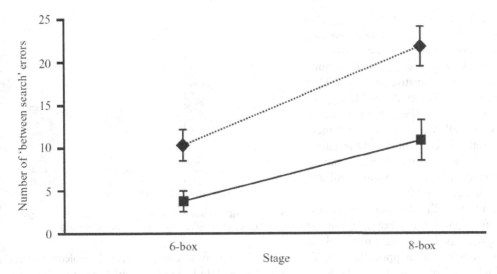

Mean number of 'between-search' errors (◆······◆, ADHD; ■——■, controls) committed during performance of the 6-box and 8-box stages of the spatial working memory task. (Bars represent ±1 s.e.m.)

Figure 9.1B Performance of adults with ADHD and healthy controls on the CANTAB spatial working memory task.

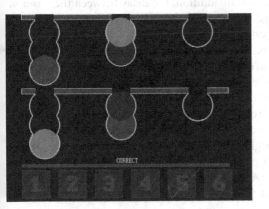

Figure 9.2A CANTAB stockings of Cambridge test of planning.

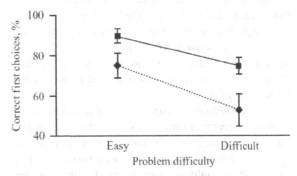

Figure 9.2B Performance of adults with ADHD and healthy controls on the CANTAB stockings of Cambridge task.

easily be perceived as stacks of colored balls held in stockings or socks suspended from a beam. At the bottom of the screen is a row of numbers from 1 to 6. Subjects are required to compute "in their mind's eye" the minimum number of moves needed to rearrange the colored balls in the bottom array to match the top array. The subject then has to select from the digits presented at the bottom of the screen the number of moves required. The time taken to respond and the number of moves selected are taken as measures of the subject's planning ability. This test of spatial planning is based on the Tower of London task (Owen et al., 1995). As can be seen in Figure 9.2B, adult ADHD patients performed significantly more poorly

than controls; patients with ADHD were approximately 20% less accurate than controls in calculating the minimum number of moves required to correctly match the upper and lower arrays. Notably, no increase in latency was observed in the ADHD group. Further evidence of neurocognitive dysfunction involving the prefrontal cortex was provided by the finding of impairments on a test of cognitive flexibility (the CANTAB attentional set-shifting task), which is derived from the Wisconsin Card Sorting Test. Performance on this CANTAB test has been associated with left anterior and right dorsolateral prefrontal cortex activity in functional brain imaging studies. In addition, the ADHD patients were significantly slower to respond to target stimuli on a go/no-go test (McLean et al., 2004).

In contrast, the ADHD and control groups performed equivalently on a test of decision making, which is thought to involve orbitofrontal activation, and on a test of visual pattern recognition memory, which has been shown to be sensitive to temporal but not frontal lobe damage (Owen et al., 1995), suggesting that there is specificity in the pattern of cognitive abnormalities. Overall, the profile of impairment is consistent with pathological abnormality in lateral frontostriatal circuitry and is similar to the pattern of dysfunction observed in medication-naïve children with ADHD (Kempton et al., 1999).

Performance on tests of EFs is dependent on several distinct cognitive faculties. For example, the test of spatial planning described earlier requires working memory, the ability to withhold inappropriate impulsive actions, and tolerance of delay during deliberation. As noted earlier, it has been suggested (Clark et al., 2007) that some or all the deficits in ADHD manifested on various cognitive tasks may stem from a common "core" cognitive deficit (or deficits) rather than being distinct deficits. One proposal of such a core cognitive deficit relates to response inhibition. The term "response inhibition" is used to describe the ability to withhold inappropriate responses, and the construct may relate closely to that of behavioral impulsivity in ADHD.

An established measure of response inhibition is stop-signal reaction time (SSRT), which measures the time it takes to internally suppress a response (see Fig. 9.3A; Aron et al., 2003). In one version of this task, a left- or right-pointing arrow stimulus appears

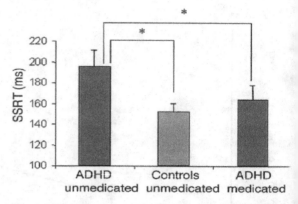

Figure 9.3B Performance on the SSRT task of healthy volunteers and adults with ADHD both on and off methylphenidate.

on the computer screen in each trial. Subjects respond by a left or right key press as quickly as possible ("go" task), unless they hear a beep (randomly presented in 25% of trials) when they must attempt to withhold (i.e. stop) a response. A median go reaction time (GRT) is obtained. In addition, the delay between the onset of the go and stop signals is varied to obtain and identify the stop-signal delay (SSD), at which the participant can reliably withhold responding for 50% of the trials (Aron et al., 2003). The SSRT is calculated by subtracting the SSD from the GRT. SSRT performance has been shown to be disrupted by damage to the right inferior frontal gyrus, whereas brain activation correlating with successful inhibitory control has been shown in the right inferior prefrontal cortex (Rubia et al., 2003). SSRT performance is impaired in adults (and children) with ADHD and is independent of simple reaction times (see Fig. 9.3B; Aron et al., 2003; Bedard et al., 2003).

In a recent study, SSRT performance was found to be significantly associated with search errors on the SWM task in both patients with adult ADHD and patients with right frontal lesions (Clark et al., 2007). In the right frontal patients, impaired performance on both variables was correlated with the volume of damage to the inferior frontal gyrus. Therefore it was postulated that response inhibition and working memory impairments in ADHD may emerge from a common neuropathological process. Such pathology could relate to right frontal cortex abnormalities in ADHD.

A 2004 meta-analysis of 33 studies concluded that neurocognitive deficits in adults with ADHD are found across a range of domains, in particular involving attention, behavioral inhibition, and memory, with normal performance for simple reaction times

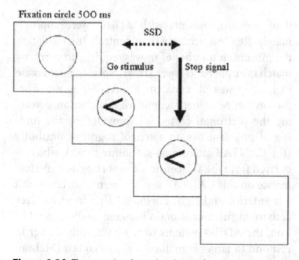

Figure 9.3A The stop-signal reaction time task.

(Harvey, Epstein, & Curry, 2004). More recent studies in adults with ADHD have reported impairments in a wider range of functions, including continuous performance and gambling tasks (Malloy-Diniz et al., 2007), reaction time and a stop-signal task (Lampe Konrad et al., 2007), verbal and visual memory, set shifting and speed of visuomotor search (Müller et al., 2007), working memory (Schweitzer, Hanford, & Medoff, 2006), and "interference control" (King et al., 2007). Future factor analytic studies using multidomain neurocognitive batteries will help clarify whether common mechanisms underlie performance deficits on tests of nominally distinct cognitive processes. Such analyses will also help determine whether any such processes (e.g. response inhibition) should be considered "primary" or "core" deficits. Additionally, as overarching statements about the presence or absence of a deficit in ADHD based on group averages may fail to recognize important subgroups in this population, future studies could also usefully identify subgroups with clinically meaningful performance deficits by referencing test performance against appropriate normative data, controlling for factors known to influence cognitive function such as age, estimated premorbid IQ, and gender. A recent study in adults using a battery of neurocognitive tests reported associations with four candidate genes associated with ADHD (Boonstra et al., 2008).

Confounding variables in studying neurocognition in adults with ADHD

Understanding the neurocognitive profile of adult ADHD is complicated not only by heterogeneity of symptom presentation but also by other variables, which should be controlled in clinical and research assessments. The following section provides a nonexhaustive list of such "confounding variables."

Assessment and diagnosis

The various reports of neurocognitive performance in groups of subjects with a diagnosis of ADHD have reflected a range of diagnostic procedures and diagnostic thresholds.

Comorbidity

Most children and adults with ADHD have clinically significant comorbidity, including various neurocognitive disorders, such as problems with reading, writing, mathematics, and language (Sachdev, 1999;

Wender et al., 2001). Common comorbid disorders in adults include *DSM-IV* Cluster B personality disorders, substance-related disorders, and mood disorders (Sachdev, 1999). As these disorders have also been associated with various neurocognitive deficits (Bazanis et al., 2002; Elliott et al., 1998; Iddon et al., 1998; Kurtz & Morey, 1999; Owen et al., 1990; Purcell et al., 1998; Rubinsztein et al., 2000; Veale et al., 1996), comorbidity is an important confounding variable in studies of the neurocognitive characteristics of ADHD.

Adult ADHD commonly co-occurs with *DSM-IV* borderline personality disorder (BPD; Sachdev, 1999), and there have been several reports of neurocognitive impairments in patients with BPD, involving attention, verbal and visual memory, planning and information processing, as well as problems with cognitive inflexibility, poor self-monitoring, and perseveration (O'Leary, 2000; O'Leary et al., 1991; Stein, Hollander, & Liebowitz, 1993; Stein et al., 1994; Van Reekum, 1993). Further, self-harm in BPD patients has been associated with deficits in attention and memory (Burgess, 1991). However, a study that compared three groups of subjects – 19 adults selected on the basis of ADHD, 19 adult patients selected on the basis of BPD, and 19 nonclinical controls – found that the ADHD group, but not the BPD group, had significant impairment of CANTAB SWM performance relative to nonclinical controls (Dowson et al., 2004). These results were consistent with the claim that aspects of working memory are "particularly impaired" in adult ADHD, compared with other psychiatric disorders that also affect frontal-lobe-mediated EFs. In addition, two studies involving children with ADHD found that working memory deficits were associated with language impairments (Jonsdottir et al., 2005; Tirosh & Cohen, 1998).

ADHD subtypes

There have been several reports in both children and adults of differences in neurocognitive performance among *DSM-IV* types of ADHD (Levy et al., 2005; Nigg et al., 2002; O'Driscoll et al., 2005), although there were no subtype differences in various EF measures in a study of adolescents (Martel, Nikolas, & Nigg, 2007) and in working memory in adults (Schweitzer et al., 2006). For example, when children with ADHD that included hyperactivity were compared with those without hyperactivity, 60% of the latter had a comorbid developmental reading or arithmetic disorder, in contrast to none of the comparison group (Hynd, Lorys, et al., 1991). Yet 40% of the former group had comorbid conduct disorder. Another report, of 177 children, found that those with the hyperactive-impulsive type of ADHD had no difficulty with certain tasks compared with the other subtypes (Harrier & De Ornellas, 2004), whereas a study of boys aged 11–14 found that the combined type but not the inattentive type was associated with impairments in motor planning and response inhibition (Dunn, Robbins, & Harris, 2001). Differences among the *DSM-IV* ADHD types have also been reported for adults (Dunn et al., 2001) and may contribute to neurocognitive variations among published studies of ADHD, as different samples may reflect varying proportions of ADHD subtypes.

Age, gender, and IQ

A 7-year follow-up study to young adulthood found that various EF deficits were stable over time (Biederman et al., 2007), although a meta-analysis in relation to inhibitory motor control, which found a significant difference between ADHD patients and matched controls in SSRT for both children and adults, also reported some differences between children and adults: reaction time was significantly longer in children but not in adults, and there was a significant interaction between the elongation of the latency to stop and to respond in adults, but not in children (Lijffijt et al., 2005). Although effects of age on some measures of EF were not found in other studies in children with ADHD (Biederman et al., 2007; Dunn et al., 2001; Harrier & De Ornellas, 2004; Seidman et al., 2005), associations with age have been reported for some measures of EF (Dreschler et al., 2005; Nigg et al., 2002).

In a study of children with ADHD, gender was not associated with performance in planning and "reconstitution" tasks (Harrier & De Ornellas, 2004) or with performance in all but one of several EF tasks (Seidman et al., 2005). However, a 45% rate of "language problems" was reported in a large series of 3,208 children, and this comorbidity was more prevalent among girls (Levy et al., 2005). It was significantly related to sequencing and short-term memory performance.

IQ is another possible confounding factor, and it was found to be associated with performance on some neurocognitive tasks in a sample of 177 children with ADHD (Harrier & De Ornellas, 2004).

Effects of pharmacological treatments for ADHD on neurocognitive functions

Methylphenidate (MPH)

MPH, a dopaminergic and noradrenergic reuptake inhibitor, is currently the main treatment of choice for ADHD in children and adults (Faraone et al., 2004; Kinsbourne et al., 2001; Solanto, 1998). Moreover, it has been reported that, following stimulant medication, both children and adults with ADHD show a variety of improvements in performance involving tests of response inhibition, working memory, motor speed, processing speed, attention, and vigilance (Aron et al., 2003; Kempton et al., 1999; Mehta, Goodyer, & Sahakian, 2004; Rapoport et al., 1980; Riordan et al., 1999; Solanto, 1998). Although an effect of MPH was not found in healthy elderly volunteers (Turner et al., 2003), improved neurocognitive performances have been reported in younger volunteers (Elliott et al., 1997). This finding suggests that MPH usually produces improvements in neurocognitive performance in nonclinical samples (i.e. those containing subjects most of whom do not have ADHD).

A single case study of an adult with ADHD indicated that MPH may have a potential for improving SWM in such patients (Mehta, Calloway, & Sahakian, 2000). This finding was consistent with the hypothesis of impaired catecholaminergic modulation of neurocognitive processes involving the prefrontal cortex in ADHD (Bor et al., 2003; Mehta, Owen, et al., 2000; Owen, Evans, & Petrides, 1996; Postle et al., 2000; Solanto, 2002; Swanson et al., 1998). A subsequent study of 18 adults with ADHD examined whether such subjects would show the same neurocognitive responses to MPH as children with ADHD and healthy young volunteers (Turner et al., 2005). The effects of MPH on SWM and attention were assessed using a double-blind placebo-controlled crossover design. The neurocognitive battery was designed to assess working memory and sustained attention, using tasks that have been used previously to explore the effects of MPH in children with ADHD, healthy volunteers, and the case study report in adult ADHD noted earlier (Elliott et al., 1997; Mehta, Calloway, et al., 2000; Mehta et al., 2004; Turner et al., 2003). The tasks had been shown to be sensitive to frontostriatal damage and to catecholamine manipulations in healthy adults (Coull et al., 1995; Elliott et al., 1997; Mehta, Owen, et al., 2000; Mehta et al., 1999; Rogers et al., 1999). MPH resulted in an improvement in SWM performance and sustained attention, together with a faster response time, which was a similar neurocognitive response to MPH to that previously reported for childhood ADHD. Another study of 13 adults with ADHD and controls found that SSRT was significantly improved with a single dose of MPH (see Fig. 9.3B; Aron et al., 2003).

Another study, with a double-blind, placebo-controlled crossover design and involving 43 adults with ADHD, found that MPH was associated with medication effects for commission errors, standard error of mean reaction time on a continuous performance task (CPT), mean reaction time on the CPT, and response reengagement speed on a change task. MPH also had a large effect on a measure of SSRT in a subgroup with relatively slow SSRT performance on placebo (Boonstra et al., 1999).

Atomoxetine

A promising treatment alternative to stimulant medications is atomoxetine, a selective noradrenaline uptake inhibitor (Pliszka, 2005). Atomoxetine gives 24-hours-a-day coverage when effective, although the full effects of a given dose may take up to 12 weeks to develop.

Two studies of adults with ADHD (Ns = 280 and 256) examined the effects of atomoxetine on a Stroop task performance in double-blind, placebo-controlled, parallel designs. Atomoxetine was associated with improved performance, and the results supported a previous claim that this drug improved inhibitory capacity (Faraone et al., 2005). In addition, in a study of 22 adults with DSM-IV ADHD, who received a single oral dose of atomoxetine in a placebo-controlled double-blind crossover design, atomoxetine improved response inhibition (Chamberlain et al., 2007). It was suggested that this improvement may have been via noradrenically mediated augmentation of prefrontal cortex functions.

Modafinil

Recent evidence has indicated that the novel wake-promoting agent modafinil may be effective in the treatment of ADHD. Children with ADHD have been reported to show reductions in hyperactivity, inattention, and impulsivity with modafinil. A comparison of the efficacy of modafinil versus dextroamphetamine in the treatment of adults with ADHD showed that both

drugs resulted in a significant reduction in ADHD symptoms (Taylor & Russo, 2000). Only minimal neurocognitive testing was included in this study, although trends toward improvement were seen on a Stroop task, digit span, and verbal fluency. In addition, two company-sponsored, double-blind placebo-controlled trials, assessing the longer term effects of modafinil in 246 children with ADHD (Reeves, 2003), reported significant improvements in ADHD behavior using a teacher-rated measure.

In a recent study, modafinil improved motor response inhibition on the stop-signal task in healthy adult volunteers (Turner et al., 2003a), whereas SSRT, which has been correlated with clinical aspects of impulsivity in children with ADHD (Schachar et al., 1995), was improved by MPH in adults (Aron et al., 2003) and children (Bedard et al., 2003; Tannock et al., 1989) with ADHD. In the study in adult volunteers (Turner et al., 2003a), modafinil also improved neurocognitive performance on measures of spatial planning, recognition memory, and digit span, together with a slowing in response latency on several tasks. It was suggested that modafinil might serve to improve accuracy by enhancing reflection before response initiation (Kagan, 1966; Kagan & Scholten, 1985).

In another study that examined whether the beneficial effects of modafinil on response inhibition and other cognitive domains extended to adult patients with ADHD, 20 adult patients with a DSM-IV diagnosis of ADHD were entered in a double-blind, randomized, placebo-controlled crossover study using a single 200-mg dose of modafinil (Turner et al., 2004). Modafinil produced a similar pattern of cognitive enhancement to that observed in healthy adults, with improvements on tests of short-term memory span, visual memory, spatial planning, and stop-signal motor inhibition. On several measures, increased accuracy was accompanied by slowed response latency. This alteration in the speed–accuracy trade-off may also indicate that modafinil increases the ability to "reflect" on problems while decreasing impulsive responding. Improvements were also seen in sustained attention, which was unaffected by medication in healthy subjects.

If these benefits are shown to be maintained with chronic administration, modafinil may have potential as a therapy for adult ADHD, with a similar effect to stimulants such as MPH in improving stop-signal response inhibition, but without the side effects commonly experienced with stimulant drugs.

Role of neurocognitive assessments in clinical practice

As noted earlier, a *DSM-IV* diagnosis of ADHD, which involves obtaining a history considered to be compatible with an onset in childhood and with clinically significant features of ADHD in adulthood, partly depends on a clinician's judgment based on information from the subject and informants. Although groups of subjects with a diagnosis of ADHD have been associated with a range of neurocognitive deficits, at present there are insufficient data to justify the use of neurocognitive assessments as a diagnostic instrument for an individual diagnosis (McGough & Barkley, 2004) – even though the results of four memory tests have been claimed to correctly identify 81% of a group of adults with ADHD (Dige & Wik, 2005). However, a combination of tests may eventually provide reliable predictive validity in relation to etiology and response to medication (Perugini et al., 2000).

Nevertheless, performance on a range of tasks that have been reported to be impaired in ADHD – such as response inhibition and working memory – can provide a profile that helps identify a patient's strengths and weaknesses. This information may be of value when advising a patient about suitable employment and appropriate domains in which to develop adaptive strategies.

Further, neurocognitive assessment may be of value by identifying a general measure of cognitive abilities such as IQ, as well as specific comorbid learning difficulties. Again, this information may help the clinician give appropriate advice.

For neurocognitive assessment to play a greater role in diagnostic procedures and monitoring for adult ADHD, tests must show a relationship to underlying abnormalities of brain function. In addition, performance on such tests should relate to occupational or social functioning and/or the response to treatment. Such tests should be easily administered and have good psychometric properties such as test-retest and inter-rater reliability. Additionally, the resulting data output must be easy to interpret by comparisons with a well-defined normative database.

Conclusions

Groups of adults with a diagnosis of ADHD are associated with a range of neurocognitive deficits. How-ever, previous reports have used a variety of assessment methods, and the diagnosis of *DSM-IV* ADHD in adults is confounded by comorbidities (Sachdev, 1999). Despite attempts to identify one core neurocognitive deficit related to ADHD, impairments have been found in several domains, including attention, working memory, response inhibition, motivation, temporal information processing, and regulation of activation (Pennington, 2005). There is evidence implicating various neural networks, including fronto-cerebellar and, in particular, frontostriatal connections (Nigg, 2005; Nigg & Casey, 2005).

Although a diagnosis of ADHD in an adult, or a decision to prescribe a trial of medication, cannot yet be based on a profile of neurocognitive performances, such information may help the clinician provide appropriate advice and, occasionally, make the diagnosis of clinically significant ADHD unlikely on the basis of exceptionally good performances on tests of EF. Assessment of IQ and common comorbid learning disabilities may also be useful when setting appropriate educational, occupational, and social goals.

Future neurocognitive research, using relatively reliable methodology to obtain a profile of neurocognitive performances, may play an important part in identifying subtypes based on the neurobiological substrates of this etiologically heterogeneous syndrome (American Psychiatric Association, 2004). These subtypes may prove to have predictive validity for the effects of medication regimes. Various possible neurocognitive endophenotypes have been suggested, including various performances on EF tasks and combinations of impairments (Diamond, 2005; Nigg et al., 2005). The common comorbidities of ADHD will continue to be confounding variables in neurocognitive assessments of adults with ADHD.

References

American Psychiatric Association. (1994). *Diagnostic and Statistical Manual of Mental Disorders.* 4th ed. Washington, DC: American Psychiatric Press.

American Psychiatric Association. (2000). *Diagnostic and Statistical Manual of Mental Disorder: DSM-IV-R.* 4th ed. text rev. Washington, DC: American Psychiatric Press.

Aron AR, Dowson JH, Sahakian BJ, Robbins TW. (2003). Methylphenidate improves response inhibition in adults with attention-deficit/hyperactivity disorder. *Biol Psychiatry* 54:1465–8.

Baker SC, Rogers RD, Owen AM, et al. (1996). Neural systems engaged by planning: a PET study of the Tower of London task. *Neuropsychologia* **34**(6):515–26.

Banerjee TD, Middleton F, Faraone SV. (2007). Environmental risk factors for attention-deficit/hyperactivity disorder. *Acta Paediatr* **96**(9):1269–74.

Barbaresi WJ, Katusic SK, Colligan RC, et al. (2002). How common is attention-deficit/hyperactivity disorder? Incidence in a population-based birth cohort in Rochester, Minn. *Arch Paediatr Adolesc Med* **156**(3):209–10.

Barkley RA, Grodzinsky G, DuPaul GJ. (1992). Frontal lobe functions in attention deficit disorder with and without hyperactivity: a review and research report. *J Abnorm Child Psychol* **20**:163–88.

Barnett R, Maruff P, Vance A, Luk ES, Costin J, Wood C, Pantelis C. (2001). Abnormal executive function in attention deficit hyperactivity disorder: the effect of stimulant medication and age on spatial working memory. *Psychol Med* **31**:1107–15.

Bazanis E, Rogers RD, Dowson JH, et al. (2002). Neurocognitive deficits in decision-making and planning of patients with DSM-III borderline personality disorder. *Psychol Med* **32**:1395–1405.

Bedard AC, Ickowicz A, Logan GD, Hogg-Johnson S, Schachar R, Tannock R. (2003). Selective inhibition in children with attention-deficit hyperactivity disorder off and on stimulant medication. *J Abnorm Child Psychol* **31**(3):315–27.

Bekker EM, Overtoom CC, Kooij JJ, Buitelaar JK, Verbaten MN, Kenemans JL. (2005). Disentangling deficits in adults with attention-deficit/hyperactivity disorder. *Arch Gen Psychiatry* **62**(10): 1129–36.

Bekker EM, Overtoon CC, Kenemans JL, et al. (2005). Stopping and changing in adults with ADHD. *Psychol Med* **35**(6):807–16.

Biederman J, Mick E, Faraone SV. (2000). Age-dependent decline of symptoms of attention-deficit/hyperactivity disorder: Impact of remission definition and symptom type. *Am J Psychiatry* **157**:816–18.

Biederman J, Petty CR, Fried R, Doyle AE, Spencer T, Seiderman LJ, et al. (2007). Stability of executive function deficits into young adult years: a prospective longitudinal follow-up study of grown-up males with ADHD. *Acta Psychiatr Scand* **116**(2):129–36.

Boonstra AM, Kooij JJ, Buitelaar JK, Oosterlaan J, Sergeant JA, Heister JG, et al. (2008). An exploratory study of the relationship between four candidate genes and neurocognitive performance in adult ADHD. *Am J Med Genet B Neuropsychiatr Genet* **147**(3): 397–402.

Boonstra AM, Kooij JJ, Oosterlaan J, Serjeant JA, Buitelaar JK. (2005). Does methylphenidate improve inhibition and other cognitive abilities in adults with childhood-onset ADHD? *J Clin Exp Neuropsychol* **27**(3):278–98.

Boonstra AM, Oosterlaan J, Sergeant JA, Buitelaar JK. (2005). Executive functioning in adult ADHD: a meta-analytic review. *Psychol Med* **35**(8):1097–1108.

Bor D, Duncan J, Wiseman RJ, Owen AM. (2003). Encoding strategies dissociate prefrontal activity from working memory demand. *Neuron* **37**:361–7.

Burden MJ, Mitchell DB. (2005) Implicit memory development in school-aged children with attention deficit hyperactivity disorder (ADHD): conceptual processing deficit? *Dev Neuropsychol* **28**(3):779–807.

Burgess JW. (1991). Relationship of depression and cognitive impairment to self-injury in borderline personality disorder. *Psychiatry Res* **31**:77–87.

Castellanos FX, Giedd JN, Eckburg P, et al. (1994). Quantitative morphology of the caudate nucleus in attention deficit hyperactivity disorder. *Am J Psychiatry* **151**:1791–1976.

Castellanos FX, Giedd JN, Marsh WL, et al. (1996). Quantitative brain magnetic resonance imaging in attention-deficit hyperactivity disorder. *Arch Gen Psychiatry* **53**(7):607–16.

Castellanos FX, Sonuga-Barke EJ, Schers A, Di Martino A, Hyde C, Walters JR. (2005). Varieties of attention-deficit/hyperactivity disorder-related intra-individual variability. *Biol Psychiatry* **57**(11):1416–23.

Castellanos FX, Tannock R. (2002). Neuroscience of attention-deficit/hyperactivity disorder: the search for endophenotypes. *Nat Rev Neurosci* **3**(8):617–28.

Chamberlain SR, Del Campo N, Dowson J, Muller U, Clark L, Robbins TW, Sahakian BJ. (2007). Atomoxetine improved response inhibition in adults with attention-deficit/hyperactivity disorder. *Biol Psychiatry* **62**(9):977–84.

Clark L, Blackwell AD, Aron AR, Turner DC, Dowson J, Robbins TW, Sahakian BJ. (2007). Association between response inhibition and working memory in adult ADHD: A link to right frontal cortex pathology? *Biol Psychiatry* **61**(12):1395-401.

Coull JT, Sahakian BJ, Middleton HC, et al. (1995). Differential effects of clonidine, haloperidol, diazepam and tryptophan depletion on focused attention and attentional search. *Psychopharmacology (Berl)* **121**:222–30.

Diamond A. (2005). Attention-deficit disorder (attention deficit/hyperactivity disorder without hyperactivity). *Dev Psychopathol* **17**(3):807–25.

Dige N, Wik G. (2005). Adult attention deficit hyperactivity disorder identified by neuropsychological testing. *Int J Neurosci* 115(2):169–83.

Dowson JH, McLean A, Bazanis E, et al. (2004). Impaired spatial working memory in adults with attention-deficit/hyperactivity disorder: comparisons with performance in adults with borderline personality disorders and in control subjects. *Acta Psychiatr Scand* 109:1–10.

Doyle AE, Faraone SV Seidman LJ, et al. (2005). Are endophenotypes based on measures of executive functions useful for molecular genetic studies of ADHD? *J Child Psychol Psychiatry* 46(7):774–803.

Dreschler R, Brandeis D, Foldengi M, Imhof K, Steinhausen HC. (2005). The course of neuropsychological functions in children with attention deficit hyperactivity disorder from late childhood to early adolescence. *J Child Psychol Psychiatry* 46(8):824–36.

Dunn WM, Robbins NC, Harris CL. (2001). Adult attention-deficit/hyperactivity disorder: neuropsychological correlates and clinical presentation. *Brain Cogn* 46(1–2):114–21.

Elliott R, Sahakian BJ, Matthews K, Bannerjea A, Rimmer J, Robbins TW. (1997). Effects of methylphenidate on spatial working memory and planning in healthy young adults. *Psychopharmacology (Berl)* 131:196–206.

Elliott R, Sahakian BJ, Michael A, Paykel ES, Dolan RJ. (1998). Abnormal neural response to feedback on planning and guessing tasks in patients with unipolar depression. *Psychol Med* 28:559–71.

Faraone SV, Biederman J, Spencer T, Michelson D, Adler L, Reimherr F, Seidman L. (2005). Atomoxetine and Stroop task performance in adult attention-deficit/hyperactivity disorder. *J Child Adolesc Psychopathol* 15(4):664–70.

Faraone SV, Biederman J, Spencer T, Wilens T, Seidman LJ, Mick E, Doyle AE. (2000). Attention-deficit/hyperactivity disorder in adults: an overview. *Biol Psychiatry* 48:9–20.

Faraone SV, Spencer T, Aleardi M, Pagano C, Biederman J. (2004). Meta-analysis of the efficacy of methylphenidate for treating adult attention-deficit/hyperactivity disorder. *J Clin Psychopharmacol* 24:24–9.

Gallagher R, Blader J. (2001). The diagnosis and neuropsychological assessment of adult attention/deficit disorder. *Ann N Y Acad Sci* 931:148–71.

Geeraerts S, Lafosse C, Vaes N, Vandenbussche E, Verfaille K. (2007). Dysfunction of right-hemisphere attentional networks in attention deficit hyperactivity disorder. *J Clin Exp Neuropsychol* Mar 12:1–11 [Epub ahead of print].

Giedd JN, Blumenthal J, Molloy E, Castellanos FX. (2001). Brain imaging of attention deficit/hyperactivity disorder. *Ann N Y Acad Sci* 931:33–49.

Grodzinsky G, Diamond R. (1992). Frontal lobe functioning in boys with attention deficit hyperactivity disorder. *Dev Neuropsychol* 8:427–45.

Harrier LK, De Ornellas K. (2004). Performance of children diagnosed with ADHD on selected planning and reconstitution tests. *Appl Neuropsychol* 12(2):106–19.

Harvey AS, Epstein JN, Curry JF. (2004). Neuropsychology of adults with attention-deficit/hyperactivity disorder: a meta-analytic review. *Neuropsychology* 18(3):485.

Himelstein J, Newcorn JH, Halperin JM. (2000). The neurobiology of attention-deficit hyperactivity disorder. *Front Biosci* 5:D461–78.

Hynd GW, Hern KL, Novey ES, et al. (1993). Attention-deficit-hyperactivity disorder and asymmetry of the caudate nucleus. *J Child Neurol* 8:339–47.

Hynd GW, Lorys AR, Semrud-Clikeman M, Nieves N, Hueltner MI, Lakey BB. (1991). Attention deficit disorder without hyperactivity: a distinct behavioural and neurocognitive syndrome. *J Child Neurol* 6(suppl):537–43.

Hynd GW, Semrud-Clikeman M, Lorys AR, Novey ES, Eliopulos D. (1990). Brain morphology in developmental dyslexia and attention deficit disorder/hyperactivity. *Arch Neurol* 47:919–26.

Hynd GW, Semrud-Clikeman M, Lorys AR, Novey ES, Eliopulos D, Lyytinen H. (1991) Corpus callosum morphology in attention-deficit-hyperactivity disorder: morphometric analysis of MRI. *J Learn Disabil* 24:141–6.

Iddon JL, McKenna PJ, Sahakian BJ, Robbins TW. (1998). Impaired generation and use of strategy in schizophrenia: evidence from visuospatial and verbal tasks. *Psychol Med* 28:1049–62.

Johnson DE, Epstein JN, Waid LR, Latham PK, Veronin KE, Anton RF. (2001). Neuropsychological performance deficits in adults with attention-deficit/hyperactivity disorder. *Arch Clin Neuropsychol* 16:587–604.

Jonsdottir S, Bouna A, Sergeant JA, Scherder EJ. (2005). The impact of specific language impairment on working memory in children with ADHD combined subtype. *Arch Clin Neuropsychol* 20(4):443–56.

Kagan J. (1966). Reflection-impulsivity: the generality and dynamics of conceptual tempo. *J Abnorm Psychol* 71:17–24.

Kagan JA, Scholten CA. (1985). On resource strategy limitations in hyperactivity: cognitive impulsivity reconsidered. *J Child Psychol Psychiatry* 26:97–109.

Kelly AM, Margulies DS, Castellanos FX. (2007). Recent advances in structural and functional brain imaging studies of attention-deficit/hyperactivity disorder. *Curr Psychiatry Rep* **9**(5):401–7.

Kempton S, Vance A, Maruff P, Luk E, Costin J, Pantelis C. (1999). Executive function and attention deficit hyperactivity disorder: stimulant medication and better executive function performance in children. *Psychol Med* **29**:527–38.

Kessler RC, Adler L, Barkley R, Biederman J, Conners CK, Demler O, et al. (2006). The prevalence and correlates of adult ADHD in the United States. *Am J Psychiatry* **163**(4):716–23.

King JA, Colla M, Brass, Hensen I, von Cramen D. (2007). Inefficient cognitive control in adult ADHD. *Behav Brain Funct* **3**:42–52.

Kinsbourne M, De Quiros GB, Tocci Rufo D. (2001). Adult ADHD. Controlled medication assessment. *Ann N Y Acad Sci* **931**:287–96.

Kovner R, Budman C, Frank Y, Sison C, Lesser M, Halperin J. (1998). Neuropsychological testing in adult attention-deficit/hyperactivity disorder: a pilot study. *Int J Neurosci* **96**:225–35.

Kuntsi J, McLoughlin G, Asherson P. (2006). Attention deficit hyperactivity disorder. *Neuromolecular Med* **8**(4):461–84.

Kuntsi J, Oosterlaan J, Stevenson J. (2001), Psychological mechanisms in hyperactivity. *J Child Psychol Psychiatry* **42**(2):199–210.

Kurtz JE, Morey LC. (1999). Verbal memory dysfunction in depressed outpatients with and without borderline personality disorder. *J Psychopathol Behav Assess* **21**:141–56.

Lampe Konrad K, Kroener S, Fast K, Kunert HJ, Herpertz SC. (2007). Neuropsychological and behavioural disinhibition in adult ADHD compared to borderline personality disorder. *Psychol Med* May 17:1–13 [Epub ahead of print].

Levy F, Hay DA, Bennett KS, McStephen M. (2005). Gender differences in ADHD subtype comorbidity. *J Am Acad Child Adolesc Psychiatry* **44**(4):368–76.

Levy F, Hay DA, McStephen M, Wood C, Waldman I. (1997). Attention-deficit hyperactivity disorder: a category or a continuum? Genetic analysis of a large-scale twin study. *J Am Acad Child Adolesc Psychiatry* **36**(6):737–44.

Lijffijt M, Kenemans JL, Verboten MN, von Engelund H. (2005). A meta-analysis review of stopping performance in attention-deficit/hyperactivity disorder: deficient inhibitory motor control? *J Abnorm Psychol* **114**(2):216–22.

Lou HC, Henriksen L, Bruhn P. (1984). Focal cerebral hypoperfusion in children with dysphasia and/or attention deficit disorder. *Arch Neurol* **41**:825–29.

Lou HC, Henriksen L, Bruhn P, Borner H, Nielsen JB. (1989). Striatal dysfunction in attention deficit and hyperkinetic disorder. *Arch Neurol* **46**: 48–52.

Makris N, Buka SL, Biederman J, Papadimitriou GM, Hodge SM, Valera EM, et al. (2007). Attention and executive system abnormalities in adults with childhood ADHD: a DT-MRI study of connections. *Cerebr Cortex* Sept 30 [Epub ahead of print].

Malloy-Diniz L, Fuentes D, Leite WB, Correa H, Bechara A. (2007). Impulsive behaviour in adults with attention-deficit/hyperactivity disorder. *J Int Neuropsychol Soc* **13**(4):693–8.

Manes F, Sahakian B, Clark L, et al. (2002). Decision-making processes following damage to the pre-frontal cortex. *Brain* **125**(3):624–39.

Martel M, Nikolas M, Nigg JT. (2007). Executive function in adolescents with ADHD. *J Am Acad Child Adolesc Psychiatry* **46**(11):1437–44.

McGough JU, Barkley RA. (2004). Diagnostic controversies in adult attention deficit hyperactivity disorder. *Am J Psychiatry* **61**(11):1948–56.

McLean A, Dowson J, Toone B, et al. (2004). Characteristic neurocognitive profile associated with adult attention-deficit/hyperactivity disorder. *Psychol Med* **34**:681–92.

Mehta MA, Calloway P, Sahakian BJ. (2000). Amelioration of specific working memory deficits by methylphenidate in a case of adult attention deficit/hyperactivity disorder. *J Psychopharmacol* **14**(3):299–302.

Mehta MA, Goodyer IM, Sahakian BJ. (2004). Methylphenidate improves working memory and set-shifting in AD/HD: relationships to baseline memory capacity. *J Child Psychol Psychiatry* **45**: 293–305.

Mehta MA, Owen AM, Sahakian BJ, Mavaddat N, Pickard JD, Robbins TW. (2000). Methylphenidate enhances working memory by modulating discrete frontal and parietal lobe regions in the human brain. *J Neurosci* **20**:RC65(1–6).

Mehta MA, Sahakian BJ, McKenna PJ, Robbins TW. (1999). Systemic sulpiride in young adult males simulates the profile of cognitive deficits in Parkinson's disease. *Psychopharmacology (Berl)* **146**:162–74.

Müller BW, Gimbel K, Keller-Pliessing A, Sartary G, Gastpar M, Davids E. (2007). Neuropsychological assessment of adult patients with attention-deficit/hyperactivity disorder. *Eur Arch Psychiatry Clin Neurosci* **257**(2):12–119.

Nigg JT. (2005). Neuropsychological theory and findings in attention-deficit/hyperactivity disorder. *Biol Psychiatry* **57**(11):1424–35.

Nigg JT, Blaskey LG, Huang-Pollock CL, Rappley MD. (2002). Neuropsychological executive functions and DSM-IV ADHD subtypes. *J Am Acad Child Adolesc Psychiatry* **41**(1):59–66.

Nigg JT, Casey BJ. (2005). An integrative theory of attention-deficit/hyperactivity disorder based on the cognitive and affective neurosciences. *Dev Psychopathol* **17**(3):785–806.

Nigg JT, Willcutt EG, Doyle AE, Sonuga-Barke EJ. (2005). Causal heterogeneity in attention-deficit/hyperactivity disorder: do we need neuropsychologically impaired subtypes? *Biol Psychiatry* **57**(11):1224–30.

O'Driscoll GA, Départie L, Holahan AL, Savion-Lemieux T, Barr RG, Jolicoeur C, et al. (2005). Executive functions and methylphenidate response in subtypes of attention-deficit/hyperactivity disorder. *Biol Psychiatry* **57**(11):1452–60.

O'Leary KM. (2000). Borderline personality disorder. Neuropsychological testing results. *Psychiatr Clin North Am* **23**:41–60.

O'Leary KM, Brauwers P, Gardiner DL, Cowdry RW. (1991). Neuropsychological testing of patients with borderline personality disorder. *Am J Psychiatry* **148**:106–11.

Oosterlaan J, Scheres A, Sergeant JA. (2005). Which executive functioning deficits are associated with ADHD, ODD/CD and comorbid ADHD+ODD/CD? *J Abnorm Child Psychol* **33**(1):69–85.

Owen AM, Downes JJ, Sahakian BJ, Polkey CE, Robbins TW. (1990). Planning and spatial working memory following frontal lobe lesions in man. *Neuropsychologia* **28**(10):1021–34

Owen AM, Evans AC, Petrides M. (1996). Evidence for a two-stage model of spatial working memory processing within the lateral frontal cortex: a positron emission tomography study. *Cerebr Cortex* **6**:31–8.

Owen AM, Sahakian BJ, Semple J, Polkey CE, Robbins TW. (1995). Visuo-spatial short-term recognition memory and learning after temporal lobe excisions, frontal lobe excisions and amygdalo-hippocampectomy in man. *Neuropsychologia* **33**(1):1–24.

Pennington BF. (2005). Towards a new neuropsychological model of attention-deficit/hyperactivity disorder: subtypes and multiple deficits. *Biol Psychiatry* **57**(11):1221–3.

Pennington BF, Ozonoff S. (1996). Executive functions and developmental psychopathology. *J Child Psychol Psychiatry* **37**:51–87.

Perugini EM, Harvey EA, Lovejoy DW, Sandstone K, Webb AM. (2000). The predictive power of combined neuropsychological measures for attention-deficit/hyperactivity disorder in children. *Child Neuropsychol* **6**(2):101–14.

Pliszka SR. (2005). The neuropsychopharmacology of attention-deficit/hyperactivity disorder. *Biol Psychiatry* **57**:1385–90.

Postle BR, Stern CE, Rosen BR, Corkin S. (2000). An fMRI investigation of cortical contributions to spatial and nonspatial visual working memory. *Neuroimage* **11**:409–23.

Purcell R, Maruff P, Kyrios M, Pantelis C. (1998). Neuropsychological deficits in obsessive-compulsive disorder. *Arch Gen Psychiatry* **55**:415–23.

Rapoport JL, Buchsbaum MS, Weingarten H, Zahn TP, Ludlow C, Mikkelsen EJ. (1980). Dextroamphetamine. Its cognitive and behavioural effects in normal and hyperactive boys and normal men. *Arch Gen Psychiatry* **37**:933–43.

Reeves K. (2003). Modafinil treats symptoms of ADHD in children. *Progr Neurol Psychiatry* **14**:9.

Rhodes SM, Coghill DR, Matthews K. (2005). Neuropsychological functioning in stimulant-naïve boys with hyperkinetic disorder. *Psychol Med* **35**(8):1109–20.

Riordan HJ, Flashman LA, Saykin AJ, Frutiger SA, Carroll KE, Huey L. (1999). Neuropsychological correlates of methylphenidate treatment in adult ADHD with and without depression. *Arch Clin Neuropsychol* **14**:217–33.

Rogers RD, Blackshaw AJ, Middleton HC, et al. (1999). Tryptophan depletion impairs stimulus-reward learning while methylphenidate disrupts attentional control in healthy young adults: implications for the monoaminergic basis of impulsive behaviour. *Psychopharmacology (Berl)* **146**:482–91.

Rubia K, Smith AB, Brammer MJ, Taylor E. (2003). Right inferior prefrontal cortex mediates response inhibition while mesial prefrontal cortex is responsible for error detection. *Neuroimage* **20**(1):351–8.

Rubinsztein JS, Michael A, Paykel ES, Sahakian BJ. (2000). Cognitive impairment in remission in bipolar affective disorder. *Psychol Med* **30**:1025–36.

Rugino TA, Copley TC. (2001). Effects of modafinil in children with attention-deficit/hyperactivity disorder: an open-label study. *J Am Acad Child Adolesc Psychiatry* **40**:230–5.

Rugino TA, Samsock TC. (2003). Modafinil in children with attention-deficit hyperactivity disorder. *Paediatr Neurol* **29**:136–42.

Sachdev P. (1999). Attention deficit hyperactivity disorder in adults. *Psychol Med* **29**(3):507–14.

Sanuga-Barke EJ, Castellanos FX. (2005). A common core dysfunction in attention-deficit/hyperactivity disorder: A scientific red herring? *Behav Brain Sci* **28**(3):443–4.

Schachar R, Tannock R, Marriott M, Logan G. (1995). Deficient Inhibitory control in attention deficit hyperactivity disorder. *J Abnorm Childhood Psychol* **23**(4):411–37.

Schweitzer JB, Hanford RB, Medoff DR. (2006). Working memory deficits in adults with ADHD: is there evidence for subtype difference? *Behav Brain Funct* **2**: 43–54.

Seidman LJ, Biederman J, Faraone SV, Wilber W, Ouellette C. (1997). Toward defining a neuropsychology of attention deficit-hyperactivity disorder: performance of children and adolescents from a large clinically-referred sample. *J Comorbidity Clin Psychol* **65**(1):150–60.

Seidman LJ, Biederman J, Monuteaux MC, Valera E, Doyle A, Faraone SV. (2005). Impact of gender and age on executive functioning: do girls and boys with and without attention deficit hyperactivity disorder differ neuropsychologically in preteens and teenage years. *Dev Neuropsychol* **27**(1):79–105.

Sergeant JA. (2005). Modelling attention-deficit/hyperactivity disorder: a critical appraisal of the cognitive-energetic model. *Biol Psychiatry* **57**(11):1248–55.

Solanto MV. (1998). Neuropsychopharmacological mechanisms of stimulant drug action in attention-deficit hyperactivity disorder: a review and integration. *Behav Brain Res* **94**:127–52.

Solanto MV. (2002). Dopamine dysfunction in AD/HD: integrating clinical and basic neuroscience research. *Behav Brain Res* **130**:65–71.

Sonuga-Barke EJ. (2005). Causal models of attention-deficit/hyperactivity disorder: from common simple deficits to multiple developmental pathways. *Biol Psychiatry* **57**(11):1231–8.

Stein DJ, Hollander E, Cohen L, et al. (1994). Neuropsychiatric impairment in impulsive personality disorders. *Psychiatry Res* **48**:257–66.

Stein DJ, Hollander E, Liebowitz MR. (1993). Neurobiology of impulsivity and the impulse control disorders. *J Neuropsychiatry Clin Neurosci* **5**: 9–17.

Swanson JM. (2003). Role of executive function in ADHD. *J Clin Psychiatry* **64**(suppl):35–39.

Swanson J, Castellanos FX, Murias M, LaHoste G, Kennedy J. (1998). Cognitive neuroscience of attention deficit hyperactivity disorder and hyperkinetic. *Curr Opin Neurobiol* **8**:263–71.

Tannock R, Ickowicz A, Schachar R. (1995). Differential effects of methylphenidate on working in ADHD children with and without comorbid anxiety. *J Am Acad Child Adolesc Psychiatry* **34**:886–96.

Tannock R, Schachar RJ, Carr RP, Logan GD. (1989). Dose-response effects of methylphenidate on academic performance and overt behaviour in hyperactive children. *Pediatrics* **84**:648–57.

Taylor FB, Russo J. (2000). Efficacy of modafinil compared to dextroamphetamine for the treatment of attention deficit hyperactivity disorder in adults. *J Child Adoles Psychopharmacol* **10**:311–20.

Thapar A, Langley K, Owen MJ, O'Donovan MC. (2007). Advances in genetic findings on attention deficit hyperactivity disorder. *Psychol Med* **37**(12): 1681–92.

Tirosh E, Cohen A. (1998). Language deficit with attention-deficit disorder: a prevalent comorbidity. *J Child Neurol* **13**(10):493–7.

Toplak ME, Tannock R. (2005) Tapping and anticipation performance in attention deficit hyperactivity disorder. *Percept Mot Skills* **100**(3):659–75.

Tsal Y, Shalev L, Mevorach C. (2005). The diversity of attention deficits in ADHD: the prevalence of four cognitive factors in ADHD versus controls. *J Learn Disabil* **38**(2):142–7.

Turner DC, Blackwell AD, Dowson JH, McLean A, Sahakian BJ. (2005). Neurocognitive effects of methylphenidate in adult attention-deficit/hyperactivity disorder. *Psychopharmacology (Berl)* **178**(2–3): 286–95.

Turner DC, Clark L, Dowson J, Robbins TW, Sahakian BJ. (2004). Modafinil improves cognition and response inhibition in adult attention-deficit/hyperactivity disorder. *Biol Psychiatry* **15**(10):1031–40.

Turner DC, Robbins TW, Clark L, Aron AR, Dowson JH, Sahakian BJ. (2003a) Cognitive enhancing effects of modafinil in healthy volunteers. *Psychopharmacology (Berl)* **165**(3):260–9.

Turner DC, Robbins TW, Clark L, Aron AR, Dowson J, Sahakian BJ. (2003b). Relative lack of cognitive effects of methylphenidate in elderly male volunteers. *Psychopharmacology (Berl)* **168**:455–64.

Vaidya CJ, Austin G, Kirkorian G, et al. (1998). Selective effects of methylphenidate in attention deficit hyperactivity disorder: functional magnetic resonance study. *Proc Natl Acad Sci USA* **95**:14494–9.

Van Reekum R. (1993). Acquired and developmental brain dysfunction in borderline personality disorder. *Can J Psychiatry* **38**(suppl 1):S4–S10.

Veale DM, Sahakian BJ, Owen AM, Marks IM. (1996). Specific cognitive defects in tests sensitive to frontal lobe dysfunction in obsessive-compulsive disorder. *Psychol Med* **26**:1261–9.

Wender PH, Wolf LE, Wasserstein J. (2001). Adults with ADHD. An overview. *Ann N Y Acad Sci* **931**:1–16.

Willcutt EG, Doyle AE, Nigg JT, Faraone SV, Pennington BF. (2005). Validity of the executive function theory of attention-deficit/hyperactivity disorder: a meta-analysis review. *Biol Psychiatry* 57(11):1336–46.

Williams D, Stott CM, Goodyer IM, Sahakian BJ. (2000). Specific language impairment with or without hyperactivity: neuropsychological evidence for frontostriatal dysfunction. *Dev Med Child Neurol* 42:368–75.

Woods SP, Lovejoy DW, Ball JD. (2002). Neuropsychological characteristics of adults with ADHD: a comprehensive review of initial studies. *Clin Neuropsychol* 16:12–34.

Yang B, Chan RC, Zou X, Jing J, Mai J, Li J. (2007). Time perception deficit in children with ADHD. *Brain Res* Jul 17 (Epub ahead of print).

Chapter

10

Adult ADHD and mood disorders

Thomas E. Brown

Most discussions of comorbidity between ADHD and mood disorders proceed from a categorical approach, simply describing the percentage of individuals with ADHD who are also diagnosed with various types of mood disorder. This approach is consistent with current diagnostic criteria, which recognize no overlap between symptoms of mood disorders and ADHD. However, there are sound clinical and theoretical reasons for thinking about ADHD and mood disorders using a more dimensional perspective. A spectrum of severity of mood regulatory problems is found among persons with ADHD, and there is a spectrum of ADHD problems found in varying degrees among individuals diagnosed with disorders on the mood disorders spectrum. Both mood disorders and ADHD tend to be dimensional; comorbidity between ADHD and mood disorders is not cleanly categorical!

This chapter describes the spectrum of mood disorders associated with ADHD, the incidence of overlap between these two diagnostic categories, and implications of such overlap for research and clinical practice. I begin with the proposal that most individuals with ADHD suffer from some degree of chronic difficulty in regulating emotion; I argue that impairments of emotional regulation may be an overlooked core feature of ADHD. Yet, although mood regulatory problems, in varying degrees, may be clinically significant in many individuals with ADHD, there is clear evidence that some individuals with ADHD suffer from mood regulatory problems sufficiently severe to warrant an additional diagnosis of mood disorder. This chapter describes the continuum of mood disorders often found comorbid with ADHD; it also discusses how clinical care and treatment of individuals with ADHD may need to be modified to address problems with mood regulation, whether these problems are sufficiently severe to warrant a separate diagnosis or not.

Role of emotion in cognition and in ADHD

Currently established diagnostic criteria for ADHD include no reference to problems with emotional regulation, yet numerous investigators have reported that persons with ADHD tend to have chronic problems in regulating emotions. Wender's (1995) Utah Criteria for ADHD include "affective liability," "hot temper," and "overreacts" among symptoms of ADHD. Conners' Adult ADD Rating Scale includes 2 items related to anger regulation ("still throw tantrums" "short-fuse/hot temper") and 2 items related to depressive feelings ("lack faith in my abilities" and "hard to believe in myself") in the ADHD Index that comprises that scale's 12 statistically best items for identifying adults with ADHD (Conners, Erhardt, & Sparrow, 1999). Data from the Brown ADD Scales for Adults (1996) indicate positive correlations between responses to items related to emotional regulation (e.g. "excessively impatient," "sensitive to criticism," "easily irritated," "depressed mood") and the total score for the combination of all five clusters of ADHD-related impairments of executive function. Clinical data obtained from various samples and theoretical arguments described by Barkley (2010) suggest that problems in emotional regulation constitute a significant aspect of the core problems of persons with ADHD that has been overlooked in the *DSM-IV* criteria for ADHD.

Over the past 15 years increasing numbers of researchers have recognized that emotion and processing of information are inseparable in the human mind. Dodge argued that information processing is never without emotion: "All information processing is emotional, in that emotion is the energy level that drives, organizes, amplifies, and attenuates cognitive

ADHD in Adults: Characterization, Diagnosis and Treatment, ed. Jan Buitelaar, Cornelis Kan and Philip Asherson.
Published by Cambridge University Press. © Cambridge University Press 2011.

activity (1991, p. 159)." Neuroscientists have demonstrated that emotion plays an essential role in activating the brain, assigning priorities to cognitive inputs and activities, and sustaining motivation for behavior (e.g. Damasio, 1994; Roll, 1999). Research on the role of emotion in cognitive functioning has also highlighted the fact that much of the influence of emotion on cognition is instantaneous and outside the realm of conscious experience (e.g. LeDoux, 1996; Phelps, 2005). Emotion plays an implicit but powerful role in guiding executive functions of the brain.

Yet the interaction of emotion and executive functions (EFs) of the brain is bidirectional. Executive functions are not only activated and sustained by emotion but they also are involved in modulating emotion and in managing its impact on behavior. As Denckla (1996) has noted, a very basic element in the evolution of an individual's capacity for self-control, from preschool years onward, is development of the ability to inhibit and modulate expression of emotion so that intense emotion does not intrude excessively on important cognitive tasks or spill over into impulsive behaviors that may be hurtful or otherwise maladaptive. Cognitive and neurophysiological factors influencing the cognitive control of emotion have been reviewed by Green, Cahill, and Malhi (2007).

For many persons with ADHD, a syndrome characterized by developmental impairment of EFs, this "top-down" regulation of emotions is chronically problematic. Models of executive function formulated by Barkley (1997, 2006) and me (1996, 2000, 2005, 2009) propose a broader phenotype for the ADHD syndrome than is included in the current *DSM*. Both our models include regulation of alertness and activation as well as regulation of and by emotion. We contend that these elements are essential to executive functioning and that impairments in these emotion-related functions are an essential component of the EF impairments of the syndrome of ADHD.

Although impairments of emotional regulation may be an important aspect of the ADHD syndrome, similar impairments are also characteristic of many other psychiatric disorders, some of which are essentially characterized by more severe forms of such impairments. Thus the question arises: what is the relationship between impairments in emotional regulation often found in persons with ADHD and impairments in regulation of emotion observed in persons diagnosed with mood disorders, anxiety disorders, and the like? Banaschewski, Hollis,

Oosterlaan, and others (2005) have proposed a useful way to address this question, suggesting that "many deficits [of ADHD] are shared with other disorders and some differences between ADHD and other disorders may be *quantitative* rather than *qualitative* (p. 136, italics added)."

An example of such quantitative differences can be found in the research of Mick and colleagues (2005), who studied 274 children with ADHD to assess levels of irritability in those with and without mood disorder diagnoses. Using data from three modules of the KSADS, they identified three intensity levels for irritability: (1) "extreme explosive irritability," (2) "clinically significant irritability lacking an explosive or extreme impairment," and (3) a less impairing level of irritability identified as "ODD-type irritability, low frustration tolerance." These researchers then evaluated protocols to determine how ratings of these levels of irritability were associated with ADHD and with mood disorder diagnoses.

Results indicated that, although 76% of the total sample of ADHD children had been rated as manifesting ODD-type irritability (easily annoyed, loses temper, angry, or resentful), there were clear differences in the level of severity of irritability between those with and without comorbid mood disorders. Among those who were not mood-disordered, 67% had shown irritability at the least severe level compared to 85% of those diagnosed with unipolar depression and 90% of those diagnosed with bipolar disorder. More severe but moderate levels of irritability were found in 17% of those without mood disorder, 57% of those with unipolar depression, and 83% of those with bipolar disorder. The most severe level of irritability (super-angry/grouchy/cranky) was found in only 8% of those without mood disorder, 16% of those with unipolar depression, and 77% of those diagnosed with bipolar disorder (Mick et al., 2005, p. 578). These data illustrate how some mood regulatory symptoms – in this case, irritability – may be seen as an aspect of ADHD at one level of severity, and then, at a level significantly more severe and impairing, those symptoms may be seen as warranting an additional diagnosis (e.g. a comorbid mood disorder).

Incidence of mood disorders among adults with ADHD

Before describing the incidence of mood disorders among adults with ADHD, it should be recognized that overlaps or comorbidity of one psychiatric disorder with another is described in a variety of ways. Some reports of diagnostic overlap are cross-sectional, identifying only those individuals with ADHD who are seen as having another disorder within a specified time frame (e.g. within the past year). Other reports of overlap refer to lifetime comorbidity; under this rubric an individual who had a diagnosed problem with cannabis abuse for one year at age 20 would be counted as having a comorbid substance use disorder at age 45, even if he had no problem with substance abuse in the intervening 25 years. Lifetime estimates should be considered with this limitation in mind because, as Rutter, Kim-Cohen, and Maughan (2006) pointed out, psychopathology manifest in earlier years of life does not always persist throughout a lifetime.

Most discussions of comorbidity do not include what Lahey et al. (2002) referred to as "dynamic comorbidity." This term refers to the tendency of some psychiatric disorders to wax and wane over an individual's life span, possibly in response to situational influences, the presence or absence of specific stressors or supports, or unfolding developmental factors. Much psychiatric comorbidity is dynamic in this sense. Therefore, when considering reports of psychiatric comorbidity, both in research and in clinical practice, it is important to be clear about the way it is being defined.

Another factor to be considered in evaluating reports of comorbidity is the sample selection. Most estimates of psychiatric comorbidity are based on clinical samples, groups of individuals who have sought treatment for one or more psychiatric problems. Rates of comorbidity in clinical samples are likely to be considerably higher than in the general population because persons with more severe and complicated impairments are more likely to seek treatment. Clinical samples do not include individuals in the community who may have similar disorders with less severe levels of impairment but who have not sought treatment or who have obtained private treatment where their records are less likely to be included in research. In contrast, epidemiological samples may underreport psychopathology, with or without comorbidity, because persons approached in such studies may have less willingness to disclose the full extent of their personal difficulties. Differences between clinical and epidemiological sampling are illustrated later in this chapter.

Although many types of mood disorders are described in *DSM-IV-TR* (American Psychiatric Association, 2000), the mood disorders reported in studies of comorbidity generally include the following types:

Major depressive disorder (MDD): characterized by one or more major depressive episodes (i.e. at least 2 weeks of depressed mood or loss of interest) accompanied by at least four additional symptoms of depression. This disorder is associated with high mortality; up to 15% of individuals with severe major depressive disorder die by suicide.

Dysthymic disorder: characterized by chronically depressed mood that occurs for most of the day, more days than not, for at least 2 years. To qualify for diagnosis, this chronically depressed mood must be accompanied by at least two other symptoms specified in the diagnostic criteria.

Bipolar disorder (BPD): manifest in either of two primary types: Type I, which includes one or more manic episodes or episodes of mania mixed with depression, or Type II, which is characterized by one or more major depressive episodes accompanied by at least one hypomanic episode. Both manic episodes and hypomanic episodes are defined as distinct periods during which there is abnormally and persistently elevated expansive or irritable mood, accompanied by at least three additional symptoms from a list including decreased need for sleep, flight of ideas, and excessive involvement in pleasurable activities with a high potential for painful consequences.

The primary difference between manic and hypomanic episodes is the level of severity of impairment. Manic episodes cause severe impairment in social or occupational functioning, may have psychotic features, and often require hospitalization. Hypomanic episodes are significantly impairing, but not severe enough to cause marked impairment in social or occupational functioning, are not accompanied by psychotic features, and do not generally require hospitalization.

Several symptoms differentiate unipolar depression from bipolar disorders. One of these is severe irritability and anger. Perlis, Smoller, et al. (2004) studied outpatients with MDD or BPD and found that anger attacks were significantly more common among bipolar (62%) than unipolar (26%) depressed individuals. Logistic regression found that the presence of anger attacks emerged as a significant predictor of bipolarity.

In a subsequent study comparing a large number of nonpsychotic outpatients with unipolar or bipolar disorders, Perlis, Brown, et al. (2006) found that fears were more common in bipolar patients, whereas sadness, insomnia, somatic complaints, and depressed behavior were more common in patients with unipolar depression. That study also showed that bipolar disorder was more often associated with a family history of BPD, earlier age of onset, and more depressive episodes.

Although major depressive disorder and bipolar disorder can be differentiated, in recent years considerable evidence has been found that these two types of mood disorder exist on a dimensional spectrum (Akiskal, 2005, 2006; Benazzi, 2006; Cassano et al., 2004) in which both may have similar symptoms, but increased impairment is associated with the bipolar syndromes.

Overlap is also often found between mood disorders and anxiety disorders. Consistent with Nemeroff's (2002) observation of strong positive correlations between measures of severity of depressive symptoms and anxiety symptoms, Simon et al. (2004) reported that more than 50% of the first 500 patients in the Systematic Treatment Enhancement Program (STEP) for Bipolar Disorder had one or more comorbid anxiety disorders. This overlap tended to be associated with earlier age of onset, decreased likelihood of recovery, poorer role functioning and quality of life, less euthymic time, and greater likelihood of suicide.

Although major depressive disorder is relatively common in the general population, the incidence of bipolar disorders is relatively low. Kessler et al. (2005) reported on the replication of the National Comorbidity Study, a nationally representative epidemiological sample of 9282 English-speaking adults in the US population. This study found the following lifetime rates of mood disorders: major depressive disorder: 16.6%; dysthymia: 2.5%; bipolar I–II disorders: 3.9%; and any mood disorder: 20.8%.

In contrast, Millstein et al. (1997) found a much higher incidence of mood disorders in a clinical sample of adults with ADHD. Among those with combined-type ADHD, they found an incidence of 63% for major depressive disorder, 23% for dysthymia, and 17% for bipolar disorder (I–II combined). For predominantly inattentive-type subjects, that group obtained identical incidence rates for major depression, but lower rates for dysthymia (11%) and for bipolar disorder (3%).

A different clinical sample was described by McGough et al. (2005). In their sample of parents diagnosed with persistent ADHD who had two or more offspring with ADHD, these researchers found incidence rates of comorbid mood disorders very similar to those obtained by Millstein et al. (1997) in their predominantly inattentive ADHD subgroup: 59% with major depression, 15% with dysthymia, and 4% with bipolar disorder.

A relatively high incidence of overlap between ADHD and bipolar disorder is not found only in samples of persons initially diagnosed with ADHD. Nierenberg et al. (2005) reported that, among the first 1000 adults in the STEP study, overall lifetime prevalence of ADHD was 9.5%, more than double the estimated rate of ADHD in the general population of adults. Among these bipolar adults, lifetime incidence of ADHD followed the same gender ratio often reported for ADHD in children: approximately three males to each female.

Nierenberg and colleagues' (2005) report on the STEP study also indicated that those patients with both ADHD and BPD tended to be more severely ill than those whose BPD was not accompanied by ADHD. Those with both disorders had onset of their mood disorder about 5 years earlier, had shorter periods of wellness, and were more frequently depressed. They also had a greater number of other comorbid psychiatric diagnoses with substantially higher rates of several anxiety disorders and alcohol and substance abuse and dependence.

These findings from the STEP study are consistent with a report from Wilens, Biederman, et al. (2003) who compared adults with both ADHD and bipolar disorder to adults diagnosed with ADHD and no mood disorder. Those patients who had both ADHD and BPD tended to have combined-type ADHD (96% vs. 59%), had poorer global functioning, and more comorbid disorders. Most of these comorbid patients had type II BPD (88%); manic symptoms were predominantly euphoric in 22%, predominantly irritable in 45%, and mixed euphoric/irritable in 33%.

It is not uncommon for patients with BPD to have a history of childhood psychiatric disorders. In a sample of adults diagnosed with BPD, Henin and colleagues (2007) found a significantly higher incidence of ADHD, oppositional-defiant disorder, conduct disorder, childhood anxiety, and enuresis compared to patients without mood disorders. This finding suggests that, among individuals with more severe mood disorders, problems with emotional regulation do not await adult onset; they often appear in diagnosable forms during childhood or adolescence.

More detailed information about the age of onset and clinical course of mood disorders was provided in a study by Perlis, Miyahara, et al. (2004), who surveyed the first 1000 patients in the STEP study of BPD to compare clinical course, comorbidity, functional status, and quality of life for groups of patients with bipolar disorder with differing ages of onset. Among those patients 27.7% had onset of BPD before 13 years, and 37.6% had onset between 13 and 18 years. Earlier onset was associated with greater rates of comorbid anxiety disorders, more substance abuse, more recurrences, shorter periods of euthymia, greater likelihood of suicide attempts, and more violence. These findings led those researchers to suggest that earlier age of onset of BPD tends to herald a more severe course of disease and higher rates of comorbidity.

Among persons with various types of mood disorders there is considerable variability in course and outcome. At least 60% of individuals with major depressive disorder, single episode, can be expected to have a second episode. Individuals who have had a second episode have a 70% chance of having a third, and individuals who have had three episodes have a 90% chance of experiencing a fourth. For those with recurrent episodes, there may be depression-free periods of many years or multiple episodes of depression closely spaced. About 40% of those with major depressive episodes continue to have symptoms that fully meet diagnostic criteria for major depression one year later, whereas 40% have no continuing depressive symptoms at that time (American Psychiatric Association, 2000).

Among bipolar patients who entered the STEP study symptomatic, more than half (58.4%) subsequently achieved recovery. During the subsequent 2 years of follow-up, 48.5% of these patients experienced recurrences, most (34.7%) developed depressive episodes, and 13.8% developed manic, hypomanic, or mixed episodes. The time until 25% of the individuals experienced a depressive episode was 21.4 weeks; until 25% experienced a manic/hypomanic/mixed episode it was 85 weeks (Perlis, Ostacher, et al., 2006).

Treatment of mood problems associated with ADHD in adults

When an adult is found to have both ADHD and a mood disorder, it is important for the evaluating clinician to assess carefully current impairments and the relative urgency of each of these syndromes. In some cases, the mood disorder clearly demands priority for treatment; for example, when the patient is suffering from serious disruptions of eating and/or sleeping or is experiencing suicidal intentions or serious suicidal ideation, psychotic symptoms, and/or acute agitation or aggression suggestive of developing mania. Such cases generally warrant immediate treatment of the mood disorder and then a reassessment of ADHD impairments once the mood problems have been adequately stabilized by appropriate treatment.

In other cases, impairment of mood regulation may be less acute, less dangerous, and more chronic. Mood symptoms in these cases may be characterized more by demoralization and dysthymic symptoms that lack the severity or change from the individual's previous baseline functioning expected for a diagnosis of major depressive episode. Or the patient may manifest a long-term pattern of chronic hyperactivity/impulsivity that is relatively stable, without the "distinct period of abnormally and persistently elevated, expansive or irritable mood" specified in *DSM-IV* diagnostic criteria for mania and hypomania.

In cases where the patient's problems with mood regulation are less acute and more chronic, these problems may be an aspect of or a reaction to their chronic ADHD impairments. For such patients, the clinician may choose to begin with the usual treatment interventions for ADHD to determine whether effective treatment of the ADHD symptoms may help significantly to alleviate the patient's dysthymic and/or hyperactive/impulsive symptoms. If this approach is taken, the clinician will want to monitor the patient's responses to treatment very carefully, especially in the early phases, so that an appropriate change of intervention strategy can be made promptly if the patient responds to the ADHD treatment with increased severity of depressive or escalating symptoms of mania. Carlson and Meyer (2009) have described considerations for the use of ADHD medications with patients who have symptoms of comorbid bipolar disorder.

For patients with ADHD who also have significant problems with depressive mood, the clinician may wish to consider a trial of a tricyclic antidepressant (TCA) to treat both the ADHD symptoms and the depressive symptoms. Wilens and colleagues (1995, 1996) have reported on clinical trials that demonstrated moderate effectiveness of TCAs for treatment of ADHD in adults over a 1-year period. Prince et al.

(2006) have noted that, in some cases, these TCA treatments for ADHD in adults have been augmented by the concurrent use of stimulants or other adjunctive medications. Because TCAs have also been demonstrated to be effective for dysthymia and major depressive disorder, they may provide effective treatment for both ADHD and comorbid depressive symptoms.

Selective serotonin reuptake inhibitors (SSRIs) have not been found to be effective for the alleviation of ADHD symptoms, but they do tend to be effective for treatment of unipolar depression. Another option for patients with both ADHD and dysthymia or major depressive disorder is to stabilize treatment of the patient's ADHD symptoms using stimulants or atomoxetine and then, if depressive symptoms continue to be problematic to the patient, to add an SSRI to address the depressive symptoms.

There is a risk in treating patients who have a mood disorder, with or without ADHD, using TCA or SSRI medications. Either of these types of antidepressants can cause excessive activation or "switching" in patients whose depressive symptoms are accompanied by an underlying bipolar disorder. If a patient with ADHD and depressive symptoms shows no significant symptoms or history of bipolar disorder, an antidepressant medication might be started, before or after stabilization on ADHD medication treatment. However, such treatments should be closely monitored by the clinician for indicators of agitation or increased activation. If these symptoms occur in response to medication treatments for either ADHD or depressive symptoms, those medications should be discontinued until the mood problems have been stabilized with appropriate medication (Prince et al., 2006).

Another option for treatment of patients with ADHD and BPD was tested by Wilens, Prince, et al. (2003). In an open trial with patients diagnosed with ADHD and a current or lifetime history of either BPD-I (10%) or BPD-II (90%), treatment with buproprion-SR over 6 weeks produced significant reductions in ADHD symptoms and in both manic and depressive symptoms. Buproprion was not associated with manic activation. The authors concluded that buproprion might have a role in the treatment of ADHD with BPD.

Some clinicians routinely treat bipolar patients with a combination of an antidepressant and a mood stabilizer, presumably to alleviate both manic and depressive symptoms. However, Sachs et al. (2007) reported a study of bipolar patients treated with this combination versus bipolar patients treated with a mood stabilizer and placebo. Results challenged the assumption that this combined treatment is always preferable. Twenty-three percent of those treated with the combination of antidepressant and mood stabilizer had a durable recovery, in contrast to 27% of those treated with mood stabilizer and placebo. Given the narrow difference between the groups on these interventions, it seems reasonable to conclude that the combination of mood stabilizers and antidepressants is helpful for some bipolar patients, but not more helpful than a mood stabilizer alone for others.

One way of deciding whether to use or continue the mood stabilizer/antidepressant combination was proposed by Hartouche, Akiskal, and colleagues (2005), based on data from a French study of adults with unipolar depression. From their data sorting out good responders to antidepressants versus poor responders, these researchers urged that poor responders to antidepressants and those who do not respond well to the combination of mood stabilizer and antidepressant should promptly be taken off the antidepressant and treated with a mood stabilizer alone. However, Rihmer and Akiskal (2006) argued that judicious use of antidepressant medications augmented by mood stabilizers, atypical neuroleptics, or benzodiazepine may be more helpful in preventing suicide attempts in depressed patients than some studies and conventional policy might suggest. Clinical judgment is required for each individual case.

For those patients with diagnosed BPD, published expert consensus guidelines for treatment (American Psychiatric Association, 2002; Bauer et al., 1999; Sachs et al., 2000) recommend use of a mood stabilizer and urge avoidance of monotherapy with antidepressants. Yet, an analysis of data on bipolar patients in the replication of the National Cormobidity Study found that, although most people with BPD receive lifetime professional treatment for emotional problems, use of antimanic medications is uncommon, especially in general medical settings (Merikangas et al., 2007).

Data reported by Simon et al. (2004) from the first 1000 patients in the STEP study indicated that, on entry, only 59% of those patients had received at least "minimally adequate" treatment with a mood stabilizer medication. Although 72% of those bipolar patients met diagnostic criteria for at least one additional psychiatric disorder, few were being treated with the combination of mood stabilizer and an additional medication recognized as effective for treating that comorbid disorder. Within that STEP sample only 9% of those who currently met diagnostic criteria for ADHD had received any medication with demonstrated efficacy for ADHD. That study concluded that "both bipolar disorder itself and associated comorbidities are currently undertreated with pharmacotherapy" (Simon et al., 2004, p. 518).

Much remains to be learned about the treatment of adults whose ADHD is complicated by a mood disorder. There is, at present, little research to guide the clinician as to which types of treatment, especially which combinations of medications, are most helpful and least problematic for patients with this comorbidity, which appears in a variety of forms that are often concurrent to additional comorbid disorders. However, it is clear that, although both ADHD and any of the various mood disorders can, in themselves, cause significant impairment, the combination of ADHD and a mood disorder is likely to be severely impairing and, in some cases, may be life threatening.

When both ADHD and a mood disorder are present in an adult patient, it is important to assess very carefully the relative severity of each and to plan carefully to prioritize and provide optimal treatment for each of the disorders, taking fully into account characteristics of the individual patient and any additional comorbidities that may be present. It is also essential to monitor these complex patients carefully on an ongoing basis so that treatment outcome can be optimized.

References

Akiskal HS. (2005). Searching for behavioral indicators of bipolar II in patients presenting with major depressive episodes. *J Affect Disord* **84**(2–3):279–90.

Akiskal HS. (2006). The DSM-IV and ICD-10 categories of recurrent (major) depression and bipolar II disorders: evidence that they lie on a dimensional spectrum. *J Affect Disord* **92**(1):45–54.

American Psychiatric Association. (2000). *Diagnostic and Statistical Manual of Mental Disorders*. 4th ed., text rev. Washington, DC: American Psychiatric Press.

American Psychiatric Association. (2002). Practice guidelines for the treatment of patients with bipolar disorder (revision). *Am J Psychiatry* **159**(4 suppl):1–50.

Banaschewski T, Hollis C. Oosterlaan J, Roeyers H, Rubia K, Willcutt E, et al. (2005). Towards an understanding of unique and shared pathways in the psychopathophysiology of ADHD. *Dev Sci* **8**(2): 132–40.

Barkley RA. (1997). *ADHD and the Nature of Self-Control*. New York: Guilford Press.

Barkley RA. (2006). *Attention-Deficit Hyperactivity Disorder: A Handbook for Diagnosis and Treatment*. 3rd ed. New York: Guilford Press.

Barkley RA. (2010). Deficient emotional self-regulation is a core component of attention-deficit/hyperactivity disorder. *J ADHD Rel Disord* **1**(2): 5-37.

Bauer M, Callahan A, Jampala C, et al. (1999). Clinical practice guidelines for bipolar disorder from the Dept. of Veterans Affairs. *J Clin Psychiatry* **60**(1):9–21.

Benazzi F. (2006). A continuity between bipolar II depression and major depressive disorder? *Prog Neuro-Psychopharmacol Biol Psychiatry* **30**(6):1043–50.

Brown TE. (1996). *Brown Attention Deficit Disorder Scales for Adolescents and Adults*. San Antonio: Psychological Corporation.

Brown TE. (2000). Emerging understandings of attention deficit disorders and comorbidities. In: Brown TE, ed. *Attention Deficit Disorders and Comorbidities in Children, Adolescents and Adults*. Washington, DC: American Psychiatric Press: 3–55.

Brown TE. (2005). *Attention Deficit Disorder: The Unfocused Mind in Children and Adults*. New Haven: Yale University Press.

Brown TE. (2009). Developmental complexities of attentional disorders. In: Brown TE, ed. *ADHD Comorbidities: Handbook for ADHD Complications in Children and Adults*. Washington, DC: American Psychiatric Press: 3–22.

Carlson GA, Meyer SE. (2009). ADHD with mood disorders In: Brown TE, ed. *ADHD Comorbidities: Handbook for ADHD Complications in Children and Adults* (pp. 97–130). Washington, DC: American Psychiatric Press.

Cassano GB, Rucci P, Frank E, Fagiolini A, Dell'Osso L, Shear MK, et al. (2004). The mood spectrum in unipolar and bipolar disorder: arguments for a unitary approach. *Am J Psychiatry* **161**:1264–9.

Conners CK, Erhardt D, Sparrow EP. (1999). *Conners' Adult ADHD Rating Scales*. North Tonawanda, NY: Multi-Health Systems.

Damasio AR. (1994). *Descartes' Error: Emotion, Reason, and the Human Brain*. New York: G. P. Putnam's Sons.

Denckla MB. (1996). A theory and model of executive function. In **Lyon GR, Krasnegor NA**, eds. *Attention, Memory, and Executive Function*. Baltimore: Paul H. Brookes: 263–78.

Dodge KA. (1991). Emotion and social information processing. In Garber J, Dodge KA, eds. *Development of Emotion Regulation and Dysregulation*. New York: Cambridge University Press: 159–81.

Green MJ, Cahill CM, Malhi GS. (2007). The cognitive and neurophysiological basis of emotion dysregulation in bipolar disorder. *J Affect Disord* 103: 29-42.

Hartouche EG, Akiskal HS, Lancrenon S, Chatenet-Duchene L. (2005). Mood stabilizer augmentation in apparently "unipolar" MDD: predictors of response in the naturalistic French national EPIDEP study. *J Affect Disord* 84:243-9.

Henin A, Biederman J, Mick E, et al. (2007). Childhood antecedent disorders to bipolar disorders in adults: a controlled study. *J Affect Disord* 99:51-7.

Kessler RC, Berglund P, Demler O, Jin R, Merikangas KR, Walters EE. (2005). Lifetime prevalence and age-of-onset distributions of DSM-IV disorders in the National Comorbidity Survey Replication. *Arch Gen Psychiatry* 62:593-602.

Lahey BB, Loeber R, Burke J, Rathouz P, McBurnett K. (2002). Waxing and waning in concert: dynamic comorbidity of conduct disorder with other disruptive and emotional problems over 7 years among clinic-referred boys. *J Abnorm Psychol* 111(4):556-67.

LeDoux J. (1996). *The Emotional Brain*. New York: Simon & Schuster.

McGough JJ, Smalley SL, McCracken JT, Yang M, Del'Homme M, Lynn, DE, et al. (2005). Psychiatric comorbidity in adult attention deficit hyperactivity disorder: findings from multiplex families. *Am J Psychiatry* 162(9):1621-7.

Merikangas K, Akiskal H, Angst J, Greenberg PE, Hirshfeld RMA, Petukhova M, et al. (2007). Lifetime and 12-month prevalence of bipolar spectrum disorder in the National Comorbidity Survey Replication. *Arch Gen Psychiatry* 64:543-52.

Mick E, Spencer T, Wozniak J, Biederman J. (2005). Heterogeneity of irritability in attention-deficit/hyperactivity disorder subjects with and without mood disorders. *Biol Psychiatry* 58:576-82.

Millstein RB, Wilens TE, Biederman J, Spencer TJ. (1997). Presenting ADHD symptoms and subtypes in clinically referred adults with ADHD. *J Atten Disord* 2(3):159-66.

Nemeroff CB. (2002). Comorbidity of mood and anxiety disorders: the rule, not the exception. *Am J Psychiatry* 159(1): 3-4.

Nierenberg AA, Miyahara S, Spencer T, Wisniewski SR, Otto MW, Simon N, et al. (2005). Clinical and diagnostic implications of lifetime attention-deficit/hyperactivity disorder comorbidity in adults with bipolar disorder: data from the first 1000 STEP-BD participants. *Biol Psychiatry* 57(11):1467-73.

Perlis RH, Brown E, Baker RW, Nierenberg AA. (2006). Clinical features of bipolar depression versus major depressive disorder in large multicenter trials. *Am J Psychiatry* 163(2):225-31.

Perlis RH, Miyahara S, Marangell LB, Wisniewski SR, Ostacher MJ, DelBello MP, et al. (2004). Long-term implications of early onset in bipolar disorder: data for the first 1000 participants in the Systematic Treatment Enhancement Program for Bipolar Disorder. *Biol Psychiatry* 55(9):875-81.

Perlis RH, Ostacher MJ, Patel J, Marangell LB, Zhang H, Wisniewski SR, et al. (2006). Predictors of recurrence in bipolar disorder: primary outcomes from the Systematic Treatment Enhancement Program for Bipolar Disorder. *Am J Psychiatry* 163(2): 217-24.

Perlis RH, Smoller J, Fava M, Rosenbaum JF, Nierenberg AA, Sachs GS. (2004). The prevalence and clinical correlates of anger attacks during depressive attacks in bipolar disorder. *J Affect Disord* 79(1-3):291-5.

Phelps E. (2005). The interaction of emotion and cognition: the relationship between the human amygdala and cognitive awareness. In Hassin R, Uleman J, Bargh JA, eds. *The New Unconscious*. New York: Oxford University Press: 61-76.

Prince JB, Wilens TE, Spencer TJ, Biederman J. (2006). Pharmacotherapy of ADHD in adults. In Barkley RA, ed. *Attention-Deficit Hyperactivity Disorder: A Handbook for Diagnosis and Treatment*. New York: Guilford Press: 704-38.

Rihmer Z, Akiskal H. (2006). Do antidepressants t(h)reat(en) depressives? Toward a clinically judicious formulation of the antidepressant-suicidality FDA advisory in light of declining national suicide statistics from many countries. *J Affect Disord* 94(1-3): 3-13.

Roll ET. (1999). *The Brain and Emotion*. New York: Oxford University Press.

Rutter M, Kim-Cohen J, Maughan B. (2006). Continuities and discontinuities in psychopathology between childhood and adult life. *J Child Psychol Psychiatry* 47:276-95.

Sachs GS, Nierenberg AA, Calabrese JR, Marangell LB, Wisniewski SR, Gyulai, L., et al. (2007). Effectiveness of adjunctive antidepressant treatment for bipolar depression. *N Engl J Med* 356(17):1711-22.

Sachs GS, Printz D, Kahn D, et al. (2000). The Expert Consensus Guideline Series: Medication treatment of bipolar disorder 2000. *Postgrad Med*, 1-204.

Simon N, Otto MW, Weiss RD, Bauer MS, Miyahara S, Wisniewski SR, et al. (2004). Pharmacotherapy for bipolar disorder and comorbid conditions. *J Clin Psychopharmacol* 24(5):512-20.

Wender PH. (1995). *Attention-Deficit Hyperactivity Disorder in Adults*. New York: Oxford University Press.

Wilens TE, Biederman J, Prince J, Spencer TJ, Faraone SV, Warburton R, et al. (1996). Six-week, double blind, placebo-controlled study of desipramine for adult attention deficit hyperactivity disorder. *Am J Psychiatry* **153**:1147–53.

Wilens TE, Biederman J, Spencer T. (1995). A systematic assessment of tricyclic antidepressants in the treatment of adult attention-deficit hyperactivity disorder. *J Nerv Ment Dis* **184**:48–50.

Wilens TE, Biederman J, Wozniak J, Gunawardene S, Wong S, Monuteaux MC. (2003). Can adults with attention-deficit/hyperactivity disorder be distinguished from those with comorbid bipolar disorder? Findings from a sample of clinically referred adults. *Biol Psychiatry* **54**:1–8.

Wilens TE, Prince JB, Spencer T, Van Patten SL, Doyle R, Girard K, et al. (2003). An open trial of bupropion for the treatment of adults with attention deficit/hyperactivity disorder and bipolar disorder. *Biol Psychiatry* **54**:9–16.

Attention-deficit hyperactivity disorder and anxiety disorders in adults

Margaret Weiss, Christopher Gibbins, and Julia D. Hunter

Introduction

In the past it was commonly believed that ADHD and anxiety were mutually exclusive. It was assumed that anxiety would necessarily mitigate the impulsive, novelty-seeking, daredevil behaviors we associated with ADHD. These assumptions are interesting, because clinical observation and later research have increased awareness that problems with attention, working memory, executive function, and an uncomfortable form of inner restlessness commonly co-occur. We hypothesize that these comorbidities occur in excess of what would occur by chance. We suggest that the cognitive impairments associated with ADHD are anxiety producing and that anxiety in turn exacerbates problems with attention.

Anxious patients describe being "edgy" or "jittery." ADHD adult patients are often "twitchy." They have "nervous habits" like jiggling their knees (the Wender sign; Paul Wender, personal communication) or "picking." When successfully medicated, both groups of patients use the word "calm" to describe the improvement. Recent observations that anxiety sometimes improves with medication for ADHD such as atomoxetine (Sumner et al., 2005) raises new questions. Is improvement in anxiety with treatment of ADHD driven by the improvement in ADHD or by an unexpected anxiolytic effect of the drug on a distinct comorbid disorder independent of ADHD? Are all anxiety symptoms equally responsive?

ADHD and executive dysfunction are overlapping but distinct problems (Biederman et al., 2006). Anxiety and executive dysfunction are also overlapping but distinct problems (Bedard et al., 2004). Working memory is a critical component of the impairment experienced in ADHD (Bedard et al., 2004; McInnes et al., 2007), anxiety disorders (Manassis et al., 2007), and the comorbid condition (Schatz & Rostain, 2006). When

all three problems are prominent both developmentally and currently, it becomes evident that attention, anxiety, and problems with working memory are intertwined. These disabilities create a vicious circle. Anxiety increases the risk of attention problems, attention deficits are anxiogenic (Roth et al., 2004), and both are driven by and cause difficulty with working memory.

The objective of this chapter is to review the literature on comorbidity, differential diagnosis, and treatment response of ADHD and anxiety disorders in adults.

Can ADHD and anxiety coexist?

The *DSM-IV-TR* (American Psychiatric Association, 2000) has by tradition grouped a family of disorders together as anxiety disorders, although the empirical base for this grouping is not well defined. Anxiety disorders include generalized anxiety disorders (GAD), post traumatic stress disorder (PTSD), panic disorder, obsessive-compulsive disorder, phobias, and social anxiety disorder. Unfortunately the checklists used to measure the severity of these disorders often include a preponderance of nonspecific problems such as pain, impaired sleep, and somatic complaints. For the purposes of identifying clinically salient aspects of these wide-ranging disorders' relationship with ADHD, we prefer to emphasize those aspects of each of these disorders that can be considered pathognomonic.

Cognitive-behavior therapy is a mainstay of treatment for anxiety disorders. One would think that this would inspire a revision of the diagnostic criteria for anxiety to place a stronger emphasis on pathognomonic cognitions and less emphasis on nonspecific somatic complaints. We have been slow to acknowledge that the core of each of the anxiety disorders is found in a unique attribute: worry (GAD), terror (PTSD), panic, fear (phobia), or being watched (social

ADHD in Adults: Characterization, Diagnosis and Treatment, ed. Jan Buitelaar, Cornelis Kan and Philip Asherson.
Published by Cambridge University Press. © Cambridge University Press 2011.

anxiety). The fact that these attributes often overlap or occur together has led some investigators to classify anxiety disorders by the presence of more than one of these problems on their own (Spencer, Biederman, & Wilens, 1999). Making the differential diagnosis between ADHD and the anxiety disorders is facilitated by differentiating those symptoms most specific to each anxiety disorder, rather than somatic complaints common to both or medication side effects such as insomnia, agitation, headache, appetite, or irritability.

Attention-deficit hyperactivity disorder (ADHD) is classified into the inattentive, hyperactive-impulsive, and combined types. Just as the grouping of anxiety disorders may be explained more by tradition than by evidence, so this may be true for the ADHD subtypes. The empirical literature has determined that approximately 75% of a clinic population and 50% of a community population will have the combined type, meaning they will have difficulty with both disruptive behavior and attention (Carlson & Mann, 2000; Carlson, Shin, & Booth, 1999; Faraone et al., 1998, 2000). This would suggest that disruptiveness in children drives a referral bias. Children are referred by others, and disruptive behavior is what bothers other people most.

By contrast review of the demographic characteristics of the adult clinic trials has consistently shown that a little more than half of the patients are combined type (Belendiuk et al., 2007). There are several possible explanations for this difference between ADHD in children and in adults. Adults are more likely to be self-referred and have good insight into their own problems with attention (Biederman et al., 2007). Furthermore, although frank hyperactivity diminishes with time, attention deficits do not (Biederman, Mick, & Faraone, 2007; Faraone, Biederman, & Mick, 2006). Because there is evidence that anxiety disorders are more prominent in patients with inattentive type (March et al., 2000; MTA Cooperative Group, 1999a, 1999b) and because comorbid anxiety may also be more common in women with ADHD (Biederman, 2004), it is possible that residual difficulty with cognition, attention, and anxiety becomes a more prominent aspect of the psychopathology associated with ADHD with age.

There is no lack of opportunity for the family of anxiety disorders characterized by worry, fear, trauma, and terror to overlap with the family of ADHD syndromes characterized by problems with attention

with and without obvious hyperactivity or impulsivity. Living with ADHD is "nerve wracking." If you know you are going to perform badly on a test, anxiety may be appropriate. If you know you are going to blurt out offensive comments at a party, social anxiety may be appropriate. If you know you cannot manage activities of daily living, separation anxiety from a caregiver may be quite reasonable.

Subjective aspects of ADHD and anxiety can be impossible to differentiate. Patients with both disorders describe a subjective feeling of restlessness, being unable to turn their thoughts off, or feeling "jittery." The subjective experience of ADHD in adults and the subjective experience of anxiety can be similar.

Research into the interplay of ADHD and anxiety is limited, difficult to interpret, and inconsistent. For example, Pliszka found that anxiety inhibited impulsivity (Pliszka, 1989, 1998, 2000, 2003; Pliszka et al., 1999), but this finding was not replicated using a different method (Oosterlaan & Sergeant, 1998). There is considerable research to show that anxiety has a negative impact on attention (Manassis et al., 2007; Pliszka, 2000) and very limited research to show that inattention increases anxiety (Roth et al., 2004).

Empirical research into the epidemiology of ADHD and anxiety in children suggests that up to one-third of patients with ADHD have a comorbid anxiety disorder (Biederman, Faraone, & Lapey, 1992), and the same has been found for adults (Kessler et al., 2005, 2006; McGough et al., 2005). This exceeds what would be found by chance alone and is consistent with the hypothesis that ADHD is a risk factor for an anxiety disorder.

We also know that, although the relatives of ADHD probands may have increased risk for anxiety, the two disorders do not co-segregate (Perrin & Last, 1996). This suggests that both disorders have a genetic component and may coexist, but are transmitted independently.

In summary, we conclude that there is a reciprocal increase of risk for patients with ADHD to have problems with anxiety and for patients with anxiety to suffer from ADHD that is not explained by an overlap in symptoms (Milberger et al., 1995).

Clinical presentation of ADHD and anxiety disorders

Biederman and colleagues have examined the correlates of ADHD and anxiety using a definition of anxiety disorders as the presence of two or more anxiety disorders identified in well-validated diagnostic interviews such as the Semi-Structured Diagnostic Interview for DSM-IV (SCID-IV) or the Kiddie Schedule for Affective Disorders and Schizophrenia (KSADS). This has been an effective method of finding those patients with distinct, severe, and impairing anxiety and effectively excluding those patients who might have relatively trivial and common problems such as a simple phobia. However, this method may also exclude patients who have a single but severe anxiety disorder such as serious panic attacks or obsessive-compulsive disorder. Yet, Biederman's definition of two anxiety disorders has reinforced our awareness of the extent to which one anxiety disorder presents a risk factor for other anxiety disorders.

ADHD and generalized anxiety disorder (ADHD/GAD)

Patients with ADHD have more to worry about. They are often in trouble. They make mistakes and are often criticized. People take offense at their errors and behaviors and attribute an intent that is often not present. Not all people with ADHD "care" about pleasing other people, and those that do not may be less vulnerable to negative feedback. This may explain why anxiety does seem to protect against conduct problems (Jensen, 2001). For those individuals who do "care," who have strong prosocial skills, and who want to be liked, or are perfectionistic, the awareness that they are likely to get into trouble combines with the uncertainty that they cannot anticipate when they will get into trouble to create uncertainty and secondary anxiety. This is a double bind: you cannot succeed (ADHD), you cannot fail (performance anxiety), and you cannot avoid the problem (daily life). Once anxiety is established it is immediate, a source of focus, and emotionally salient – all of which will make return to the task at hand very difficult. What then starts as an appropriate worry becomes an overvalued idea that cannot be easily shed.

The same type of vicious cycle is evident for impulsive behaviors – it can be anxiogenic to never know what you will do next. The question that patients with generalized anxiety get stuck on is the "What if?" Because this is a question that never has an answer, it becomes a source of hyperfocus that can dominate cognition to the complete exclusion of the boring and mundane here and now.

ADHD and post traumatic stress disorder (ADHD/PTSD)

It is well established that ADHD in adults is associated with an increased risk for accidents, driving accidents, extreme sports, and substance use (Biederman & Faraone, 2004). Each of these in turn would be expected to present an increased risk for trauma, leading to the possibility that adults with ADHD can be expected to have greater exposure to trauma and so an increased likelihood of PTSD. This has been found to be the case in adults (Adler et al., 2004), but not in children (Wozniak et al., 1999), suggesting that increased risk for PTSD in patients with ADHD may represent a comorbidity that develops over time.

PTSD increases the risk for ADHD, indicating that when trauma does exist it may be complicated by attention difficulties or disruptive behaviors as well as a range of other psychiatric problems (Famularo et al., 1996). This relationship has important implications for differential diagnosis. It has been suggested that in children with a history of serious trauma such as sexual or physical abuse, there is a risk of misinterpreting the symptoms as being ADHD rather than PTSD (Weinstein, Staffelbach, & Biaggio, 2000). The presence of trauma is not an exclusion for ADHD, especially if ADHD antedates the traumatic experience.

ADHD and obsessive-compulsive disorder (ADHD/OCD)

Patients with ADHD are at increased risk for OCD (Arnold et al., 2005; Geller et al., 2002, 2003, 2004; Masi et al., 2006), and when both disorders are present impairment is additive (Sukhodolsky et al., 2005). Both disorders require treatment. It has been suggested that this comorbidity is counterintuitive given that we think of obsessive behaviors as a preoccupation with details and ADHD as a lack of attention to detail. OCD is characterized by rigidity, control, neatness, cleanliness, and extremes of organization. In contrast, ADHD is characterized by oblivious attitudes to time, random and impulsive behaviors, messiness, and disorganization. What is missed in these diagnostic caricatures is their similarity: both ADHD and OCD represent opposing ends of a common disability. This becomes most evident when we think of how OCD patients often have "a messy drawer" and ADHD patients are often intensely attached to a collection that they enjoy organizing and reorganizing or are obsessed with a compulsive behavior such as using the computer, playing videogames, going shopping, or using pornography, etc. This common underlying psychopathology is also evident when we observe adults with ADHD who develop rigid and intractable schedules or habits as a coping strategy. To become organized they have to set up a steel structure that precludes flexibility, because the capacity to hold the structure in mind in the face of a temporary challenge is still not present.

ADHD and social anxiety disorder (ADHD/SAD)

ADHD is sometimes associated with excessive familiarity with others in childhood. However, this does not mean it is incompatible with social anxiety disorder. Social anxiety represents a performance anxiety related to being watched by others. It is certainly true that many patients with ADHD enjoy being in the public limelight and are free from even usual degrees of shyness. Yet it is also true that individuals with ADHD who do become self-conscious may experience burning embarrassment as they realize that they suffer from social blindness. The social anxiety that results may then be somewhat atypical in that it is not without cause. It is then useful to ask patients if they avoid social situations because they are concerned about being inappropriate, talking too much, and exhibiting verbal impulsivity and other symptoms associated with ADHD. In this case we can conceptualize the social anxiety disorder as secondary to ADHD, although it would be naïve to assume that this implies that the SAD does not then require treatment in its own right.

ADHD can also predispose to SAD in that we see patients with ADHD who simply have lost all relationships and so find themselves socially isolated. Adults with severe ADHD often have lost touch with their family. They do not participate or do well in community activities. They have no friends. They cannot play team sports. After a while, forced social isolation, even in someone who likes people, will lead to fear of social contact. What differentiates patients with ADHD/SAD who have been marginalized from those with SAD alone is that the former have more to fear than fear itself. Even if they overcome their fear of people, if they do not have the skills to be

with people they will still have a severe problem with socialization.

ADHD and separation anxiety (ADHD/SA)

ADHD is a disorder of performance not ability, and the domain of impairment that is often affected most profoundly encompasses activities of daily living. This means that otherwise highly intelligent patients become incapacitated by poor self-care, self-directed activity, and simple tasks like managing money, cooking, driving, or cleaning up their room. In childhood and adolescence this incapacity represents a real dilemma for parents, who often give in to doing these things for their children, rather than taking on the endless effort required to get them to do these things independently. It is also quite painful to stand by and watch someone try to tidy a room without getting distracted or to get out of bed and get dressed in less than an hour. The result is that people with ADHD excel at getting other people to do these things for them. The relationships that emerge out of this disability are often characterized by dependency, but it is not a psychological dependency. ADHD patients actually depend on someone else to function as an attention system, and to provide the working memory to accomplish basic life skills. When left on their own, as for example happens when they go off to college, they experience anxiety – but it is may be differentiated from separation anxiety based on attachment in that the fear is less of being left alone than of being unable to manage without the parent or partner who has previously provided assistance.

Treatment

The literature described in this chapter suggests that anxiety disorders and ADHD represent independent disorders, each of which contributes to increasing comorbidity with independent and additive contributions to morbidity. There is suggestive evidence that ADHD is anxiogenic and that anxiety exacerbates problems with working memory and attention; there is inconsistent evidence suggesting that anxiety in the presence of ADHD may act as a modest brake on disinhibition and impulsivity (Manassis et al., 1996, 2000, 2007). Patients who are anxious to please others may be protected against willful wrongdoing and conduct problems (MTA Cooperative Group, 1999b), but this behavior is distinct from attention problems.

Does anxiety moderate response to stimulants?

The empirical literature on this question remains inconsistent. A thorough review of this literature is needed that is well beyond the scope of this chapter. Early studies consistently found that anxious children had a mitigated response to stimulants (Pliszka, 1989, 1998; Tannock, Ickowicz, & Schachar, 1995), but this finding was not replicated in later studies (Diamond, Tannock, & Schachar, 1999). Without an in-depth review of the methodology of these different studies, it is premature to conclude that the discrepancies between these studies are well understood or that more recent findings necessarily supersede older studies.

Most recently, the Multimodal Treatment of ADHD study (MTA) found that the subset of children who had both an anxiety disorder and ADHD did not show diminished response of ADHD to stimulant medication. This comorbid group showed a modest differential added benefit from combination and behavioral interventions as compared to medication alone. This finding further reinforces the clinical interpretation that morbidity in ADHD and anxiety is driven by both disorders and that treatment of ADHD will lead to improvement in core ADHD symptoms, but treatment of anxiety in its own right is necessary for anxiety itself to improve. It is interesting that the same was not found in looking at sequential, combined treatment with selective serotonin reuptake inhibitors (SSRIs) and stimulants in comorbid anxiety both in children (Abikoff et al., 2005) and adults (Weiss & Hechtman, 2006). In both studies combination pharmacotherapy did not lead to greater overall benefit as compared with monotherapy. It may be that combination treatment of stimulant and behavioral management of anxiety lead to more added benefit than the combination of two medications.

Future research

It has been suggested that anxiety and ADHD represent a distinct subset of ADHD patients (Jensen et al., 2001) and, when comorbid, may present a significant moderator of treatment outcome (Jensen et al., 2001; March et al., 2000). This is a very important clinical issue. We know the most about ADHD as a primary disorder as it has been the subject of many clinical trials in children. Although the MTA has done a great deal to heighten awareness of differential responses to treatment for children with various comorbid conditions, each of these unique diagnostic groups requires further research in its own right. This research needs to look at much more than improvement of the ADHD core symptoms. We need empirical data on every aspect of assessment and treatment. For example, we know more about how anxiety affects ADHD outcome with medication than we know about how problems with attention affect the outcome of anxiety.

The MTA found that a combination of medication and psychological treatment offered some differential benefit over medication alone in comorbid ADHD with anxiety. This may be even more likely to be the case with adults. Adult patients are looking for coping strategies, they have already experimented with them, and they are self-referred and self-motivated. Adults with ADHD and anxiety may be able to use "thinking" strategies better than children. They may be a fraction less impulsive, better able to reason, and better able to observe the impact of the psychological interventions they employ.

At the present time many practicing clinicians rely on symptom screeners for ADHD, but do not routinely use broad-band scales that will highlight other diagnostic issues. Every clinical assessment needs to look at subthreshold but impairing symptoms outside the core symptoms, possible important differentials, and multiple comorbidities and their interaction. For clinicians using a *DSM*-based system it is useful to use *DSM*-based checklists such as symptom inventories (Gadow, Sprafkin, & Weiss, 1999, 2004) or a broad based scale such as the Strengths and Difficulites Questionnaire (www.sdqinfo.com) (Goodman, 2001).

Awareness of both the adult's perception of symptoms and the report of others immediately alerts clinicians to important treatment issues for which our evidence base is full of holes. Which treatment do I start with? Will treatment for one disorder help the other disorder? Are medication treatments for both disorders going to be of added benefit? Alternatively, is there a risk for medication treatment for one disorder to have a negative impact on the other? For example, is it possible that SSRI treatment for anxiety would disinhibit and exacerbate ADHD, or conversely is it possible that stimulant treatment would increase a patient's anxiety? Lastly, how does the presence of two disorders affect differential risk over the life cycle?

In reviewing these empirical questions it becomes apparent that we are going to need methodological innovations to study comorbidity. Such research will need large sample sizes, naturalistic designs, methods for evaluating treatment sequence, and broad measures of functional outcome (March et al., 2005; Weiss, Gadow, & Wasdell, 2006). Clinical trials in ADHD have emphasized external observables (disruptiveness) more than subjective feeling states, partly because children are poor informants on how they feel. Work with adults with ADHD and anxiety may provide a window into the internal world experienced by children with the same comorbidity. Adults with ADHD and anxiety describe "scattered minds" as a chief complaint – perhaps children feel the same intangible and invisible difficulty.

Summary

Anxiety and ADHD are distinct but mutually disabling disorders. When both disorders are present together, both need to be assessed and treated. Future research is needed to determine both whether anxiety is a moderator of ADHD treatment and whether attention is a moderator of anxiety treatment. Given that we have established that adults with anxiety have an increased likelihood of having had childhood attention problems (Safren et al., 2001) and that adults with ADHD are at increased risk of anxiety (Kessler et al., 2006), we need effective treatment strategies for the specific difficulties associated with this comorbid condition (Young & Bramham, 2007). Specific pharmacological (Weiss, Walkup, & Garland, 1997; Weiss et al., 2006) and psychological therapies (Ramsay & Rostain, 2007; Safren, 2006; Weiss & Hechtman, 2006), which are not evident by studying each disorder as a unique disorder, may be indicated to treat ADHD in the presence of anxiety.

References

Abikoff H, McGough J, Vitiello B, et al. (2005). Sequential pharmacotherapy for children with comorbid attention-deficit/hyperactivity and anxiety disorders. *J Am Acad Child Adolesc Psychiatry* 44(5):418–27.

Adler LA, Kunz M, Chua HC, Rotrosen J, Resnick SG. (2004). Attention-deficit/hyperactivity disorder in adult patients with posttraumatic stress disorder (PTSD): is ADHD a vulnerability factor? *J Atten Disord* 8(1):11–16.

American Psychiatric Association. (2000). *Diagnostic and Statistical Manual of Mental Disorders*. 4th ed., text rev. Washington: American Psychiatric Press.

Arnold PD, Ickowicz A, Chen S, Schachar R. (2005). Attention-deficit hyperactivity disorder with and without obsessive-compulsive behaviours: clinical characteristics, cognitive assessment, and risk factors. *Can J Psychiatry* 50(1):59–66.

Bedard AC, Martinussen R, Ickowicz A, Tannock R. (2004). Methylphenidate improves visual-spatial memory in children with attention-deficit/hyperactivity disorder. *J Am Acad Child Adolesc Psychiatry* 43(3):260–8.

Belendiuk KA, Clarke TL, Chronis AM, Raggi VL. (2007). Assessing the concordance of measures used to diagnose adult ADHD. *J Atten Disord* 10(3):276–87.

Biederman J. (2004). Impact of comorbidity in adults with attention-deficit/hyperactivity disorder. *J Clin Psychiatry* 65(suppl 3):3–7.

Biederman J, Faraone SV. (2004). A controlled study of functional impairments in 500 ADHD adults. Paper presented at: Annual Meeting of the American Psychiatric Association; May 5: New York.

Biederman J, Faraone SV, Lapey K. (1992). Comorbidity of diagnosis in attention deficit hyperactivity disorder. *Child Adolesc Psychiatr Clin North Am* 1(2): 335–60.

Biederman J, Mick E, Faraone SV. (2000). Age-dependent decline of symptoms of attention deficit hyperactivity disorder: impact of remission definition and symptom type. *Am J Psychiatry* 157(5):816–18.

Biederman J, Petty C, Fried R, et al. (2006). Impact of psychometrically defined deficits of executive functioning in adults with attention deficit hyperactivity disorder. *Am J Psychiatry* 163(10):1730–8.

Biederman J, Wilens TE, Spencer TJ, Adler LA. (2007). Diagnosis and treatment of adults with attention-deficit/ hyperactivity disorder. *CNS Spectr* 12(4 suppl 6):1–15.

Carlson CL, Mann M. (2000). Attention-deficit/ hyperactivity disorder, predominantly inattentive subtype [in process citation]. *Child Adolesc Psychiatr Clin N Am* 9(3):499–510, vi.

Carlson CL, Shin M, Booth J. (1995). The case for DSM-IV subtypes in ADHD. *Ment Retard Dev Disabil Res Rev* 5:199–206.

Diamond IR, Tannock R, Schachar RJ. (1999). Response to methylphenidate in children with ADHD and comorbid anxiety. *J Am Acad Child Adolesc Psychiatry* 38(4): 402–9.

Famularo R, Fenton T, Kinscherff R, Augustyn M. (1996). Psychiatric comorbidity in childhood post traumatic stress disorder. *Child Abuse Negl* 20(10):953–61.

Faraone SV, Biederman J, Friedman D. (2000). Validity of DSM-IV subtypes of attention-deficit/hyperactivity disorder: a family study perspective. *J Am Acad Child Adolesc Psychiatry* 39(3):300–7.

Faraone SV, Biederman J, Mick E. (2006). The age-dependent decline of attention deficit hyperactivity disorder: a meta-analysis of follow-up studies. *Psychol Med* **36**(2):159–65.

Faraone SV, Biederman J, Weber W, Russell RL. (1998). Psychiatric, neuropsychological, and psychosocial features of DSM-IV subtypes of attention-deficit/hyperactivity disorder: results from a clinically referred sample. *J Am Acad Child Adolesc Psychiatry* **37**(2):185–93.

Gadow K, Sprafkin J, Weiss M. (2004). *Manual for the Adult Self Report Inventory and Adult Symptom Inventory.* Stony Brook, NY: Checkmate Plus.

Gadow K, Sprafkin J, Weiss MD. (1999). *Adult Symptom Inventory.* New York: Checkmate Plus.

Geller DA, Biederman J, Faraone SV, Cradock K, Hagermoser L, Zaman N, et al. (2002). Attention-deficit/hyperactivity disorder in children and adolescents with obsessive-compulsive disorder: fact or artifact? *J Am Acad Child Adolesc Psychiatry* **41**(1): 52–8.

Geller DA, Biederman J, Faraone S, Spencer T, Doyle R, Mullin B, et al. (2004). Re-examining comorbidity of Obsessive Compulsive and Attention-Deficit Hyperactivity Disorder using an empirically derived taxonomy. *Eur Child Adolesc Psychiatry* **13**(2): 83–91.

Geller DA, Coffey B, Faraone S, et al. (2003). Does comorbid attention-deficit/hyperactivity disorder impact the clinical expression of pediatric obsessive-compulsive disorder? *CNS Spectr* **8**(4): 259–64.

Goodman R. (2001). Psychometric properties of the strengths and difficulties questionnaire. *J Am Acad Child Adolesc Psychiatry* **40**(11):1337–45.

Jensen PS. (2001). Introduction – ADHD comorbidity and treatment outcomes in the MTA. *J Am Acad Child Adolesc Psychiatry* **40**(2):134–6.

Jensen PS, Hinshaw SP, Kraemer HC, et al. (2001). ADHD comorbidity findings from the MTA study: comparing comorbid subgroups. *J Am Acad Child Adolesc Psychiatry* **40**(2):147–58.

Kessler RC, Adler L, Barkley R, et al. (2006). The prevalence and correlates of adult ADHD in the United States: results from the National Comorbidity Survey Replication. *Am J Psychiatry* **163**(4):716–23.

Kessler RC, Berglund P, Demler O, Jin R, Walters EE. (2005). Lifetime prevalence and age-of-onset distributions of DSM-IV disorders in the National Comorbidity Survey Replication. *Arch Gen Psychiatry* **62**(6):593–602.

Manassis K, Tannock R, Barbosa J. (2000). Dichotic listening and response inhibition in children with comorbid anxiety disorders and ADHD. *J Am Acad Child Adolesc Psychiatry* **39**(9):1152–9.

Manassis K, Tannock R, Masellis M. (1996). Cognitive differences between anxious, normal, and ADHD children on a dichotic listening task. *Anxiety* **2**(6):279–85.

Manassis K, Tannock R, Young A, Francis-John S. (2007). Cognition in anxious children with attention deficit hyperactivity disorder: a comparison with clinical and normal children. *Behav Brain Funct* **3**:4.

March JS, Silva SG, Compton S, Shapiro M, Califf R, Krishnan R. (2005). The case for practical clinical trials in psychiatry. *Am J Psychiatry* **162**(5):836–46.

March JS, Swanson JM, Arnold LE, et al. (2000). Anxiety as a predictor and outcome variable in the multimodal treatment study of children with ADHD (MTA). *J Abnorm Child Psychol* **28**(6):527–41.

Masi G, Millepiedi S, Mucci M, Bertini N, Pfanner C, Arcangeli F. (2006). Comorbidity of obsessive-compulsive disorder and attention-deficit/hyperactivity disorder in referred children and adolescents. *Compr Psychiatry* **47**(1):42–7.

McGough JJ, Smalley SL, McCracken JT, et al. (2004). Psychiatric comorbidity in adult attention deficit hyperactivity disorder: findings from multiplex families. *Am J Psychiatry* **162**(9):1621–7.

McInnes A, Bedard AC, Hogg-Johnson S, Tannock R. (2007). Preliminary evidence of beneficial effects of methylphenidate on listening comprehension in children with attention-deficit/hyperactivity disorder. *J Child Adolesc Psychopharmacol* **17**(1):35–49.

Milberger S, Biederman J, Faraone SV, Murphy J, Tsuang MT. (1995). Attention deficit hyperactivity disorder and comorbid disorders: issues of overlapping symptoms. *Am J Psychiatry* **152**(12):1793–9.

MTA Cooperative Group. (1999a). A 14-month randomized clinical trial of treatment strategies for attention-deficit/hyperactivity disorder: the MTA Cooperative Group Multimodal Treatment Study of Children with ADHD [see comments]. *Arch Gen Psychiatry* **56**(12):1073–86.

MTA Cooperative Group. (1999b). Moderators and mediators of treatment response for children with attention-deficit/hyperactivity disorder: the Multimodal Treatment Study of children with attention-deficit/hyperactivity disorder [see comments]. *Arch Gen Psychiatry* **56**(12):1088–96.

Oosterlaan J, Sergeant JA. (1998). Response inhibition and response re-engagement in attention-deficit/hyperactivity disorder, disruptive, anxious and normal children. *Behav Brain Res* **94**(1):33–43.

Perrin S, Last CG. (1996). Relationship between ADHD and anxiety in boys: results from a family study. *J Am Acad Child Adolesc Psychiatry* **35**(8):988–96.

Pliszka SR. (1989). Effect of anxiety on cognition, behavior, and stimulant response in ADHD. *J Am Acad Child Adolesc Psychiatry* **28**(6):882–7.

Pliszka SR. (1998). Comorbidity of attention-deficit/hyperactivity disorder with psychiatric disorder: an overview. *J Clin Psychiatry* **59**(suppl 7):50–8.

Pliszka SR. (2000). Patterns of psychiatric comorbidity with attention-deficit/hyperactivity disorder. *Child Adolesc Psychiatr Clin North Am* **9**(3):525–40, vii.

Pliszka SR. (2003). Psychiatric comorbidities in children with attention deficit hyperactivity disorder: implications for management. *Paediatr Drugs* **5**(11):741–50.

Pliszka SR, Carlson CL, Swanson JM. (1999). *ADHD with Comorbid Disorders: Clinical Assessment and Management*. New York: Guilford Press.

Ramsay JR, Rostain AL. (2007). *Cognitive Behavioral Therapy for Adult ADHD: An Integrative Psychosocial and Medical Approach*. New York: Routledge.

Roth RM, Wishart HA, Flashman LA, Riordan HJ, Huey L, Saykin AJ. (2004). Contribution of organizational strategy to verbal learning and memory in adults with attention-deficit/hyperactivity disorder. *Neuropsychology* **18**(1):78–84.

Safren SA. (2006). Cognitive-behavioral approaches to ADHD treatment in adulthood. *J Clin Psychiatry* **67**(suppl 8):46–50.

Safren SA, Lanka GD, Otto MW, Pollack MH. (2001). Prevalence of childhood ADHD among patients with Generalized Anxiety Disorder and a comparison condition, Social Phobia. *Depress Anxiety* **13**(4):190–1.

Schatz DB, Rostain AL. (2006). ADHD with comorbid anxiety: a review of the current literature. *J Atten Disord* **10**(2):141–9.

Spencer T, Biederman J, Wilens T. (1999). Attention-deficit/hyperactivity disorder and comorbidity. *Pediatr Clin North Am* **46**(5):915–27, vii.

Sukhodolsky DG, do Rosario-Campos MC, Scahill L, et al. (2005). Adaptive, emotional, and family functioning of children with obsessive-compulsive disorder and comorbid attention deficit hyperactivity disorder. *Am J Psychiatry* **162**(6):1125–32.

Sumner C, Sher L, Sutton V, Bakken R, Paczkowski M, Kelsey D. (2005). Atomoxetine treatment for pediatric patients with ADHD and comorbid anxiety. Paper presented at: AACAP; October 23; Toronto.

Tannock R, Ickowicz A, Schachar R. (1995). Differential effects of methylphenidate on working memory in ADHD children with and without comorbid anxiety. *J Am Acad Child Adolesc Psychiatry* **34**(7):886–96.

Weinstein D, Staffelbach D, Biaggio M. (2000). Attention-deficit hyperactivity disorder and posttraumatic stress disorder: differential diagnosis in childhood sexual abuse. *Clin Psychol Rev* **20**(3):359–78.

Weiss MD, Gadow K, Wasdell MB. (2006). Effectiveness outcomes in attention-deficit/hyperactivity disorder. *J Clin Psychiatry* **67**(suppl 8):38–45.

Weiss M, Hechtman L. (2006). A randomized double-blind trial of paroxetine and/or dextroamphetamine and problem-focused therapy for attention-deficit/hyperactivity disorder in adults. *J Clin Psychiatry* **67**(4):611–9.

Weiss M, Walkup J, Garland EJ. (1997). Stimulants and SSRIs. *Child Adolesc Psychopharmacol News* **2**:11–2.

Weiss M, Wasdell M, Faulkner L, et al. (2006). Atomoxetine in clinical practice. *Future Neurol* **1**(3):249–58.

Wozniak J, Crawford MH, Biederman J, et al. (1999). Antecedents and complications of trauma in boys with ADHD: findings from a longitudinal study. *J Am Acad Child Adolesc Psychiatry* **38**(1):48–55.

Young S, Bramham J. (2007). *ADHD in Adults, A Psychological Guide to Practice*. Sussex, England: Wiley and Sons.

Chapter 12

Attention-deficit hyperactivity disorder and the substance use disorders

Timothy E. Wilens

Introduction

The overlap between attention-deficit hyperactivity disorder (ADHD) and alcohol or drug abuse or dependence (referred to here as substance use disorders [SUD]) in adolescents and adults has been an area of increasing clinical, research, and public health interest worldwide. ADHD (the term "ADHD" used here also refers to previous definitions of the disorder) has an onset in early childhood and affects from 6–8% of juveniles worldwide (Faraone et al., 2003) and 4–5% of adults (Kessler et al., 2006). Longitudinal data suggest that childhood ADHD persists in around 75% of cases into adolescence and in approximately one-half of cases into adulthood (for a review, see Weiss, 1992). Substance use disorders (SUD) usually have their onset in adolescence or early adulthood and affect between 10–30% of US adults and a less defined but sizable number of juveniles (Ross, Glaser, & Germanson, 1988; Kessler et al., 1994). As reviewed, the literature demonstrates a bidirectional overlap between ADHD and SUD (Levin, Evans, & Kleber, 1999; Schubiner et al., 1995; Wilens, 2004a).

The study of comorbidity between SUD and ADHD is relevant to both research and clinical practice in developmental pediatrics, psychology, and psychiatry, with implications for diagnosis, prognosis, treatment, and health care delivery. The identification of specific risk factors of SUD within ADHD may permit more targeted treatments for both disorders at earlier stages of their expression – potentially dampening the morbidity, disability, and poor long-term prognosis in adolescents and adults with this comorbidity (Mannuzza et al., 1993; Weiss, 1992). In the following sections, we review data relevant to understanding the overlap between ADHD and SUD with an emphasis on tangible factors mediating this association.

ADHD in adolescents and adults with SUD

In adolescents three recent studies have incorporated structured psychiatric diagnostic interviews assessing ADHD and other disorders in substance-abusing groups. In an early study, DeMilio (1989) and associates, applying *DSM-III* criteria, reported that one-quarter of 57 inpatient adolescents with SUD had current ADHD with conduct and mood disorders also present. Similarly, in Canadian juvenile offenders there were significantly higher rates of ADHD in those with SUD (23%) than in non-SUD juveniles (0%; Milin et al., 1991). Additionally, higher rates of ADHD were reported in juveniles with drug abuse compared to alcohol abuse (Milin et al., 1991). In another study of psychiatric comorbidity in 52 inpatient adolescents with SUD, 31% had ADHD, with no differences among the various substances of abuse reported (Hovens et al., 1994). In these studies, there was an overrepresentation of both mood and conduct disorders, with from 60–90% of SUD adolescents having a conduct disorder.

Studies in SUD adults are similar to those in adolescents. For example, studies of alcohol abusers yielded rates of between 35–71% of adult alcoholics with childhood-onset and persistent ADHD (Goodwin et al., 1975; Wilens, Spencer, & Biederman, 1995). Including both alcohol and drug addiction, from 15–25% of adult addicts and alcoholics have current ADHD (Wilens, 1998). For example, Schubiner et al. (2000) found that 24% of 201 inpatients in a substance abuse treatment facility had ADHD, and two-thirds also had conduct disorder. However, the importance of careful diagnosis has been demonstrated by Levin, Evans, and Kleber (1998), who found that, although

ADHD in Adults: Characterization, Diagnosis and Treatment, ed. Jan Buitelaar, Cornelis Kan and Philip Asherson.
Published by Cambridge University Press. © Cambridge University Press 2011.

10% of cocaine-dependent adults met strict criteria for ADHD (clear childhood and adult ADHD), another 11% were found to have ADHD symptoms only as adults.

Adults with ADHD and SUD have been reported to have an earlier onset of SUD relative to adults without ADHD (Wilens, Biederman, Mick, et al., 1997). Additionally, more severe SUD has been reported in ADHD adults compared to adults without ADHD (Carroll & Rounsaville, 1993; Levin et al., 1997; Schubiner et al., 2000). For example, Carroll and Rounsaville (1993) showed that, compared to cocaine abusers without ADHD, those with ADHD were younger at presentation for treatment and manifested an earlier onset and more frequent and more severe cocaine use.

ADHD as a risk factor for SUD

The association of ADHD and SUD is particularly compelling from a developmental perspective, as ADHD manifests earlier than SUD; therefore, SUD as a risk factor for ADHD is unlikely. Thus, it is important to evaluate to what extent ADHD is a precursor of SUD. Longitudinal studies of children with ADHD or of children who develop SUD provide the most compelling data supporting this developmental hypothesis.

Longitudinal studies: ADHD

Prospective studies of ADHD children have provided evidence that the group with conduct or bipolar disorders co-occurring with ADHD has the poorest outcome with respect to developing SUD and major morbidity (Biederman et al., 1997; Lambert et al., 1987; Lynskey & Fergusson, 1995; Mannuzza et al., 1993; Weiss et al., 1985). For example, in 5- and 8-year follow-up studies, more alcohol use was shown among hyperactive and largely conduct-disordered ADHD adolescents compared to non-ADHD controls (Blouin, Bornstein, & Trites, 1978; Satterfield, Hoppe, & Schell, 1982). Moreover, as part of an ongoing prospective study of ADHD, risk for SUD in ADHD mid-adolescents (mean age 15 years) compared to non-ADHD controls was largely accounted for by comorbid conduct or bipolar disorders (Biederman et al., 1997). However, it is of interest that, in the older siblings of these probands, ADHD is an independent risk factor for the development of an SUD (Milberger, Biederman, Faraone, Wilens, & Chu, 1997). Our findings were confirmed by Katusic and associates

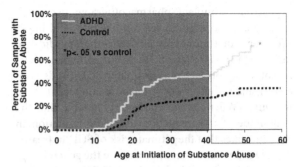

Figure 12.1 Risk for SUD in untreated adults with ADHD.

(2003) in their large case-controlled study of 363 youth with ADHD compared to 726 matched controls followed from age 5 to mid-adolescence. They reported that ADHD was associated with a threefold risk for SUD and that there was an earlier onset of SUD in the ADHD group. Similarly, work by Molina and Pelham (2003) showed the risk ADHD confers on SUD in later adolescence.

These data support retrospectively derived data from untreated adults with ADHD that indicate a higher risk for SUD and an earlier age of SUD onset in ADHD adults (mean age of full SUD at 19 years) compared to non-ADHD controls (mean age 22 years, p < 0.01), which are notable in the presence of comorbid conduct or bipolar disorder (Wilens, Biederman, Mick, et al., 1997; see Fig. 12.1).

ADHD treatment and SUD

Clarification of the critical influence of ADHD treatment in youth on later SUD remains hampered by methodological issues. Because prospective studies in ADHD youth are naturalistic and hence not randomized for treatment, attempts to disentangle positive or deleterious effects of treatment from the severity of the underlying condition(s) are hampered by serious confounds. Although concerns about the abuse liability and potential kindling of specific types of abuse (i.e. cocaine) secondary to early stimulant exposure in ADHD children have been raised (Drug Enforcement Administration, 1995; Vitiello, 2001), the preponderance of clinical data do not appear to support such a contention.

To reconcile findings in this important area, we conducted a meta-analysis of the literature (Wilens et al., 2003), including a large prospective study underway in Germany (Huss, 1999). We analyzed seven studies examining the later risk of SUD in children exposed to stimulant pharmacotherapy: two studies into adolescence and five studies into adulthood. We found that stimulant pharmacotherapy did not increase the risk for later SUD. In fact, stimulant pharmacotherapy protected against later SUD (odds ratio of 1.9), and the effect was stronger in adolescents than in adults (Wilens et al., 2003). It is notable that the magnitude of risk reduction (e.g. 50% reduction in risk) indicates that the ultimate risk of SUD in treated ADHD individuals may approximate the general population risk in individuals without ADHD.

Higher risk for SUD has been consistently observed in studies of ADHD adults compared to non-ADHD adults. For example, we previously reported that in never-treated adults with ADHD the risk of SUD developing over the life span is twofold compared to non-ADHD adults (52% vs. 27%, respectively; Biederman et al., 1995). Whereas psychiatric comorbidity with bipolar or juvenile conduct disorder clearly increases that risk (Mannuzza et al., 1991, 1993, 1998; Weiss et al., 1985), ADHD itself appears to be a risk factor for marijuana, nicotine, and alcohol use (independent of conduct disorder) and for full SUD (Biederman et al., 1995; Wilens, Biederman, Mick, et al., 1997). Adults with ADHD + SUD have the added burden of increased risk for other psychiatric disorders compared to those with either condition alone (Wilens, Kwon, et al., 2005). In adults with SUD, we found no differences in the selection of substances (Biederman et al., 1995). Hence, the literature strongly indicates a bidirectional overrepresentation of SUD and ADHD among subjects with these disorders and that adults with ADHD plus SUD are at risk for other psychiatric comorbidity and a longer course of SUD.

SUD pathways associated with ADHD

Cigarette smoking in youth is often a gateway to more severe alcohol and drug use disorders (Kandel & Faust, 1975; Kandel & Logan, 1984). In this context, an increasing body of literature shows an intriguing association between ADHD and cigarette smoking. In an early report (Milberger, Biederman, Faraone, Chen, & Jones, 1997), we found in boys that ADHD was a significant predictor for early initiation of cigarette smoking (before age 15) and higher risk for cigarette use, even after adjusting for potential confounding variables (e.g. socioeconomic status, IQ, and psychiatric comorbidity). In addition, ADHD youth with conduct, mood, and anxiety disorders had especially high rates

of cigarette smoking. Higher rates of ADHD in adults smokers have also been reported (Pomerleau et al., 1995). Similarly, this same group reported that ADHD adults were less likely to quit smoking than those adult smokers without ADHD. The effect of ADHD treatment on cigarette cessation remains untested.

The presence of ADHD also appears to influence the transition into and out of SUD. Recent work indicates that ADHD and related comorbidities accelerate the transition from less severe drug or alcohol abuse to more severe dependence (1.2 years in ADHD versus 3 years in non-ADHD controls; Wilens, Biederman, Mick, et al., 1997); reflecting recent work demonstrating a linear trend to more psychiatric comorbidity in adults with ADHD, SUD (compared to controls), or ADHD + SUD (compared to adults with either ADHD or SUD or controls) (Wilens, unpublished data). Important pathways appear operant. For example, preliminary work indicated that half of ADHD youth who smoke will develop a SUD in young adulthood (Biederman et al., 2005). Furthermore, ADHD may heighten the risk for a drug use disorder, particularly in individuals with an alcohol use disorder (Biederman et al., 2000).

Moreover, ADHD may affect remission from SUD. Whereas early investigations suggested that adolescents and young adults with ADHD were more likely to have a briefer course of SUD than matched controls (Hechtman & Weiss, 1986), we reported contrary findings. In a study of 130 referred adults with ADHD + SUD and 71 SUD adults without ADHD, the rate of remission and duration of SUD differed between ADHD subjects and controls (Wilens, Biederman, & Mick, 1998). The median time to SUD remission was more than twice as long in ADHD than in control subjects (Fig. 12.1B), with the SUD lasting more than 3 years longer in the ADHD adults compared to their non-ADHD peers (Wilens et al., 1998). Hence, the aggregate data indicate that ADHD and associated conditions developmentally influence the initiation, transition, and recovery from SUD.

Familial relationships between ADHD and SUD

Family studies are highly informative about the nature of the association between two co-occurring disorders. For instance, if the relationship between ADHD and SUD is of a familial nature, then family members of individuals (probands) with SUD or ADHD should

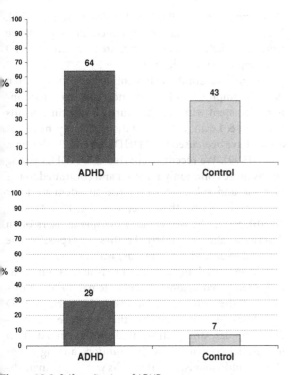

Figure 12.2 Self-medication of ADHD symptoms.

be at elevated risk for the other disorder. The available literature shows that adolescent and adult offspring of SUD parents are at increased risk not only for SUD but also for aggressive and antisocial behaviors (Chassin, Rogosch, & Barrera, 1991; Mathew et al., 1993; Moss et al., 1995; Nunes et al., 1998; Sher et al., 1991; Tarter & Edwards, 1988). In controlled studies, children of substance-abusing parents have also been reported to have abnormal cognitive and behavioral traits, including shorter attention spans and higher impulsivity, aggressiveness, hyperactivity, and rates of ADHD compared to nonaffected children (Aronson & Gilbert, 1963; Fine et al., 1976; Stanger et al., 1999; Steinhusen, Gobel, & Nestler, 1984; Wilens, 1994). For example, in a classic study, Earls and associates (1988) found elevated rates of ADHD in children of alcoholics compared to children of controls; this relationship was more robust when both parents were affected by SUD. We recently reported in a pilot study that the risk for ADHD in children of parents with SUD was elevated relative to controls (Wilens, Hahesy, et al., 2005; see Fig. 12.2). Moreover, we found that approximately half of the school-aged offspring of parents with SUD plus ADHD had ADHD – necessitating screening for ADHD in the children of

parents with SUD plus ADHD (Wilens, Hahesy, et al., 2005). Although familial risk is clearly operant in mediating ADHD and SUD, exposure of vulnerable adolescents to parental SUD also increases the risk for subsequent SUD (Biederman et al., 2000).

The link between ADHD in children and SUD has been noted for many years to aggregate in families. Independent studies by Morrison and Stewart (1971) and Cantwell (1972) found elevated rates of alcoholism in the parents of youth with ADHD. The transmission of SUD in ADHD families remains under study, with family studies showing a preferentially elevated risk for SUD in relatives of ADHD children with conduct disorder (Biederman et al., 1990; Milberger, Biederman, Faraone, Wilens, & Chu, 1997) and independent transmission of ADHD and SUD in families (Milberger et al., 1998).

Although the influence of prenatal substance exposure is confounded by many factors (Griffith, Azuma, & Chasnoff, 1994; Richardon & Day, 1994), several reports have documented an increased risk of postnatal complications, including neuropsychiatric abnormalities, in the offspring of predominantly alcohol-dependent mothers (Abel & Sokol, 1989; Finnegan, 1976; Steinhausen, Willms, & Spohr, 1993; Volpe, 1992). For example, in one of the few follow-up studies of children diagnosed with fetal alcohol syndrome, high rates of psychiatric disturbance including ADHD were found in more than two-thirds of 33 adolescents (Steinhausen et al., 1993). Data in cocaine-exposed youth are complex, suggesting that confounding variables may also be a major factor leading to ADHD-like symptoms (Griffith et al., 1994; Richardson & Day, 1994). In addition, because family data are generally lacking, to what extent reported outcomes are due to exposure to substances versus the contribution of parental psychopathology (indexing familial genetic/environmental risks) is unknown (Merikangas et al., 1998; Tsuang et al., 1996).

Discussion

A review of the literature indicates the following important associations between ADHD and SUD: (1) there is a clinical and statistical bidirectional overlap of ADHD and SUD; (2) the familial risks for ADHD and SUD have been found to be increased in studies of both ADHD and SUD individuals; (3) ADHD is a risk factor for earlier onset SUD; however, co-occurring conduct and bipolar disorders confer a much greater risk for very early onset SUD independently and when comorbid with ADHD; (4) pharmacotherapy of ADHD reduces the risk for SUD to that in the general population; and (5) adults with ADHD have a more prolonged course of SUD. Thus, although the literature supports a robust relationship between ADHD and SUD, the nature of this association remains unclear.

Combined data from retrospective accounts of adults and prospective observations of youth would suggest that juveniles with ADHD are at increased risk for cigarette smoking during adolescence. ADHD youth with conduct or bipolar disorder (particularly adolescent onset) are at risk for very early cigarette use and SUD (i.e. < 16 years of age), whereas the typical age of risk for the onset of SUD accounted for by ADHD itself is probably in young adulthood: between 17 to 22 years of age. ADHD individuals disproportionately become involved with cigarettes, alcohol, and then drugs (Biederman et al., 2000; Milberger, Biederman, Faraone, Chen, & Jones, 1997). ADHD accelerates the transition from less severe alcohol or drug abuse to more severe dependence (Wilens et al., 1998). Conduct or bipolar disorder co-occurring with ADHD tends to further heighten the risk for SUD and accelerate the process. Hence, young adults with ADHD leaving home for independent living or college should be informed about the concerns of SUD dependence.

The precise mechanism(s) mediating the expression of SUD in ADHD remains to be seen. In studies of drug- and alcohol-dependent populations, the self-medication of anxiety, depressive, and aggressive symptoms has been forwarded as a plausible explanation for SUD (Khantzian, 1997). Even though similar efforts have not been systematically undertaken for ADHD (Bukstein, Brent, & Kaminer, 1989; Kaminer, 1992), this self-medication hypothesis is compelling in ADHD given that the disorder is chronic and often associated with demoralization and failure (Biederman et al., 1993; Mannuzza et al., 1993; Weiss, 1992), factors frequently associated with SUD in adolescents (Kandel & Logan, 1984; Yamaguchi & Kandel, 1984).

Despite a paucity of systematically derived data, evidence exists that a subgroup of ADHD individuals are self-medicating. For example, one study has suggested a developmental progression from ADHD to conduct disorder and eventual SUD that is related to demoralization and failure (Mannuzza et al., 1989). Other evidence of self-medication includes data indicating that both ADHD adolescents (Gittelman et al., 1985; Hartsough & Lambert, 1987) and adults

(Biederman et al., 1995) prefer drugs over alcohol. Moreover, ADHD adults with nicotine dependence were less likely to quit relative to their non-ADHD counterparts (Pomerleau et al., 1995).

Of interest, adults with nicotine dependence often describe improved attention and executive functioning, consistent with the literature on nicotinic agents (Rezvani & Levin, 2001), and more recently, nicotinic agents have been used for ADHD (Wilens, Biederman, et al., 1999). We recently reported that ADHD young adults more commonly initiated and continued to use nicotine and substances of abuse to attenuate their mood and improve their sleep (see Fig. 12.2; Wilens, 2004b). Similarly, young adult marijuana users often describe a calming of internal restlessness (possibly the decay of hyperactive symptoms) with marijuana.

The potential importance of self-medication needs to be tempered against more systematic data showing that the strongest relationship between ADHD and SUD is mediated by the presence of conduct, bipolar, and antisocial disorders in addition to familial contributions. In addition, among drug-abusing individuals, ADHD adults were indistinguishable from their non-ADHD peers in the type of substance abused (Biederman et al., 1995). Contrary to anecdotal reports (Khantzian, 1983), systematic data indicate that cocaine and stimulant abuse are not overrepresented in ADHD; in fact, as is the case in non-ADHD abusers, marijuana continues to be the most commonly abused agent (Biederman et al., 1995). Furthermore, SUD in ADHD youth may be accounted for largely by a family history of SUD (Milberger et al., 1998).

The robust findings from family studies on the nature of the relationship between ADHD and SUD, coupled with findings of postsynaptic dopamine DAT, D2, and D4 receptor polymorphisms associated with ADHD (Cook et al., 1995; Faraone et al., 1999; LaHoste et al., 1996), suggest that a polygenic mechanism may be operant. It may also be that ADHD and early-onset SUD may represent variable expressivity of a shared risk factor (Comings et al., 1991; Ebstein et al., 1996). Clearly, more work needs to be done examining the contribution of psychiatric symptoms and deficits to explain the relationship of SUD and ADHD.

Diagnosis and treatment guidelines

Evaluation and treatment of comorbid ADHD and SUD should be part of a plan in which consideration s given to all aspects of the adult's life. Any intervention in this group of patients should occur only after a careful evaluation of the patient, including psychiatric, addiction, social, cognitive, educational, and family assessment. A thorough history of substance use, including past and current usage and treatments, should be obtained. Careful attention should be paid to the differential diagnosis, including medical and neurological conditions whose symptoms may overlap with ADHD (hyperthyroidism) or be a result of SUD (i.e. protracted withdrawal, intoxication, hyperactivity). Current psychosocial factors contributing to the clinical presentation need to be explored thoroughly. Although no specific guidelines exist for evaluating the patient with active SUD, in our experience at least one month of abstinence is useful in accurately and reliably assessing for ADHD symptoms. Semi-structured psychiatric interviews or validated rating scales of ADHD (Adler & Cohen, 2004) are invaluable aids for the systematic diagnostic assessments of this group.

ADHD symptoms in SUD adults – namely inattention (majority), impulsivity, and hyperactivity – appear to be developmentally related to those in children (Millstein et al., 1997). In addition, patients may have associated stubbornness, low frustration tolerance, and chronic conflicts in social relations with peers and authorities. ADHD-related impulsivity appears to be especially problematic in SUD adolescents and adults because it may be a major obstacle in addiction treatment (Tarter & Edwards, 1988).

The treatment needs of individuals with SUD and ADHD need to be considered simultaneously; however, the SUD needs to be addressed initially (Riggs, 1998). If the SUD is active, immediate attention needs to be paid to *stabilization of the addiction(s)*. Depending on the severity and duration of the SUD, adolescents or adults may require inpatient treatment. Self-help groups are an effective treatment modality for many with SUD. In tandem with addiction treatment, SUD patients with ADHD require intervention(s) for the ADHD (and, if applicable, comorbid psychiatric disorders). Education of the individual, family members, and other caregivers is a useful initial step in improving recognition of the ADHD.

Although the efficacy of various psychotherapeutic interventions for ADHD or SUD remains to be established, pilot data suggest efficacy of behavioral and cognitive therapies for adults with ADHD (McDermott & Wilens, 2000; Safren et al., 2005; Wilens, McDermott, et al., 1999). Effective psychotherapy for

this comorbid group combines the following elements: structured and goal-directed sessions, proactive therapist involvement, and knowledge of SUD and ADHD (McDermott & Wilens, 2000). Often, SUD and ADHD therapeutics are completed in tandem with other addiction modalities (i.e. Alcoholic and Narcotics Anonymous, rational recovery) including pharmacotherapy.

Medication serves an important role in reducing the symptoms of ADHD and other concurrent psychiatric disorders. Effective agents for adults with ADHD include the psychostimulants, noradrenergic agents, and catecholaminergic antidepressants (Wilens, 2003). Findings from open and controlled trials suggest that medications used in adults with ADHD plus SUD effectively treat the ADHD, but have little effect on substance use or cravings (see Table 12.1) and are plagued by high attrition.

We recently conducted a meta-analysis of the role of pharmacological treatment for ADHD in adolescents and adults with ADHD plus SUD (Wilens, Monuteaux, et al., 2005). We identified four studies in adolescents and six in adults (two controlled and eight open). We found that treating ADHD pharmacologically in individuals with ADHD plus SUD has a moderate impact on ADHD and SUD that is not observed in controlled trials and does not result in worsening of SUD or adverse interactions specific to SUD.

In adults with ADHD+SUD, the nonstimulant agents (atomoxetine), antidepressants (bupropion), and extended-release or longer acting stimulants (DEA, 1995; Jaffe, 2002; Langer et al., 1986) with lower abuse liability and diversion potential are preferable (Riggs, 1998). Although of particular interest because of its broad spectrum of activity in ADHD in adults (Michelson et al., 2003) and lack of abuse liability (Heil et al., 2002), atomoxetine remains untested in this group. When choosing antidepressants, one should be mindful of potential drug interactions with substances of abuse, as has been reported between tricyclic antidepressants and marijuana (Wilens, Biederman, et al., 1997). In individuals with SUD and ADHD, there should be frequent monitoring of pharmacotherapy, including evaluation of compliance with treatment, random toxicology screens as indicated, and coordination of care with addiction counselors and other caregivers.

Of interest, no evidence exists that treating ADHD pharmacologically exacerbates the SUD. In particular, bupropion did not increase use or craving of

Table 12.1 Pharmacological efficacy in adults with comorbid ADHD and substance use disorders

Study (year)	N	Design	SUD sample	Medication	Duration	Daily dose (range)	Retention	Outcome	Concurrent treatment
Levin et al., (1998)	12	Open	Cocaine dependence	MPH	12 weeks	68 mg (40–80 mg)	8/12	Improvements in ADHD' Decrease in self-reported cocaine use and positive urines.	Individual weekly relapse prevention therapy
Upadhyaya et al., 2001	10	Open	Alcohol and/or cocaine ab/dep	Venlafaxine	12 weeks	300 mg	4/10	Significant improvements in ADHD and in alcohol craving and frequency	Weekly and then monthly psychotherapy
Levin et al., 2002	11	Open	Cocaine dependence	Bupropion	12 weeks	(250–400 mg)	10/11	Reductions in ADHD and cocaine cravings (p's<.01)	Individual weekly relapse prevention therapy; weekly meetings
Prince et al., 2002	32	Open	Mixed SUD	Bupropion SR	6 weeks	326 mg (100–400 mg)	19/32	Improvements in ADHD (−46%), substance use severity (−22%, p<.01)	No additional therapy
Schubiner et al., 2002	48	Double blind, placebo controlled	Cocaine abuse	MPH	13 weeks	90 mg	25/48 58% – placebo 45% – MPH	Trend to improved hyperactive-impulsive sx; No difference in cocaine use (self-reported or urines)	Twice weekly group CBT for SUD; Weekly individual CBT for ADHD
Somoza et al., 2004	41	Open	Cocaine Abuse	MPH	10 weeks	60 mg	29/41	Improvement in both cocaine dependence and ADHD sxs.	Individual SUD therapy throughout trial.
TOTAL (N = 6)	154	Double blind = 1 Open = 5	ADHD and mixed SUD	Bupropion = 2 MPH = 3 Venlafaxine = 1	6–13 weeks	Moderate doses	95/154 (62%)	Significant reduction in ADHD symptoms in 4/5 studies; Mild reduction of SUD	The majority of subjects received concurrent therapy

Abbreviations used: Ab = abuse, AE = adverse event, CBT = cognitive-behavioral therapy, Dep = dependence, MPH = methylphenidate, SUD = substance use disorder, Sx = symptom.

substance use, in general, or cocaine use, in particular. Moreover, subjective as well as objective data have shown that MPH use was not associated with increased cocaine use or cocaine craving. These findings are consistent with those of Grabowski et al. (1997, 2004), who systematically evaluated MPH as a potential cocaine-blocking agent by studying cocaine addicts without ADHD and administering MPH or placebo. Although MPH was not effective in reducing cocaine use or craving compared to placebo, there was no evidence that it exacerbated any aspect of the cocaine addiction. Similar findings have been reported in a pilot study using dextroamphetamine in adult amphetamine abusers in which no exacerbation of the stimulant abuse or craving emerged during the 12-week randomized and controlled trial (Shearer et al., 2001).

Mechanistically, Volkow and colleagues have completed a series of studies in non-ADHD adults that have, among other findings, helped elucidate the mechanism of action of MPH (Volkow et al., 1995) and why MPH does not have the same abuse liability as cocaine (Volkow et al., 1998). In one study, this group demonstrated that intravenous MPH had a slower dissociation than cocaine from the sites of action of sympathomimetics, the dopamine transporter protein (Volkow et al., 1995). Orally administered MPH had slower uptake into the striatum, as well as slower binding and dissociation with the dopamine transporter protein relative to cocaine (Volkow et al., 1999, 2001, 2002). Likewise, orally administered MPH had low euphorogenic properties relative to intravenous cocaine (Volkow et al., 2001). These aggregate findings suggest the low abuse liability of stimulants in ADHD adults without an addiction and should alleviate fears that inadvertent administration of therapeutic oral doses of stimulants to current addicts would uniformly worsen their addiction. The topic of diversion of stimulants is further discussed by Kollins in Chapter 21.

Summary

In summary, there is a strong literature supporting a relationship between ADHD and SUD. Clearly, ADHD adolescents with conduct or bipolar disorder as part of their clinical picture are at the highest risk for SUD. ADHD without comorbidity appears to confer an intermediate risk factor for SUD that is manifested in young adults/ college-aged students. Both family-genetic and self-medication influences may be

operational in the development and continuation of SUD in ADHD subjects; however, systematic data are lacking. Patients with ADHD and SUD require multimodal intervention incorporating addiction and mental health treatment. Pharmacotherapy in ADHD and SUD individuals needs to take into consideration abuse liability, potential drug interactions, and compliance concerns.

Although the existing literature has provided important information on the relationship of ADHD and SUD, it also points to a number of areas in need of further study. The mechanism by which untreated ADHD leads to SUD, as well as the risk reduction of ADHD treatment on later SUD, needs to be better understood. The influence of the adequateness of treatment of ADHD on later SUD needs to be delineated. Given the prevalence and major morbidity and impairment caused by SUD and ADHD, prevention and treatment strategies for these patients need be further developed and evaluated.

Acknowledgments

This research was supported by NIDA: DA14419- and NIH K24 DA016264 to T. Wilens, MD

References

Abel EL, Sokol RJ. (1989). Alcohol consumption during pregnancy: the dangers of moderate drinking. In: Goedde HW, Agarwal DP, eds. *Alcoholism: Biomedical and Genetic Aspects.* Oxford: Pergamon Press: 228–37.

Adler L, Cohen J. (2004). Diagnosis and evaluation of adults with ADHD. *Psychiatr Clin North Am* 27(2):187–201.

Aronson H, Gilbert A. (1963). Preadolescent sons of male alcoholics: an experimental study of personality patterning. *Arch Gen Psychiatry* 8:235–41.

Biederman J, Faraone SV, Keenan K, Knee D, Tsuang MT. (1990). Family-genetic and psychosocial risk factors in DSM-III attention deficit disorder. *J Am Acad Child Adolesc Psychiatry* 29:526–33.

Biederman J, Faraone SV, Monuteaux MC, Feighner JA. (2000). Patterns of alcohol and drug use in adolescents can be predicted by parental substance use disorders. *Pediatrics* 106(4):792–7.

Biederman J, Faraone SV, Spencer T, Wilens TE, Norman D, Lapey KA, et al. (1993). Patterns of psychiatric comorbidity, cognition, and psychosocial functioning in adults with attention deficit hyperactivity disorder. *Am J Psychiatry* 150:1792–8.

Biederman J, Monuteaux M, Mick E, Wilens T, Fontanella J, Poetzl KM, et al. (2006). Is cigarette smoking a gateway drug to subsequent alcohol and illicit drug use disorders? A controlled study of youths with and without ADHD. *Biol Psychiatry* 59(3):258–64.

Biederman J, Wilens T, Mick E, Faraone S, Weber W, Curtis S, et al. (1997). Is ADHD a risk for psychoactive substance use disorder? Findings from a four year follow-up study. *J Am Acad Child Adolesc Psychiatry* 36:21–9.

Biederman J, Wilens TE, Mick E, Milberger S, Spencer TJ, Faraone SV. (1995). Psychoactive substance use disorders in adults with attention deficit hyperactivity disorder (ADHD): effects of ADHD and psychiatric comorbidity. *Am J Psychiatry* 152(11):1652–8.

Blouin A, Bornstein R, Trites R. (1978). Teenage alcohol use among hyperactive children: a five year follow-up study. *J Pediatr Psychology* 3:188–94.

Bukstein OG, Brent DA, Kaminer Y. (1989). Comorbidity of substance abuse and other psychiatric disorders in adolescents. *Am J Psychiatry* 146:1131–41.

Cantwell D. (1972). Psychiatric illness in the families of hyperactive children. *Arch Gen Psychiatry* 27: 414–17.

Carroll KM, Rounsaville BJ. (1993). History and significance of childhood attention deficit disorder in treatment-seeking cocaine abusers. *Compr Psychiatry* 34:75–82.

Chassin L, Rogosch F, Barrera M. (1991). Substance use and symptomatology among adolescent children of alcoholics. *J Abnorm Psychol* 100(4):449–63.

Comings D, Comings B, Muhleman D, Dietz G, Shahbahrami B, Tast D, et al. (1991). The dopamine D2 receptor locus as a modifying gene in neuropsychiatric disorders. *JAMA* 266:1793–1800.

Cook EH, Stein MA, Krasowski MD, Cox NJ, Olkon DM, Kieffer JE, et al. (1995). Association of attention deficit disorder and the dopamine transporter gene. *Am J Hum Genet* 56:993–8.

DeMilio L. (1989). Psychiatric syndromes in adolescent substance abusers. *Am J Psychiatry* 146:1212–14.

Drug Enforcement Administration. (1995). *Methylphenidate Review Document*. Washington, DC: Office of Diversion Control, Drug and Chemical Evaluation Section.

Earls F, Reich W, Jung KG, Cloninger CR. (1988). Psychopathology in children of alcoholic and antisocial parents. *Alcohol Clin Exp Res* 12(4):481–7.

Ebstein R, Novick O, Umansky r, Priel B, Osher Y, Blaine D, et al. (1996). Dopamine D4 receptor exon III polymorphism associated with the human personality trait of novelty seeking. *Nat Genet* 12:78–80.

Faraone S, Biederman J, Weiffenbach B, Keith T, Chu M, Weaver A, et al. (1999). Dopamine D4 gene 7-repeat allele and attention-deficit hyperactivity disorder. *Am J Psychiatry* 156(5):768–70.

Faraone SV, Sergeant J, Gillberg C, Biederman J. (2003) The worldwide prevalence of ADHD: is it an American condition? *World Psychiatry* 2(2):104–13.

Fine EW, Yudin LW, Holmes J, Heinemann S. (1976). Behavioral disorders in children with parental alcoholism. *Ann N Y Acad Sci* 273:507–17.

Finnegan LP. (1976). Clinical effects of pharmacologic agents on pregnancy, the fetus and the neonate. *Ann N Y Acad Sci* 281:74–89.

Gittelman R, Mannuzza S, Shenker R, Bonagura N. (1985). Hyperactive boys almost grown up, I: Psychiatric status. *Arch Gen Psychiatry* 42:937–47.

Goodwin DW, Schulsinger F, Hermansen L, Guze SB, Winokur G. (1975). Alcoholism and the hyperactive child syndrome. *J Nerv Ment Dis* 160:349–53.

Grabowski J, Roache JD, Schmitz JM, Rhoades H, Creson D, Korszun A. (1997). Replacement medication for cocaine dependence: methylphenidate. *J Clin Psychopharmacol* 17(6):485–8.

Grabowski J, Shearer J, Merrill J, Negus SS. (2004). Agonist-like, replacement pharmacotherapy for stimulant abuse and dependence. *Addict Behav* 29(7):1439–64.

Griffith DR, Azuma SD, Chasnoff IJ. (1994). Three-year outcome of children exposed prenatally to drugs. *J Am Acad Child Adolesc Psychiatry* 33:20–7.

Hartsough CS, Lambert NM. (1987). Pattern and progression of drug use among hyperactives and controls: a prospective short-term longitudinal study. *J Child Psychol Psychiatry* 28:543–53.

Hechtman L, Weiss G. (1986). Controlled prospective fifteen year follow-up of hyperactives as adults: non-medical drug and alcohol use and anti-social behaviour. *Can J Psychiatry* 31:557–67.

Heil SH, Holmes HW, Bickel WK, Higgins ST, Badger GJ, Laws HF, et al. (2002). Comparison of the subjective, physiological, and psychomotor effects of atomoxetine and methylphenidate in light drug users. *Drug Alcohol Depend* 67(2):149–56.

Hovens JG, Cantwell DP, Kiriakos R. (1994). Psychiatric comorbidity in hospitalized adolescent substance abusers. *J Am Acad Child Adolesc Psychiatry* 33(4):476–83.

Huss M. (1999). ADHD and substance abuse. Paper presented at: IX Annual European Congress of Psychiatry; Hamburg.

Jaffe SL. (2002). Failed attempts at intranasal abuse of Concerta. *J Am Acad Child Adolesc Psychiatry* 41(1):5.

Kaminer Y. (1992). Clinical implications of the relationship between attention-deficit hyperactivity disorder and psychoactive substance use disorders. *Am J Addict* 1:257–64.

Kandel D, Faust R. (1975). Sequence and stages in patterns of adolescent drug use. *Arch Gen Psychiatry* 32:923–32.

Kandel DB, Logan JA. (1984). Patterns of drug use from adolescence to young adulthood: I. Periods of risk for initiation, continued use, and discontinuation. *Am J Public Health* 74:660–6.

Katusic SK, Barbaresi WJ, Colligan RC, Weaver A, Mrazek DA, Jacobsen SJ. (2003). Substance abuse among ADHD cases: A population-based birth cohort study. Paper presented at: Pediatric Academic Society; Seattle, WA.

Kessler RC, Adler L, Barkley R, Biederman J, Conners CK, Demler O, et al. (2006). The prevalence and correlates of adult ADHD in the United States: Results from the

Kessler RC, McGonagle KA, Zhao S, Nelson CB, Hughes M, Eshleman S, et al. (1994). Lifetime and 12-month prevalence of DSM- III-R psychiatric disorders in the United States. *Arch Gen Psychiatry* 51:8–19.

Khantzian EJ. (1983). An extreme case of cocaine dependence and marked improvement with methylphenidate treatment. *Am J Psychiatry* 140:784–5.

Khantzian EJ. (1997). The self-medication hypothesis of substance use disorders: a reconsideration and recent applications. *Harv Rev Psychiatry* 4:231–44.

LaHoste GJ, Swanson JM, Wigal SB, Glabe C, Wigal T, King N, et al. (1996). Dopamine D4 receptor gene polymorphism is associated with attention deficit hyperactivity disorder. *Mol Psychiatry* 1:121–4.

Lambert N, Hartsough C, Sassone D, Sandoval J. (1987). Persistence of hyperactivity symptoms from childhood to adolescence and associated outcomes. *Am J Orthopsychiatry* 57(1):22–32.

Langer DH, Sweeney KP, Bartenbach DE, Davis PM, Menander KB. (1986). Evidence of lack of abuse or dependence following pemoline treatment: results of a retrospective survey. *Drug Alcohol Depend* 17:213–27.

Levin FR, Evans S, Kleber HD. (1998). Prevalence of adult attention-deficit/hyperactivity disorder among cocaine abusers seeking treatment. *Drug Alcohol Depend* 52:15–25.

Levin FR, Evans SM, Kleber HD. (1999). Practical guidelines for the treatment of substance abusers with adult attention-deficit hyperactivity disorder. *Psychiatr Serv* 50(8):1001–3.

Levin FR, Evans SM, McDowell DM, Brooks DJ, Nunes E. (2002). Bupropion treatment for cocaine abuse and adult attention-deficit/hyperactivity disorder. *J Addict Dis* 21(2):1–16.

Levin FR, Evans SM, McDowell DM, Kleber HD. (1998). Methylphenidate treatment for cocaine abusers with adult attention-deficit/hyperactivity disorder: a pilot study. *J Clin Psychiatry* 59(6):300–5.

Levin, Evans SM, Rosenthal M, Kleber HD. (1997). Psychiatric comorbidity in cocaine abusers in outpatient settings or a therapeutic community. Paper presented at: Annual Meeting of CPDD; Nashville.

Low KG, Gendaszek AE. (2002). Illicit use of psychostimulants among college students: a preliminary study. *Psychol Health Med* 7(3):283–7.

Lynskey M, Fergusson D. (1995). Childhood conduct problems, attention deficit behaviors and adolescent alcohol, tobacco, and illicit drug use. *J Abnorm Child Psychol* 23(3):281–302.

Mannuzza S, Gittelman-Klein R, Konig PH, Giampino TL. (1989). Hyperactive boys almost grown up: IV. Criminality and its relationship to psychiatric status. *Arch Gen Psychiatry* 46:1073–9.

Mannuzza S, Klein RG, Bessler A, Malloy P, LaPadula M. (1993). Adult outcome of hyperactive boys: educational achievement, occupational rank, and psychiatric status. *Arch Gen Psychiatry* 50:565–76.

Mannuzza S, Klein R, Bessler A, Malloy P, LaPadula M. (1998). Adult psychiatric status of hyperactive boys grown up. *Am J Psychiatry* 155(4):493–8.

Mannuzza S, Klein RG, Bonagura N, Malloy P, Giampino TL, Addalli KA. (1991). Hyperactive boys almost grown up. V. Replication of psychiatric status. *Arch Gen Psychiatry* 48:77–83.

Mathew RJ, Wilson WH, Blazer DG, George LK. (1993). Psychiatric disorders in adult children of alcoholics: data from the epidemiologic catchment area project. *Am J Psychiatry* 150(5):793–800.

McCabe SE, Teter CJ, Boyd CJ.(2004). The use, misuse and diversion of prescription stimulants among middle and high school students. *Subst Use Misuse* 39(7):1095–116.

McDermott SP, Wilens TE. (2000). Cognitive therapy for adults with ADHD. In: Brown T, ed. *Subtypes of Attention Deficit Disorders in Children, Adolescents, and Adults.* Washington, DC: American Psychiatric Press: 569–606.

Merikangas K, Stolar M, Stevens D, Goulet J, Preisig M, Fenton B, et al. (1998). Familial transmission of substance use disorders. *Arch Gen Psychiatry* 55(11):973–9.

Michelson D, Adler L, Spencer T, Reimherr FW, West S, Allen AJ, et al. (2003). Atomoxetine in adults with ADHD: two randomized, placebo-controlled studies. *Biol Psychiatry* 53:112–20.

Milberger S, Biederman J, Faraone S, Chen L, Jones J. (1997). ADHD is associated with early initiation of cigarette smoking in children and adolescents. *J Am Acad Child Adolesc Psychiatry* **36**:37–44.

Milberger S, Biederman J, Faraone S, Wilens T, Chu M. (1997). Associations between ADHD and psychoactive substance use disorders: findings from a longitudinal study of high-risk siblings of ADHD children. *Am J Addict* **6**:318–29.

Milberger S, Faraone S, Biederman J, Chu M, Wilens T. (1998). Familial risk analysis of the association between attention-deficit/hyperactivity disorder and psychoactive substance use disorders. *Arch Pediatr Adolesc Med* **152**:945–51.

Milin R, Halikas JA, Meller JE, Morse C. (1991). Psychopathology among substance abusing juvenile offenders. *J Am Acad Child Adolesc Psychiatry* **30**(4):569–74.

Millstein RB, Wilens TE, Biederman J, Spencer TJ. (1997). Presenting ADHD symptoms and subtypes in clinically referred adults with ADHD. *J Attent Disord* **2**(3):159–66.

Molina B, Pelham W. (2003). Childhood predictors of adolescent substance use in a longitudinal study of children with ADHD. *J Abnorm Psychol* **112**(3):497–507.

Morrison JR, Stewart MA. (1971). A family study of the hyperactive child syndrome. *Biol Psychiatry* **3**:189–95.

Moss H, Vanyukov M, Majumder PP, Kirisci L, Tarter R. (1995). Prepubertal sons of substance abusers: influences of parental and familial substance abuse on behavioral disposition, IQ, and school achievement. *Addict Behav* **20**(3):345–58.

Musser CJ, Ahmann PA, Theye FW, Mundt P, Broste SK, Mueller-Rizner N. (1998). Stimulant use and potential for abuse in Wisconsin as reported by school administrators and longitudinally followed children. *J Dev Behav Pediatr* **19**(3):187–92.

Nunes EV, Weissman MM, Goldstein RB, McAvay G, Seracini AM, Verdeli H, et al. (1998). Psychopathology in children of parents with opiate dependence and/or major depression. *J Am Acad Child Adolesc Psychiatry* **37**(11):1142–51.

Pomerleau O, Downey K, Stelson F, Pomerleau C. (1995). Cigarette smoking in adult patients diagnosed with attention deficit hyperactivity disorder. *J Subst Abuse* **7**:373–8.

Poulin C. (2001). Medical and nonmedical stimulant use among adolescents: from sanctioned to unsanctioned use. *Can Med Assoc J* **165**(8):1039–44.

Prince J, Wilens T, Waxmonsky J, Hammerness P, Monuteaux M, Goldman S, et al. (2002). An open study of sustained-release bupropion in adults with ADHD and substance use disorders. In: Scientific Proceedings of the American Psychiatric Association; Philadelphia; NR 222.

Rezvani AH, Levin ED. (2001). Cognitive effects of nicotine. *Biol Psychiatry* **49**(3):258–67.

Richardson GA, Day NL. (1994). Detrimental effects of prenatal cocaine exposure: illusion or reality? *J Am Acad Child Adolesc Psychiatry* **33**:28–34.

Riggs PD. (1998). Clinical approach to treatment of ADHD in adolescents with substance use disorders and conduct disorder. *J Am Acad Child Adolesc Psychiatry* **37**(3):331–2.

Ross HE, Glaser FB, Germanson T. (1998). The prevalence of psychiatric disorders in patients with alcohol and other drug problems. *Arch Gen Psychiatry* **45**:1023–31.

Safren SA, Otto MW, Sprich S, Winett CL, Wilens TE, Biederman J. (2005). Cognitive-behavioral therapy for ADHD in medication-treated adults with continued symptoms. *Behav Res Ther* **43**(7):831–42.

Satterfield JH, Hoppe CM, Schell AM. (1982). A prospective study of delinquency in 110 adolescent boys with attention deficit disorder and 88 normal adolescent boys. *Am J Psychiatry* **139**:795–8.

Schubiner H, Saules KK, Arfken CL, Johanson CE, Schuster CR, Lockhart N, et al. (2002). Double-blind placebo-controlled trial of methylphenidate in the treatment of adult ADHD patients with comorbid cocaine dependence. *Exp Clin Psychopharmacol* **10**(3):286–94.

Schubiner H, Tzelepis A, Isaacson JH, Warbasse LH, Zacharek M, Musial J. (1995). The dual diagnosis of attention-deficit/hyperactivity disorder and substance abuse: case reports and literature review. *J Clin Psychiatry* **56**(4):146–50.

Schubiner H, Tzelepis A, Milberger S, Lockhart N, Kruger M, Kelley BJ, et al. (2000). Prevalence of attention-deficit/hyperactivity disorder and conduct disorder among substance abusers. *J Clin Psychiatry* **61**(4):244–51.

Shearer J, Wodak A, Mattick R, Van Beek I, Lewis JE, Hall WG, et al. (2001). Pilot randomized controlled study of dexamphetamine substitution for amphetamine dependence. *Addiction* **96**:1289–96.

Sher KJ, Walitzer KS, Wood PK, Brent EE. (1991). Characteristics of children of alcoholics: putative risk factors, substance use and abuse, and psychopathology. *J Abnorm Psychol* **100**:427–48.

Somoza EC, Winhusen TM, Bridge TP, Rotrosen JP, Vanderburg DG, Harrer JM, et al. (2004). An open-label pilot study of methylphenidate in the treatment of cocaine dependent patients with adult attention deficit/hyperactivity disorder. *J Addict Dis* **23**(1):77–92.

Stanger C, Higgins S, Bickel W, Elk R, Grabowski J, Schmitz J, et al. (1999). Behavioral and emotional problems among children of cocaine- and opiate-dependent parents. *J Am Acad Child Adolesc Psychiatry* 38(4):421–8.

Steinhausen H, Gobel D, Nestler V. (1984). Psychopathology in the offspring of alcoholic parents. *J Am Acad Child Adolesc Psychiatry* 23:465–71.

Steinhausen HC, Willms J, Spohr HL. (1993). Long-term psychopathological and cognitive outcome of children with fetal alcohol syndrome. *J Am Acad Child Adolesc Psychiatry* 32:990–4.

Carter RE, Edwards K. (1988). Psychological factors associated with the risk for alcoholism. *Alcohol Clin Exp Res* 12:471–80.

Tsuang MT, Lyons MJ, Eisen SA, Goldberg J, True W, Lin N, et al. (1996). Genetic influences on DSM-III-R drug abuse and dependence: a study of 3,372 twin pairs. *Am J Med Genet* 67(5):473–7.

Upadhyaya HP, Brady KT, Sethuraman G, Sonne SC, Malcolm R. (2001). Venlafaxine treatment of patients with comorbid alcohol/cocaine abuse and attention-deficit/hyperactivity disorder: a pilot study. *J Clin Psychopharmacol* 21(1):116–18.

Vitiello B. (2001). Long-term effects of stimulant medications on the brain: possible relevance to the treatment of attention deficit hyperactivity disorder. *J Child Adolesc Psychopharmacol* 11(1):25–34.

Volkow ND, Ding Y, Fowler JS, Wang G, Logan J, Gatley JS, et al. (1995). Is methylphenidate like cocaine? Studies on the pharmacokinetics and distribution in the human brain. *Arch Gen Psychiatry* 52:456–63.

Volkow N, Wang G, Fowler J, Gatley S, Logan J, Ding Y, et al. (1998). Dopamine transporter occupancies in the human brain induced by therapeutic doses of oral methylphenidate. *Am J Psychiatry* 155(10):1325–31.

Volkow N, Wang G, Fowler J, Hitzemann R, Angrist B, Gatley S, et al. (1999). Association of methylphenidate-induced craving with changes in right striatoorbitofrontal metabolism in cocaine abusers: implications in addictions. *Am J Psychiatry* 156(1):19–26.

Volkow ND, Wang GJ, Fowler JS, Logan J, Franceschi D, Maynard L, et al. (2002). Relationship between blockade of dopamine transporters by oral methylphenidate and the increases in extracellular dopamine: therapeutic implications. *Synapse* 43(3):181–7.

Volkow ND, Wang GJ, Fowler JS, Logan G, Gerasimov M, Maynard L, et al. (2001). Therapeutic doses of oral methylphenidate significantly increase extracellular dopamine in human brain. *J Neurosci* 21:RC121.

Volpe JJ. (1992). Effect of cocaine use on the fetus. *N Eng J Med* 327:399–406.

Weiss G. (1992). *Attention-Deficit Hyperactivity Disorder*. Philadelphia: W. B. Saunders.

Weiss G, Hechtman L, Milroy T, Perlman T. (1985). Psychiatric status of hyperactives as adults: a controlled prospective 15 year followup of 63 hyperactive children. *J Am Acad Child Adolesc Psychiatry* 24:211–20.

Wilens TE. (1994). The child and adolescent offspring of drug-and alcohol-dependent parents. *Curr Opin Psychiatry* 7:319–23.

Wilens T. (1998). Alcohol and other drug use and attention deficit/hyperactivity disorder. *Alcohol Health Res World* 22(2):127–30.

Wilens T. (2003). Drug therapy for adults with attention-deficit hyperactivity disorder. *Drugs* 63(22):2395–411.

Wilens T. (2004a). Attention-deficit/hyperactivity disorder and the substance use disorders: the nature of the relationship, subtypes at risk and treatment issues. *Psychiatr Clin North Am* 27(2):283–301.

Wilens T. (2004b). Subtypes of ADHD youth at risk for substance abuse. Paper presented at: 157th Annual Meeting of the American Psychiatric Association; May 1–6; New York.

Wilens T, Biederman J, Mick E. (1998). Does ADHD affect the course of substance abuse? Findings from a sample of adults with and without ADHD. *Am J Addict* 7:156–63.

Wilens TE, Biederman J, Mick E, Faraone SV, Spencer T. (1997). Attention deficit hyperactivity disorder (ADHD) is associated with early onset substance use disorders. *J Nerv Ment Dis* 185(8):475–82.

Wilens TE, Biederman J, Spencer TJ. (1997). Case study: adverse effects of smoking marijuana while receiving tricyclic antidepressants. *J Am Acad Child Adolesc Psychiatry* 36:45–8.

Wilens TE, Biederman J, Spencer TJ, Bostic J, Prince J, Monuteaux MC, et al. (1999). A pilot controlled clinical trial of ABT-418, a cholinergic agonist, in the treatment of adults with attention deficit hyperactivity disorder. *Am J Psychiatry* 156(12):1931–7.

Wilens T, Faraone S, Biederman J, Gunawardene S. (2003). Does stimulant therapy of ADHD beget later substance abuse: a metanalytic review of the literature. *Pediatrics* 11(1):179–85.

Wilens T, Hahesy A, Biederman J, Bredin E, Tanguay S, Kwon A, et al. (2005). Influence of parental SUD and ADHD on ADHD in their offspring: preliminary results from a pilot controlled family study. *Am J Addict* 14(2):179–87.

Wilens T, Kwon A, Tanguay S, Chase R, Faraone S, Biederman J. (2005). Characteristics of adults with attention deficit hyperactivity disorder plus substance use disorder: the role of psychiatric comorbidity. *Am J Addict* 14(4):319–28.

Wilens T, McDermott S, Biederman J, Abrantes A, Hahesy A, Spencer T. (1999). Cognitive therapy in the treatment of adults with ADHD: a systematic chart review of 26 cases. *J Cogn Psychother* **13**(3):215–26.

Wilens T, Monuteaux M, Snyder L, Moore BA. (2005). The clinical dilemma of using medications in substance abusing adolescents and adults with ADHD: what does the literature tell us? *J Child Adolesc Psychopharmacol* **15**(5):787–98.

Wilens T, Spencer T, Biederman J. (1995). Are attention-deficit hyperactivity disorder and the psychoactive substance use disorders really related? *Harv Rev Psychiatry* **3**:260–2.

Yamaguchi K, Kandel DB. (1984). Patterns of drug use from adolescence to young adulthood: III. Predictors of progression. *Am J Public Health* **74**:673–81.

Adult ADHD and organic brain disorders (including psychotic symptoms and tics)

Asko Niemela

Organic brain syndromes are conditions that can be traced to brain diseases, injuries, other factors affecting brain activity, or diseases of other organs or organ systems. The fact that the *DSM-IV-TR* classification of diseases (American Psychiatric Association, 2000) does not recognize a class termed "organic brain syndromes" may be attributed to the associated implication that "nonorganic" mental disturbances do not have any biological basis at all. Instead the *DSM-IV-TR* places organic brain syndromes in three groups: (1) delirium, dementia, amnestic disorders, and other cognitive disorders; (2) mental disorders due to a general medical condition; and (3) substance-related disorders. The last group is considered in Chapter 12.

No problems are normally encountered in the differential diagnosis between organic brain syndromes and attention-deficit hyperactivity disorder (ADHD) because the latter is a developmental disorder, so that, although manifested as such at an adult age, its symptoms must have been visible throughout the individual's life. Of the other syndromes listed here, delirium is brought about rapidly in response to some particular etiological factor and generally disappears when that factor is treated, whereas dementia involves increasing memory and functional difficulties in a person who has previously had no problems in these areas. In the case of traumatic brain injury a distinct impact on the central nervous system and time of occurrence are usually known, and it is possible to point to the resulting changes in concentration, activity, impulsiveness, and other cognitive and executive functions.

Although psychotic disturbances differ markedly from ADHD, a considerable period of time may elapse before occurrence of the psychotic phase of schizophrenia; during this period aberrations (referred to as prodromal symptoms) that have many features in common with ADHD symptoms may be noted in the subject's actions. Likewise there are many similarities between ADHD and Tourette syndrome, although the serious tics in the latter are clearly distinguishable from the symptoms of ADHD. A genetic connection between the two has nevertheless been emphasized by Comings (2000), who regards both ADHD and Tourette syndrome as a single manifestation of ADHD, whereas other researchers believe that there is a group of patients in whom ADHD and Tourette syndrome are linked together and other groups in whom the conditions are not linked.

As far as medication is concerned, it is interesting that the drugs used to treat ADHD can also be effective in treating other conditions; conversely, some drugs developed for treating other diseases have come to be used for ADHD as well, or at least the possibility of using them is under investigation. All told, among the drugs affecting the central nervous system, those that improve cognitive or functional skills or capacities are also potentially useful for treating ADHD.

Delirium

The background to states of delirium may lie in somatic disturbances, the effects of chemical substances or withdrawal symptoms, or possibly combinations of several etiologies. Patients with delirium may present with attentional problems typical of ADHD – in the form of reduced capacities for focusing, maintaining, or shifting attention or in changes in psychomotor activity – but a state of delirium always involves other symptoms that are not present in ADHD. In addition, delirious symptoms tend to develop very quickly, in a matter of hours or days, and are typically accompanied by a blurring of consciousness and diurnal variations in the state of delirium, in which patients may be fully conscious at one

ADHD in Adults: Characterization, Diagnosis and Treatment, ed. Jan Buitelaar, Cornelis Kan and Philip Asherson.
Published by Cambridge University Press. © Cambridge University Press 2011.

moment and disoriented and confused the next, with reduced awareness of their surroundings in terms of time, place, and person. Patients suffering from delirium can experience alterations in intellectual capabilities (e.g. memory or perceptual problems) that cannot be attributed to dementia symptoms. A decline in their knowledge of recently learned things can occur, whereas their long-term memory may well remain intact.

Whereas the hyperactivity symptoms characteristic of ADHD occur repeatedly in the same form, patients with delirium typically undergo rapid fluctuations in psychomotor activity from hypoactivity to hyperactivity. Similarly, their stream of speech may be intensified or reduced, or they may overreact to external stimuli. Disturbances of the sleep-wakefulness cycle, including insomnia, may occur.

Dementia and amnestic disorders

The essential feature of dementia is memory disturbance, although debilitation may be observed in many other cognitive functions. The principal problem lies in the learning of new information or the recall of things that have been learned recently, although patients may also experience difficulties in registering, storing, and recovering information. Deficits may be found in linguistic abilities and motor functions, even though the actual locomotory mechanisms as such may be intact. Patients may find it difficult to recognize or observe things in spite of well-preserved sensory functions (agnosia).

Patients may also experience some deficiency in executive functions; in general there is a decline in thought processes, problem-solving ability, orientation, attention, concentration, and judgment without any loss of consciousness. Dementia may also involve decreases in emotional capacity and emotional stability, irritability, apathy, and eccentricities in social behavior. It is usually a progressive disease and should be recognizable as a decline in functional ability relative to a previous level. It may or may not be accompanied by behavioral symptoms. Moderate or serious dementia has a considerable impact on the ability to cope independently in everyday activities, but in a mild form it may create problems and difficulties without actually preventing the patient from managing activities of daily living.

One interesting question is the extent to which the medications used to treat patients with dementia can also be effective for treating ADHD. Acetylcholinesterase blockers, such as donepezil, rivastigmine, and galantamine, and N-methyl-D-aspartic acid (NMDA) antagonists such as memantine relieve the symptoms of dementia and help patients manage in their everyday lives, but only a few reports are available at present on their use for treating ADHD, and even in those studies the numbers of patients have been very limited. Wilens et al. (2005) conducted a 12-week open trial to determine whether donepezil as an adjuvant to stimulant medication would relieve the residual symptoms of ADHD and associated deficiencies in functional control of executive functions. All the patients, seven children and six adults, were stabilized on a stimulant medication, but no clinically or statistically significant differences on the ADHD Rating Scale or Executive Function Checklist were documented in the seven subjects who completed the trial. After a 12-week double-blind comparison of galantamine medication with a placebo, Biederman et al. (2006) concluded that this drug was of no clinical benefit to adult ADHD patients.

According to the *DSM-IV-TR* (American Psychiatric Association, 2000) definition, amnestic disturbances are attributable either to the direct physiological consequences of a general medical condition, the continued use of intoxicants or drugs, or exposure to toxic substances, or the cause may remain entirely unresolved. The result may be an inability to learn new things or to remember what has just been learned. If the condition has existed for a month or less, it is customary to speak of a short-term syndrome, but if it continues for more than a month the condition may be regarded as chronic.

Traumatic brain injury

The postconcussional syndrome that arises from traumatic brain injury (TBI) typically involves memory and attention symptoms. In addition the patient may complain of pain and unpleasant feelings (e.g. headache or dizziness). Frequent accompanying emotional changes are irritability, emotional instability, depression, and/or anxiety. Patients may also complain of problems in concentration and in performing specific tasks and of memory difficulties. Other typical symptoms are insomnia and reduced alcohol tolerance.

Given that stimulants play an important role in the treatment of ADHD, their applicability has also been studied in postconcussional syndrome. Whyte et al. (2004) conducted a double-blind, repeated crossover, placebo-controlled trial with 34 adult patients having moderate to serious brain damage to assess the effect of methylphenidate on their attention problems; they found considerable improvements in the speed of processing information, attentiveness during individual work tasks, and other people's estimates of their attention faculties, whereas no improvement was noted in divided attention, sustained attention, or susceptibility to distraction.

In a trial reported by Kim et al. (2006) 18 brain-injured patients were given either 20 mg methylphenidate or a placebo on a double-blind basis. The effects on the working memory and visuospatial attention tasks were assessed in terms of accuracy of response and reaction time. The methylphenidate group showed significant improvements in accuracy of response for both the working memory and visuospatial attention tasks relative to the placebo group. A significant decrease in reaction time was observed for the task of working memory in the methylphenidate group.

In his review on this topic, Siddall (2005) found 10 papers assessing the efficacy and safety of methylphenidate in adult and childhood TBI patients and noted that the results point to its potential for improving memory, attention, concentration, and mental processing, but that no conclusion can be reached regarding the drug's behavioral effects. He also observed that more extensive double-blind, placebo-controlled trials would be needed to assess the optimal dosage and the stage at which medication should be started. It is also clear that information is needed on the duration of treatment and its long-term effects in cases of mild, moderate, and serious TBI.

The effects on cognitive performance of cholinergic augmentation of the medication provided for brain-injury patients have also been examined recently. Zhang et al. (2004) observed that augmentation with donepezil improved short-term memory performance and maintenance of attention in these patients. In a comparison of the effects of donepezil, galantamine, and rivastigmine on susceptibility to fatigue, amnesia, attention difficulties, and lack of initiative in a series of 111 outpatients based on the patients' own assessments, Tenovuo (2005) failed to find any significant differences in either efficacy or tolerance among the three drugs; the clearest benefit reported among those who experienced any benefit at all was improved vigilance and attention.

Psychotic symptoms

The most common symptoms experienced by psychotic patients are an impaired sense of reality, hallucinations, and delusions. Their speech may be incoherent, and they may feel that their thoughts re-echo in their heads, that ideas are being put into their heads that are not their own, or that their ideas are being taken from them. These symptoms are often associated with a feeling that someone external to them is able to influence their thoughts or actions against their will. Neologisms or breaks may occur in their speech, and they may have delusions that are also connected with external control and influence or simply with passivity, an inability to cope. Patients usually experience auditory hallucinations as voices that comment on their actions and order them to do certain things, or else the voices may be talking about them. Their behavior can be disorganized or even catatonic. All the symptoms just described are referred to as positive symptoms of psychosis, whereas the negative symptoms include blunting of the emotions, impoverishment of speech, a marked lack of self-will or initiative, apathy, and an inability to experience sensations of pleasure. The negative symptoms depart markedly from those of ADHD.

In the *DSM-IV-TR* classification (American Psychiatric Association, 2000), psychotic diseases include schizophrenia, other schizophreniform disorder, schizoaffective disorder, delusional disorder, brief psychotic disorder, shared psychotic disorder, psychotic disorder due to a general medical condition, substance-induced disorder, and psychotic disorder not otherwise specified. The most interesting of these conditions as far as ADHD is concerned is schizophrenia, the essential features of which are functional deterioration and the occurrence of the positive and/or negative symptoms listed earlier. The symptoms may also be divided into prodromes, acute-stage symptoms, and sequelae.

Although it is not usually difficult to distinguish between ADHD and psychotic symptoms, schizophrenia is sometimes slow to set in, and its prodromal symptoms can resemble depressive disorders, anxiety disorders, and the symptoms of ADHD. Symptoms associated with the prodromal stage of schizophrenia include anxiety, restlessness, irritability, anger, depression, inability to experience enjoyment, ideas of self-destruction, mood fluctuations, apathy, inability to concentrate, loss of appetite, and insomnia; a weakened ability for conceptual thought, absorption in one's own thoughts, obsessions, compulsive actions, bizarre speech, delusions, and withdrawal may also be observed. As Cohen, Gotowiec, and Seeman (2000) noted in their paper, the prodromal symptoms may progress for years before the first psychotic evidence of schizophrenia emerges. It is also evident that attention deficits may be linked with those symptoms of behavioral, cognitive, and affective decline as additional prodromal features (Hambrecht et al., 2002).

Thus attention deficit is an aspect common to both ADHD and schizophrenia. In his review of attention problems associated with schizophrenia and ADHD, Barr (2001) treated those problems as two separate forms, each representing a complex syndrome. The most clearly distinguishable deviation in schizophrenia seems to be a difficulty in maintaining the focus of attention, and many authors have pointed to a disturbance in the direction and control of attention, reporting findings such as heightened distractibility, a failure to maintain mental functions, and an abnormal level of arousal. Thus neuropsychological studies of schizophrenia and ADHD have pointed both to attention deficit findings of a similar kind and differences between the two groups in certain subclasses of the attention faculty. Both diseases entail distractibility and difficulties in maintaining the focus of attention, but persons who are disposed to development of a psychosis are likely to experience a milder decline in perceptual sensitivity and the processing of information relative to those suffering from ADHD (Barr 2001).

Some neurophysiological research has also explored similarities between ADHD and schizophrenia. One of the few comparative studies of event-evoked potentials in schizophrenia and ADHD patients has demonstrated that patients with schizophrenia fail to inhibit the P50 auditory event-evoked response, whereas those with ADHD and controls do not (Olincy et al. 2000); on the basis of this finding the authors concluded that the mechanism of the attention deficit may be different in these two diseases.

ADHD patients may also have psychotic symptoms, of course. In their report on 241 consecutively referred patients with ADHD and/or autistic spectrum disorders (ASDs), Stahlberg et al. (2004) noted that 5% of the ADHD patients had a bipolar disturbance

with psychotic symptoms and 5% had schizophrenia or some other psychotic disorder. Meanwhile Elman et al. (1998), in a comparison of patients suffering from both schizophrenia and ADHD with patients having schizophrenia alone, reported that those who had ADHD diagnosed in childhood had had more obvious developmental disturbances at that age. The progress of schizophrenia had been more insidious, the response to neuroleptics had been poorer, and the general outcome of treatment had been less satisfactory than in those patients with schizophrenia alone.

One of the crucial problems concerning concurrent AHDH and psychotic symptoms is that the typical drugs prescribed for ADHD – stimulants – can trigger psychotic symptoms. Tossell et al. (2004) and Pine et al. (1993) have reported on the treatment of patients with psychotic and simultaneous ADHD symptoms with psychostimulant supplementation of ongoing neuroleptic therapy, but additional well-controlled trials are needed in this area. Nevertheless the results of their studies give us reason to assume that ADHD occurring concurrently with psychotic symptoms can be treated once the latter have been stabilized.

Tic symptoms

Tic symptoms cover a wide variety of involuntary nonrythmic, stereotyped motor movements ranging from mild, transient forms to extremely serious cases of Tourette syndrome, which include vocal tics that involve the production of sounds as well. The most common forms of tics affect the head and facial area, the hands, or the feet, and the vocal forms can range from whines, growls, and clearings of the throat to distinct speech sounds, words, and even sentences. Tourette syndrome, first described by Gilles de la Tourette in 1885, can involve both vocal and complex motor movements simultaneously. It is customarily regarded as a rare disease and one that is difficult to treat, but the increased interest shown in it in more recent times has revealed milder forms.

The cause of Tourette syndrome is unknown, but certain areas of the brain, most notably the basal ganglia and frontal lobe, have been implicated. No special tests have been devised for establishing its presence, and diagnosis is based on a case history together with clinical symptoms and observations. It most commonly begins in childhood, at a mean age of 6.4 years as shown in one large international multicenter survey of 3500 cases, and with a male:female ratio of 4.3:1 (Freeman et al., 2000).

Tic symptoms of various kinds occur in children much more frequently than does Tourette syndrome, with 297 (6.6%) of a total of 4479 Swedish children aged 7–15 years studied having had tic symptoms at the time of examination or during the preceding year (Khalifa & von Knorring, 2003); in this study the prevalence of Tourette syndrome in the population as a whole was 0.6%, another 0.8% had chronic motor tics, and 0.5% had chronic vocal tics.

The prevalence of Tourette syndrome is better known in children than in adults and was estimated at around 1% among children aged 5–16 years in the review article of Robertson (2003), although higher rates have been quoted in community studies. Mason et al. (1998) obtained a figure of 3% among 13- to 14-year-old children in a school, and Burd et al. (1986), who asked all the doctors in North Dakota to report on patients with Tourette syndrome in their care, reached estimated prevalence figures of 0.22 per 10,0000 women and 0.77 per 10,000 men, although the prevalence in children was again higher than in adults.

The prognosis for the disease is difficult to estimate, but in most cases it seems to become milder with advancing age. Thus, in the series of 58 patients aged between 15 and 25 years studied by Erenberg, Cruse, and Rothner (1987), 26% reported that the symptoms disappeared by late youth or early adulthood, and a further 47% said that they had become very much milder, the remainder being of the opinion that the symptoms had remained the same (14%) or worsened (also 14%).

Spencer et al. (2001) observed tic symptoms in 12% of their ADHD patients, as opposed to 4% of the control group, and so few cases of Tourette syndrome occurred that they were treated simply as one group of tic cases. In their epidemiological study, Apter et al. (1993) reported that 8.3% of the young people aged 16–17 years with Tourette syndrome that they studied had ADHD, whereas Comings (2000) claimed that 25–85% of all Tourette syndrome carriers have concurrent ADHD or ADD (ADHD without hyperactivity and/or impulsiveness).

The most significant diseases occurring concurrently with Tourette syndrome are obsessive-compulsive disease (OCD), ADHD, and learning difficulties. The connection between Tourette syndrome and OCD, especially at an adult age, has been emphasized in recent years, and Peterson et al. (2001), in their extensive follow-up study, reported significant correlations both between tic symptoms and OCD and between OCD and ADHD. They investigated the relationships among tic symptoms, OCD, and ADHD both longitudinally and cross-sectionally in a random sample of 976 children aged 1–10 years in families in northern New York State by means of interviews and followed up 776 of these cases 8, 10, and 15 years later. Tic symptoms in childhood, youth, or early adulthood were predictive of increased tic symptoms of this kind in late youth and early adulthood, ADHD symptoms in youth predicted more OCD symptoms in early adulthood, and OCD in youth predicted increased ADHD symptoms in adulthood.

Clinically ADHD can usually be clearly distinguished from Tourette syndrome. Even though stimulants may exacerbate tic symptoms, the current recommendation is to treat moderate to severe ADHD with concurrent mild to moderate tic symptoms with stimulants, but to use alternative medication if the tic symptoms are problematic.

References

American Psychiatric Association. (2000). *Diagnostic and statistical manual of mental disorders.* 4th ed. text. rev. Washington, DC: American Psychiatric Association.

Apter A, Pauls DL, Bleich A, Zohar AH, Kron S, Ratzoni G, et al. (1993). An epidemiologic study of Gilles de la Tourette's syndrome in Israel. *Arch Gen Psychiatry* 50(9):734–8.

Barr WB. (2001). Schizophrenia and attention deficit disorder: two complex disorders of attention. *Ann N Y Acad Sci* 931:239–50.

Biederman J, Mick E, Faraone S, Hammerness P, Surman C, Harpold T, et al. (2006). A double-blind comparison of galantamine hydrogen bromide and placebo in adults with attention-deficit/hyperactive disorder: a pilot study. *J Clin Psychopharmacol* 26(2):163–6.

Burd L, Kerbeshian J, Wikenheiser M, Fisher W. (1986). Prevalence of Gilles de la Tourette's syndrome in North Dakota adults. *Am J Psychiatry* 143:787–8.

Cohen RZ, Gotowiec A, Seeman MV. (2000). Duration of pretreatment phases in schizophrenia: women and men. *Can J Psychiatry* 45(6):544–7.

Comings DE. (2000). Attention-deficit/hyperactivity disorder with Tourette syndrome. In: Brown TE, ed. *Attention Deficit Disorders and Comorbidities in Children, Adolescents, and Adults.* Washington, DC: American Psychiatric Press: 363–92.

Elman I, Sigler M, Kronenberg J, Lindenmayer JP, Doron A, Mendlovic S, Gaoni P. (1998). Characteristics of patients with schizophrenia successive to childhood attention deficit hyperactivity disorder (ADHD). *Isr J Psychiatry Relat Sci* **35**(4):280–6.

Erenberg G, Cruse RP, Rothner AD. (1987). The natural history of Tourette syndrome: a follow-up study. *Ann Neurol* **22**(3):383–5.

Freeman RD, Fast DK, Kerbeshian J, et al. (2000). An international perspective on Tourette syndrome: selected findings from 3500 individuals in 22 countries. *Dev Med Child Neurol* **42**(7):436–47.

Hambrecht M, Lammertink M, Klosterkotter J, Matuschek E, Pukrop R. (2002). Subjective and objective neuropsychological abnormalities in a psychosis prodrome clinic. *Br J Psychiatry* **43**(suppl):30–7.

Khalifa N, von Knorring AL. (2003). Prevalence of tic disorders and Tourette syndrome in a Swedish school population. *Dev Med Child Neurol* **45**(5): 315–9.

Kim YH, Ko MH, Na SY, Park SH, Kim KW. (2006). Effects of single-dose methylphenidate on cognitive performance in patients with traumatic brain injury: a double-blind placebo-controlled study. *Clin Rehabil* **20**(1):24–30.

Mason A, Banerjee S, Eapen V, et al. (1998). The prevalence of Tourette syndrome in a mainstream school population. *Dev Med Child Neurol* **40**(12):847–8.

Olincy A, Ross RG, Harris JG, Young DA, McAndrews MA, Cawthra E, et al. (2000). The P50 auditory event-evoked potential in adult attention-deficit disorder: comparison with schizophrenia. *Biol Psychiatry* **47**(11):969–77.

Peterson BS, Pine DS, Cohen P, Brook JS. (2001). Prospective, longitudinal study of tic, obsessive-compulsive, and attention-deficit/ hyperactivity disorders in an epidemiological sample. *J Am Acad Child Adolesc Psychiatry* **40**(6):685–95.

Pine DS, Klein RG, Lindy DC, Marshall RD. (1993). Attention-deficit hyperactivity disorder and comorbid psychosis: a review and two clinical presentations. *J Clin Psychiatry* **54**(4):140–5.

Robertson MM. (2003). Diagnosing Tourette syndrome: is it a common disorder? *J Psychosom Res* **55**(1):3–6.

Siddall OM. (2005). Use of methylphenidate in traumatic brain injury. *Ann Pharmacother* **39**(7–8):1309–13.

Spencer TJ, Biederman J, Faraone S, Mick E, Coffey B, Geller D, et al. (2001). Impact of tic disorders on ADHD outcome across the life cycle: findings from a large group of adults with and without ADHD. *Am J Psychiatry* **158**;611–7.

Stahlberg O, Soderstrom H, Rastam M, Gillberg C. (2004). Bipolar disorder, schizophrenia, and other psychotic disorders in adults with childhood onset AD/HD and/or autism spectrum disorders. *J Neural Trans* **111**(7):891–902.

Tenovuo O. (2005). Central acetylcholinesterase inhibitors in the treatment of chronic traumatic brain injury – clinical experience in 111 patients. *Prog Neuropsychopharmacol Biol Psychiatry* **29**(1):61–7.

Tossell JW, Greenstein DK, Davidson AL, Job SB, Gochman P, Lenane M, et al. (2004). Stimulant drug treatment in childhood-onset schizophrenia with comorbid ADHD: an open-label case series. *J Child Adolesc Psychopharmacol* **14**:448–54.

Whyte J, Hart T, Vaccaro M, Grieb-Neff P, Risser A, Polansky M, Coslett HB. (2004). Effect of methylphenidate on attention deficits after traumatic brain injury: a multidimensional, randomized, controlled trial. *Am J Phys Med Rehabil* **83**(6):401–20.

Wilens TE, Waxmonsky J, Scott M, Swezey A, Kwon A, Spencer TJ and Biederman J. (2005). An open trial of adjunctive donepezil in attention-deficit/hyperactive disorder. *J Child Adolesc Psychopharmacol* **15**(6):947–55.

Zhang L, Plotkin RC, Wang G, Sandel ME, Lee S. (2004). Cholinergic augmentation with donepezil enhances recovery in short-term memory and sustained attention after traumatic brain injury. *Arch Phys Med Rehabil* **85**(7):1050–5.

Chapter

14

Overlap between ADHD and autism spectrum disorder in adults

Christopher Gillberg, I. Carina Gillberg, Henrik Anckarsäter, and Maria Råstam

Introduction

Autism was long considered to be a very rare disorder, the best defined in child psychiatry (Rutter & Schopler, 1992), and one that occurred in isolation, often with no comorbidity (except, possibly, mental retardation) and presumably with one etiology. It is now clear that autism in its classic variant is but part of a broader spectrum of disorders that include not only "autistic disorder" (as defined by *DSM-IV*) but also a number of conditions, including Asperger disorder and so-called pervasive developmental disorders not otherwise specified (PDDNOS)/atypical autism (Wing & Potter, 2002). It has also become generally accepted that these "autism spectrum disorders" (ASDs, including autistic disorder) are much more common than previously assumed, with overall childhood prevalence usually reported at just under 1% (Gillberg et al., 2006). To complicate things, genetic studies have shown that ASDs extend into "lesser variants" and "broader phenotypes" with some characteristic autism features but with little or no clinical impairment. Population studies suggest that such lesser variants or features of autism occur in several percent of children (Briskman, Happé, & Frith, 2001; Constantino & Todd, 2003; Posserud et al., 2006).

The comorbidity issue in autism has not been resolved, and authorities in the field still argue about whether autism can be associated with other disorders, including ADHD. Both the *DSM-IV* and ICD-10 include a section of the diagnostic criteria that is difficult to interpret but that would tend to make researchers and clinicians loathe to diagnose coexisting/comorbid ADHD in ASD.

Conversely, ADHD has long been agreed to be a common type of childhood behavior disorder and one that does blend into normality. Its prevalence has long been agreed to be around or more than 5% of the childhood population. Even with a high prevalence of ASD (say 1%), only a small proportion of all individuals with ADHD could have comorbid ASD. This would be true even if all individuals with ASD had ADHD, which would be unlikely to be the case on theoretical grounds and is not borne out by clinical experience.

Very few empirical studies have ever addressed the issue of whether ADHD – or the symptoms considered typical of the disorder – shows some overlap/comorbidity with ASD. A small number of child studies exist, but no formal studies, other than those from our own group, have ever been published looking at the phenomenon in adults.

In this chapter we briefly review the limited data that exist in the field, starting with what is known in children. Given that both ADHD and ASD show a strong tendency to persist from childhood into adult life, it is important for understanding the overlap of the two categories in adulthood to have a good knowledge base of their childhood comorbidity. A summary of the evidence that exists in adults follows. We end by summing up what the overlap of ASD with ADHD might mean, clinically and neurobiologically, and what the projected child findings infer in terms of adult outcome. The chapter also includes a brief survey of interventions that might be helpful.

Diagnostic boundaries in ASDs

Before considering the issue of whether features of autism occur in ADHD, there is a need to be clear about some of the diagnostic boundaries and problems in the field.

First, in this context, we disregard the hierarchical criteria of the diagnosis of autism/ASD (such as those of the ICD-10); that is, we assume that ASD can occur in ADHD and that, at this point in time, it is not clear that one type of disorder or problem takes

---

ADHD in Adults: Characterization, Diagnosis and Treatment, ed. Jan Buitelaar, Cornelis Kan and Philip Asherson.
Published by Cambridge University Press. © Cambridge University Press 2011.

precedence over another. This issue of precedence is especially important in these disorders, as ASDs are generally regarded as the more severe diagnosis that may override ADHD, and ADHD is amenable to pharmacological treatment, whereas ASDs are not.

Second, even though clinical impairment is assumed as part of the diagnostic categories of both ADHD and ASD, we recognize that they are not clearly defined conditions with a precise cut-off point, neither in terms of symptoms nor degree of clinical impairment.

Third, although we accept the symptomatic diagnostic criteria of *DSM*/ICD for most of the named conditions, we mostly disregard them for Asperger syndrome because as, in clinical practice, it is very difficult to find individuals who *truly* match the criteria for this disorder according to *DSM*/ICD.

Fourth, ASD is used as an umbrella term to refer to all conditions meeting *DSM*/ICD criteria for pervasive developmental disorders, except Asperger syndrome for which the criteria of Gillberg and Gillberg (1989) are used. We use the term "autism features" for conditions that do not meet full diagnostic criteria for ASD, but do meet several of the *DSM*/ICD symptom criteria of autistic disorder (in most instances 3 or more of the 12 listed).

Finally, it needs to be recognized that the term "autism" is sometimes regarded as synonymous with "social communication problems," which may or may not be pathogenetically linked to the so-called core syndrome of autism. At present, it is unclear whether all the symptoms listed for autism in the diagnostic manuals are specific to autism or whether some represent more general social communication problems.

Diagnostic criteria for ASDs

There are at least four different clinically important variants of ASDs and possibly one subclinical variant of the condition.

Autistic disorder/childhood autism is usually considered to be the most severe variant of ASD, with onset in the first 3 years of life and presenting with a triad of problems in reciprocal social interaction, reciprocal communication (including language), and the ability to vary the behavioral repertoire, which is believed by some (Wing & Gould 1979) to be linked to reduced imagination skills (American Psychiatric Association, 1994). Autistic disorder is almost always

associated with severe cognitive deficits, and 80% are diagnosed as suffering from mental retardation or a learning disability. Associated medical conditions such as fragile X syndrome, tuberous sclerosis, Chromosome 22q11 deletion syndrome CATCH 22, or chromosomal aberrations may be documented in at least 25% of cases (for an overview, see Gillberg & Coleman, 2000), and up to 90% have unspecific symptoms of brain pathology such as epilepsy (Steffenburg, 1991). These proportions are much lower in the other forms of ASD, although larger than in the general population (Rutter et al., 1994) (ref).

However, it has not been clearly documented that the "autism" (i.e. the basic social-communication deficit), is any less severe in so-called *Asperger syndrome* than in autistic disorder. It is possible that the main (or only) difference between autistic disorder and Asperger syndrome is that IQ is much lower in the former condition and that it is the learning disability rather than the autism per se that contributes to the overall clinical impression of a more severe disorder. Asperger syndrome – according to *DSM-IV-TR* (American Psychiatric Association, 2000) and ICD-10 (WHO, 1993) – is diagnosed by the same general criteria as autistic disorder, with the important differences that development in the first 3 years of life should have been normal and there is no insistence that reciprocal communication problems be present.

However, there is now widespread agreement that cases meeting those criteria either do not exist in real life or are so rare as to make the diagnostic entity clinically almost meaningless (Leekam et al., 2000) or the diagnostic criteria are so far removed from physicians' own cases of Asperger syndrome that the individuals they described do not meet them (Miller & Ozonoff, 1997). If the ICD-10 or *DSM-IV* criteria for Asperger syndrome (which are almost identical) are stringently applied, fewer than 2% of all individuals with an ASD can be expected to meet them (Leekam et al., 2000). In clinical practice and in many research studies, the criteria for Asperger syndrome published by Gillberg and Gillberg (1989) and elaborated in Gillberg (1991) – which are based on the original case reports by Hans Asperger (1944) – are often used instead (Table 14.1). Asperger syndrome is sometimes referred to as "high-functioning autism." However, this term is misleading, given that it is not the autism that is high functioning. If used at all, a more appropriate phrase is "high-functioning (or normally intelligent) individuals with autism."

Table 14.1 Gillberg's criteria for Asperger's disorder

All of the following six criteria must be met for confirmation of diagnosis:

1. Severe impairment in reciprocal social interaction (at least two of the following):
   1. inability to interact with peers
   2. lack of desire to interact with peers
   3. lack of appreciation of social cues
   4. socially and emotionally inappropriate behavior

2. All-absorbing narrow interest (at least one of the following):
   1. exclusion of other activities
   2. repetitive adherence
   3. more rote than meaning

3. Imposition of routines and interests (at least one of the following):
   1. on self, in aspects of life
   2. on others

4. Speech and language problems (at least three of the following):
   1. delayed development
   2. superficially perfect expressive language
   3. formal, pedantic language
   4. odd prosody, peculiar voice characteristics
   5. impairment of comprehension including misinterpretations of literal/implied meanings

5. Nonverbal communication problems (at least one of the following):
   1. limited use of gestures
   2. clumsy/gauche body language
   3. limited facial expression
   4. inappropriate expression
   5. peculiar, stiff gaze

6. Motor clumsiness: poor performance on neurodevelopmental examination

Atypical autism, albeit rather loosely defined in the ICD-10, is the term applied in triad cases not meeting full criteria for autistic disorder or Asperger syndrome. Some authors (e.g. Billstedt, Gillberg, & Gillberg, 2005) have suggested that for this diagnosis to be made individuals would have to meet at least 5 of the 12 ICD-10 symptoms for childhood autism, at least one of which must come from the social domain of the triad, but criteria for autism/Asperger syndrome are not met. Atypical autism is roughly equivalent to the *DSM-IV-TR* category "pervasive developmental disorder not otherwise specified (PDDNOS)," which the manual describes even more vaguely than atypical autism.

The fourth established variant of ASD is *disintegrative disorder of childhood*, an extremely rare condition with regression and triad symptoms appearing only after about 3 years or more of normal or near-normal development.

Finally, there is the usually subclinical, *broader behavioral phenotype of autism* roughly equivalent to

autistic features. These are categories that are not yet official diagnostic entities but have been shown to be common mild presentations of triad problems in the extended families of individuals with diagnosed autism.

Unfortunately, Rett syndrome is included as a particular variant of an ASD or PDD both in the ICD-10 and *DSM-IV*. This categorization does not make sense, given that Rett syndrome is but one of the many medical disorders (including tuberous sclerosis, Moebius syndrome, and fragile X syndrome) that have a large subgroup of patients with marked autistic features/autism. Why only Rett syndrome and none of the others should be considered an ASD has never been motivated (Gillberg, 1994).

Childhood studies of the overlap of ADHD and ASDs

ASD in ADHD

An early population-based study from our group on 7-year-old children born in the early 1970s (Gillberg, 1983) indicated that impairing attention deficit disorder (ADD) – diagnosed according to the *DSM-III*, but equivalent to DSM-IV ADHD in about 85% of cases (Rasmussen & Gillberg, 2000) – at least when combined with motor perceptual problems (or in recent parlance "developmental coordination disorder [DCD]"), is often associated with autistic symptoms. Twenty-five years ago these symptoms were often referred to as "psychotic behavior," but they were actually indistinguishable from autism "triad" symptoms (i.e. the social, communication, and behavioral problems considered to be at the core of the autistic syndrome). Several of the individuals with such "psychotic behavior" were demonstrated to meet full diagnostic criteria for Asperger syndrome on follow-up in adolescence (Hellgren et al., 1994) and early adulthood (Rasmussen & Gillberg, 2000), and the remainder would all have fit under the current umbrella concept of ASD. This group of children with the combination of ADD/ADHD, DCD, and ASD (including Asperger syndrome) constituted 0.67% of the general population of 7-year-olds. It is interesting to note that this figure corresponds very well with recent estimates of the overall prevalence of ASD (e.g. Chakrabarti & Fombonne, 2005; Gillberg, 2006). In addition, the findings, albeit based on a relative small general population sample of about 5000 children, indicated that the majority of children with ASD in the general population have additional ADD/ADHD and DCD problems. Interestingly, children with milder variants of ADD/ADHD with DCD did not show autistic features at all (Gillberg, 1983; Gillberg & Gillberg, 1989; Gillberg & Wing, 1999).

This early study was followed by Swedish general population sample surveys in Mariestad (Landgren et al., 1996) and Karlstad (Kadesjo & Gillberg, 1998), which roughly replicated its results. The Karlstad study found an interactive effect of DCD on ADHD in predicting a high rate of autistic features (including Asperger syndrome), speech and language problems, and academic failure (Kadesjo & Gillberg, 1999). As in the early study, the more recent Swedish studies showed that ADHD without DCD was not associated with autistic features. Similar conclusions were drawn by an Australian group, which reported that autism and ADHD often clinically co-occur, but that the link between the two may be mediated by DCD (Piek & Dyck, 2004). In the Karlstad study both autistic features and ADHD showed considerable stability over a few years, but follow-up into adult age was not done.

In a UK study from the 1990s, a very high proportion (65–80% according to parent report) of children with ADHD had autistic features/empathy problems (Clark et al., 1999).

A number of recent studies have looked at the effects of central stimulants in children with ADHD who also meet criteria for an ASD or have a high load of autistic features (e.g. Gillberg et al., 1997). In several of these studies it is unclear which – if any – is considered the "primary" disorder and which should be counted as "comorbid." Of course, this distinction can usually not be determined retrospectively or perhaps not even prospectively. However, the publication of a number of studies of this type in recent years is indirect testimony to the growing realization that ADHD/ASD coexistence in one and the same individual is not an extremely rare phenomenon.

Several studies have demonstrated the common co-occurrence of social interaction problems in ADHD. However, they have generally attributed these problems to the comorbidity of ADHD with oppositional-defiant disorder (ODD) and/or conduct disorder. One recent study (Green et al., 2000) showed that, in some instances, ODD and ASDs overlap. Given the possible association of ODD with ADHD on the one hand and with ASDs on the other, this overlap could be taken to suggest that the link between

ODD and ASDs is mediated by ADHD. However, such a link was not demonstrated in the study, which did not set out specifically to examine ADHD.

There is good evidence that having few or no friends is a common feature of ADHD (Barkley, 1998; Bauermeister et al., 2005). It is also a cardinal symptom in ASDs. Conclusions on the basis of this finding can only be tentative because of the high prevalence of friendship problems across the board of severe child psychiatric disorders, not just in ADHD and ASDs.

ASD in tic disorders with ADHD

Clinically impairing tic disorders, particularly Tourette syndrome, are very often comorbid with ADHD and obsessive-compulsive disorder (OCD; Comings & Comings, 1990, Robertson, 2000). Most individuals diagnosed with Tourette syndrome who are functionally disabled have ADHD, OCD, or both, and it is usually the presence of OCD or ADHD that mediates the high degree of clinical impairment.

Comings and Comings (1991) suggested the comorbidity of tic disorders with ASDs. Several single and multiple case reports have documented the coexistence of Tourette syndrome and Asperger syndrome (Berthier et al., 2003; Kerbeshian, Burd, & Fisher, 1990; Ringman & Jankovic, 2000).

A population and clinic study of Tourette syndrome (Kadesjo & Gillberg, 2000) documented the presence of ADHD in 64% and OCD in 38% of 58 cases. The vast majority of those with ADHD also had "major social interaction problems," including a large subgroup with Asperger syndrome or several DSM-IV symptoms of autistic disorder. It was not possible (because of the small number of cases) to determine on the basis of the findings from that study whether the link with autistic features was mediated by ADHD or OCD or by Tourette syndrome "in itself."

ASD and ADHD in certain genetic behavioral phenotype syndromes

A number of genetically well-delineated syndromes are associated with a fairly persistent clinical behavioral presentation ("behavioral phenotype syndromes"). Tuberous sclerosis, the fragile X syndrome and the 22q11 deletion syndrome are the (most frequent and) best researched of these conditions, and a high rate of ADHD and ASDs has been repeatedly documented in all three. Very often, in these behavioral phenotype syndromes, ADHD and ASD occur together in the same individual. For instance, in the 22q11 deletion syndrome, 30% of all affected individuals meet diagnostic criteria for ADHD, and about one in three also meet criteria for an ASD (Niklasson et al., 2001, 2002, 2005, 2009). In tuberous sclerosis, the link between ADHD and ASD appears to be even stronger, with the vast majority of those meeting behavioral criteria for one of these disorders also meeting criteria for the other (IC Gillberg, Gillberg, & Ahlsen, 1994; Hunt & Dennis, 1987). Males with the fragile X syndrome often meet diagnostic criteria for ADHD and ASD. Sometimes ASD is the diagnostic category that applies early in life, and criteria for ADHD are met only later in childhood. In other individuals, both disorders coexist throughout childhood and adolescence (Hagerman 1999).

ADHD in ASD

There have been no more than a handful of studies formally addressing the issue of ADHD in autism and Asperger syndrome. There have been slightly more studies looking at noncategorically diagnosed attention deficits and hyperactivity/impulsivity symptoms in people diagnosed in the autism spectrum.

Ehlers and Gillberg (1993) found a very high rate of ADHD (usually with DCD) in a population study of Asperger syndrome. Interestingly, the comorbidity was most often seen in individuals with Asperger syndrome who also had tics. A similarly high rate of ADHD in Asperger syndrome was reported later by Ghaziuddin, Weidmer-Mikhail, and Ghaziuddin (1998).

Baron-Cohen and co-workers (1990) reported that 6.5% of 447 individuals with ASDs met criteria for definite or probable Gilles de la Tourette syndrome. Many of these patients also had ADHD.

Goldstein and Schwebach (2004) reported that 74% of a clinical group of cases with ASDs ("PDDs") also met diagnostic criteria for ADHD according to a retrospective clinical chart review. Very similar findings were obtained by Yoshida and Uchiyama (2004), who found that 85% of those with Asperser's disorder and 58% of those with autistic disorder met criteria for ADHD. A recent Swedish study reported that about three-quarters of all children with PDD and normal levels of intelligence also met criteria for ADHD and deficits in attention, motor control, and perception (DAMP; Sturm, Fernell, & Gillberg, 2004). Gadow

et al. (2004) also found a high rate of ADHD in PDD, but not more often than in other clinical psychiatric disorders. Finally, a high rate of ADHD in autism spectrum disorders was recently reported by Keen and Ward (2004).

ASD in adults with ADHD

To our knowledge, no studies have been published looking at the occurrence of ASDs in ADHD in representative samples of adults. Nevertheless, follow-up into early adulthood of the children in the Gillberg (1983) study suggested that at least 75% of those children who had shown ADHD (+DCD) with ASD at age 7 years continued to meet criteria for Asperger syndrome or atypical autism at age 22 years (Rasmussen & Gillberg, 2000). If these findings are generalized to other populations, one would expect that at least 0.5% of the general population of young adults would show the combination of ADHD (+DCD) and ASD.

A large-scale study of adult psychiatric patients with attention deficit and social interaction problems found a considerable degree of overlap between ASD and ADHD. Of 273 patients (aged 18–60 years, the majority in their late twenties and early thirties), roughly 41% had ADHD as the "major" clinical diagnosis, 47% had ASDs as the major diagnosis, and 12% had other diagnoses. Almost 40% of those with ASDs also met criteria for ADHD. The vast majority of all the patients with ASDs or ADHD also met criteria for one or more (often several) personality disorders (Anckarsäter et al., 2006). A small number (29 in the total group of 273) had psychotic conditions (schizophrenia, bipolar disorder; Stahlberg et al., 2004). The findings cannot be generalized to other adult psychiatric patients, given the potential risk of referral bias in the sample. However, they do underscore the not infrequent coexistence of ASD with ADHD in adult psychiatric cases and that, at least in all patients showing attention deficits and major social interaction problems, both diagnoses should be considered.

Are social impairments and communication problems part of ADHD?

Clinically, it is evident that many individuals with ADHD have severe social impairment. The type of social interaction problems associated with oppositional-defiant disorder (ODD) is generally accepted as a coexisting problem in more than half of all individuals with a diagnosis of ADHD. It is not clear whether they are two separate disorders or if ADHD with ODD is a severe form of ADHD with social interaction aberrations. Whether there is a link between ODD and ASD has not been established (Green et al., 2000). Some authors (e.g. Kadesjo et al., 2003) have argued that certain symptoms currently believed to be essential for diagnosing ODD are, in effect, more typical of severe ADHD.

Similarly, both clinical experience and several formal studies have shown that speech and language/communication (particularly pragmatic) problems are commonly associated with ADHD (Ramberg et al., 1996; Rasmussen & Gillberg, 1983). However, it is not clear whether such problems should be regarded as part of the syndrome of ADHD, a complication of ADHD, or an altogether separate set of dysfunctions.

Are attention deficits and/or hyperactivity part of ASDs?

Clinical experience and some systematic studies suggest that attention deficits are almost universal in Asperger syndrome (e.g. Ehlers & Gillberg 1993) and are very common indeed in classic cases of autistic disorder. However, it is not clear that these attention deficits are of the type most consistently encountered in ADHD. In ASDs, inattention is more commonly of the "not listening" and "difficulty shifting" type, rather than the "short attention span" and "distractibility" type often assumed to be characteristic of clinically diagnosed ADHD. Nevertheless, the distinction is not clear, and many studies directly or indirectly suggest that executive function deficits, believed by many to be essential for the development of ADHD, are also characteristic of ASDs (see the later discussion).

Hyperactivity is a very common presenting symptom in autism. Formal study as to the possible early comorbidity of ASD with hyperkinesia is lacking. However, the extreme hyperactivity seen in many young children with autism, a type of hyperkinetic behavior that is usually greatly reduced when the child with autism is placed in an "autism-friendly" environment, could be seen as a reaction to the breakdown of communication and sense-making in children with ASDs who have not been properly recognized.

Are ADHD and autism on a spectrum?

Gillberg and Gillberg (1989) and Gillberg (1990) suggested that, at least in a subgroup of cases with autism, the condition exists on a spectrum with "deficits in attention, motor control, and perception (DAMP)" and, hence, with ADHD. It is not extremely rare for a child to present with ADHD/DAMP symptoms early in life and then to go on to develop the full-blown clinical phenotype of Asperger syndrome or even autism. There is widespread clinical agreement that severe levels of hyperactivity in a preschool-aged child should always prompt suspicion that the "underlying" disorder might be autism. It is not unheard of for a child suspected of suffering from severe ADHD (because of extremes of early-onset hyperactivity and impulsivity) to be treated with a stimulant and for autistic features to emerge in the course of such treatment. In the past, such autistic features were often believed to be a side effect of the treatment per se. Although that is a real possibility, a more common link might be the suppression of severe hyperactivity leading to the "unmasking" or "surfacing" of the ASD that was always present but hidden under the more conspicuous symptoms associated with extreme hyperactivity.

Conversely, a sizable group of children who present early in life with major social impairments and who raise suspicion of suffering from autism will meet criteria for ADHD and not for autism a few years later (Gillberg et al., 1990).

Is there a shared biological, neuropsychological, or psychosocial background of risk factors in ADHD and autism spectrum disorders? Surprisingly little has been published in terms of the overlap of ADHD and ASDs at the familial/clinical level, despite the now widely held assumption that these types of problems often segregate in the same extended families (Cederlund & Gillberg, 2004). Some studies in the early 1990s did suggest a strong familial overlap of the conditions (e.g. Gillberg, 1991, Gillberg, Gillberg, & Steffenburg, 1992), but conclusions will have to await larger scale systematic studies.

However, there is, perhaps unexpectedly, already rather more to suggest a biological link between the two diagnosed conditions at the molecular genetic level. Thus, for instance, genome scan studies of autism have suggested certain chromosomal regions of interest for autism susceptibility genes, and genome scan studies of ADHD have demonstrated that some of these regions (e.g. on chromosomes 2q, 15q, and 16p) are also susceptibility sites for ADHD (e.g. Bakker et al., 2003; Fisher et al., 2002; Ogdie, 2003; Smalley et al., 2002). In addition, the serotonin transporter gene has been suggested to be down-regulated in both ADHD and ASDs (Murphy et al., 2004).

Neuroanatomy and neurophysiology

However, at the brain biological level, the evidence linking the two conditions is highly contradictory. On the one hand there are many studies suggesting brainstem, cerebellar, basal ganglia, and frontal dysfunction in both conditions (Coleman, 2005; Sowell et al., 2003), even though it is not clear that the types of dysfunction are shared across them. On the other hand, some studies do suggest markedly different brain pathologies in the two disorders. For instance, in systematic studies, autism is quite often associated with macrocephalus (in about 20% of the cases; Bolton et al., 2001; Gillberg & de Souza, 2002; Miles et al., 2000), whereas ADHD is often reported to be linked to smaller overall brain size (Castellanos et al., 2002; Rapoport et al., 2001; Seidman, Valera & Makris, 2005). Nevertheless, there are cases of ADHD with macrocephalus (Gillberg & de Souza, 2002), and a reasonable hypothesis for testing in empirical study is that macrocephalus (and the underlying reason for it) might be one of the links between ADHD and autism.

Studies of a number of behavioral phenotype syndromes have revealed a strong link between ADHD and ASD. As noted earlier, this link may be particularly strong with 22q11 deletion syndrome, tuberous sclerosis, and fragile X syndrome. These three syndromes have a very high rate of documented neuroanatomical and neurophysiological frontal and frontotemporal lobe abnormality, which could be a marker for the underlying brain link between the two diagnostic entities.

Neuropsychology

Neuropsychologically, there is mounting evidence that autism and ADHD may be on a spectrum in a proportion of cases. For instance, studies comparing children with autism, Asperger syndrome, and ADHD (e.g. Ehlers et al., 1997) have indicated that Asperger syndrome represents the "middle ground" between autism and ADHD when it comes to WISC-R test profiles. Executive function deficits in autism and Asperger syndrome are both similar and dissimilar from such deficits documented in ADHD (Booth et al.,

2003; Nyden, Hjelmquist, & Gillberg, 2000). One study showed shared executive function deficits across ASD and ADHD, but central coherence problems only in the former group. This finding could be taken to mean that ADHD symptoms in both types of disorders are mediated through executive function deficits and that central coherence deficits underlie the ASD. Another recent study (Geurts et al., 2004) documented executive function deficits in both disorders, even though they tended to be more profound in ASD than in ADHD.

Psychosocial factors

ADHD is strongly linked to low social class and psychosocial adversity (e.g. Biederman et al., 1998; Gillberg, 1983; Taylor et al., 2004). Most authors regard the psychosocial risk factors to be some of the mediators of associated psychiatric/behavioral problems and poor outcome in ADHD rather than being primary or causal risk factors in themselves. ASDs are not linked to social class or psychosocial adversity. Overall, according to the literature published to date, there is little, if anything, in the realm of psychosocial background that can account for the variance of a possible association of ASD with ADHD.

Who should receive the dual diagnosis of ADHD and ASD?

We have argued throughout that ADHD is sometimes associated with ASD. The current ICD-10 criteria do not allow dual diagnosis of the two types of disorder. The exclusionary criteria of *DSM-IV* are less stringent, specifying that the "other" diagnosis should only be excluded if its symptoms are better accounted for by the diagnosis already established.

It is our recommendation that the next versions of these diagnostic manuals reconsider the wording of the exclusionary criteria as regards these two groups of disorder. ASD, when clinically important, should be diagnosed in cases with clinically impairing ADHD and vice versa.

Hyperactivity should not automatically lead to assessment with a view to diagnosing possible ADHD. Severe and impairing hyperactivity should always prompt suspicion that the individual might instead be suffering from a "primary" disorder of autism (or severe learning disability or, more rarely, Tourette or bipolar disorder). Severe attention deficits in a an

163

individual might well signal Asperger syndrome rather than ADHD, but the comorbidity of both is no rare phenomenon, so clinically impairing symptoms in this domain should lead to consideration of the possibility of both disorders being present.

Persons already diagnosed as suffering from an ASD are at high risk of also having ADHD. Therefore, during follow-up of individuals with diagnoses of autism and, perhaps particularly, Asperger syndrome/PDDNOS, clinicians need to be aware of the need to assess for ADHD symptoms. Effective treatment (including medication) for such symptoms is available in many cases and should not be withheld for reasons of strict adherence to ill-founded diagnostic algorithms.

ASD symptoms in a child diagnosed as suffering from ADHD are not extremely rare, and again, clinicians catering to the follow-up needs of children with ADHD need to be aware of the possible association and be prepared to diagnose and intervene on account of autism symptomatology. Structured education and behavior modification in an autism-friendly setting may be needed in such cases.

Conclusion and overall clinical implications

ADHD is a common disorder, and ASDs, relatively speaking, are much less prevalent. Thus, despite a sizable association between ADHD and ASDs, the vast majority of children with the former diagnosis will not have autism, Asperger syndrome, or even marked autistic features. Nevertheless, an important minority of all patients with ADHD do have clinically impairing ASDs that need to be diagnosed and acted on. Clinicians need to be aware that it may be difficult to make the distinction between ADHD and ASDs in early life and that some children diagnosed under one of these categories in the preschool years may later have symptoms and problems better accounted for under the diagnostic label of the other. Setting up diagnostic and treatment teams specifically to cater to the needs of individuals with either label may not be the best way forward in the field. Given the very considerable comorbidity of ADHD with other conditions, and the very considerable comorbidity of ASDs with other conditions, it would seem a better idea for services to target persons with neuropsychiatric/neurodevelopmental disorders more broadly

than to launch new "autism only" or "ADHD only" services.

Summary

Only a very limited number of studies have addressed the issue of overlap between autism spectrum disorders and ADHD. The number of studies that have investigated this topic in adults is even smaller. ASDs are not commonly encountered in ADHD, given the rather low prevalence of the former group of disorders and the very high population rate of the latter condition. Nevertheless, an important minority of individuals with ADHD, particularly of those with associated developmental coordination disorder and other learning disabilities, do have ASDs to a degree that meet/correspond to diagnostic criteria, and a larger number have autistic features. The rate of ADHD in ASDs is probably much higher than hitherto acknowledged. Some recent studies suggest that in adults presenting with personality disorders, both ASDs and ADHD need to be carefully screened for. In addition, specialists working in ADHD clinics and those working in autism clinics need to be well aware of the possible overlap with the "other" type of disorder.

References

American Psychiatric Association. (1994). *Diagnostic and Statistical Manual of Mental Disorders: DSM-IV*. 4th ed. Washington, DC: American Psychiatric Association.

American Psychiatric Association. (2000). *Diagnostic and Statistical Manual of Mental Disorders: DSM-IV-TR*. 4th ed. text. rev. Washington, DC: American Psychiatric Association.

Anckarsäter H, Stahlberg O, Larsson T, Hakansson C, Jutblad S-B, Niklasson L, et al. (2006). The impact of ADHD and autism spectrum disorders on temperament character and personality development. *Am J Psychiatry* 163: 1239–44.

Asperger H. (1944). Die "Autistischen psychopathen" in Kindesalter. *Archive für Psychiatrie und Nervenkrankheiten* 117:76–136. Translated by Frith U, ed. (1991). *Autism and Asperger Syndrome*. Cambridge: Cambridge University Press: 37–92.

Bakker SC, Van Der Meulen EM, Buitelaar JK, Sandkuijl LA, Pauls DL, Monsuur AJ, et al. (2003). A whole-genome scan in 164 Dutch sib pairs with attention-deficit/hyperactivity disorder: suggestive evidence for linkage on chromosomes 7p and 15q. *Am J Hum Genet* 72(5):1251–60.

Barkley RA. (1998). *Attention Deficit Hyperactivity Disorder: A Handbook for Diagnosis and Treatment.* 2nd ed. New York: Guilford Press.

Baron-Cohen S, Scahill VL, Izaguirre J, Hornsey H, Robertson MM. (1999). The prevalence of Gilles de la Tourette syndrome in children and adolescence with autism: a large scale study. *Psychol Med* 29:1151–9.

Bauermeister JJ, Matos M, Reina G, Salas CC, Martinez JV, Cumba E, Barkley RA. (2005).Comparison of the DSM-IV combined and inattentive types of ADHD in a school-based sample of Latino/Hispanic children. *J Child Psychol Psychiatry* 46(2):166–79.

Berthier ML, Kulisevsky J, Asenjo B, Aparicio J, Lara D. (2003). Comorbid Asperger and Tourette syndromes with localized mesencephalic, infrathalamic, thalamic, and striatal damage. *Dev Med Child Neurol* 45(3):207–12.

Biederman J, Wilens TE, Mick E, Faraone SV, Spencer T. (1998). Does attention-deficit hyperactivity disorder impact the developmental course of drug and alcohol abuse and dependence? *Biol Psychiatry* 44:269–73.

Billstedt E, Gillberg IC, Gillberg C. Autism after adolescence: population-based 13–22-year follow-up study of 120 individuals with autism diagnosed in childhood. *J Autism Dev Disord* 35:351–60.

Bolton PF, Roobol M, Allsopp L, Pickles A. (2001). Association between idiopathic infantile macrocephaly and autism spectrum disorders. *Lancet* 358(9283):726–7.

Booth R, Charlton R, Hughes C, Happe F. (2003). Disentangling weak coherence and executive dysfunction: planning drawing in autism and attention-deficit/hyperactivity disorder. *Philos Trans R Soc Lond B Biol Sci* 358(1430):387–92.

Briskman J, Happé F, Frith U. (2001). Exploring the cognitive phenotype of autism: weak "central coherence" in parents and siblings of children with autism: II. Real-life skills and preferences. *J Child Psychol Psychiatry* 42:309–16

Castellanos FX, Lee PP, Sharp W, Jeffries NO, Greenstein DK, Clasen LS, et al. (2002). Developmental trajectories of brain volume abnormalities in children and adolescents with attention-deficit/hyperactivity disorder. *JAMA* 288:1740–8.

Cederlund M, Gillberg C. (2004). One hundred males with Asperger syndrome: a clinical study of background and associated factors. *Dev Med Child Neurol* 46(10):652–60.

Chakrabarti S, Fombonne E. (2005). Pervasive developmental disorders in preschool children: confirmation of high prevalence. *Am J Psychiatry* 162(6):1133–41.

Clark T, Feehan C, Tinline C, Vostanis P. (1999). Autistic symptoms in children with attention deficit-hyperactivity disorder. *Eur Child Adolesc Psychiatry* 8(1):50–5.

Coleman M, ed. (2005). *The Neurology of Autism.* New York: Oxford University Press.

Comings DE, Comings BG. (1990). A controlled family history study of Tourette's syndrome, I: Attention-deficit hyperactivity disorder and learning disorders. *J Clin Psychiatry* 51:275–80.

Comings DE, Comings BG. (1991). Clinical and genetic relationships between autism-pervasive developmental disorder and Tourette syndrome: a study of 19 cases. *Am J Med Genet* 39:180–91.

Constantino J, Todd RD. (2003). Autistic traits in the general population: a twin study. *Arch Gen Psychiatry* 60:524–30.

Ehlers S, Gillberg C. (1993). The epidemiology of Asperger syndrome. A total population study. *J Child Psychol Psychiatry* 34:1327–50.

Ehlers S, Nyden A, Gillberg C, Sandberg AD, Dahlgren SO, Hjelmquist E, Oden A. (1997). Asperger syndrome, autism and attention disorders: a comparative study of the cognitive profiles of 120 children. *J Child Psychol Psychiatry* 38(2):207–17.

Fisher SE, Francks C, McCracken JT, McGough JJ, Marlow AJ, MacPhie IL, et al. (2002). A genomewide scan for loci involved in attention-deficit/hyperactivity disorder. *Am J Hum Genet* 70:1183–96.

Gadow KD, DeVincent CJ, Pomeroy J, Azizian A. (2004). Psychiatric symptoms in preschool children with PDD and clinic and comparison samples. *J Autism Dev Disord* 34:379–93.

Geurts HM, Verte S, Oosterlaan J, Roeyers H, Sergeant JA. (2004). How specific are executive functioning deficits in attention deficit hyperactivity disorder and autism? *J Child Psychol Psychiatry* 45:836–54.

Ghaziuddin M, Weidmer-Mikhail E, Ghaziuddin N. (1998). Comorbidity of Asperger syndrome: a preliminary report. *J Intellect Disabil Res* 42(pt 4):279–83.

Gillberg C. (1983). Perceptual, motor and attentional deficits in Swedish primary school-children. Some child psychiatric aspects. *J Child Psychol Psychiatry* 24:377–403.

Gillberg C. (1989). Asperger syndrome in 23 Swedish children. *Dev Med Child Neurol* 31:520–31.

Gillberg C. (1990). Autism and pervasive developmental disorders. *J Child Psychol Psychiatry* 31:99–119.

Gillberg C. (1991). Clinical and neurobiological aspects of Asperger syndrome in six family studies. In: Frith U, ed. *Autism and Asperger Syndrome.* Cambridge: Cambridge University Press: 122–46.

Gillberg C. (1994). Debate and argument: Having Rett syndrome in the ICD-10 PDD category does not make sense. *J Child Psychol Psychiatry* 35:377–8.

Gillberg C, Carlström G, Rasmussen P. (1983). Hyperkinetic disorders in seven- year-old children with perceptual, motor and attentional deficits. *J Child Psychol Psychiatry* 24:233–46.

Gillberg C, Cederlund M, Lamberg K, Zeijlon L. (2006). The autism epidemic. The registered prevalence of autism in a Swedish urban area. *J Autism Dev Disord* 36(3): 429–35.

Gillberg C, Coleman M. (2000). *The Biology of the Autistic Syndromes*. 3rd ed. London: MacKeith Press.

Gillberg C, de Souza L. (2002). Head circumference in autism, Asperger syndrome, and ADHD: a comparative study. *Dev Med Child Neurol* 44:296–300.

Gillberg C, Ehlers S, Schaumann H, Jakobsson G, Dahlgren SO, Lindblom R, et al. (1990). Autism under age 3 years: a clinical study of 28 cases referred for autistic symptoms in infancy. *J Child Psychol Psychiatry* 31:921–34.

Gillberg C, Gillberg IC, Steffenburg S. (1992). Siblings and parents of children with autism: a controlled population-based study. *Dev Med Child Neurol* 34(5):389–98.

Gillberg C, Melander H, von Knorring AL, Janols LO, Thernlund G, Hagglof B, et al. (1997). Long-term stimulant treatment of children with attention-deficit hyperactivity disorder symptoms. A randomized, double-blind, placebo-controlled trial. *Arch Gen Psychiatry* 54:857–64.

Gillberg C, Wing L. (1999). Autism: not an extremely rare disorder. *Acta Psychiatr Scand* 99:399–406.

Gillberg IC, Gillberg C. (1989). Asperger syndrome – some epidemiological considerations: a research note. *J Child Psychol Psychiatry* 30:631–8.

Gillberg IC, Gillberg C, Ahlsen G. (1994). Autistic behaviour and attention deficits in tuberous sclerosis: a population-based study. *Dev Med Child Neurol* 36(1):50–6.

Goldstein S, Schwebach AJ. (2004). The comorbidity of pervasive developmental disorder and attention deficit hyperactivity disorder: results of a retrospective chart review. *J Autism Dev Disord* 34:329–39.

Green J, Gilchrist A, Burton D, Cox A. (2000). Social and psychiatric functioning in adolescents with Asperger syndrome compared with conduct disorder. *J Autism Dev Disord* 30:279–93.

Hagerman R. (1999). Fragile X syndrome. In: Hagerman R, ed. *Neuro-Developmental Disorders: Diagnosis and Treatment*. New York: Oxford University Press: 61–132.

Hellgren L, Gillberg IC, Bagenholm A, Gillberg C. (1994). Children with deficits in attention, motor control and perception (DAMP) almost grown up: psychiatric and personality disorders at age 16 years. *J Child Psychol Psychiatry* 35:1255–71.

Hunt A, Dennis J. (1987). Psychiatric disorder among children with tuberous sclerosis. *Dev Med Child Neurol* 29(2):190–8.

Kadesjo B, Gillberg C. (1998). Attention deficits and clumsiness in Swedish 7-year-old children. *Dev Med Child Neurol*. 40(12):796–804.

Kadesjo B, Gillberg C. (1999). Developmental coordination disorder in Swedish 7-year-old children. *J Am Acad Child Adolesc Psychiatry* 38(7):820–8.

Kadesjo B, Gillberg C. (2000). Tourette's disorder: epidemiology and comorbidity in primary school children. *J Am Acad Child Adolesc Psychiatry* 39(5):548–55.

Kadesjo C, Hägglöf B, Kadesjo B, Gillberg C. (2003). Attention-deficit-hyperactivity disorder with and without oppositional defiant disorder in 3- to 7-year-old children. *Dev Med Child Neurol* 45(10):693–9.

Keen D, Ward S. (2004). Autistic spectrum disorder: a child population profile. *Autism* 8(1):39–48.

Kerbeshian J, Burd L, Fisher W. (1990). Asperger's syndrome: to be or not to be? *Br J Psychiatry* 156:721–5.

Landgren M, Pettersson R, Kjellman B, Gillberg C. (1996). ADHD, DAMP, and other neurodevelopmental/psychiatric disorders in 6-year-old children: epidemiology and comorbidity. *Dev Med Child Neurol* 38:891–906.

Leekam SR, Libby S, Wing L, Gould J, Gillberg C. (2000). Comparison of ICD-10 and Gillberg's criteria for Asperger syndrome. *Autism* 4:11–28.

Miles JH, Hadden LL, Takahashi TN, Hillman RE. (2000). Head circumference is an independent clinical finding associated with autism. *Am J Med Genet* 95(4):339–50.

Miller JN, Ozonoff S. (1997). Did Asperger's cases have Asperger disorder? A research note. *J Child Psychol Psychiatry* 38(2):247–51.

Murphy DL, Lerner A, Rudnick G, Lesch KP. (2004). Serotonin transporter: gene, genetic disorders, and pharmacogenetics. *Mol Interv* 4(2):109–23.

Niklasson L, Rasmussen P, Oskarsdottir S, Gillberg C. (2001). Neuropsychiatric disorders in the 22q11 deletion syndrome. *Genet Med* 3(1):79–84.

Niklasson L, Rasmussen P, Oskarsdottir S, Gillberg C. (2002). Chromosome 22q11 deletion syndrome (CATCH 22): neuropsychiatric and neuropsychological aspects. *Dev Med Child Neurol* 44(1):44–50.

Niklasson L, Rasmussen P, Oskarsdottir S, Gillberg C. (2005). Attention deficits in children with 22q.11 deletion syndrome. *Dev Med Child Neurol* **47**(12):803–7.

Niklasson L, Rasmussen P, Oskarsdottir S, Gillberg C. (2009). Autism, ADHD, mental retardation and behavior problems in 100 individuals with 22q11 deletion syndrome. *Res Dev Disabil* **30**(4):763–73.

Nyden A, Hjelmquist E, Gillberg C. (2000). Autism spectrum and attention-deficit disorders in girls. Some neuropsychological aspects. *Eur Child Adolesc Psychiatry* **9**(3):180–5.

Ogdie MN. (2003). A genomewide scan for attention-deficit/hyperactivity disorder in an extended sample: suggestive linkage on 17p11. *Am J Hum Genet* **72**(5):1268–79.

Piek JP, Dyck MJ. (2004). Sensory-motor deficits in children with developmental coordination disorder, attention deficit hyperactivity disorder and autistic disorder. *Hum Mov Sci* **23**(3–4):475–88.

Posserud M-B, Astri J, Lundervold, Gillberg C. (2006). Autistic features in a total population of 7–9-year-old children assessed by the ASSQ (Autism Spectrum Screening Questionnaire. *J Child Psychol Psychiatry* **47**(2):167–75.

Ramberg C, Ehlers S, Nyden A, Johansson M, Gillberg C. (1996). Language and pragmatic functions in school-age children on the autism spectrum. *Eur J Disord Commun* **31**(4):387–413.

Rapoport JL, Castellanos FX, Gogate N, Janson K, Kohler S, Nelson P. (2001). Imaging normal and abnormal brain development: new perspectives for child psychiatry. *Aust N Z J Psychiatry* **35**(3):272–81.

Rasmussen P, Gillberg C. (1983). Perceptual, motor and attentional deficits in seven-year-old children. Paediatric aspects. *Acta Paediatr Scand* **72**(1):125–30.

Rasmussen P, Gillberg C. (2000). Natural outcome of ADHD with developmental coordination disorder at age 22 years: a controlled, longitudinal community-based study. *J Am Acad Child Adolesc Psychiatry* **39**:1424–31.

Ringman JM, Jankovic J. (2000). Occurrence of tics in Asperger's syndrome and autistic disorder. *J Child Neurol* **15**(6):394–400.

Robertson MM. (2000). Tourette syndrome, associated conditions and the complexities of treatment. *Brain* **123**(pt 3):425–62.

Rutter M, Bailey A, Bolton P, Le Couteur A. (1994). Autism and known medical conditions: myth and substance. *J Child Psychol Psychiatry* **35**(2):311–22.

Rutter M, Schopler E. (1992). Classification of pervasive developmental disorders: some concepts and practical considerations. *J Autism Dev Disord* **22**(4): 459–82.

Seidman LJ, Valera EM, Makris N. (2005). Structural brain imaging of attention-deficit/hyperactivity disorder. *Biol Psychiatry* **57**:1263–72.

Sowell ER, Thompson PM, Welcome SE, Henkenius AL, Toga AW, Peterson BS. (2003). Cortical abnormalities in children with attention-deficit hyperactivity disorder. *Lancet* **362**: 1699–1707.

Smalley SL, Kustanovich V, Minassian SL, Stone JL, Ogdie MN, McGough JJ, et al. (2002). Genetic linkage of attention-deficit/hyperactivity disorder on chromosome 16p13, in a region implicated in autism *Am J Hum Genet* **71**:959–63.

Stahlberg O, Soderstrom H, Rastam M, Gillberg C. (2004). Bipolar disorder, schizophrenia, and other psychotic disorders in adults with childhood onset ADHD and/or autism spectrum disorders. *J Neural Transm* **111**(7):891–902.

Steffenburg S. (1991). Neuropsychiatric assessment of children with autism: a population-based study. *Dev Med Child Neurol* **33**(6):495–511.

Sturm H, Fernell E, Gillberg C. (2004). Autism spectrum disorders in children with normal intellectual levels: associated impairments and subgroups. *Dev Med Child Neurol* **46**(7):444–7.

Taylor E, Dopfner M, Sergeant J, Asherson P, Banaschewski T, Buitelaar J, et al. (2004). European clinical guidelines for hyperkinetic disorder – first upgrade. *Eur Child Adolesc Psychiatry* **13**(suppl 1): I7–30.

WHO (World Health Organization). (1993). *The ICD-10 Classification of Mental and Behavioural Disorders. Diagnostic Criteria for Research*, 1993 Geneva: WHO.

Wing L, Gould J. (1979). Severe impairments of social interaction and associated abnormalities in children: epidemiology and classification. *J Autism Dev Disord* **9**:11–29.

Wing L, Potter D. (2002). The epidemiology of autistic spectrum disorders: is the prevalence rising? *Ment Retard Dev Disabil Res Rev* **8**(3):151–61.

Yoshida Y, Uchiyama T. (2004). The clinical necessity for assessing Attention Deficit/Hyperactivity Disorder (ADHD) symptoms in children with high-functioning Pervasive Developmental Disorder (PDD). *Eur Child Adolesc Psychiatry* **13**(5):307–14.

Chapter 15

ADHD in adults with intellectual disabilities

Kiriakos Xenitidis, Eleni Paliokosta, Vangelis Pappas, and Jessica Bramham

Introduction

ADHD is a neurodevelopmental syndrome, and its diagnostic validity in adults has only recently been established (Toone, 2004; Zwi & York, 2004). There is considerable controversy around the exact prevalence of the condition in adults, but rates from 2.9–16.4% have been reported (Faraone & Biederman, 2005) depending, among other factors, on the diagnostic criteria used. Comorbidity is the norm rather than the exception and includes oppositional-defiant disorder, conduct disorder, specific learning disabilities, and tic disorders in childhood. In the adult ADHD population, anxiety and depressive disorders, substance abuse, and personality disorders are the most common comorbidities (Kutcher et al., 2004). The coexistence of ADHD with intellectual disabilities (ID; mental retardation, general learning disability) represents a special case of ADHD comorbidity.

The reported prevalence of ADHD in adults with ID varies widely. This variability is accounted for by the range of definitions and diagnostic criteria used for ID, in addition to the factors contributing to the variability of ADHD prevalence rates in adults in general. Rates of ADHD in children and adults with ID vary from 4–42% depending on the target population, sampling methodology, the severity of ID, and the context in which each study was conducted (Dekker & Koot, 2003; Fox & Wade, 1998; Hardan & Sahl, 1997; Rojan et al., 1993). Emerson (1993) performed a secondary analysis of the 1999 Office for National Statistics survey of the Mental Health of Children and Adolescents in Great Britain and estimated the prevalence of ADHD as increased eightfold in children with ID compared to children without ID. Prevalence rates of 15% in adults are commonly quoted, and an "ADHD-positive" rate of 16.9% has recently been reported in a small sample of adults with ID of a wide range of severity (La Malfa et al., 2008)

Kuntsi et al. (2004) showed that ADHD and low IQ co-occurrence has genetic origins, as genes that influence both ADHD and IQ accounted for 86% of the phenotypic correlation between ADHD symptom scores and IQ, and 100% of the phenotypic correlation between ADHD research diagnosis and IQ. However, there are no data regarding individuals with ADHD whose IQ falls in the ID range.

Classification issues

The issues surrounding diagnostic criteria for ADHD in adulthood in the two major classification systems, *DSM-IV* and ICD-10, are discussed elsewhere in this book. The main issue involves extrapolating from childhood diagnostic criteria into adulthood.

It is often presumed that ADHD symptoms are inherent to developmental disorders, and this has promoted a culture that has generally discouraged identification of the disorder as a comorbidity to conditions like ID or autism. Thus "diagnostic overshadowing" – the attribution of any behavioral or psychological symptoms to the underlying ID rather than a coexisting mental condition – is affecting the diagnosis of ADHD in this population (Reiss & Szyszko, 1983). According to *DSM-IV* (American Psychiatric Association, 1994) criteria, for the diagnosis of ADHD to be made in the context of ID, the observed behavior must be "inconsistent with the developmental level" of the subject. Even if diagnostic criteria are themselves relatively straightforward to apply in children with developmental disorders because they are based on observable behaviors such as distractibility and fidgetiness, difficulties arise in determining whether the observed behavior is inconsistent with the child's

ADHD in Adults: Characterization, Diagnosis and Treatment, ed. Jan Buitelaar, Cornelis Kan and Philip Asherson.
Published by Cambridge University Press. © Cambridge University Press 2011.

developmental level (Tonge, 2000). Although *DSM-IV* clearly highlights the importance of a differential ADHD diagnosis in children with low IQ, it provides little guidance on how to determine if the symptoms are excessive (Seager & O'Brien, 2003).

Application of this criterion to adults with ID is more complicated. ADHD may manifest differently in people with milder versus more severe levels of ID and with more cognitive symptoms such as inattention in mild to moderate ID or with more motor features of ADHD such as excessive movement in more severe levels of ID (Pearson, 1993). The diagnosis is only to be applied where the overall picture is in excess of that expected on the basis of the severity of intellectual impairment. Diagnosis is further complicated for people with ID and autism spectrum disorder. In *DSM-IV*, pervasive developmental disorders are exclusionary criteria for ADHD diagnosis, although the major deficits characterizing the two disorders are quite distinct.

Clinical presentation and diagnosis

The scientific literature suggests that clinicians feel more confident about making a diagnosis of ADHD in patients without ID (Reiss & Szyszko, 1983; Sevin et al., 2003; White et al., 2005) This may be related to the failure to take into account developmental issues, including developmentally consistent levels of activity and of attention. Buckley et al. (2006) investigated the diagnosis of ADHD in people with ID by sending questionnaires to consultants working in general adult psychiatry, child and adolescent psychiatry, and intellectual disability psychiatry. Overall, respondents were more confident about making a diagnosis of ADHD in people without ID. Those working with children were significantly more confident than those working with adult populations in diagnosing and treating ADHD, irrespective of the level of ID.

Because ID has typically been used as an exclusionary diagnostic criterion in ADHD research, the literature about the clinical presentation in this population is limited. In addition, due to the traditional stance that children and adolescents grow out of their ADHD symptoms, clinical data are limited in the adult population. However, a number of studies following different research approaches have supported the validity of the ADHD diagnosis in people with intellectual disabilities (Antshel et al., 2006). Studies using factor analysis of items reflecting a range of psychological

symptoms in both adults and children with intellectual disabilities have identified hyperactivity subscales for several behavior rating questionnaires (Aman et al., 1996; Freund & Reiss, 1991; Reiss & Valenti-Hein, 1994). Studies comparing the psychological characteristics of children with ADHD with and without intellectual disabilities have suggested that their clinical presentation is similar (Fee, Matson, & Benivadez, 1994). When the activity behaviors and attention problems of children with ID with and without high levels of ADHD symptoms were compared, significant differences were found: children with ID and ADHD were found to have lower levels of on-task behavior and elevated levels of fidgeting (Handen et al., 1998) as well as deficits in visual selective attention, and they also made fewer correct target detections and more error commissions on a vigilance task (Pearson et al., 1996). Children with both ID and ADHD had significantly more symptoms in seven of nine behavioral/emotional subscales of the Personality Inventory for Children-Revisited (Pearson et al., 2000). Studying teachers' perspectives about ADHD presentations in ID children, Fee et al. (1994) concluded that a subset of intellectually impaired children show a typical pattern of ADHD behavior; thus criteria for diagnosing ADHD in normal-IQ children are likely to be applicable to children with ID. More recently, Simonoff et al. (2007) studied adolescents with mild intellectual disabilities using the parents' and teachers' Strengths and Difficulties Questionnaire; they identified a negative linear relationship between ADHD symptoms and IQ. Neither the profiles of ADHD symptoms nor the comorbidity with emotional/behavioral problems differed according to the presence of ID.

The identification of differences between ID groups with and without ADHD and the similarities of ADHD symptoms in children irrespective of the presence of ID justify the validity of ADHD comorbidity and raise questions about the ecological validity of the *DSM-IV* diagnostic criteria restrictions. However, empirical data about the clinical presentation of ADHD in ID adults are sparse. La Malfa et al. (2008) applied an ADHD screening rating scale, the Conners' Adult ADHD Rating Scales (CAARS) screening version, to 46 adults with mild to severe ID. The resulting prevalence of ADHD-positive cases was 19.6%. These data are in accord with results reported in the general adult literature. Statistical analysis established that the degree of ID influenced all the test scores, except for the inattentive subscale. However, the authors emphasized that all of the participants with positive ADHD total scores (tot > 70) reached the cut-off score in the inattentive subscale as well. Perhaps this finding is due to the fact that hyperactive behavior is present either in ADHD or in the most severe levels of ID, but difficulties in attention are present in people with ADHD and ID to an extent not attributable to their cognitive impairment.

Children and adults with ID are expected to present with limited coping skills and adaptive functioning. They are less able to learn from experience regarding the impact of their symptoms and behavior. As a result their impairment due to their ADHD symptoms will probably be more prominent, and any intervention that could address these difficulties could have a significant impact on the quality of life of their caregivers and of themselves. It should be emphasized that people with ID often do not raise any concerns about their difficulties and their symptoms and that their caregivers/teachers often actually initiate the referral and the assessment process.

Management and treatment

There is growing evidence from childhood studies that ADHD can be successfully treated in people with ID (Handen et al., 1999; Pearson et al., 2003). The main treatment approaches are pharmacological, using stimulant (methylphenidate, amphetamine) and non-stimulant (e.g, atomoxetine) medication.

As when treating ADHD in the general population (Arnold et al., 1997), methylphenidate is an efficacious treatment for both cognitive and behavioral symptoms in ADHD in people with ID. However, the rate of response may be reduced, whereas the rate of adverse effects may be increased (Posey et al., 2005). Handen et al. (1977) recontacted the families of 51 children with ID and ADHD 12–62 months after their participation in a double-blind study of methylphenidate. They found that children with ID+ADHD continued to present behavioral difficulties at follow-up. Children with a higher IQ were more likely to be prescribed methylphenidate at follow-up. Although ADHD-related symptoms decreased with age, 68% of the children with ID+ADHD continued to manifest significant deficits in attention span, impulsivity, and activity level at follow-up and appeared to be at risk for an inpatient psychiatric hospitalization.

Amphetamine is a stimulant drug that has been shown to be as effective as methylphenidate for the treatment of ADHD (Elia et al., 1991). It is prescribed either as the D-isomer (dexamphetamine) or as a mixture of L- and D-isomers (mixed amphetamine salts). Although the majority of studies have been performed in people without ID, there are limited reports that suggest its efficacy in children with ID and comorbid ADHD (Alexandris & Lundell, 1968; Payton et al., 1989).

Although there is a lack of research examining ADHD treatment in adults with ID, one study that examined ADHD medication use in these populations yielded promising results (Jou et al., 2004). These researchers conducted a retrospective chart review of patients treated in a clinic that specialized in developmental disabilities. Improvement was assessed using the Aberrant Behavior Checklist-Community Version (ABC-C) and the global improvement item of the Clinical Global Impression scale. Five of ten consecutive adult outpatients who were treated with either methylphenidate or amphetamine were judged to be responders, based on impressions from chart review and the ABC-C. Significant improvements were observed in the hyperactivity and irritability subscales of the ABC-C. Adverse events were minimal, and no patients required treatment termination. The authors concluded that psychostimulants might be effective in the treatment of ADHD in adults with ID.

Atomoxetine is a noradrenaline reuptake inhibitor used for the treatment of ADHD (Kratochvil et al., 2006; Wilens et al., 2006). It has also been used for the treatment of ADHD symptoms in children with pervasive developmental disorders (Arnold et al., 2006). Risperidone is an atypical antipsychotic drug that appears to be generally safe, well tolerated, and effective for treating severely disruptive behaviors such as aggression and destructive behavior in children with ID or borderline intellectual functioning (Reyes et al., 2006). Risperidone's effectiveness in ADHD symptoms has been supported by some research findings (Aman et al., 2004; Correia Filho et al., 2005), but is not generally supported (NICE 2008). There are no data on the use or efficacy of risperidone or atomoxetine in adults with ADHD and ID, although limited anecdotal clinical evidence in the UK exists of this usage.

However, the fact that available clinical evidence is based mostly on small open-label trials or retrospective studies and is not derived from randomized controlled trials or meta-analyses represents a drawback in developing rigorous guidelines for the management of ADHD in this population. Currently, three

Cochrane Review Protocols are under preparation, analyzing data from existing studies, aiming to systematically current information, evaluate its importance, and identify review areas for future research (Thompson et al., 2008a, 2008b, 2008c).

Conclusion

Clinical and empirical data support the validity of ADHD diagnosis in people with ID. The importance of diagnosing ADHD in adults with ID arises from the frequency of inattentive and hyperactive/impulsive symptoms in this population, the additional impairment these symptoms may be associated with, and the potential to alleviate symptoms and improve functioning with appropriate treatment and management. There is some evidence (at least in children) that multi-axial comorbidity itself (Angold et al., 1999) or even the presence of psychiatric symptoms that do not amount to a syndromic diagnosis may increase psychosocial stress and maladaptation across the whole range of intellectual functioning (Gjaerum & Bjornerem, 2003).

As ADHD symptomatology is at least as common in adults with ID as in their nondisabled counterparts, ADHD needs to be carefully considered in individuals with ID presenting in a variety of settings. Identification of ADHD in this population can be difficult because of issues of diagnostic overshadowing, among other factors. Clinical presentation may be different in patients with different intellectual levels and may be atypical in individuals with ID (Brown et al., 2004). However, it is important that the diagnosis be made when appropriate, as ADHD can contribute synergistically with ID to increase occupational, interpersonal, and educational impairment. The diagnosis is particularly important in light of available pharmacological and psychosocial treatments. Recent government (Hart & Pettingell, 2005) documentation in the United Kingdom has highlighted the need for people with ID to have access to mental health care services that are available to nondisabled individuals.

References

Alexandris A, Lundell FW. (1968). Effect of thioridazine, amphetamine and placebo on the hyperkinetic syndrome and cognitive area in mentally deficient children. *Can Med Assoc J* **98**(2):92–6.

Aman MG, Binder C, et al. (2004). Risperidone effects in the presence/absence of psychostimulant medicine in children with ADHD, other disruptive behavior disorders, and subaverage IQ. *J Child Adolesc Psychopharmacol* **14**(2):243–54.

Aman MG, Tasse MJ, et al. (1996). The Nisonger CBRF: a child behavior rating form for children with developmental disabilities. *Res Dev Disabil* **17**(1):41–57.

Angold A, Costelo EJ, et al. (1999). Comorbidity. *J Child Psychol Psychiatry* **40**:57–88.

Antshel K, Phillips M, et al. (2006). Is ADHD a valid disorder in children with intellectual delays? *Clin Psychol Rev* **26**(5):555–72.

Arnold LE, Abikoff HB, et al. (1997). National Institute of Mental Health Collaborative Multimodal Treatment Study of Children with ADHD (the MTA). Design challenges and choices. *Arch Gen Psychiatry* **54**(9): 865–70.

Arnold LE, Aman MG, et al. (2006). Atomoxetine for hyperactivity in autism spectrum disorders: placebo-controlled crossover pilot trial. *J Am Acad Child Adolesc Psychiatry* **45**(10):1196–205.

Brown EC, Aman MG, et al. (2004). Empirical classification of behavioral and psychiatric problems in children and adolescents with mental retardation. *Am J Ment Retard* **109**(6):445–55.

Buckley S, Dodd P, et al. (2006). Diagnosis and management of attention-deficit hyperactivity disorder in children and adults with and without learning disability. *Psychiatr Bull* **30**:251–3.

Correia Filho AG, Bodanese R, et al. (2005). Comparison of risperidone and methylphenidate for reducing ADHD symptoms in children and adolescents with moderate mental retardation. *J Am Acad Child Adolesc Psychiatry* **44**(8):748–55.

Dekker MC, Koot HM. (2003). DSM-IV disorders in children with borderline to moderate intellectual disability. I: Prevalence and impact. *J Am Acad Child Adolesc Psychiatry* **42**(8):916–22.

Elia J, Borcherding BG, et al. (1991). Methylphenidate and dextroamphetamine treatments of hyperactivity: are there true nonresponders? *Psychiatry Res* **36**(2): 141–55.

Emerson E. (2003). Prevalence of psychiatric disorders in children and adolescents with and without intellectual disability. *J Intellect Disabil Res* **47**(pt 1):51–8.

Faraone SV, Biederman J. (2005). What is the prevalence of adult ADHD? Results of a population screen of 966 adults. *J Atten Disord* **9**(2):384–91.

Fee VE, Matson JL, & Benavidez DA. (1994). Attention deficit-hyperactivity disorder among mentally retarded children. *Res Dev Disabil* **15**(1):67–79

Fox RA, Wade EJ. (1998). Attention deficit hyperactivity disorder among adults with severe and profound mental retardation. *Res Dev Disabil* **19**(3):275–80.

Freund LS, Reiss AL. (1991). Rating problem behaviors in outpatients with mental retardation: use of the Aberrant Behavior Checklist. *Res Dev Disabil* 12(4):435–51.

Gjaerum B, Bjornerem H. (2003). Psychosocial impairment is significant in young referred children with and without psychiatric diagnoses and cognitive delays – applicability and reliability of diagnoses in face of co-morbidity. *Eur Child Adolesc Psychiatry* 12(5):239–48.

Handen B, McAuliffe S, et al. (1998). A playroom observation procedure to assess children with mental retardation and ADHD. *J Abnorm Child Psychol* 26(4):269–77.

Handen BL, Feldman HM, et al. (1999). Efficacy of methylphenidate among preschool children with developmental disabilities and ADHD. *J Am Acad Child Adolesc Psychiatry* 38(7):805–12.

Handen BL, Janosky J, et al. (1997). Long-term follow-up of children with mental retardation/borderline intellectual functioning and ADHD. *J Abnorm Child Psychol* 25(4):287–95.

Hardan A, Sahl R. (1997). Psychopathology in children and adolescents with developmental disorders. *Res Dev Disabil* 18(5):369–82.

Hart S, Pettingell J. (2005). Valuing people with learning disabilities. *J Roy Soc Health* 125(1):16–17.

Jou R, Handen B, et al. (2004). Psychostimulant treatment of adults with mental retardation and attention-deficit hyperactivity disorder. *Aust Psychiatry* 12(4): 376–9.

Kratochvil CJ, Wilens TE, et al. (2006). Effects of long-term atomoxetine treatment for young children with attention-deficit/hyperactivity disorder. *J Am Acad Child Adolesc Psychiatry* 45(8):919–27.

Kuntsi J, Eley TC, et al. (2004). Co-cccurrence of ADHD and low IQ has genetic origins. *Am J Med Genet B Neuropsychiatr Genet* 124b:41–7.

Kutcher S, Aman M, et al. (2004). International Consensus statement on attention-deficit/hyperactivity disorder (ADHD) and disruptive behaviour disorders (DBDs): clinical implications and treatment practice suggestions. *Eur Neuropsychopharmacol* 14:11–28.

La Malfa G, Lassi S, et al. (2008). Detecting attention-deficit/hyperactivity disorder (ADHD) in adults with intellectual disability: the use of Conners' Adult ADHD Rating Scales (CAARS). *Res Dev Disabil* 29(2): 158–64.

Payton JB, Burkhart JE, et al. (1989). Treatment of ADDH in mentally retarded children: a preliminary study. *J Am Acad Child Adolesc Psychiatry* 28(5):761–7.

Pearson DA. (1993). Dual diagnosis in children: attention deficit hyperactivity disorder. *S Q Rev* 1:1–3.

Pearson DA, Lahar D, et al. (2000). Patterns of behavioral adjustment and maladjustment in mental retardation: comparison of children with and without ADHD. *Am J Ment Retard* 105(4):236–51.

Pearson DA, Santos CW, et al. (2003). Treatment effects of methylphenidate on behavioral adjustment in children with mental retardation and ADHD. *J Am Acad Child Adolesc Psychiatry* 42(2):209–16.

Pearson DA, Yaffee LS, et al. (1996). Sustained and selective attention in children with mental retardation: A comparison of children with and without ADHD. *Am J Ment Retard* 100:592–607.

Posey DJ, Aman MG, et al. (2005). Randomized, controlled, crossover trial of methylphenidate in pervasive developmental disorders with hyperactivity. *Arch Gen Psychiatry* 62(11):1266–74.

Reiss S, Szyszko J. (1983). Diagnostic overshadowing and professional experience with mentally retarded persons. *Am J Ment Defic* 87(4):396–402.

Reiss S, Valenti-Hein D. (1994). Development of a psychopathology rating scale for children with mental retardation. *J Consult Clin Psychol* 62(1):28–33.

Reyes M, Croonenberghs J, et al. (2006). Long-term use of risperidone in children with disruptive behavior disorders and subaverage intelligence: efficacy, safety, and tolerability. *J Child Adolesc Psychopharmacol* 16(3):260–72.

Rojan J, Borthwick-Duffy SA, et al. (1993). The association between psychiatric diagnosis and severe behaviour problems in mental retardation. *Ann Clin Psychiatry* 5:163–70.

Seager MC, O'Brien G. (2003). Attention deficit hyperactivity disorder: review of ADHD in learning disability: the Diagnostic Criteria for Psychiatric Disorders for use with adults with learning disabilities/mental retardation [DC-LD] criteria for diagnosis. *J Intellect Dis Res* 47(suppl 1):26–31.

Sevin JA, Bowers-Stephens C, et al. (2003). Psychiatric disorders in adolescents with developmental disabilities: longitudinal data on diagnostic disagreement in 150 clients. *Child Psychiatry Hum Dev* 34(2):147–63.

Simonoff E, Pickles A, et al. (2007). ADHD symptoms in children with mild intellectual disability. *J Am Acad Child Adolesc Psychiatry* 46(5):591–600.

Thomson AB, Maltezos S, et al. (2008a). Amfetamine for attention deficit hyperactivity disorder in people with learning disabilities (protocol). *Cochrane Database Syst Rev* (1).

Thomson AB, Maltezos S, et al. (2008b). Amoxetine for attention deficit hyperactivity disorder in people with learning disabilities (protocol). *Cochrane Database Syst Rev* (1).

Thomson AB, Maltezos S, et al. (2008c). Risperidone for attention deficit hyperactivity disorder in people with learning disabilities (protocol). *Cochrane Database Syst Rev* (1).

Tonge BJ, ed. (2000). Psychiatric and behaviour disorders among mentally retarded children and adolescents In: Gelder MG., Lopez-Ibor JJ, Andreasen NC, eds. *New Oxford Textbook of Psychiatry*. New York: Oxford University Press.

Toone B. (2004). Attention deficit hyperactivity disorder in adulthood. *J Neurol Neurosurg Psychiatry* 75:523–5.

White P, Chant D, et al. (2005). Prevalence of intellectual disability and comorbid mental illness in an Australian community sample. *Aust N Z J Psychiatry* 39: 395–400.

Wilens TE, Newcorn JH, et al. (2006). Long-term atomoxetine treatment in adolescents with attention-deficit/hyperactivity disorder. *J Pediatr* 149(1):112–9.

Zwi M, York A. (2004). Attention-deficit hyperactivity disorder in adults: validity unknown. *Adv Psychiatr Treat* 10:248–59.

Chapter 16

ADHD, personality, and its disorders

Fiona E. van Dijk and Henrik Anckarsäter

Introduction

From clinical, neurocognitive, and neurobiological perspectives, ADHD is regarded as a meaningful diagnosis today, in childhood as well as in adulthood (Faraone, 2005). However, the adult symptom profile and ADHD's complex pattern of overlap with other mental health problem constellations have yet to be detailed and clarified (McGough & Barkley, 2004; Nigg, Blaskey, et al., 2002). So far, relatively little attention has been paid to the relationship of ADHD to maladaptive personality traits and personality disorders in adults (Lewinsohn et al., 1997; Nigg, John, et al., 2002), most probably because of the theoretical hiatus between the fields of child neuropsychiatry and adult personality and its disorders. Yet the coexistence of ADHD and personality disorders certainly does matter, not only for longitudinal prediction but specifically for a deeper understanding of adult problem arrays, for better phenotype characterization in neurobiological research, and for the development of new treatment strategies.

ADHD is the term chosen for the fourth edition of the *Diagnostic and Statistical Manual of Mental Disorders* (American Psychiatric Association, 1994), whereas the two earlier editions – *DSM-III* (American Psychiatric Association, 1980) and *DSM-III-R* (American Psychiatric Association, 1987) – contained related diagnostic definitions focusing on the inattentive facet of the syndromatic disorder. In *DSM-IV*, ADHD is diagnosed on the basis of problems with attention (inattentive subtype), action and impulse control (hyperactive subtype), *or* both (combined subtype). The current version of the International Classification of Diseases (ICD-10; WHO, 1990) includes a definition based on hyperactivity – hyperkinetic disorder – in which inattention is seen as a frequently complicating, coexisting problem rather than as an aspect of the

syndrome. As this textbook sets out from the ADHD concept, we consistently use the term "hyperactivity," which thus covers also the description of hyperkinesia.

According to *DSM-IV*, the essential feature of a personality disorder is "an enduring pattern of inner experience and behavior that deviates markedly from what is expected in the individual's culture." This definition contains several problems. Inner experiences are difficult to operationalize into diagnostic criteria, whereas diagnosing personality disorders on the basis of behavioral patterns may short-circuit attempts to "explain" behaviors by personality traits. At the same time, systematic definitions of behaviors are the most readily available features and will remain central among diagnostic criteria as long as interrater agreement is a priority. In this situation, it is important to recognize behaviorally defined disorders for what they are – relatively stable phenotypes for the study of cognitive, biological, and/or social covariates.

Although Axis II of *DSM-IV* is theoretically available to record personality disorders at all ages (with the exception of antisocial personality disorder), these disorders are rarely diagnosed before young adulthood (i.e. at an age when a more stable personality organization is being developed). Conversely, disorders classified as "usually first diagnosed in infancy, childhood, or adolescence" are not often assessed in adults. There is, however, every reason to assume that personality traits – or such differences in reaction patterns (temperaments) that form the basis on which adult traits develop – are discernible at a very early stage of child development (Caspi et al., 2003). By tradition, temperaments and personality are defined on the basis of the variance in the whole population, whereas psychiatric diagnoses, such as ADHD or personality disorders, focus on small groups of persons with disabling or distressful symptoms; these different perspectives

---

ADHD in Adults: Characterization, Diagnosis and Treatment, ed. Jan Buitelaar, Cornelis Kan and Philip Asherson.
Published by Cambridge University Press. © Cambridge University Press 2011.

have made it difficult to understand that different designations may refer to similar underlying phenomena. The growing awareness of "childhood" disorders, such as ADHD, among adults, of temperament differences already in infancy, and of manifestations of some Axis II disorders at least by adolescence (Lewinsohn et al., 1997) certainly calls for a cross-disciplinary reexamination of data and definitions.

ADHD and personality disorders

Antisocial personality disorder

A number of diagnostic definitions have been proposed to capture specific personality traits among persistently aggressive, destructive and dishonest persons, children as well as adults. These definitions have mainly relied on behavioral criteria, such as those in the DSM system, which define ASPD as a pervasive and stable pattern of aggressive and/or covert antisocial behaviors with onset before the age of 15, corresponding to the diagnostic criteria for conduct disorder (CD). As an "intermediary" diagnosis between ADHD and CD, the DSM system has included oppositional-defiant disorder (ODD) to describe severely oppositional attitudes and provocative behaviors. The combination of early-onset disruptive behaviors with deficient emotional reactions to others and to the consequences of one's own behavior, as well as with dishonest and dominance-seeking interpersonal strategies, has been described as "psychopathy," first in the European psychiatric tradition of personality disorders and then in North America, based on Cleckley's 1951 book, The Mask of Sanity. This proposed syndrome has not been included in the ICD or DSM classifications, even if the ICD-10 dissocial personality disorder includes more criteria reflecting interpersonal and emotional aspects than the more behavior-based DSM-IV definition of ASPD. However, this proposed syndrome has had considerable impact on research on personality in association with criminal behaviors, especially violence, not least because of its operationalization in the Psychopathy Checklist (PCL-R; Hare, 1980).

Factor analyses of the items in this checklist demonstrated a three-factor structure comprising "destructive and impulsive behavioral patterns" (factor 3), "blunted emotional integration of morally charged cognitions" (factor 2), and "a glib, dominance-seeking and dishonest interpersonal style" (factor 1; Cooke & Michie, 2001); Hare later proposed that the behavioral factor be split in two, distinguishing impulsive behaviors from outright norm-breaking. By comparing this factor structure to ADHD and other childhood-onset neuropsychiatric problems, we hope to add clarity to the nosology of these factors. The behavioral, third factor of the PCL-R and DSM-IV diagnostic criteria for ASPD and childhood disruptive behavior disorders, especially CD and ODD but also ADHD, all contain items that reflect impulsive, aggressive, or self-promoting behaviors with negative consequences that are not sufficiently evaluated before action takes place. However, the different diagnoses are based on criteria describing such behaviors in relation to heterogeneous settings or situations that occur at different stages of development, so that hyperactivity can be noted in an infant, whereas norm-breaking demands at least a basic understanding of what norms are meant to be. Inattention is defined by behaviors in task-related situations that require painstaking control, ODD by interpersonal norm-breaking, and CD by infractions of social norms for behavior during childhood, getting farther and farther into the realm of criminal acts as the perpetrator gets older.

There is no lack of longitudinal, prospective studies assessing the long-term development of ADHD or related conditions. Longitudinal studies that have used clinical diagnostic definitions are briefly reviewed in Table 16.1. Because they require diagnostics, the studies presented are mostly based on clinic referrals. In addition, several population-based studies have followed representative cohorts and are informative about longitudinal development and associations between symptom assessments at various stages and outcomes; for example, studies from San Francisco (Babinski et al., 1999), Pittsburgh (Loeber et al., 1998), Dunedin (Moffitt & Caspi, 2001), Sweden (Klinteberg et al., 1993) and London (Farrington, 2000). We reference these population-based studies in the following sections when appropriate, but let us start by summarizing the main findings from the clinical studies; and then examine a number of methodological problems that need to be considered when interpreting and using the results.

Comparisons of children identified as hyperactive to controls clearly and consistently show increased risks for CD, ASPD, and criminality later in life (Table 16.2). It may even be concluded with reasonable confidence that a majority of clinic-referred children with hyperactive ADHD (i.e. combined or

Table 16.1 The main reviewed prospective longitudinal studies on the association between childhood hyperactivity (using clinical diagnostic categories at inclusion) and antisocial personality disorder

Study, Main reference	Approximate years of inclusion	Cases	Controls	Treatment	Follow-up
Clinic-referred study groups					
Montreal *Weiss et al., 1985* *Hechtman & Weiss, 1986*	1962–5	104 (95 boys and 9 girls) long-term hyperactive children (aged 6–12)	45 matched "hypernormal"[a] school-mate controls	4 received psychostimulants, and 20 a conventional high-dose neuroleptic	59% were followed up after 15 years at 21–33 years of age, by blind and nonblind clinical assessments, court records, and, for those lost to follow-up, by parental contacts, contacts over the phone, etc.
New York Group 1 *Gittelman et al., 1985* *Mannuzza et al., 1993* Group 2 *Mannuzza et al., 1991* *Mannuzza et al., 1998* Group 1 & 2 *Mannuzza et al., 2004*	1970–7	115 (Group 1) and 111 (Group 2) hyperactive boys (aged 6–12)	178 matched hypernormal nonpsychiatric outpatient controls	All subjects had "medication and/or behavior therapy"	About 90% were followed after a mean interval of 16 and 17 years at mean ages 26, 24 and 24, by blind structured assessments and, for the first group, by official files
Boston *Biederman et al., 1992, 1996*	1992	140 referred or recruited boys with ADHD (aged 6–17)	120 unmatched control boys from outpatient services or recruited by advertisements	89% had a lifetime history of treatment with psychostimulants, 44% during the follow-up period	>80% were followed-up after 4 years by blind/semiblind new assessments
Los Angeles *Satterfield, Hoppe, & Schell, 1982*	1970–2	110 hyperactive boys between (aged 6–12)	75 matched paid public school controls, 13 non-ADHD brothers of cases	"Most" or "all" subjects had CS medication	81% were followed up until age 25 through official records
Wisconsin *Barkley et al., 2004* *Fischer et al., 2002*	1979–80	158 consecutive hyperactive children (144 boys, 14 girls, aged 4–12)	81 matched nonhyperactive controls recruited among the subjects' friends	22% vs. 0% had treatment with stimulants during the high school years	≥90% were followed up after a mean interval of 14 years at between 19–25 years old through structured interviews and official records
Developmental Trends Study *Loeber et al., 2000*	1987	177 outpatient boys at three clinics, (aged 7–12), 75% of whom were referred for disruptive behaviors	No controls	Medication in an unknown proportion[b] but required to discontinue two days prior to assessments	About 90% remained in the study and were followed by blind structured assessments yearly until ages 18–19
Population-based study					
Rasmussen & Gillberg, 2000	1977	61 7-year-old children (47 boys, 14 girls) with ADD with or without DCD, most of whom met *DSM-IV* criteria for AD/HD	51 population-based controls (27 boys, 24 girls) matched for SES and age	No one had medication with psychostimulants	90% were followed up with blind structured assessments and official files at 22 years of age

Note: Several well-known longitudinal studies are referred in the text but not included in the table as they did not use clinical diagnostics at baseline (e.g. the Dunedin and the Philadelphia studies). For a more comprehensive table including these studies and meta-analyses of results, please see Hofvander et al., 2009.
[a] Hypernormal, meaning that controls have been selected on a number of criteria, such as not being hyperactive, and are therefore not representative for the general population.
[b] When stated that no information is provided, this is based on the main references as cited. Some of these studies are published in a large number of papers and chapters, and even though we scrutinized this literature to the best of our ability, we may have missed some sources of information.

Table 16.2 Adult or follow-up outcomes of children initially identified with hyperactivity or related diagnoses vs. controls

Study	Persistence of AD/HD	Conduct disorder	Antisocial personality disorder	Criminality (various measures)	Incarceration
Montreal	36% vs. 2% had "at least one moderately or severely disabling symptom"	"about 10% ... antisocial disturbed"	23% vs. 2%	Court appearances 18% vs. 5% Any offense: 68% vs. 59% Nontheft convictions: 5% vs. 0%	None mentioned
New York Group 1 Group 2 Group 1 & 2	8% vs. 1% (group 1) 4% vs. 0% (group 2)	27–32% vs. 8%	18% vs. 2% (group 1) 12% vs. 3% (group 2)	Arrested: 39% vs. 20%, Convicted: 28% vs. 11% Aggressive crimes 6% vs. 2% (group 1)	5% vs. 0% (group 1) 2% vs. 0% (group 2)
Boston	58% vs. 6% "full or subthreshold" ADHD, more common when combined with ODD/CD	23% vs. 3%	Not within range of follow-up	Not within range of follow-up	Not within range of follow-up
Los Angeles	Not assessed	Not assessed	Not assessed	Juvenile arrests: 46% vs. 11% Felony arrests: 21% vs. 1% Recidivism: 9% vs. 0%	Institutionalized as adolescents: 25% vs. 1% Incarcerated as adults: 12% vs. 0%
Wisconsin	5% vs. 0%	31% vs. 11% developed CD at some stage	21% vs. 4%	Arrested ≥2 times: 39% vs. 12%	None mentioned
Gothenburg	Severe hyperactivity-impulsivity: 15% vs. 2% Severe inattention: 44% vs. 7% Combination of both: 9% vs. 0%	Not assessed	18% vs. 2%	Any criminal conviction: 15% vs. 0%	None mentioned

hyperactive subtype), at least during some phase, exhibit oppositional-defiant attitudes and behaviors, that at least one-third develop an early-onset CD, and that at least one-fifth go on to develop adult ASPD, according to a recent meta-analysis based on all longitudinal, prospective studies providing prevalence figures among index cases and controls (Hofvander et al., 2009). Another salient finding was that only small subgroups of those initially identified with hyperactivity or ADHD still met criteria for these diagnoses at follow-up. Longitudinal studies invariably have to deal with attrition, but the majority of the studies discussed here have high follow-up rates, and even in the single study with the highest attrition, the one from Montreal, indirect information from parents and official records supported that those retained in the study were representative of the whole initial group, at least regarding criminal histories (Weiss et al., 1985).

To avoid leaving the longitudinal literature with an oversimplified view of the findings, we must examine some methodological problems in these studies. Let us start with the manner of recruitment and the inclusion criteria for both index subjects and controls. The longitudinal studies' samples are either clinic referred or population based. Clinic-referred children may not be representative of the hyperactive children in the general population. This is difficult to establish as the reports often omit more specific information on how and by whom the subjects were referred. Criteria for study inclusion have included "minimal brain dysfunction (MBD)," "hyperkinesia," "hyperactivity/impulsivity," or ADHD, often casually understood as ADHD in its broadest sense. Having found no study where attention-deficit disorder without hyperactivity (ADD or ADHD inattentive type) has been specifically investigated in relation to ASPD or associated features, we conclude that inattention is not confirmed as a risk factor in this context. Population-based studies generally provide more detailed information on the background population and ways of selection, but use broader definitions to describe traits rather than conditions and often have arbitrary cut-offs within the assumed normal distribution of problems (such as the lowest or highest quartile or ratings below or above two standard deviations from the mean) to yield proxies for diagnoses.

As hyperactivity is a common phenomenon among children, group comparisons between index subjects and controls thought to form a representative sample from the general population (including hyperactives) will differ from those using controls selected to be "hypernormal" (i.e. without signs of this or that), and thus they are no longer "normal" in a statistical sense. Controls recruited among children referred for other mental health problems will naturally differ from controls recruited among friends or from school registers. We also know that subjects with hyperactivity or ADHD more often than not have other concomitant behavioral or mental problems. It is therefore crucial to know whether such problems precluded inclusion in the first place and whether the included children were seen as representative of all hyperactive children or only of subgroups with or without some specific combination of problem areas. For example, in the study of outcome in the form of conduct problems, criminality, or diagnoses including such behaviors, the extent to which index children had these or similar problems already at inclusion and which definitions were used at follow-up are essential information.

Longitudinal studies also challenge our capacity to keep the effects of time on the studied phenomena constantly in mind. For the developmental problems of interest to us, the degree of overlap between behavior types and thereby between disorders depends on the age at which the cross-section is done. Unfortunately, the majority of studies used broad age ranges already at inclusion, often recruiting small children as well as prepubertal or pubertal adolescents. Operational criteria for categorical diagnoses often mix current symptoms with lifetime problem histories, which may obscure both developmental features and the role of subsyndromal problems. Our targeted conditions are also most likely to represent problems that follow a waxing and waning course and thereby may oscillate over and under any diagnostic cut-off (Biederman et al., 2001; Lahey et al., 2002). These methodolog-

ical problems have to be considered when reassessing whether ADHD in the absence of early-onset conduct deviance is really a risk factor for adult antisocial behaviors (Lilienfeld & Waldman, 1990).

The Montreal study, which did not exclude children with conduct problems at inclusion, demonstrated that *all* subjects who eventually developed ASPD had an early onset of conduct problems as noted at the initial screening or at the first follow-up (Herrero, Hechtman, & Weiss, 1994). In the Wisconsin study, adult "predatory-overt" criminality was predicted by teenaged CD only (Barkley et al., 2004). In the Developmental Trends Study, in which boys referred to outpatient clinics had annual assessments, ADHD in the absence of conduct problems at inclusion did not predict the later onset of CD (Loeber et al., 1995). In the Los Angeles study, the absence of childhood conduct problems indicated a very low risk for later CD and criminality, as illustrated by 16 children with hyperactivity but no conduct problems who committed only minor adolescent offenses in two cases and no adult offenses at follow-up (Satterfield & Schell, 1997). The Pittsburgh study showed that "callous unemotional behaviors," depression, and onset of marijuana use between 13 and 17 years of age predicted antisocial personality development, whereas ODD and ADHD in the absence of conduct problems showed no such association (Loeber et al., 2002). In the London-based study, 8- and 9-year-old boys were classified according to the presence or absence of hyperactivity-impulsivity and conduct problems. Follow-up results indicated that both factors were independently predictive for adolescent convictions (age 10–16), whereas for adult convictions (age 17–25), conduct problems alone remained a significant predictor (Farrington, 2000). A cluster analysis of teacher assessments of 13-year-old boys in Sweden followed until ages 18–23 documented an increased risk for criminality in the aggression-hyperactivity-inattention cluster, but not in the hyperactivity-inattention cluster (Bergman & Magnusson, 1986). In several of the studies, it was noted that the presence of even one single behavioral problem in childhood (e.g. fighting, stealing, or lying) was an important risk factor for subsequent antisocial development (e.g. Montreal, Los Angeles). The risk of antisocial development was also higher in subjects with persistent hyperactivity than in those who had remitted during the follow-up period. Children who did not display any behavioral risk factors generally fared well (Herrero et al., 1994).

However, some studies have reported conflicting findings and claim that there is a direct relationship between ADHD and ASPD, even in the absence of early-onset CD. The New York City longitudinal study tried to establish study groups of children with hyperactivity but no conduct problems at inclusion. Again, the increased risk of adolescent CD and antisocial personality development was significantly associated with previously noted, even low-grade, conduct problems, just as in the Montreal study; however, in the New York study increased risk was seen also among children who had reportedly shown no conduct problems at inclusion. Hyperactivity in itself, even in the absence of early conduct problems, was therefore claimed to constitute a risk factor for the later development of antisocial behaviors and/or ASPD (Mannuzza et al., 2004). This claim is problematic as conduct problems were not systematically assessed at inclusion, especially not in the first New York study group. Included boys were reported not to have aggressive behaviors as the "primary reason for referral" (Mannuzza et al., 1993) or "clinically significant presenting problems involving aggression or other antisocial behaviors" (Mannuzza et al., 1998). A report from the San Francisco study also portrayed hyperactivity-impulsivity as an independent predictor of adult criminality, which actually was the case only for some categories of less severe crimes among males only. Crimes against people were again only predicted by conduct problems (Babinski et al., 1999).

Many longitudinal studies have also included children of considerably varying ages at the "baseline" assessments. In the New York City study discussed earlier, children were included from the age of 6, and in the San Francisco study from the age of 5, which means that no matter how carefully conduct problems were assessed at inclusion, it would be possible for subgroups of children to develop an early-onset CD *after* inclusion in the study, but before the age of 10 (which is the *DSM* definition for early-onset CD) or at least the onset of puberty, and then go on to have adult problems. The Pittsburgh study also included first, fourth, and fifth graders, which may have influenced the authors' perspective on overlap between hyperactivity-impulsivity and conduct problems. The Boston study demonstrated that, in children with ADHD, CD almost always developed before the age of 12 (Biederman et al., 1996), and it has been reported that the mean age at onset of CD may be early in childhood (Kim-Cohen et al., 2005); however, we

actually know little about the development of CD in relation to prepuberty. The best hypothesis therefore remains that ADHD is a precursor to early-onset conduct problems and aggression and then, and only then, constitutes a major risk factor for adulthood severe criminality and ASPD.

As for the nosological status of ODD, Loeber and co-workers (2002) proposed that ODD symptoms act as an independent risk factor in addition to ADHD and CD or as an intermediary state between those conditions. In most of the reviewed studies (e.g. New York City, Developmental Trends, and Boston), however, ODD did not predict CD development in a statistical sense, probably as it is so common among children with ADHD at some stage. ADHD-based ODD and CD instead seem to represent two sequential developmental complications of hyperactivity and may, of course, result from interacting or additional risk factors in the form of genetic factors associated with aggression or environmental factors related to criminality. This does not make them "independent" disorders. In the Boston and New York studies, virtually all children with ADHD who developed CD had already developed ODD, and early-onset CD almost always develops out of a condition marked by hyperactivity or the like (Lahey & Loeber, 1997).

Support for this notion also comes from twin studies that demonstrate common genetic mechanisms underlying hyperactivity and oppositional/conduct problems (Nadder et al., 2002; Silberg et al., 1996). A recent twin study examined possible explanatory models for the overlap between ADHD and CD and found that a model with "three different disorders" could be rejected, as both common genetic and environmental effects for ADHD and CD could be identified (Rhee et al., 2008).

We have now arrived at the question of prediction. Is there any reliable way to assess traits or features that give a valid prediction of later antisocial outcome among children? Despite the number of studies presented, no predictive model has yet been established, and in view of the figures presented, it seems reasonable to assume that the increased risks are so unspecific that predictions will overinclude children to such a degree that they become of little practical value. No other feature is as predictive as early-onset antisocial behaviors ("nothing predicts behavior as behavior"), and this effect precludes additions of predictive value from other factors in statistical models, even if it could be interesting to study more detailed characteristics of childhood behavior, such as age at onset or severity. Underlying this continuity of aggression and antisocial behaviors, genetic effects explain between 65% and 70% of the interindividual variance in aggression (Burt, 2009; Frisell et al., 2010), and some of these effects are common with ADHD (Rhee et al., 2008).

Another salient feature that seems to be associated with poor outcomes of ADHD is its persistence or that of some of its symptoms, such as restlessness, into adulthood. In both the Montreal and New York studies, the risk of antisocial behaviors was associated with the persistence of ADHD or of ADHD-related symptoms. This, however, is not of much use for prediction. Lynam's (1996) suggestion that the combination of ADHD and CD identifies a group of "fledgling psychopaths" may be consistent with the literature to the extent that this combination represents the most risk-laden subgroup, but as we have seen, at least one-third of all children with ADHD also develop CD, and a considerable proportion, between one-third and one-half in the cited studies, of these children will *not* go on to be antisocial or criminal in adulthood. Note that the definitions of "criminality" are also quite loose and seldom include severe violent crimes. Figures on the group level may also be elusive, as when 160 of 174 nontheft crimes in the Montreal study were perpetrated by four subjects (Hechtman & Weiss, 1986). Of course, it would have been of societal good to be able to identify these 4 among the initial 104 kids, but research at its current level is very far from being able to do so.

ADHD and the early-onset progression into ODD and CD ending up in ASPD thus explain the third, behavioral factor of the proposed psychopathy construct. The second factor of psychopathy describes deficient handling of stimuli and words related to concepts such as "guilt," "responsibility," "love," and "fear" without appropriate accompanying emotional resonance, indicating both that the person has a reduced or aberrant understanding of their meaning and will not have the same access to emotions to guide behavioral reactions as others. This was already referred to as "semantic blindness" by Cleckley (1951), who thought that it was a core deficit in the condition he described. It is reflected by the operational criteria for ASPD and has been demonstrated in many psychophysiological research models (Hofvander et al., 2009). This emotional deficit facet of psychopathy or ASPD was also associated both with ADHD and childhood autistic traits in a retrospective study of adult offenders (Soderstrom et al., 2005) and may be the result of autistic-like

traits interacting with impulsive disruptivenes on the ADHD-ODD-CD spectrum.

Finally on treatment, there is a striking contrast between our relatively detailed knowledge about the longitudinal outcome of hyperactivity and the means available for treatment aimed at preventing or changing a destructive development. The established treatment for ADHD, psychostimulants, does not have documented efficacy for treating either ODD or CD and nearly all the longitudinal studies have included children who have actually *been* treated with stimulants (Table 16.1). More recently, atypical neuroleptics have been used to treat disruptiveness, but are so far not recommended for general use because of their considerable side effects and the lack of evidence for efficacy from controlled trials. Other therapeutic measures for ADHD or CD, such as cognitive-behavior therapy, group therapies, and psychoeducative measures or training, are equally untested in the longitudinal developmental frame discussed in this chapter.

Borderline personality disorder

BPD is a complex and seriously disabling mental disorder. It is estimated to occur in about 1% or 2% of the general population (Torgersen, Kringlen, & Cramer, 2001), and it is the most common personality disorder in psychiatric clinical settings. Studies commonly suggest a three-factor structure consisting of a pervasive pattern of disturbed relations to other persons, affective or emotional dysregulation, and behavioral dyscontrol or impulsivity (Sanislow, Grilo, & McGlashan, 2000). These factors are thought to express core dimensions of borderline psychopathology, which may reflect underlying abnormal neurobiological processes involving genetic and developmental susceptibility. The three factors are conspicuously analogous to the factor solution proposed for psychopathy, again capturing the triad of maladaptive interpersonal attitudes, deficient emotional processing, and behavior dyscontrol. Even if this structure may merely represent one common to personality disorders, there is an obvious overlap between ADHD and BPD for at least the impulsivity of the third factor, and it is also evident from a clinical point of view that patients with ADHD, ASPD and BPD share symptoms of impulsivity. Of course, a common trait such as this one may cause artifactual coexistence and obscure the aspects that really are specific for the conditions.

Over the past years, a few studies have addressed a possible relationship between ADHD and BPD. In contrast to the high-quality prospective follow-up studies that have assessed the association between ADHD and ASPD, studies on ADHD and BPD have generally relied on clinical cross-sectional designs. BPD is mainly diagnosed in women and seems to have a presumed gender ratio that is the reverse of that for ASPD (American Psychiatric Association, 1994). In addition, as familial associations between ASPD and BPD are well demonstrated (Goldman, D'angelo, & DeMaso, 1993), a closer investigation of the relationship between ADHD and BPD seems well justified. In contrast to the previous section, here we review the literature chronologically. Again we have to take into account several methodological problems when interpreting the results. Ways of recruitment and inclusion of subjects and controls, small sample sizes, and the definitional vagaries that were already discussed have to be kept in mind.

Research on ADHD symptomatology and BPD started in the early 1980s. Andrulonis and co-workers identified three distinct subtypes of BPD in a group of 106 hospitalized adult borderline patients: those with no history of organicity; those with a history of trauma, encephalitis, or epilepsy; and those with a history of attention deficits or learning disabilities. They reported a considerable overlap (about 25%) between the latter two subtypes and minimal brain dysfunction (a term that was abandoned in 1980 when ADD was introduced in the *DSM*, with a considerable conceptual overlap between MBD and ADD). The patients with minimal brain dysfunction consisted mainly of males with early developmental difficulties. They were characterized by aggressive and hyperactive behavior, academic difficulties during childhood, and antisocial acting out with drug/alcohol abuse during adolescence (Andrulonis et al., 1981, 1982). These studies showed that a significant subgroup of borderline patients have a "spectrum" disorder on an organic brain dysfunction continuum, which includes symptoms that have later been referred to the ADHD domain.

At least a decade later, looking for antecedents of personality disorders in childhood, Rey and co-workers examined continuities between Axis I disorders in adolescents and personality disorders in young adults. They found that the adolescents with disruptive disorders were more likely at follow-up to have a personality disorder on the dramatic/impulsive cluster, which includes both BPD and ASPD, than those

with emotional disorders. All disruptive disorders were associated with a wide range of personality psychopathology in adulthood. Specific associations were found between CD and ASPD and between ADHD (with hyperactivity) and BPD. The authors suggested that disruptive disorders in childhood might be reconceptualized as disorders of personality rather than as Axis I diagnoses (Rey et al., 1995). Thus the studies of both Andrulonis and Rey attempted to put BPD into a developmental context and suggested a significant relationship between ADHD features and BPD.

Fossati and co-workers tried to overcome some limitations of these pioneer studies by evaluating the presence of specific associations between retrospectively assessed childhood ADHD symptoms and adult BPD in a controlled design. They administered the Wender Utah Rating Scale (WURS), a self-report instrument, to 42 consecutive BPD subjects and four control groups: admitted subjects (1) with any cluster B personality disorder diagnosis, (2) with any cluster A or cluster C personality disorder diagnosis, (3) with no personality disorder diagnosis, and (4) nonclinical volunteers. This study showed a significant relationship between the presence and severity of childhood ADHD symptoms and adult BPD. No less than 60% of the BPD subjects had probably met criteria for ADHD in childhood, even after controlling for ASPD (Fossati et al., 2002). Such figures have to be interpreted as suggesting the etiological heterogeneity of both disorders, and it remains unclear which characteristics are specifically related, possibly expressing the same underlying susceptibility, and which are not.

The specificity of clinical ADHD characteristics in adults with BPD has also been investigated using the self-report Attention Deficit Scale for Adults (ADSA). The statements in the ADSA relate to a wider range of characteristics than those found in the *DSM-IV*, including mood lability, temper, disorganization, and impulsivity. Dowson and co-workers showed that seven of the nine scales of the ADSA discriminated between ADHD and BPD, despite the overlap of clinical features involved in the two syndromes. The seven scales showing significant intergroup differences involved attention, organization, and persistence. Impaired task and goal persistence were the main discriminators between those with ADHD and those with BPD, with the ADHD group being the more impaired. Nonsignificant differences were found for two scales that were related to impatience, examples of aggression, taking undue risks, and failure to take the likely results of actions into account (Dowson et al., 2004). These findings seem to be in line with earlier results, but they also provide some indication that symptoms referring to the inattention domain of ADHD are to be specially considered in the relationship between ADHD and BPD. A limitation of this study may be that ADHD was not excluded from the BPD group nor was BPD excluded from the ADHD group.

In contrast to these studies, Kooij and co-authors used semi-structured clinical interviews in the assessment procedure in their study on the relationship between ADHD and coexisting BPD and ASPD. Their results showed that, among 53 referred ADHD patients, 11% presented with a subthreshold diagnosis and only 4% with a full BPD diagnosis. The most frequent symptom overlap was found for affective instability and inappropriate anger, symptoms that have been identified as ADHD-associated features (Kooij et al., unpublished data). The authors explained the difference between the prevalence of subthreshold and full diagnostic occurrence of BPD by the use of a clinical interview to establish the ADHD diagnosis, a more restrictive scoring system than relying on self-report scores only.

Data from ongoing research on the relationship between adult ADHD (i.e. meeting ADHD criteria in childhood as well as in adulthood, also using semi-structured clinical interviews) and BPD in 103 clinically referred female adults showed that 33% of a group of 63 patients with BPD also have ADHD and that 15% of 40 adult ADHD female patients also meet criteria for BPD (Van Dijk et al., unpublished data). Trying to further clarify the relationship between ADHD and BPD, the investigators used latent class analyses (LCA; McCutcheon, 1987) of the ADHD and BPD symptoms. LCA is a statistical technique that generates hypotheses and may thus supplement standard diagnostic categories. Four mutually exclusive classes of patients were identified: one with only ADHD symptoms; one with BPD symptoms and ADHD symptoms of hyperactivity; one with BPD symptoms and ADHD symptoms of inattention, hyperactivity, and impulsivity; and one with BPD symptoms and ADHD symptoms of inattention and hyperactivity. The hyperactive symptoms were relatively high across all classes, indicating that this is an unspecific symptom domain with poor differentiating value between ADHD and BPD. A transition model, associating the adult classes with retrospective childhood ADHD symptomatol-

ogy, showed, in addition to the expected associations between adult and childhood ADHD symptomatology, a remarkable probability that an outcome characterized by both ADHD and BPD symptoms in adulthood might be associated with a childhood without any significant ADHD symptomatology (i.e. subclinical hyperactivity), whereas an adult outcome with predominantly BPD symptoms could be traced back to combined ADHD symptoms in childhood. These data would fit a model in which the ADHD subtypes are not viewed as discrete categories that are permanent over time; they are also in line with the previously discussed findings of heterotypic diagnoses at adult follow-up in the longitudinal studies (Table 16.2) or in the Dunedin study, in which a follow-up at age 26 found formerly disruptive children across all adult diagnostic categories without the expected specificity (Kim-Cohen et al., 2003).

Although identifying a subgroup of patients with both ADHD and BPD may lead to an alternative, more beneficial treatment, research on the consequences of coexisting ADHD and borderline personality disorder is limited. Two case reports have shown possible subjective and neurocognitive benefits from a psychostimulant (methylphenidate) in two patients with BPD and ADHD (Hooberman & Stern, 1984; Van Reekum & Links, 1994). Schulz and co-workers used amphetamine to investigate the hypothesis that patients with BPD are prone to psychosis following ingestion of a dopamine agonist, but found that patients with a borderline diagnosis without comorbidity instead improved in their general clinical condition (Schulz et al., 1988). Considering the lack of research in this area, studies of pharmacotherapeutical alleviation of ADHD symptoms in patients presenting with personality disorders are urgently needed.

Dimensional personality traits

As we have seen, in the *DSM* system, personality disorders are recorded on a separate axis and, in accordance with the ICD system, are defined categorically. Both principles are controversial and disputed by most experts because empirical data lend no support for a delineation of personality disorders from other mental disorders or for a categorical structure of personality traits (Livesley, 2001). To overcome the limitations of the currently used diagnostic categories, Widiger has proposed that dimensional models of personality may be helpful in addressing problems of excessive co-occurrence, heterogeneity among persons with the same diagnosis, and artifactual or epiphenomenal diagnostic distinctions (Widiger, 2005). Categorical and dimensional perspectives on personality disorders may also be seen as complementary, and each offers valuable insights (Pickles & Angold, 2003).

A variety of alternative dimensional models have been proposed to replace the categorical *DSM-IV* personality disorders in future versions of the manual (for an overview see Widiger & Simonsen, 2005). However, there is still considerable debate about which dimensional system is most valid and useful (Verheul, 2005). In spite of the apparent discrepancies among the competing models for describing personality structure, they have remarkable convergence on a set of three to five basic personality dimensions. The five-factor model (FFM; Widiger & Costa, 1994) and the Temperament and Character Inventory (TCI; Cloninger, Swrakic, & Przybeck, 1993) are organized explicitly with respect to five and seven higher order factors, respectively, with each broad domain further differentiated into more specific facets or subscales. These two models are the ones used most frequently in studies on dimensional models in relation to ADHD in adults. In this section we review the studies regarding empirical associations between ADHD and several personality traits.

Cloninger's model

Cloninger's biopsychosocial theory of personality is based on the assumption that personality involves four temperament dimensions and three character dimensions. The dimensions of temperament measure individual differences in basic emotional drives and are Harm Avoidance (i.e., pessimistic and anxious versus optimistic and risk-taking), Novelty Seeking (i.e. impulsive and irritable versus rigid and stoical), Reward Dependence (i.e., sociable and warm versus aloof and cold), and Persistence (i.e. persevering and ambitious versus easily discouraged and lazy). The character dimensions measure individual differences in higher cognitive processes that define a person's style of mental self-government: the character traits are described as Self-Directedness (i.e., responsible and resourceful versus blaming and inept), Cooperativeness (i.e., helpful and principled versus hostile and opportunistic), and Self-Transcendence (i.e., intuitive and insightful versus concrete and conventional; Cloninger, 1987; Cloninger et al., 1993). A self-rating

instrument, the Temperament and Character Inventory (TCI; Cloninger et al., 1993), has been developed to measure the model's seven personality dimensions. *Presence* of a personality disorder is indicated by presence of character immaturity (especially by low Self-Directedness and/or Cooperativeness), whereas the *type* of disorder is decided by the temperament configuration (Cloninger, 2000; Svrakic et al., 1993).

A few studies have investigated the TCI profiles in subjects with ADHD. Downey and colleagues (1997) used the Tri Personality Questionnaire, a precursor to the TCI, and found that ADHD subjects scored significantly higher than normal subjects on the temperament scales of Novelty Seeking and Harm Avoidance. A more recent study (Lynn et al., 2005) tested the hypothesis that Novelty Seeking and ADHD are associated and that their association is due, in part, to DNA variability at the DRD4 gene. When interpreting their results, it is important to keep in mind that the subjects in the study were parents of ADHD-affected sib pairs. Not all of them had current ADHD or a lifetime history of ADHD, and it is possible that the results cannot be generalized to other adults with ADHD. The results partly confirmed the findings of Downey and co-workers, identifying a strong role for Novelty Seeking as a predictive factor for ADHD diagnostic status. However, this association was not accounted for by the presence of a risk allele at DRD4. Consequently, it remains impossible to clarify whether Novelty Seeking increases the risk for ADHD or whether the presence of ADHD influences the development of a Novelty Seeking temperament or whether the two are merely different conceptualizations of a common phenomenon. The authors also reported the divergent finding that the temperament scale of Self-Transcendence was actually associated more strongly with ADHD than was Harm Avoidance. Further, they identified a significant role for the character dimension Cooperativeness, consistent with the notion that ADHD symptoms in childhood may hamper the maturation of character.

Another clinical study used the TCI to describe personality development and disorders in relation to ADHD symptomatology and autism spectrum disorders (ASD) among 240 subjects with neuropsychiatric disorders (of whom 147 had ADHD; Anckarsater et al., 2006). The assumption was that childhood-onset neuropsychiatric disorders would be reflected as "difficult temperaments," deficits in character maturation, and personality disorders. The self-rated personality traits in the sample differed dramatically from those reported by subjects in the general population. Extremely low scores for Self-Directedness and Cooperativeness were recorded among subjects with neuropsychiatric disorders, again consistent with the notion that these early problems form obstacles to character maturity. In addition, ADHD was specifically associated with high Novelty Seeking and high Harm Avoidance.

As these studies did not assess personality structure in subgroups of subjects with ADHD but without personality disorders, it is difficult to pin specific personality profiles to ADHD in itself. The cited ongoing study by Van Dijk and co-workers using latent class analyses (McCutcheon, 1987) on the relationship between female adult ADHD and BPD examined TCI profiles for the four latent classes of ADHD and BPD symptoms. In this study, High Novelty Seeking was found in all classes except for the class with symptoms of BPD and only the hyperactivity aspect of ADHD. The highest Novelty Seeking temperament scores were found in the class of patients with both symptoms of BPD and symptoms in all areas of ADHD. High Harm Avoidance, low Cooperativeness, and low Self-Directedness were specifically related to classes containing BPD symptoms.

An outspoken Novelty Seeking temperament suggests a vulnerability for the development of ADHD and co-occurring BPD. Contrary to patients with combined ADHD and BPD symptoms, patients with ADHD symptoms alone show normal character development.

The Five-Factor Model

The "Big Five" represents the hierarchical organization of five major dimensions of normal adult personality and provides the most widely accepted description of higher order personality traits. The five-factor model (FFM) includes the dimensions of Neuroticism, Extraversion, Openness to Experience, Conscientiousness, and Agreeableness. Each of these domains is composed of six subfactors called facets (Costa & McCrae, 1992). As in the case with Cloninger's temperament and character dimensions, only a few studies have investigated associations between the Big Five personality dimensions and ADHD.

Braaten and Rosen (1997) found that elevated self-reported *DSM-III-R* ADHD symptoms in undergraduates correlated with high Extraversion and high Neu-

roticism. The limitation here was the use of college students and assessment based on self-reports only. Nigg and co-authors (Nigg, John, et al., 2002) subsequently obtained larger and more diverse samples for the investigation of personality traits and ADHD symptoms. They used three ADHD self-report instruments, trying to overcome the limitation that the findings would be attributable to one particular approach of assessing ADHD, as well as the NEO Five Factor Inventory (NEO FFI). They found that ADHD symptoms were consistently related to low Conscientiousness, low Agreeableness, and high Neuroticism. However, these correlations did not fully explain the variation in ADHD symptoms. The data showed that attention problems were related primarily to low Conscientiousness and high Neuroticism, and hyperactivity-impulsivity was related to low Agreeableness. This study found no reliable association with ADHD for Extraversion or Openness (Nigg, John, et al., 2002).

Another study addressing the relationship of ADHD symptoms with the FFM came from Canada (Parker, Majeski, & Collin, 2004). This study used the Conners' Adult ADHD Rating Scale (CAARS) and the NEO-FFI in a sample comprised of psychology students. They used *DSM-IV* cut-off scores to categorize three groups: the inattentive ADHD type, the hyperactive-impulsive ADHD type, and non-ADHD controls. Contrary to the study of Nigg and co-workers, but in line with the work of Braaten and Rosen, the Canada study found consistent associations between high Extraversion and the hyperactive-impulsive ADHD symptoms, whereas inattentive symptoms were not related to this personality dimension. High neuroticism was instead found to be a significant predictor of both inattention and hyperactivity-impulsivity symptomatology, and again, just as in the study by Nigg and co-workers, the most powerful predictor for inattention scores was low Conscientiousness, and for hyperactivity-impulsivity it was low Agreeableness. Both personality dimensions were also significant predictors for the other symptom group and for total ADHD scores.

Even considering that these studies relied on self-reported ADHD symptom ratings, their findings nevertheless suggest substantial associations between ADHD symptoms and four of the Big Five personality dimensions: high Neuroticism, high Extraversion, low Conscientiousness, and low Agreeableness. However, Openness appeared not to be related to ADHD symptomatology. The results from research using the FFM overall seem less consistent and less specific than the TCI results that associated ADHD with high Novelty Seeking and, when there was also a personality disorder, with character immaturity.

Neurocognitive and brain domains

Its clinical presentation has suggested that ADHD is a neuropsychological disorder, and attention and executive functions have become the focus of most theories concerning its aetiological basis (Seidman et al., 2004). Both ASPD and BPD also contain domains of emotional aberrations. Deficits in theory of mind – the cognitive end result of both social understanding and emotional understanding – have been shown across these categorical definitions (Sodian, Hulsken, & Thoermer, 2003). However, the differentiation of ADHD and associated disorders on the neuropsychological level has proved much more difficult than first expected (Nigg, 2000), and many a simplified model has failed to conform to empirical data when put to the test. The executive and motivation systems of the brain may well be involved in ADHD just as in various personality traits (Nigg, Butler, et al., 2002). Executive functions have also been found to be less specific on the neuropsychological level than first assumed and seem to develop in close connection with empathy and emotional processing (Pacherie, 1997; Perner, 1998), possibly because self-restraint also boosts comprehension of others and emotional reactivity and processing are necessary elements of self-restraint. Empathy is a highly complex function based on nonlinear interactions among theory of mind, emotional mirroring, executive functions, and situational determinants (Anckarsäter & Cloninger, 2007). It is therefore obvious that prior designations of specific brain systems thought to be involved in either social functioning (especially the limbic circuitry) or executive functions (especially the prefrontal cortex) have to be reinterpreted in a wide "social brain," encompassing interactions among widely disparate systems.

Analogously, most attention in the psychiatric context has been given to the systems using monoamines as neurotransmitters, and there is indeed every reason to assume that monoamines are of central importance: almost all major psychopharmaceuticals have been shown to exert their effects through modulations of these systems. The complex phenotypes we have approached in this chapter, however, probably relate to many other transmitter systems; for example, modifications of dopamine activity may only be hoped to modify some very specific parts of the problem constellations. In contrast, it is obvious that the pharmacological angle in longitudinal research is weak and that drug response may form a key to disentangling complex phenotypes. Preliminary evidence has also implied a shared genetic origin for executive functions and personality disorders or associated features (Coolidge, Thede, & Jang, 2004).

The early "effortful control" (regulation) system in young children is thought to involve the same neural system as the executive processes related to ADHD, combined type. A critical role of this system in the developing personality is reflected in research showing that effortful control is positively related to the development of conscience and negatively to the expression of aggression (Kochanska, Murray, & Coy, 1997; Rothbart & Ahadi, 1994). The definition of temperament as individual differences in constitutionally based (emotional, motor, and attentional) reactivity and self-regulation ("effortful control") may allow us to consider both the initial state of individual differences and the early development of emotional and attentional systems (Rothbart, 2004). Multiple pathways in early development related to distinct kinds of temperamental or cognitive vulnerability might form the basis for phenotypical definitions, dimensional or categorical depending on the research models they are applied in, but clearly defined in relation to specific contexts, developmental stages, and challenges such as stimuli or tasks.

Ultimately, the pathways between early temperament and future personality (and possible psychopathology) are likely to be complex and nonlinear, because children's development unfolds on the basis of partially genetic constitutional factors through the context of social relationships, cognition, and experience. Both continuity and change must eventually be understood in such contexts (Rothbart, 2004), and it will be necessary for future research to account for all these aspects to arrive at a better understanding of the role of early neurodevelopmental variants in shaping adult personality.

Summary and conclusion

In this chapter we have dealt with complex concepts and issues concerning the relation of ADHD to personality disorders and traits. We make no pretense at completeness, but we hope to have contributed to the discussion aiming at a better understanding of ADHD in relation to personality.

Based on this literature review, we would like to propose the following distinctions as providing a plain account of the risk for ASPD and criminality carried by ADHD. Early-onset disruptive behavior disorder (corresponding to the combination of ADHD, ODD, and CD, or hyperkinetic conduct disorder) carries a sharply increased risk for later ASPD and aggressive criminality. The adult personality disorder consists of destructive behavior patterns generally accompanied by deficient or aberrant emotional processing of thought and reactions. This concept contains most of the variation in what has been called "psychopathy," which because of its moral connotations is an unsuitable term in clinical practice. The ADHD-CD-ASPD disorder is associated with an increased risk both for "hands-on" criminal acts and the remaining unique factor of psychopathy (referred to as the first factor of the PCL-R); that is, the wicked way of seeking dominance over others through manipulation and deceit. It remains an open question whether such undesired behavioral consequences should be dealt with as mental disorders. Thorough clinical diagnoses of the problem constellation in a developmental perspective are always warranted, not least as a large proportion of children with early-onset disruptive behaviors also have attention and learning problems, other forms of social interaction and communication problems that sometimes correspond to the autism spectrum definitions, and a wide range of psychiatric coexisting problems. The clinical assessment forms the basis for possible treatment strategies. In the absence of early-onset conduct problems, ADHD per se, inattentive or combined type, has not been linked to an increased risk for an adult antisocial development, and late-onset (adolescent) conduct problems do not share the same developmental basis or associations to other problem types as the early-onset form nor its grave prognosis.

With regard to associations between ADHD and BPD, systematic data are meager. Overall, the reviewed studies mainly show symptom overlap between ADHD and BPD in the disruptive hyperactivity-impulsivity domain, whereas inattention characteristics are likely to differentiate among the problem types. More, as well as more diverse, research is needed to better understand the relationship between ADHD and BPD, to clearly unravel their shared characteristics, to propose

possible pathways leading to a BPD outcome, and to improve the understanding of possible truly unique aspects of the categories.

Then, we discussed ADHD in relation to personality traits, as defined by the Big Five and Cloninger's temperament and character model. ADHD as a clinical disorder seems to express an extreme end of extroversion or novelty seeking, with possible hampered character development or decreased conscientiousness. Harm avoidance may interact in creating the risk for BPD among subjects with ADHD. However, because few studies included subgroups with ADHD in which adult personality disorders had been controlled for, it is difficult to draw specific conclusions on the delineations and overlap among ADHD, personality disorders, and personality traits.

Finally, we pointed out the critical role of early regulation and reactivity systems in the development of temperamental or cognitive vulnerability. In closing this chapter, we again want to stress the importance of the integration of theories on psychopathology, temperament, and cognition, which represents a promising future line of research.

Acknowledgments

Agneta Brimse and Monika Montell are gratefully acknowledged for their expert secretarial assistance. The study of longitudinal studies was carried out in close collaboration with Björn Hofvander and Daniel Ossowski.

References

American Psychiatric Association. (1980). *Diagnostic and statistical manual of mental disorders*. 3rd ed. Washington DC: American Psychiatric Association.

American Psychiatric Association. (1987). *Diagnostic and statistical manual of mental disorders*. 3rd ed. rev. Washington DC: American Psychiatric Association.

American Psychiatric Association. (1994). *Diagnostic and Statistical manual of mental disorders*. 4th ed. Washington DC: American Psychiatric Association.

Anckarsäter H, Cloninger CR. (2007). The genetics of empathy. In: Farrow T, Woodruff P, eds. *Empathy in Mental Illness and Health*. New York: Cambridge University Press: 261–88.

Anckarsäter H, Stahlberg O, Larson T, Hakansson C, Jutblad SB, Niklasson L, et al. (2006). The impact of ADHD and autism spectrum disorders on temperament, character, and personality development. *Am J Psychiatry* 163:1239–44.

Andrulonis PA, Glueck BC, Stroebel CF, Vogel NG. (1982). Borderline personality subcategories. *J Nerv Ment Dis* **170**:670–9.

Andrulonis PA, Glueck BC, Stroebel CF, Vogel NG, Shapiro AL, Aldridge DM. (1981). Organic brain dysfunction and the borderline syndrome. *Psychiatr Clin North Am* **4**:47–66.

Babinski LM, Hartsough CS, Lambert NM. (1999). Childhood conduct problems, hyperactivity-impulsivity, and inattention as predictors of adult criminal activity. *J Child Psychol Psychiatry* **40**:347–55.

Barkley RA, Fischer M, Smallish L, Fletcher K. (2004). Young adult follow-up of hyperactive children: antisocial activities and drug use. *J Child Psychol Psychiatry* **45**:195–211.

Bergman LR, Magnusson D. (1986). Type A behavior: a longitudinal study from childhood to adulthood 20. *Psychosom Med* **48**:134–42.

Biederman J, Faraone SV, Keenan K, Benjamin J, Krifcher B, Moore C, et al. (1992). Further evidence for family-genetic risk factors in attention deficit hyperactivity disorder. Patterns of comorbidity in probands and relatives psychiatrically and pediatrically referred samples. *Arch Gen Psychiatry* **49**:728–38.

Biederman J, Faraone SV, Milberger S, Jetton JG, Chen L, Mick E, et al. (1996). Is childhood oppositional defiant disorder a precursor to adolescent conduct disorder? Findings from a four-year follow-up study of children with ADHD. *J Am Acad Child Adolesc Psychiatry* **35**:1193–1204.

Biederman J, Mick E, Faraone SV, Burback M. (2001). Patterns of remission and symptom decline in conduct disorder: a four-year prospective study of an ADHD sample. *J Am Acad Child Adolesc Psychiatry* **40**:290–8.

Burt SA. (2009). Are there meaningful etiological differences within antisocial behavior? Results of a meta-analysis. *Clin Psychol Rev* **29**(2):163–78.

Caspi A, Harrington H, Milne B, Amell JW, Theodore RF, Moffitt TE. (2003). Children's behavioral styles at age 3 are linked to their adult personality traits at age 26. *J Pers* **71**:495–513.

Cleckley HM. (1951). The mask of sanity. *Postgrad. Med* **9**:193–7.

Cloninger CR. (1987). A systematic method for clinical description and classification of personality variants. A proposal. *Arch Gen Psychiatry* **44**:573–88.

Cloninger CR. (2000). A practical way to diagnosis personality disorder: a proposal. *J Pers Disord* **14**:99–108.

Cloninger CR, Svrakic DM, Przybeck TR. (1993). A psychobiological model of temperament and character. *Arch Gen Psychiatry* **50**:975–90.

Cooke DJ, Michie C. (2001). Refining the construct of psychopathy: towards a hierarchical model. *Psychol Assess* **13**:171–88.

Coolidge FL, Thede LL, Jang KL. (2004). Are personality disorders psychological manifestations of executive function deficits? Bivariate heritability evidence from a twin study. *Behav Genet* **34**:75–84.

Costa PT, Jr, McCrae RR. (1992). *The Revised NEO Personality Inventory (NEO-PI-R) and NEO Five-Factor Inventory (NEO-FFI) Professional Manual*. Odessa, FL: Psychological Assessment Resources.

Downey KK, Stelson FW, Pomerleau OF, Giordani B. (1997). Adult attention deficit hyperactivity disorder: psychological test profiles in a clinical population. *J Nerv Ment Dis* **185**:32–8.

Dowson JH, McLean A, Bazanis E, Toone B, Young S, Robbins TW, et al. (2004). The specificity of clinical characteristics in adults with attention-deficit/hyperactivity disorder: a comparison with patients with borderline personality disorder. *Eur Psychiatry* **19**:72–8.

Faraone SV. (2005). The scientific foundation for understanding attention-deficit/hyperactivity disorder as a valid psychiatric disorder. *Eur Child Adolesc Psychiatry* **14**:1–10.

Farrington DP. (2000). Psychosocial predictors of adult antisocial personality and adult convictions. *Behav Sci Law* **18**:605–22.

Fischer M, Barkley RA, Smallish L, Fletcher K. (2002). Young adult follow-up of hyperactive children: self-reported psychiatric disorders, comorbidity, and the role of childhood conduct problems and teen CD. *J Abnorm Child Psychol* **30**:463–75.

Fossati A, Novella L, Donati D, Donini M, Maffei C. (2002). History of childhood attention deficit/hyperactivity disorder symptoms and borderline personality disorder: a controlled study. *Compr Psychiatry* **43**:369–77.

Frisell T, Lichtenstein P, Långström N. (2010). Violent crime runs in families: a total population study of 12.5 million individuals. *Psychol Med* **25**:1–9.

Gittelman R, Mannuzza S, Shenker R, Bonagura N. (1985) Hyperactive boys almost grown up. *Arch Gen Psychiatry* **42**:937–47.

Goldman SJ, D'Angelo EJ, DeMaso DR. (1993). Psychopathology in the families of children and adolescents with borderline personality disorder. *Am J Psychiatry* **150**:1832–5.

Hare RD. (1980). A research scale for the assessment of psychopathy in criminal populations. *Pers Individ Diff* 1:111–19.

Hechtman L, Weiss, G. (1986). Controlled prospective fifteen year follow-up of hyperactives as adults: non-medical drug and alcohol use and anti-social behavior. *Can J Psychiatry* 31(6):557–67.

Herrero ME, Hechtman L, Weiss G. (1994). Antisocial disorders in hyperactive subjects from childhood to adulthood: predictive factors and characterization of subgroups. *Am J Orthopsychiatry* 64:510–21.

Hofvander B, Ossowski B, Lundström S, Anckarsäter H. (2009). Continuity of aggressive antisocial behavior from childhood to adulthood: the question of phenotype definition. *Int J Law Psychiatry* 32(4): 224–34.

Hooberman D, Stern TA. (1984). Treatment of attention deficit and borderline personality disorders with psychostimulants: case report. *J Clin Psychiatry* 45:441–2.

Kim-Cohen J, Arseneault L, Caspi A, Polo Thomás M, Taylor A, Moffitt TE. (2005). Validity of DSM-IV Conduct Disorder in $4\frac{1}{2}$-5-year-old children: a longitudinal epidemiological study. *Am J Psychiatry* 162:1108–17.

Kim-Cohen J, Caspi A, Moffitt TE, Harrington H, Milne BJ, Poulton R. (2003). Prior juvenile diagnoses in adults with mental disorder: developmental follow-back of a prospective-longitudinal cohort. *Arch Gen Psychiatry* 60:709–17.

Klinteberg B, Andersson T, Magnusson D, Stattin H. (1993). Hyperactive behavior in childhood as related to subsequent alcohol problems and violent offending: a longitudinal study of male subjects. *Pers Individ Diff* 15:381–8.

Kochanska G, Murray K, Coy KC. (1997). Inhibitory control as a contributor to conscience in childhood: from toddler to early school age. *Child Dev* 68:263–77.

Lahey BB, Loeber R. (1997). ADHD and antisocial behavior. In: Stoff DM, Breiling J, Maser JD, eds. *Handbook of Antisocial Behavior*. New York: Wiley & Sons: 243–54.

Lahey BB, Loeber R, Burke J, Rathouz PJ, McBurnett K. (2002). Waxing and waning in concert: dynamic comorbidity of conduct disorder with other disruptive and emotional problems over 7 years among clinic-referred boys. *J Abnorm Psychol* 111:556–67.

Lewinsohn PM, Rohde P, Seeley JR, Klein DN. (1997). Axis II psychopathology as a function of Axis I disorders in childhood and adolescence. *J Am Acad Child Adolesc Psychiatry* 36:1752–9.

Lilienfeld S, Waldman ID. (1990). The relation between childhood attention-deficit hyperactivity disorder and adult antisocial behavior re-examined: the problem of heterogeneity. *Clin Psychol* 10:699–725.

Livesley WJ. (2001). Commentary on reconceptualizing personality disorder categories using trait dimensions. *J Pers* 69:277–86.

Loeber R, Burke JD, Lahey BB. (2002). What are adolescent antecedents to antisocial personality disorder? *Crim Behav Ment Health* 12:24–36.

Loeber R, Farrington DP, Stouthamer-Loeber M, Moffitt TE, Caspi A. (1998). The development of male offending: key findings from the first decade of the Pittsburgh youth study. *Stud Crime Prevent*, 141–71

Loeber R, Green SM, Keenan K, Lahey BB. (1995). Which boys will fare worse? Early predictors of the onset of conduct disorder in a six-year longitudinal study. *J Am Acad Child Adolesc Psychiatry* 34:499–509.

Loeber R, Green SM, Lahey BB, Frick PJ, McBurnett K. (2000). Findings on disruptive behavior disorders from the first decade of the developmental trends study. *Clin Child Fam Psychol Rev* 3:37–60.

Lynam DR. (1996). Early identification of chronic offenders: who is the fledgling pyschopathy? *Psychol Bull* 120(2):209–34.

Lynn DE, Lubke G, Yang M, McCracken JT, McGough JJ, Ishii J, et al. (2005). Temperament and character profiles and the dopamine D4 receptor gene in ADHD. *Am J Psychiatry* 162:906–13.

Mannuzza S, Klein RG, Abikoff H, Moulton JL, III. (2004). Significance of childhood conduct problems to later development of conduct disorder among children with ADHD: a prospective follow-up study. *J Abnorm Child Psychol* 32:565–73.

Mannuzza S, Klein RG, Bessler A, Malloy P, LaPudala M. (1993). Adult outcome of hyperactive boys. Educational achievement, occupational rank, and psychiatric status. *Arch Gen Psychiatry* 50:565–76.

Mannuzza S, Klein RG, Bessler A, Malloy P, LaPudala M. (1998). Adult psychiatric status of hyperactive boys grown up. *Am J Psychiatry* 155:493–8.

Mannuzza S, Klein RG, Bonagura N, Malloy P, Giampino TL, Addalli KA. (1991). Hyperactive boys almost grown up. V. Replication of psychiatric status. *Arch Gen Psychiatry* 48:77–83.

McCutcheon AL. (1987). *Latent Class Analyses*. Newbury Park, CA: Sage.

McGough JJ, Barkley RA. (2004). Diagnostic controversies in adult attention deficit hyperactivity disorder. *Am J Psychiatry* 161:1948–56.

Moffitt TE, Caspi A. (2001). Childhood predictors differentiate life-course persistent and adolescence-limited antisocial pathways among males and females. *Dev Psychopathol* 13:355–75.

Moffitt TE, Caspi A, Harrington H, Milne BJ. (2002). Males on the life-course-persistent and adolescence-limited antisocial pathways: follow-up at age 26 years 12. *Dev Psychopathol* **14**:179–207.

Nadder TS, Rutter M, Silberg JL, Maes HH, Eaves LJ. (2002). Genetic effects on the variation and covariation of attention deficit-hyperactivity disorder (ADHD) and oppositional-defiant disorder/conduct disorder (Odd/CD) symptomatologies across informant and occasion of measurement. *Psychol Med* **32**:39–53.

Nigg JT. (2000). On inhibition/disinhibition in developmental psychopathology: views from cognitive and personality psychology and a working inhibition taxonomy. *Psychol Bull* **126**:220–46.

Nigg JT, Blaskey LG, Huang-Pollock CL, Rappley MD. (2002). Neuropsychological executive functions and DSM-IV ADHD subtypes. *J Am Acad Child Adolesc Psychiatry* **4**:59–66.

Nigg JT, Butler KM, Huang-Pollock CL, Henderson JM. (2002). Inhibitory processes in adults with persistent childhood onset ADHD. *J Consult Clin Psychol* **70**:153–7.

Nigg JT, John OP, Blaskey LG, Huang-Pollock CL, Willcutt EG, Hinshaw SP, et al. (2002). Big five dimensions and ADHD symptoms: links between personality traits and clinical symptoms. *J Pers Soc Psychol* **83**:451–69.

Pacherie E. (1997). On being the product of one's failed actions. In: Russel J, ed. *Executive Difficulties in Autism*. Oxford: Oxford University Press: 215–55.

Parker JDA, Majeski SA, Collin VT. (2004). ADHD symptoms and personality: relationships with the five-factor model. *Pers Individ Diff* **36**:977–87.

Perner J. (1998) The meta-intentional nature of executive functions and theory of mind. In: Carruthers P, Boucher J, eds. *Language and Thought: Interdisciplinary Themes*. Cambridge: Cambridge University Press: 270–83.

Pickles A, Angold A. (2003). Natural categories or fundamental dimensions: on carving nature at the joints and the rearticulation of psychopathology 3. *Dev Psychopathol* **15**:529–51.

Rassmussen P, Gillberg C. (2000). Natural outcome of ADHD with developmental coordination disorder at age 22 years: A controlled, longitudinal, community-based study. *J Am Acad Child Adolescent Psychiatry* **39**(11):1424–31.

Rey JM, Morris-Yates A, Singh M, Andrews G, Stewart GW. (1995). Continuities between psychiatric disorders in adolescents and personality disorders in young adults. *Am J Psychiatry* **152**:895–900.

Rhee SH, Willcutt EG, Hartman CA, Pennington BF, DeFries JC. (2008) Test of alternative hypotheses explaining the comorbidity between Attention-Deficit/Hyperactivity Disorder and Conduct Disorder. *J Abnorm Child Psychol* **36**:29–40.

Robbins, LN, Rutter M. (1990). *Straight and Devious Pathways from Childhood to Adulthood*. Cambridge: Cambridge University Press.

Rothbart MK. (2004). Commentary: differentiated measures of temperament and multiple pathways to childhood disorders. *J Clin Child Adolesc Psychol* **33**:82–7.

Rothbart MK, Ahadi SA. (1994). Temperament and the development of personality. *J Abnorm Psychol* **103**:55–66.

Sanislow CA, Grilo CM, McGlashan TH. (2000). Factor analysis of the DSM-III-R borderline personality disorder criteria in psychiatric inpatients. *Am J Psychiatry* **157**:1629–33.

Satterfield JH, Hoppe CM, Schell, AM. (1982). A prospective study of delinquency in 110 adolescent boys with Attention Deficit Disorder and 88 normal adolescent boys. *Am J Psychiatry* **139**:795–8.

Satterfield JH, Schell A. (1997). A prospective study of hyperactive boys with conduct problems and normal boys: adolescent and adult criminality. *J Am Acad Child Adolesc Psychiatry* **36**:1726–35.

Schulz SC, Cornelius J, Schulz PM, Soloff PH. (1988). The amphetamine challenge test in patients with borderline disorder. *Am J Psychiatry* **145**:809–14.

Seidman LJ, Doyle A, Fried R, Valera E, Crum K, Matthews L. (2004). Neuropsychological function in adults with attention-deficit/hyperactivity disorder. *Psychiatr Clin North Am* **27**:261–82.

Silberg J, Rutter M, Meyer J, Maes H, Hewitt J, Simonoff E, et al. (1996). Genetic and environmental influences on the covariation between hyperactivity and conduct disturbance in juvenile twins. *J Child Psychol Psychiatry* **37**:803–16.

Soderstrom H, Nilsson T, Sjodin AK, Carlstedt A, Forsman A. (2005). The childhood-onset neuropsychiatric background to adulthood psychopathic traits and personality disorders. *Compr Psychiatry* **46**:111–16.

Svrakic DM, Whitehead C, Przybeck TR, Cloninger CR. (1993). Differential diagnosis of personality disorders by the seven-factor model of temperament and character. *Arch Gen Psychiatry* **50**:991–9.

Torgersen S, Kringlen E, Cramer V. (2001). The prevalence of personality disorders in a community sample. *Arch Gen Psychiatry* **58**:590–6.

Van Reekum R, Links PS. (1994). N of 1 study: methylphenidate in a patient with borderline personality disorder and attention deficit hyperactivity disorder. *Can J Psychiatry* **39**:186–7.

189

Verheul R. (2005). Clinical utility of dimensional models for personality pathology. *J Pers Disord* 19: 283–302.

Weiss G, Hechtman L, Milroy T, Perlman T. (1985). Psychiatric status of hyperactives as adults: a controlled prospective 15-year follow-up of 63 hyperactive children. *J Am Acad Child Psychiatry* 24: 211–20.

Widiger TA, Costa PT, Jr. (1994). Personality and personality disorders. *J Abnorm Psychol* 103:78–91.

Widiger TA, Simonsen E. (2005). Alternative dimensional models of personality disorder: finding a common ground. *J Pers Disord* 19:110–30.

World Health Organization (WHO). (1990). *ICD-10 – International Statistical Classification of Diseases and Related Health Problems*. Geneva: WHO.

Chapter

17

Stimulant treatment of adult ADHD

Thomas Spencer and Joseph Biederman

Introduction

Adult attention-deficit hyperactivity disorder (ADHD) has been increasingly recognized in the clinical and scientific literature as a valid clinical entity (Spencer et al., 1994). Data from family aggregation, genetics, treatment response, neuropsychology, and neuroimaging studies provide compelling evidence of its neurobiological underpinnings and its syndromatic continuity with its pediatric counterpart.

Estimates of the prevalence of ADHD in adults have been based on a prevalence rate of ADHD children of 5–10% (Faraone et al., 2003) and an estimated persistence rate of 50 to 60% into adulthood (Biederman et al., 2000), which suggest that ADHD may afflict as many as 2–4% of adults. A recent replication of the National Comorbidity Study estimated the prevalence of adult ADHD among persons aged 18–44 in the US to be 4.4% (Kessler et al., 2006).

Methylphenidate

Although methylphenidate (MPH) remains the mainstay of treatment for ADHD, there are only a few controlled studies assessing its efficacy in adults with ADHD. An early literature on the subject documented equivocal responses to MPH in adults with ADHD, but these studies had methodological limitations including the use of nonstandard diagnostic methods and low daily doses of MPH (Gualtieri, Ondrusek, & Finley, 1985; Mattes, Boswell, & Oliver, 1984; Wender et al., 1985; Wood et al., 1976). For example, one of the earlier studies did not require a clear history of childhood-onset symptoms of ADHD (Wood et al., 1976), and others employed adult diagnostic criteria substantially different from those later established in DSM-III, DSM-III-R, and DSM-IV (Gualtieri et al., 1985; Mattes et al., 1984; Wender et al., 1985; Wood

et al., 1976). These criteria included symptoms of anxiety, mood, and personality disorders (e.g. affective lability, hot or explosive temper, and stress intolerance), which are now not considered to be specific to ADHD (American Psychiatric Association, 1994).

Pilot MGH methylphenidate study

To address these issues we undertook a pilot randomized, double-blind placebo-controlled clinical trial of immediate-release (IR) MPH in the treatment of 23 adults with ADHD (Spencer et al., 1995). This study used DSM-based instruments and rating scales and daily doses of MPH of 1 mg/kg/day in three divided doses, consistent with daily doses used in the pediatric literature. This study reported a robust response to MPH in adults with ADHD, which was 50% better than the findings reported in earlier studies (Wender et al., 1985) that used a much lower daily dose of MPH (average 0.6 mg/kg/day).

Because of its small sample size, our pilot study could not assess differential responses by gender, psychiatric comorbidity, or social class and could not fully assess safety and tolerability, a particularly important issue considering the robust doses used. It also relied on a crossover design, which may not be ideal to fully evaluate efficacy considering potential carryover effects. Although encouraging, our initial positive findings required confirmation from a larger, better powered parallel study using comprehensive assessments of efficacy and safety.

NIMH MGH methylphenidate study

A larger MGH study sought to address the limitations noted earlier so as to more fully assess the efficacy and safety of MPH treatment for ADHD in adulthood (Spencer et al., 2005). To do so, we recruited a

ADHD in Adults: Characterization, Diagnosis and Treatment, ed. Jan Buitelaar, Cornelis Kan and Philip Asherson.
Published by Cambridge University Press. © Cambridge University Press 2011.

large sample of adults with all subtypes of ADHD into a parallel-design protocol that included a broad range of assessments for safety and efficacy. Our main goals were to measure precisely the degree of therapeutic response and to assess safety and tolerability. Based on our previous work, we hypothesized that (1) ADHD symptoms in adults with *DSM-IV* ADHD would be responsive to optimal doses of MPH treatment (TID dosing up to 1.3 mg/kg/day); (2) neither gender, psychiatric comorbidity, nor social class would significantly affect treatment response; and (3) treatment with a higher dose of MPH than used in children would be safe and well tolerated by adults. To our knowledge, this study is the largest and most comprehensive assessment of the safety and efficacy of IR MPH in the treatment of adults with ADHD.

We recruited 146 outpatient adults with ADHD between 19 and 60 years of age. Subjects had to satisfy full diagnostic criteria for *DSM-IV* ADHD based on clinical assessment and confirmed by structured diagnostic interview. We excluded potential subjects if they had clinically unstable psychiatric conditions (i.e., bipolar disorder, psychosis, suicidality) or drug or alcohol abuse or dependence within the 6 months preceding the study; undergone a previous adequate trial of stimulant; or currently used other psychotropics.

This was a double-blind, randomized, 6-week, placebo-controlled, parallel-design study of MPH in the treatment of adult ADHD. Medication (or placebo) was prescribed under double-blind conditions in TID dosing (7:30 am, noon, and 5 pm). Study medication was titrated (forced titration) up to 0.5 mg/kg/day by week 1, 0.75 mg/kg/day by week 2, and 1.0 mg/kg/day by week 3, in TID dosing, unless adverse effects emerged. The dose was allowed to be increased to a maximum of 1.3 mg/kg by weeks 5 and 6 if efficacy was partial and treatment was well tolerated. Other psychoactive medications were not permitted during the protocol.

Of the 146 subjects enrolled in the study, 136 (93%) completed at least 2 weeks of treatment. Of those, 110 (81%) completed the full 6 weeks. The mean daily doses at week 6 were 82 $\pm$ 22 mg for MPH (1.1 $\pm$ 24 mg/kg). Under MPH treatment, ADHD symptom reduction was progressive over the 6 weeks of treatment. The MPH response attained statistical significance by the second week of treatment ($z = 3.3$, $p < 0.001$), with further improvement in ensuing weeks (z's > 4; p's < 0.001). The mean difference between MPH and placebo response constituted a 44% dif-

ference from baseline. The effect size of the difference between MPH and placebo (endpoint placebo – endpoint MPH/pooled endpoint standard deviation) was 1.41. Improvement in ADHD symptoms was equally robust for inattentive symptoms ($z = 7.2$, $p < 0.0001$) and hyperactive/impulsive symptoms ($z = 4.6$, $p < 0.0001$).

For analyses of outcome measures we included potential predictors of response as factors in random regression analyses. We found no significant associations between improvement of ADHD symptoms and gender, age, socioeconomic status, Global Assessment of Functioning (GAF) scores, or previous medication treatment. The GAF, a global measure of psychosocial functioning, was found to improve during the course of treatment ($z = 4.1$, $p < 0.0001$)

Of individual side effects reported, only MPH-associated appetite suppression, dry mouth, and mild moodiness reached our threshold for statistical significance. Weight decreased an average of 2.4 kg ($p < 0.001$) on MPH. However, weight loss was not of clinical significance in any patient.

No serious cardiovascular adverse effects were observed. However, small but statistically significant increases in pulse (7 bpm, $p < 0.001$), but not diastolic blood pressure (2 mmHg, $p < 0.06$) or systolic blood pressure (2 mmHg, $p = 0.10$) were associated with MPH treatment. In addition, the QTc interval increased slightly (0.007; week 6 vs. week 0, respectively, $p < 0.01$) in MPH patients compared with placebo. There were no statistically significant changes in the other conduction parameters (PR or QRS) on MPH. MPH levels did not correlate with dose or adverse effects or change in scores of depression and anxiety. However, MPH levels did correlate (trend) with a 30% decrease in ADHD symptoms ($z = 2.4$, $p < 0.05$).

In summary this large study of adults with ADHD demonstrated that robust MPH dosing significantly improved ADHD symptoms and functioning and was well tolerated. These results provide guidelines for the successful treatment of this condition and support for further studies of MPH using a wide range of doses over a long period of treatment.

European methylphenidate study

A European study was undertaken to test the efficacy and safety of methylphenidate in adults in an outpatient population (Kooij et al., 2004). This was a double-blind, placebo-controlled, randomized crossover trial in 45 adults with ADHD. Similar to the previously reported studies, methylphenidate was titrated from 0.5 mg/kg per day in week 1 up to 1.0 mg/kg per day in Week 3. Response rates on methylphenidate varied from 38–51% and on placebo from 7–18% depending on the outcome measure chosen. Although many subjects had side effects, those specific to methylphenidate were few and mild. The authors concluded that methylphenidate was effective and well tolerated for adults with ADHD in the short term.

Long-acting methylphenidate studies

MGH osmotic-release oral system (OROS) methylphenidate study

The objective of this study was to evaluate the safety and efficacy of once-daily osmotic-release oral system (OROS) methylphenidate in the treatment of adults with *DSM-IV* ADHD (Biederman et al., 2006). It used an identical methodology to that of the NIMH MGH methylphenidate study described earlier, replacing TID short-acting methylphenidate with once-a-day long-acting methylphenidate.

We conducted a randomized, 6-week, placebo-controlled, parallel-design study of OROS MPH in 141 adult subjects with *DSM-IV* ADHD, using standardized instruments for diagnosis. OROS MPH or placebo was initiated at 36 mg/day and titrated to optimal response, depending on efficacy and tolerability, up to 1.3 mg/kg/day. Treatment with OROS MPH was associated with clinically and statistically significant reductions in *DSM-IV* symptoms of inattention and hyperactivity-impulsivity relative to subjects treated with placebo. At endpoint, 66% of subjects (n = 44) receiving OROS MPH and 39% of subjects (n = 23) receiving placebo attained our a priori definition of response of much or very much improved on the Clinical Global Impression–Improvement scale. In addition, there was a ± 30% reduction in Adult ADHD Investigator System Report Scale scores in subjects receiving OROS MPH. OROS MPH was associated with small but statistically significant increases in systolic blood pressure (3.5 ± 11.8 mmHg), diastolic blood pressure (4.0–8.5 mmHg), and heart rate (4.5 ± 10.5 bpm). These results showed that treatment with OROS MPH in daily doses of up to 1.3 mg/kg/day was effective in the treatment of adults with ADHD. Because of the potential for increases in blood pres-

sure and heart rate, subjects receiving treatment with MPH should be monitored for changes in blood pressure parameters during treatment.

Utah OROS methylphenidate study

OROS methylphenidate is a long-acting stimulant demonstrated to be effective in the treatment of children and adolescents with ADHD. Forty-seven adults entered and 41 completed this double-blind, placebo-controlled, crossover trial of OROS methylphenidate (Reimherr et al., 2007). Each double-blind arm lasted 4 weeks. Subjects met both DSM-IV-TR and Utah Criteria for ADHD in adults. Outcome measures included the Wender-Reimherr Adult Attention Deficit Disorder Scale (WRAADDS), the adult ADHD-Rating Scale (ADHD-RS), and the Clinical Global Impressions-Improvement scale (CGI-I). At baseline, subjects were categorized as having significant emotional symptoms with the WRAADDS and/or significant oppositional-defiant symptoms using a self-report scale assessing *DSM-IV* criteria for oppositional-defiant disorder. Of the sample, 17% (N = 8) had ADHD alone, 38% (N = 18) had ADHD plus significant emotional symptoms, and 40% (N = 19) had ADHD with both significant emotional and oppositional symptoms. At a mean ± SD dose of 64.0 ± 23.3 (0.75 mg/kg), OROS methylphenidate proved superior to placebo for all clinical measures, resulting in a total WRAADDS score decrease of 42% versus 13%, respectively ($p < .001$); a total ADHD-RS score decrease of 41% versus 14%, respectively ($p = .003$); and decreases in the subscales addressing inattention, hyperactivity-impulsivity, and emotional dysregulation. OROS methylphenidate proved effective in treating adult ADHD. ADHD alone was relatively uncommon in this sample. Of note, more than 80% of the patients had ADHD with a combination of emotional and/or oppositional symptoms.

Focalin XR (dexmethylphenidate) Study

There is stereoselectivity in methylphenidate receptor site binding and its relationship to response. Moreover, recent data suggest that the d-methylphenidate isomer is the active form. This data have led to the development of a purified d threo-methylphenidate compound, Focalin®. A new extended-release dosage form of Focalin, Focalin XR®, has been developed to provide effective methylphenidate treatment for up to 12 hours. Focalin XR uses a bimodal release system, producing pharmacokinetic characteristics that, in single-dose administration, resemble those of two doses of Focalin tablets administered 4 to 5 hours apart. Focalin XR consists of a mixture of immediate- and delayed-release beads in a 50:50 ratio. The delayed release beads are coated with an absorption-delaying polymer.

Focalin XR was tested in a multicenter, randomized, fixed-dose, double-blind, placebo-controlled study in adults with ADHD (Spencer et al., 2006). Randomized adults with ADHD ($N = 221$) received once-daily d-MPH-ER 20 mg, 30 mg, or 40 mg or placebo for 5 weeks. The primary efficacy variable was change from baseline to the final visit in *DSM-IV* ADHD Rating Scale (RS) total score. Secondary efficacy parameters included the proportion of patients with improvement $\geq$30% in *DSM-IV* ADHD-RS total score, change from baseline in Inattention and Hyperactivity/Impulsivity subscale scores, and final scores on the CGI-I scale.

Of 218 evaluable patients, 184 completed the study. All d-MPH-ER doses were significantly superior to placebo in improving *DSM-IV* ADHD-RS total scores. Placebo scores improved by 7.9, in contrast to d-MPH-ER 20 mg by 13.7 ($p = .006$); 30 mg, 13.4 ($p = .012$); and 40 mg, 16.9 ($p < .001$). Improvements on the Inattentive subscale were placebo, 4.7; d-MPH-ER 20 mg, 7.7 ($p = .021$); 30 mg, 8.0 ($p = .011$); and 40 mg, 9.7 ($p < .001$). Respective improvements on the Hyperactive-Impulsive subscale were 3.2, 6.0 ($p = .005$), 5.4 ($p = .037$), and 7.2 ($p < .001$). The overall distribution of CGI-I ratings at the final visit was significantly better with each d-MPH-ER dosage than with placebo ($p = .004$, $p = .021$, $p < .001$, respectively). Safety and tolerability were as expected, based on experience with racemic MPH in adults and d-MPH in children. The authors concluded that once-daily d-MPH-ER at 20 mg, 30 mg, or 40 mg is a safe and effective treatment for adults with ADHD.

Subjects (170) in the acute trial were continued into a 6-month, open-label extension (OLE) phase. After 1 week, dosages were increased from 10 mg/d for 1 week to 20 to 40 mg/d (maintenance). Efficacy was assessed as change from baseline in ADHD Rating Scale total scores and the proportion of patients rated "very much improved" or "much improved" on the CGI-I scale. Mean changes from the end of the double-blind phase to the end of the OLE phase

in ADHD-RS total scores were −10.2 for patients switched from placebo to d-MPH-ER ($N = 20$) and −8.4 for those maintained on d-MPH-ER ($N = 82$; indicating improvement). Improvements were also observed from baseline to the end of the OLE phase, with mean changes of −22.3 and −25.9 for patients switched from placebo and those maintained on d-MPH-ER, respectively. At the end of the OLE phase, the proportion of patients who reported improvement based on CGI-I rates was 95.0% for patients switched from placebo to d-MPH-ER and 95.1% for those maintained on d-MPH-ER. D-MPH-ER was well tolerated. Most adverse events were mild to moderate. The most common (>15%) adverse events were headache, insomnia, and decreased appetite. Vital signs showed no clinically significant changes. Weight loss $\geq$7% was observed in 19.4% of patients. The authors concluded that once-daily d-MPH-ER 20 to 40 mg is safe and effective for the long-term treatment of ADHD in adult patients.

Amphetamine in adult ADHD

MGH pilot mixed amphetamine trial

We conducted a pilot study of an amphetamine in adult ADHD using the crossover design that we used in our initial pilot methylphenidate study described earlier (Spencer et al., 2001). This was a controlled trial of a mixed amphetamine salts compound (Adderall, dextroamphetamine sulfate, dextro-, levoamphetamine sulfate, dextro-, levoamphetamine aspartate, and dextroamphetamine saccharate) in the treatment of adult ADHD. It was a 7-week, randomized, double-blind, placebo-controlled, crossover study of Adderall in 27 well–characterized adults with ADHD. Medication was titrated up to 30 mg BID. Outcome measures included the ADHD Rating Scale and the Clinical Global Impression Score. Comorbid psychiatric disorders were assessed to test for potential effects on treatment outcome. Treatment with Adderall at an average oral dose of 54 mg (administered in two daily doses) was effective and well tolerated. Drug-specific improvement in ADHD symptoms was highly significant overall (42% decrease on the ADHD Rating Scale, $p < 0.001$) and sufficiently robust to be detectable in a parallel-groups comparison restricted to the first 3 weeks of the protocol ($p < 0.001$). The proportion of subjects who improved (reduction in the ADHD rating scale of $\geq$ 30%) was significantly higher with

Adderall treatment than with a placebo (70% vs. 7%; $p = 0.001$). We concluded that Adderall was effective and well tolerated in the short-term treatment of adults with ADHD.

Multisite mixed amphetamine trial

Based on our pilot results, a larger multisite trial was initiated of Adderall for adult ADHD (Weisler et al., 2004) This prospective, multisite, randomized, double-blind, placebo-controlled, parallel-group, dose-escalation study was conducted to assess the efficacy, safety, and duration of action of extended-release mixed amphetamine salts (MAS XR; Shire Pharmaceuticals Inc, Wayne, PA) in adults with ADHD, combined type. Two hundred fifty-five adults ≥18 years old were given placebo or MAS XR 20, 40, or 60 mg once daily for 4 weeks. The main outcome measures were the ADHD Rating Scale and Conners' Adult ADHD Rating Scale Short Version Self-Report (CAARS-S-S). MAS XR treatment was associated with statistically and clinically significant ADHD symptom reduction at the endpoint; mean ADHD Rating Scale scores were 18.5 for the 20-mg group ($p = .001$), 18.4 for the 40-mg group ($p < .001$), and 18.5 for the 60-mg group ($p < .001$). Adults with severe symptoms (ADHD Rating Scale score ≥32 at baseline) had significantly greater symptom reduction with the highest MAS XR dose (60 mg/day); however this dose-response relationship was determined by post hoc analysis. The mean MAS XR effect size was 0.8. Statistically significant ($p < .05$) improvements in CAARS-S-S ADHD index scores occurred at 4 and 12 hours post dose for all MAS XR groups, indicating a 12-hour duration of effect. Symptoms improved within the first treatment week. Most adverse events reported during this 4-week study were mild or moderate in intensity, and the most commonly reported adverse events were consistent with the known profile of stimulant medications. Vital signs and electrocardiograms showed no clinically significant cardiovascular changes. These results suggest that MAS XR is safe and effective in adults with ADHD and controlled ADHD symptoms for up to 12 hours.

Safety concerns

The US Food and Drug Administration (FDA) recently reviewed the prescribing information on stimulants in an effort to clarify their risks and benefits. After careful review, the only black box warning for stimulants

remains concerns over their abuse potential. Although misuse for treating fatigue can result from oral administration, abuse for euphoria typically requires insufflation, and thus there is greater risk in immediate-release formulations that can be crushed. Despite the concern that ADHD may increase the risk of abuse in adolescents and young adults (or their associates), to date there is no clear evidence that stimulant-treated ADHD children abuse prescribed medication when appropriately diagnosed and carefully monitored. Moreover, the most common abused substance in adolescents and adults with ADHD has been shown to be marijuana and not stimulants (Biederman et al., 1995). Furthermore, an additional report provides statistical evidence that the use of stimulants and other pharmacological treatments for ADHD significantly decreased the risk for subsequent substance use disorders in ADHD youth (Biederman et al., 1999).

Stimulant use has resulted in consistently documented mild increases in pulse and blood pressure of unclear clinical significance (Brown et al., 1984). Recent concerns about cardiovascular safety led to the temporary removal of Adderall-XR from the Canadian Market. In response the FDA issued the following statement:

The Canadian action was based on U.S. post-marketing reports of sudden deaths in pediatric patients. … When one considers the rate of sudden death in pediatric patients treated with Adderall products based on the approximately 30 million prescriptions written between 1999 and 2003 (the period of time in which these deaths occurred), it does not appear that the number of deaths reported is greater than the number of sudden deaths that would be expected to occur in this population without treatment. For this reason, the FDA has not decided to take any further regulatory action at this time (www.fda.gov/cder/drug/advisory/adderall.htm).

However, because it appeared that patients with underlying heart defects might be at increased risk for sudden death, the labeling for all stimulants was changed to include a warning that these patients might be at particular risk and should ordinarily not be treated with stimulants.

Although at this time there is limited concern about the general cardiovascular safety of psychostimulants, caution should be used in the treatment of patients presenting with a family history of early cardiac death or arrhythmias or a personal history of structural abnormalities, chest pain, palpitations, shortness of breath, or fainting episodes of unclear etiology, especially during exercise or during treatment with stimulants (Gutgesell et al., 1999). Before initiating treatment, patients should have a careful history to assess for the presence of preexisting cardiac disease. In such cases, consultation with a cardiologist is recommended. In addition, blood pressure and pulse should be monitored with stimulant treatment.

Conclusions

Although only recently recognized as a valid disorder in adults, the clinical picture of adult ADHD is highly reminiscent of childhood ADHD, with continued associated occupational failure and academic deficits. Similarly, many adults with ADHD suffer from antisocial, depressive, and anxiety disorders. Recent work clearly documents that, when therapeutic doses of MPH and amphetamine treatment are used in the treatment of adults with ADHD, they can lead to a robust clinical response that is highly consistent with that observed in pediatric studies using equipotent daily doses. As in childhood ADHD, medication remains a key component of treatment for adults with ADHD. More studies are needed to evaluate the efficacy and safety of stimulants over the long term and their impact on quality of life.

References

American Psychiatric Association. (1994). *Diagnostic and Statistical Manual of Mental Disorders*. 4th ed. Washington, DC: American Psychiatric Association

Biederman J, Faraone S, Mick E. (2000). Age dependent decline of ADHD symptoms revisited: Impact of remission definition and symptom subtype. *Am J Psychiatry* 157:816–17.

Biederman J, Mick E, Surman C, Doyle R, Hammerness P, Harpold T, et al. (2006). A randomized, placebo-controlled trial of OROS-methylphenidate in adults with attention-deficit/hyperactivity disorder. *Biol Psychiatry* 59:829–35.

Biederman J, Wilens T, Mick E, Milberger S, Spencer T, Faraone S. (1995). Psychoactive substance use disorder in adults with attention deficit hyperactivity disorder: effects of ADHD and psychiatric comorbidity. *Am J Psychiatry* 152:1652–8.

Biederman J, Wilens T, Mick E, Spencer T, Faraone SV. (1999). Pharmacotherapy of attention-deficit/ hyperactivity disorder reduces risk for substance use disorder. *Pediatrics* 104:e20.

Brown RT, Wynne ME, Slimmer LW. (1984). Attention deficit disorder and the effect of methylphenidate on attention, behavioral, and cardiovascular functioning. *J Clin Psychiatry* 45:473–6.

Faraone SV, Sergeant J, Gillberg C, Biederman J. (2003). The worldwide prevalence of ADHD: is it an American condition? *World Psychiatry* 2:104–13.

Gualtieri CT, Ondrusek MG, Finley C. (1985). Attention deficit disorders in adults. *Clin Neuropharmacol* 8:343–56.

Gutgesell H, Atkins D, Barst R, Buck M, Franklin W, Humes R, et al. (1999). Cardiovascular monitoring of children and adolescents receiving psychotropic drugs. *Circulation* 99:979–82.

Kessler RC, Adler L, Barkley R, Biederman J, Conners CK, Demler O, et al. (2006). The prevalence and correlates of adult ADHD in the United States: results from the National Comorbidity Survey Replication. *Am J Psychiatry* 163:716–23.

Kooij JJ, Burger H, Boonstra AM, Van Der Linden PD, Kalma LE, Buitelaar JK. (2004). Efficacy and safety of methylphenidate in 45 adults with attention-deficit/ hyperactivity disorder. A randomized placebo-controlled double-blind cross-over trial. *Psychol Med* 34:973–82.

Mattes JA, Boswell L, Oliver H. (1984). Methylphenidate effects on symptoms of attention deficit disorder in adults. *Arch Gen Psychiatry* 41:1059–63.

Reimherr FW, Williams ED, Strong RE, Mestas R, Soni P, Marchant BK. (2007). A double-blind, placebo-controlled, crossover study of osmotic release oral system methylphenidate in adults with ADHD with assessment of oppositional and emotional dimensions of the disorder. *J Clin Psychiatry* 68: 93–101.

Spencer TJ, Adler LA, McGough JJ, Muniz R, Jiang H, Pestreich L. (2006). Efficacy and safety of dexmethylphenidate extended-release capsules in adults with attention-deficit/hyperactivity disorder. *Biol Psychiatry* 61(12):1380–7.

Spencer T, Biederman J, Wilens T, Faraone S. (1994). Is attention deficit hyperactivity disorder in adults a valid disorder? *Harv Rev Psychiatry* 1:326–35.

Spencer T, Biederman J, Wilens T, Faraone SV, Doyle RD, Surman C, et al. (2005). A large, double-blind, randomized clinical trial of methylphenidate in the treatment of adults with attention-deficit/hyperactivity disorder. *Biol Psychiatry* 57:456–63.

Spencer T, Biederman J, Wilens T, Faraone S, Prince J, Gerard K, et al. (2001). Efficacy of a mixed amphetamine salts compound in adults with attention-deficit/hyperactivity disorder. *Arch Gen Psychiatry* 58:775–82.

Spencer T, Wilens T, Biederman J, Faraone SV, Ablon JS, Lapey K. (1995). A double-blind, crossover comparison of methylphenidate and placebo in adults with childhood-onset attention-deficit hyperactivity disorder. *Arch Gen Psychiatry* **52**:434–43.

Weisler R, Biederman J, Spencer TJ, et al. (2004). Mixed amphetamine salts extended release (Adderall XR®) in the treatment of adult attention-deficit/hyperactivity disorder: a randomized, controlled trial. Paper presented at: Annual Meeting of the American Psychiatric Association; New York.

Wender PH, Reimherr FW, Wood DR, Ward M. (1985). A controlled study of methylphenidate in the treatment of attention deficit disorder, residual type, in adults. *Am J Psychiatry* **142**:547–52.

Wood DR, Reimherr FW, Wender PH, Johnson GE. (1976). Diagnosis and treatment of minimal brain dysfunction in adults: a preliminary report. *Arch Gen Psychiatry* **33**:1453–60.

Chapter

18

The use of nonstimulant drugs in the treatment of adult ADHD

Wim J. C. Verbeeck and Siegfried Tuinier[†]

[†]I remember Siegfried for his formidable intellect, his breadth of interests in a wide range of topics far exceeding the realms of psychiatry, and his warm personality. He threw himself into his work with genuine enthusiasm, which translated into contributions to the field, neurodevelopment disorders in particular. Siegfried was an esteemed colleague, and inspired both clinicians and researchers through one of his personal credos: "Science[research] belongs to the coalition of the willing few".

It has been a privilege to have known Siegfried, and I hope his knowledge and wisdom will be treasured beyond the confines of Pubmed.

(Wim Verbeeck)

Introduction

To date, psychostimulants constitute the most efficacious drugs in the treatment of attention-deficit hyperactivity/impulsivity disorder (ADHD), with impressive effect sizes that are similar to what has been reported in meta-analyses of the child and adolescent literature (Faraone et al., 2004). The neurochemical mechanisms by which psychomotor stimulants such as methylphenidate (MPH) and dextroamphetamine (d-AMP) mitigate the cardinal features of ADHD are mediated, at least in part, by their ability to increase synaptic concentration of dopamine and noradrenaline (Leonard et al., 2004).

The short-acting formulations of MPH and d-AMP necessitate multiple doses per day, with an attendant impact on compliance (Biederman, Spencer, & Wilens, 2004). In addition, some individuals are sensitive to the on–off effects, and the potential risk of diversion should be considered in individuals with a history of substance abuse (Kollins et al., 2001).

Overall, these drawbacks have been eliminated by the development of extended-release preparations. Although these compounds have introduced a pharmacological renaissance in the treatment of ADHD,

their availability and affordability are restricted in certain countries.

Stimulants have compiled an impressive record of both safety end efficacy and are endorsed as the first-line medication for ADHD in adults. However, a subset of patients fail to respond to stimulants or cannot tolerate potential adverse effects such as dysphoria, anxiousness, anorexia, and exacerbations of tics (Kollins et al., 2001; Spencer et al., 2004; Wilens & Spencer, 2000). Furthermore, adults with ADHD often suffer from a comorbid disorder (depression, anxiety, tics, drug dependence) for which stimulant drugs may be inappropriate. Psychostimulants are also contraindicated in patients with glaucoma, hyperthyroidism, current use of monoamine oxidase (MAO) inhibitors, symptomatic cardiovascular diseases, uncontrolled hypertension, and drug dependence (Greenhill et al., 2002).

In view of these limitations, a variety of alternative nonstimulant medications have been explored. Agents for which evidence of efficacy has been obtained from rigorous experimental designs are listed chronologically in terms of those studies in Table 18.1. Together with these data from more robust studies, in this chapter we also describe nonrandomized studies that have reported the effectiveness of nonstimulants in the treatment of ADHD.

Although the evidence supports the descriptive, face, predictive, and concurrent validity of ADHD in adults (Spencer, Biederman, et al., 1998), we must appreciate that this transnosographical disorder still lacks a biological marker or endophenotype. In reviewing pharmacological effects on ADHD, it is crucial to bear in mind that clinical and research samples of ADHD usually represent a considerable heterogeneity of diagnoses with mixed underlying biologies (Popper, 1997), and therefore, they may have a differential

ADHD in Adults: Characterization, Diagnosis and Treatment, ed. Jan Buitelaar, Cornelis Kan and Philip Asherson. Published by Cambridge University Press. © Cambridge University Press 2011.

Table 18.1. Controlled trials of nonstimulants in adult ADHD (n = 31): 1995–2009

Author	Number	Duration (weeks)	Compound	Assessment	Comorbidity	Outcome measures	Effect	Comments
Ernst 1996*	24 (17 male)	10	Selegiline 20 mg Selegiline 60 mg	DSM-III-R Connors ATRS Utah criteria Spouse ratings in 15	Excluded	Connors ATRS CGI CPT, BDI, HAM-D, BPRS, STESS	Low and high selegiline dosage not superior to placebo	results not significant because of large placebo respons Drop outs: 12
Levin 1996	17 (15 male)	Acute dose	Nicotine skin patch 21 mg smokers 7 mg nonsmokers	DSM-IV Wender-Utah scale Connors-Wels scale	Major depression and anxiety disorders excluded	CGI (much/very much improved) SCL-90-R POMS Neuropsychol. tests	Within subjects treatment effect was significant for -severity scale $p < 0.025$ -improvement scale $p < 0.005$ -efficacy scale $p < 0.01$	
Wilens 1996	41 (21 male)	6	Desipramine 147 mg	DSM-III-R Wender-Utah Rating Scale	Bipolar disorders and substance abuse excluded	CGI ADHD RS (30%) HAM-D, HAM-A, Beck DBI	68% vs. 0% on placebo $p = 0.001$ (ADHD-RS and CGI-I)	About half of patients had a comorbid disorder Dropouts: 2
Spencer 1998*	22 (10 male)	3	Tomoxetine 76 mg	DSM-III-R	Active psychiatric disorders excluded	ADHD RS (30%) Neuropsychol. tests	Tomoxetine>placebo on ADHD-RS $p = 0.01$	Dropouts: 1
Wilens 1999*	32 (28 male)	3	ABT-418 75-mg skin patch	DSM-III-R + IV ADHD RS	44% current comorbid disorders	CGI (very much/much improved) ADHD RS (30%) Neuropsychol. tests	CGI: 40% vs. 13% placebo ($P = 0.03$) ADHD-RS 47% vs 22% placebo ($P = 0.06$)	Inattentive cluster responded better than the hyperactive/impulsive Drop outs: 3
Taylor 2000	22 (13 male)	2	Modafinil (mean 207 mg) Dexamfetamine (mean 22 mg)	DSM-IV ADHD Behavior Checklist	Excluded	DSM-IV ADHD Behavior Checklist 21 item BDI HAM-A Neuropsychol. tests	48% favorable response on modafinil 48% on amfetamine ($P < 0.001$)	No improvement on BDI, HAM-A, or tests of cognition. Dropout:1
Kuperman 2001	30 (21 male)	7	Bupropion SR max 300 mg Methylphenidate 0,9 mg/kg	DSM-IV	Excluded	CGI (very much/ much improved) ADHD-RS Neuropsychol. tests	64% on bupropion 50% on meth.phen. 27% on placebo $p = 0.14$ (CGI); $p = 0.69$ (ADHD-RS)	No significant differences in endpoint for ADHD-RS self or neuropsychological assessments. Dropouts: 5
Taylor 2001	17 (7 male)	2	Guanfacine 1.1 mg DAMP 10 mg	DSM-IV ADHD Beh. Checklist Neuropsychol. tests	Not specified	ADHD Beh. Checklist Copeland SC Neuropsychol. testing	Significant effects of both drugs ($p < 0.05$), not on Copeland SC	No effect on neuropsychol. tests, no effect on hyperactivity, marginal global effects short duration

(cont.)

Table 18.1. (cont.)

Author	Number	Duration (weeks)	Compound	Assessment	Comorbidity	Outcome measures	Effect	Comments
Levin 2001	40 (25 male)	4 weeks	-Control -Nicotine only-patch max. 10 mg/day -Methyl phenidate (Ritalin SR 20 mg/day) -Nicotine+ methylphenidate	DSM-IV Wender Utah Rating Scale Connors/Wells Adolescent and Adults Self Report CGI scale HAM-D	Excluded	CGI POMS Connors CPT ANAM	Significant improvement nicotine only vs. control (p < 0.025) and combined treatment vs. control (p < 0.05) during chronic phase on Sign. improvement nicotine alone (p < 0.05) and in combination (p < 0.005) vs. control on POMS	Small number of participants per goup Low-dosages of methyl phenidate Dropouts: 3 in control group, one in each treatment group
Wilens 2001*	40 (22 male)	6	Bupropion SR 200 mg twice daily (mean 362 mg)	DSM-III-R and DSM-IV ADHD-RS	7 comorbid disorders in 49% of patients	CGI (very much/ much improved) ADHD-FS (30%)	CGI 52% vs. 11% on placebo (p = 0.007) ADHD-RS 76% vs. 37% (p = 0.02)	Delayed onset of effect Dropouts: 2
Dorrego 2002	32 (19 male)	8	Methylphenidate 39 mg Lithium 0,68 mg/L	DSM-IV ADHD RS CAARS	No co-medication Not specified	CAARS (30%) Neuropsychol. tests Irritability Scale CPT	48% methyl phenidate 37% lithium (95% CI, −12% + 34%) for the observed difference between methylphenidate and lithium	CPT not improved Verbal memory improved Dropouts: 9
Michelson 2003a*	280 (178 male)	10	Atomoxetine 60–120 mg	DSM-IV Connors ADHD CAAR-D Sheehan scale	Excluded	CAARS CGI-S WRAADDS	0.35 effect size on primary outcome measure	Sign. reduction on CAARS and improvement on Sheehan Disability Dropouts: 61
Michelson 2003b*	256 (170 male)	10	Atomoxetine 60–120 mg	DSM-IV Connors ADHD CAAR-D Sheehan scale	Excluded	CAARS CGI-S WRAADDS	0.40 effect size on primary outcome measure	Sign. reduction on CAARS and improvement on Sheehan Disability Dropouts: 79
Turner 2004	20 (13 male)	Acute dose	Modafinil 200 mg	DSM-IV Connors ADHD	Affective disorders and substance abuse excluded	Neuropsychol. tests (CANTAB)	Significant improvement in several cognitive domains	Improved performance on tests of digit span, visual memory, spatial planning, decision making, and response inhibition.

Study	N	Duration	Drug/dose	Diagnostic criteria	Co-medication	Outcome measures	Results	Comments
Wernicke 2004*	184	Discontinuation	Atomoxetine 120 mg	DSM-IV CAAR-D	n.s.	CAARS HAMA HAMD	n.s.	No discontinuation syndrome
Wilens 2005*	162 (97 male)	8	Bupropion XL (mean 393 mg)	DSM-IV CGI-S ADHD-RS	Excluded No co-medication	ADHD-RS (30%) CGI CAARS-S:S CAARS-O:S	53% bupropion vs. 31% placebo $p = 0.003$ (CGI) $P = 0.004$ (ADHD-RS)	Former non-responders to stimulants or bupropion excluded Dropouts: 29 (16 on bupropion)
Reimherr 2005*	144	10	Atomoxetine 60–120 mg	DSM-IV Connors ADHD CAAR-D Sheehan scale	Excluded	CAARS CGI-S WRAADDS (secondary outcome measure)	WRAADS emotional dysregulation 42% vs. 19% on placebo ($p = 0.001$)	Presence of emotional dysregulation was not related to diagnostic levels of anxiety or depression
Reimherr 2005*	59 (43 male)	6 (1 week placebo lead-in)	Bupropion SR (mean 298 mg)	DSM-IV Wender Utah criteria	Excluded	CGI-I (very much/much improved) WRAADDS (50%)	CGi: ($p = 0.15$) 41% bupropion SR 22% placebo WRAADDS: ($p = 0.15$) 32% bupropion SR 11% placebo	Strict definition of improvement Unequal randomization Dropouts 12
Faraone 2005*	424	10	Atomoxetine 60–120 mg	DSM-IV Connors ADHD CAAR-D Sheehan scale	Excluded	Stroop -Color task -Word task -Color-word task	Significant main effect of medication ($p = 0.004$) and significant medication by baseline-score interaction ($p = 0.008$) for color-word score	Effect of treatment on the color-word test was significant for subjects who scored lower than the normative mean at baseline but not for subjects who scored higher. Stroop baseline and endpoint data available on 425 of 536 subjects
Adler 2006*	218	6	Atomoxetine 40 mg twice daily vs Atomoxetine 80 mg daily	DSM-IV	Excluded	TEAE CAARS-Inv.-SV ASEX Laboratory values, ECG, vital signs	No statistically significant difference between treatment groups in primary end point.	No placebo arm (?expectation bias) Primary endpoint: Likelihood of experiencing ≥ 1 of the four most commonly observed TEAE's. Dropouts: 57

(cont.)

Table 18.1. (cont.)

Author	Number	Duration (weeks)	Compound	Assessment	Comorbidity	Outcome measures	Effect	Comments
Adler 2006*	218	6	Atomoxetine 40 mg twice daily vs. atomoxetine 80 mg daily	DSM-IV CAARS CGI-ADHD-S SCID	Excluded	CAARS SF-36	Mental component summary measure SF-36 improved significantly ($p < 0.001$)	No placebo arm Dropouts : 13
Biederman 2006*	36 (18 placebo)	12	Galantamine max 24 mg (mean dose: 19.8 mg)	DSM-IV	Excluded	CGI AISRS	No significant greater reduction Galantamine vs. placebo $p = 0.5$	Possibly underdosed Dropouts: 8
Wilens 2006*	11	8 (cross over)	ABT-089 2–4–20 mg Twice daily	DSM-IV-TR	Excluded	CAARS CGI-ADHD-S HAM-A, HAM-D Computerised cognitive assessment Safety assessments	Effect sizes on the CAARS were 0.92, 0.76, and 0.71 for 2 mg, 4 mg, and 20 mg respectively	Small sample size. Homogenous study population. Most patients analysed from one study site. Relative short treatment exposure. Statistical test of efficacy one sided Of the 61 enrolled subjects, 11 completed the study.
Gehricke 2006	10	8 days	Nicotine patch (14–21 mg per day) Low doses of Methylphenidate or dextro-amphetamine	DSM-IV Wender Utah Rating Scale AHA scale Barrat Impulsivity Scale CES-D	Co-morbidity not specified	Electronic diary items assessing ADHD symptoms derived from DSM-IV criteria	Compared with placebo patch only, core symptom behavior was reduced during nicotine patch with stimulant ($p = 0.006$), nicotine patch only ($p = 0.004$), and placebo patch + stimulant medication ($p = 0.012$)	Participants received financial benefits, and aware of medication status Small sample size
Poltavski 2006	62 (all male)	6 hours	Transdermal Nicotine patch 7 mg	Self-Report Rating Scale McCarney and Anderson Current Symptoms Scale Barkley and Murphy	Not specified	Conners' CPT Stroop task WCST	Improvement Conners CPT in low attention group (errors of commission $p = 0.049$; detectability $p = 0.05$; perseverations $p = 0.025$) Impairment WCST in high attention group	Participants with attentional deficits were not necessarily diagnosed with ADHD Dropouts : 5 Inaccurate screening of attentional status.

Study	N	Duration	Medication/dose	Diagnostic criteria	Inclusion/exclusion	Scales	Results	Comments
Levin 2006	98 (56 male)	12 weeks (8 weeks at stable dose)	Methylphenidate-SR max. 80 mg/day Bupropion-SR max. 400 mg/day	Wender-Utah rating scale AARS SCID; KSCID DSM-IV	Patients with substance use disorder included	WRAADS CGI AARS Urine toxicology	21% placebo 9% methylphenidate 15% bupropion No significant group differences $p = 0.42$ (CGI, AARS)	All individuals received Cognitive Behavioral Therapy. High placebo response. Compliance was good. Dropouts: 29
Weiss 2006*	98	20 weeks	Paroxetine max. 40 mg/day Dextro-amphetamine max. 20 mg twice daily	CAARD-D Interview for DSM-IV	Inclusion of patients with SCID lifetime diagnosis of internalizing disorder	ADHD-RS-4-Inv. HAM-A HAM-D GGI-ADHD CGI-Int CGI-I	ADHD responders: $p = 0.001$ 64% dextro-amphetamine 44% paroxetine/ d-amphetamine 17% paroxetine 16% placebo Mood/anxiety responders≥: $p = 0.003$ 100% paroxetine 73% paroxetine/d-amphetamine 57% amphetamine 47% placebo	All received problem-focused therapy. ITT analysis compromised by high drop out Fixed titration schedule Dropouts: 34
Wilens 2008*	72	12 weeks	Atomoxetine 25–100 mg (mean: 89.9 mg)	DSM-IV-TR criteria for ADHD and alcohol use disorders Adult ADHD Clinician Diagnostic Scale	Exclusion of major Axis I disorders based on SCID-I, HAM-D, and HAM-A	AISRS ASRS Timeline Follow-back method OCDS CGI-ADHD-S CGI-ADHD-I	Significant improvement in atomoxetine group compared to placebo on AISRS ($p = 0.007$), CGI-ADHD-S ($P = 0.048$) and CGI-ADHD-I ($P = 0.006$)	Dropouts: 35 (atomoxetine) vs 25(placebo)
Adler 2008*	271	6 months	Atomoxetine 40–100 mg	DSM-IV-TR SCID CAADID	Excluded	CAARS-Inv: SV CAARS-O- SV CAARS-S- SV ASRS EWPS AAQoL DBS	No difference in atomoxetine vs. placebo on EWPS ($p = 0.41$) AAQoL-Life outlook subscale: atomoxetine> placebo ($p = 0.024$) DBS (observer): atomoxetine> placebo ($p = 0.011$)	Completion rate: 38% atomoxetine vs. 49% placebo

(cont.)

Table 18.1. (cont.)

Author	Number	Duration (weeks)	Compound	Assessment	Comorbidity	Outcome measures	Effect	Comments
Adler 2009*	94 47 male	6 months	Atomoxetine 25–100 mg (mean 84.5 mg)	DSM-IV-TR SCID	Exclusion of major Axis I disorders based on SCID	AISRS CAARS-Inv: SV ASRS v 1.1 CGI-ADHD-S AAQoL	Statistically superior vs. placebo on almost all post baseline visits (primary and secondary measures)	37.6% atomoxetine group vs. 44.6% placebo group completed the study 250 patients were randomized
Adler 2009*	224	14 weeks	Atomoxetine 40–100 mg	DSM-IV-TR CAARD-D Interview for DSM-IV	Specific phobias, GAD, and dysthymia allowed	CAARS-Inv: SV LSAS CGI-O-S STAI SAS AAQoL	Results are statistically significant on both CAARS-Inv: SV and LSAS; $p < 0.001$	15 dropouts during, and 82 after placebo lead-in

* Indicates industry-sponsored trials.

AAQoL = Adult ADHD Quality of Life Scale -29; AARS = Adult ADHD Rating Scale; ADHD = attention-deficit hyperactivity cisorder; ADHD-RS = Attention Deficit Disorder Rating Scale; ADHD-RS-IV-Inventory = ADHD-Rating Scale for DSM-IV, Investigator version; AISRS = ADHD Investigator Symptom Report Scale; ANAM = Automated Neuropsychological Assessment Metrics; ASEX = Arizona Sexual Experience Scale; ASRS = Adult ADHD Self Report Scale; ATRS = Abreviated Teacher Rating Scale; BPRS = Brief Psychiatric Rating Scale; CAADID = Connors Adult ADHD Diagnostic Interview for DSM-IV; CAAR-D = Connors' Adult ADHD Diagnostic Interview for DSM-IV; CAARS-InvSV = Connors' Adult ADHD Rating Scale Investigator rated; CAARS-O:S = Connors' Adult ADHD Rating Scale-Observer; CAARS-S:S = Connors' Adult ADHD Rating Scale-Self Report; CGI = Clinical Global Impression; CGI-I = CGI Improvement Scale; CGI-ADHD = CGI-I for ADHD symptoms; CGI-Int = CGI-I for mood and anxiety symptoms; CGI-O-S=CGI-Overall-Severity; CGI-S = Clinical Global Impression of Severity of illness; CPT = Continuous Performance Test; DBI = Beck Depression Inventory; DBS = Driving Behavior Survey; DSM-III-R = Diagnostic and Statistic Manual of Mental Disorders, 3rd ed., rev.; DSM-IV = Diagnostic and Statistic Manual of Mental Disorders, 4th ed.; EWPS = Endicott Work Productivity Scale; GAD = Generalized Anxiety Disorder; HAM-A = Hamilton Anxiety Scale; HAM-D = Hamilton Depression Scale; ITT = Intention to treat; KSCID = Structured Clinical Interview for DSM-IV, childhood version; LSAS = Liebowitz Social Anxiety Scale; OCDS = Obsessive Compulsive Drinking Scale; POMS = Profile of Mood States; SAS = Social Adjustment Scale-Self Report; SCID = Structured Clinical Interview for DSM-IV; SF-36 = 36-item short form health survey; SR = sustained-release; STAI = State-Trait Anxiety Inventory; STESS=Subject's Treatment Emergent Symptom Scale; TEAE = Treatment Emergent Adverse Effect; WRAADDS = Wender-Reimherr Adult Attention Deficit Disorder Scale; XL = long-acting.

response to pharmacological interventions. It should be emphasized that ADHD in this respect is not different from any other psychiatric disorder.

Tricyclic antidepressants (TCAs)

Despite extensive experience in children, including three comparative studies suggesting TCA superiority over stimulants, and in adolescents, there are only two studies of these agents in adult ADHD.

An initial chart review of TCAs for the treatment of ADHD indicated that desipramine (DES) or nortriptyline, given often in combination with other psychotropics, including stimulants, resulted in moderate improvements, which were sustained at 1 year (Wilens et al., 1995). Although this study was retrospective in nature and uncontrolled, its naturalistic nature approximates the day-to-day reality of clinical practice.

We identified one placebo-controlled trial with 41 outpatients (desipramine, $n = 19$) from an outpatient psychopharmacology clinic (Wilens et al., 1996). The mean daily dose of desipramine was 147 mg. A response was already noted during the initial 2-week titration, and progressive response was observed at weeks 4 and 6. Improvement was defined as a score of 1 or 2 ("very much" or "much" improved) on the Clinical Global Impressions-Improvement Scale (CGI-I) and a reduction on the corresponding rating scale (Attention-Deficit/Hyperactivity Disorder Rating Scale; ADHD-RS) of 30% or more. Desipramine was associated with a response in 68% of the patients versus 0% with placebo (Wilens et al., 1996).

Despite the generally robust behavioral effects of TCAs, they have weaker cognitive effects in ADHD than the psychostimulants and often leave significant residual attentional effects. The anti-ADHD effects of TCAs seem to be independent of their antidepressant effects. TCAs have a delayed onset of action of up to 4 weeks after full titration, and multiple dose adjustments are frequently required before the most effective and best tolerated dose is achieved.

In adults, desipramine has been reported to have a significantly higher risk of lethality after overdose (about 1%) than other TCAs. It induces a larger reduction in heart rate variability than imipramine, implying greater autonomic rigidity and medical risk (Popper, 2000). The pediatric literature has amplified this lingering concern during the last decade. Moreover, the fact that a handful of sudden deaths occurred

in youth who were taking DES for ADHD may have contributed to this agent's dwindling market share (Horrigan, 2001). As TCAs are metabolized by the CYP 450 system, medications that inhibit this system may raise TCA levels. In view of TCAs' potential cardiotoxicity, serial ECGs and plasma-level monitoring are mandatory.

Compared to the stimulants, TCAs have negligible abuse liability, single daily dosing, and efficacy for anxiety and depression as well (Wilens et al., 2002). They can be used in combination with stimulants to treat ADHD, either as an adjunctive treatment or to treat comorbid disorders. TCAs can also reduce stimulant-induced insomnia and weight loss (Popper, 2000). In addition, they may be a reasonable alternative for ADHD patients who have experienced tic exacerbation with stimulants (Spencer et al., 2002). Mild TCA-induced cognitive deficits, such as word-finding difficulty or "forgetting", reflecting central anticholinergic neurotoxicity, have fueled interest in other noradrenergic agents that might be effective in ADHD (Pliszka, 2001).

Norepinephrine reuptake inhibitors

Atomoxetine (formerly tomoxetine) is a specific norepinephrine transporter reuptake blocker that has minimal affinity for other receptors. It lacks the anticholinergic and antihistamine effects of TCAs (Bymaster et al., 2002; Zerbe et al., 1985). As the pharmacokinetics of atomoxetine are influenced by the polymorphic expression of cytochrome P450 2D6, dosages may have to be lowered when coadministered with CYP 2D6 inhibitors. The plasma elimination half-life of atomoxetine in poor metabolizers is approximately fourfold longer than in extensive metabolizers (20 vs. 5 hours), indicating an increased systemic exposure to atomoxetine in poor metabolizers, who subsequently may require lower dosages (Simpson & Plosker, 2004). The most frequently experienced side effects are dry mouth, insomnia, nausea, decreased appetite, constipation, and sexual problems. Like stimulants, modest increases in blood pressure and heart rate are observed, thus requiring regular monitoring of hemodynamic parameters. Atomoxetine is not associated with QT-prolongation (Wernicke et al., 2003).

Atomoxetine has been shown in a preliminary "proof of concept" controlled crossover trial to be superior to placebo. Adults experienced significant improvements in ADHD symptoms and demonstrated improvements in executive functioning (Spencer et al., 1998). The effect of atomoxetine on core symptomatology does not occur until several weeks after it is started.

More recently, two controlled multicenter studies have demonstrated the short-term efficacy of atomoxetine for the treatment of ADHD in adults. In a total of 536 adults, atomoxetine was shown to be superior to placebo. Improvements in both attentional and hyperactive-impulsive ratings were noted, with effect sizes of 0.35 and 0.40, respectively. Atomoxetine was associated with improved functioning as assessed with the Sheehan disability scale (Michelson et al., 2003). The efficacy findings of these acute studies were extended in a randomized, placebo-controlled, double-blind, 6-month trial using different efficacy measures (Adler, Spencer, et al., 2009).

Several spin-off publications resulted from these two large studies. First, combined data from these two studies demonstrated that atomoxetine produced improvement on executive functioning, as measured by the Stroop task, particularly in individuals with an executive deficit (Faraone et al., 2005). Second, it was shown that one-third of patients who met post hoc criteria for emotional dysregulation improved significantly on all measures of ADHD, including the emotional dysregulation symptoms (Reimherr, Marchant, et al., 2005).

Because ADHD typically involves extended periods of treatment, the effects of discontinuation of atomoxetine were assessed in the aftermath of two short-term studies mentioned earlier. Both gradual and abrupt discontinuation were well tolerated and did not culminate in symptom rebound or discontinuation emergent adverse effects, at least not during the 4-week observation period. Nonetheless, the authors could not rule out the possibility that outcomes could be different in patients treated over longer periods (Wernicke et al., 2004).

Three hundred and eighty-four (72%) patients who participated in the acute treatment studies (Michelson et al., 2003) and wished to continue treatment entered a 4-year open-label study with atomoxetine. The data represent the longest period of systematic pharmacological treatment yet studied in adults with ADHD, and the results support the long-term safety, efficacy, and tolerability of atomoxetine treatment, as measured by the CAARS-Inv: SV and Sheehan Disability Scale. However, it should be noted that only 69 patients completed the study (Adler, Spencer, Williams, et al., 2008).

A randomized double-blind trial compared the safety and tolerability of once- versus twice-daily atomoxetine in 218 adults with ADHD. Both dosing strategies were found to be safe, well tolerated, and efficacious, but there was a significantly greater frequency of nausea in patients treated with once-daily 80 mg atomoxetine than in patients treated with twice-daily 40 mg atomoxetine ($p = 0.007$). There is preliminary evidence supporting the switch to twice-daily dosing in a patient experiencing nausea with once-daily dosing or the switch to once-daily dosing in a patient experiencing constipation with twice-daily dosing. According to the authors, there is room for prescribers to use discretion in dosing strategies (Adler, Dietrich, et al., 2006). Additional data analysis from this trial demonstrated that amelioration of ADHD symptoms was accompanied by significant improvement in the quality of life, as measured on the CAARS and SF-36 (Adler, Sutton, et al., 2006).

After a 6-month, double-blind, placebo-controlled study with atomoxetine, adults with ADHD showed significant improvement on a disease-specific subscale of the Adult ADHD Quality of Life (AAQoL), but not on general functional outcomes, as measured by the Endicott Work Productivity Scale (EWPS). Additional functional improvements were shown in driving behavior, when rated by observers. Both treatment groups had low study endpoint completion rates (Adler, Spencer, Levine, et al., 2008).

ADHD is often associated with comorbid disorders. Two recent studies evaluated the effect of atomoxetine on the treatment of ADHD and comorbidity in adults. The first double-blind, randomized, placebo-controlled trial examining atomoxetine in adults with ADHD and comorbid alcohol abuse or dependence demonstrated clinically significant ADHD improvement, but inconsistent effects on drinking behavior. Although time-to-relapse to heavy drinking did not differ between groups, cumulative heavy drinking days were reduced 26% in atomoxetine-treated subjects versus placebo over the 12-week outpatient study. No differences were found in four other drinking measures. In view of this study's methodological limitations, these data should be considered preliminary (Wilens et al., 2008). A second, randomized, double-blind, placebo-controlled trial showed that atomoxetine monotherapy effectively improved symptoms of

ADHD and comorbid social anxiety disorder (Adler, Liebowitz, et al., 2009).

Three spontaneously reported cases (two adolescents and one child, all female) of reversible drug-induced liver injury have been identified in association with atomoxetine therapy in the 4-year post-marketing period during which approximately 4.3 million patients had been prescribed the medication. These cases are consistent with the pattern of an idiosyncratic drug reaction. Atomoxetine treatment should be discontinued in patients with jaundice or laboratory evidence of liver injury and should not be rechallenged (Bangs, Jin, et al., 2008).

A meta-analysis of 14 studies in pediatric patients suggested a potential relationship between atomoxetine use and suicidal ideation. A statistically greater incidence of suicidal ideation or behavior was observed in atomoxetine-treated pediatric patients compared with placebo-treated patients (Mantel-Haenszel incidence difference, $p = 0.01$). Suicidal attempts were rarely observed, and there were no completed suicides. Although the risk-benefit estimate for atomoxetine remains favorable, it is recommended to stay vigilant to possible suicidal ideation (Bangs, Tauscher-Wisniewski, et al., 2008). Atomoxetine carries a black box warning for suicidal ideation in children and adolescents, but there is no warning with regard to adults.

Animal studies show that atomoxetine increases extracellular levels of noradrenaline and dopamine in the prefrontal cortex, whereas in the subcortical areas it increases extracellular levels of noradrenaline but not dopamine. The lack of increase in dopamine transmission in subcortical areas such as the striatum and the nucleus accumbens may indicate a low proclivity of atomoxetine to produce tics, have psychomimetic effects, or lead to abuse (Bymaster et al., 2002). Therefore atomoxetine is clearly indicated when there is abuse potential and perhaps when comorbidities such as anxiety, depression, and tics exist (Simpson & Plosker, 2004).

Despite the elegant clinical development process of atomoxetine, there is at present a lack of head-to-head studies with unbiased methodology and thus no rational guidelines to inform the relative position of atomoxetine in the first-line treatment of ADHD (Biederman, Spencer et al., 2004).

A Medline search produced no randomized controlled trial (RCT) citations regarding the use of reboxetine or maprotiline in the treatment of ADHD. At present, the use of these noradrenergic agents remains confined to the treatment of depression.

Modafinil

Although the exact mechanism of action of modafinil is unknown, the actions of this alertness-promoting drug may be similar to that of the neuropeptides hypocretin 1 and 2, thereby promoting the release of histamine within the neuroanatomical pathways that activate internal vigilance (Ishizuka et al., 2003; Scammell et al., 2000). Unlike the psychostimulants, this hypothalamic-activating agent does not seem to influence central catecholaminergic tone in a direct manner, accounting for its reduced side effect profile and low abuse liability (Deroche-Gamonet et al., 2002). In a similar vein, it has been proposed that one of the key differences between stimulants and modafinil is their distinct effects on arousal. Two types of arousal – stimulated vigilance and normal wakefulness – exist, and each seems to be mediated by different pathways and neurotransmitters. Stimulated vigilance may be mediated by the monoamines dopamine, norepinephrine, serotonin, and acetylcholine via the ascending reticular activating system, and normal wakefulness (internal vigilance) may be mediated by ascending histaminergic neurons arising from the tuberomamillary nucleus within the hypothalamus. Stimulants exert their effects through both stimulated (catecholaminergic) arousal and normal (histaminergic) wakefulness, whereas modafinil possibly acts through selective activation of the second, more reflective type of calm wakefulness (Stahl, 2002).

The half-life of modafinil is 10 to 15 hours, which is three to five times longer than that of MPH. Its therapeutic effect does not appear to have a duration equal to its half-life. After ingestion, the effects dissipate over the next several hours at a much quicker rate than the fall in the serum concentration of the drug. Nonetheless, the effects with modafinil seem to last longer than those of stimulants (Swanson, 2003).

In a single-site, randomized, double-blind, placebo-controlled three-phase crossover trial (n = 22), modafinil produced favorable responses in 48% of patients with ADHD, similar to that achieved with amphetamine in the same study. A rather low dose of d-amphetamine was used, and the response rate to d-AMP was unusually low (48%). Minimal cognitive testing was included, with little effect shown on the Stroop Color-Word Test, the classic task associated with executive function. The investigators concluded that modafinil may be a viable alternative to conventional stimulants for the treatment of adults with ADHD (Taylor & Russo, 2000). However, results from a larger, multicenter, controlled study, sponsored by the manufacturer, failed to find any differences between three dosages of modafinil and placebo in adults with ADHD (Cephalon, 2000).

In a recent double-blind, randomized, placebo-controlled crossover design, a single 200-mg dose of modafinil produced beneficial effects on response inhibition and other cognitive domains thought to be impaired in adult patients with ADHD, but the clinical relevance of these findings needs to be confirmed in long-term administration studies (Turner et al., 2004).

Concerns have been raised by the occurrence of serious dermatological reactions to modafinil in children with ADHD (Kumar, 2008).

Cholinomimetics

Cigarette smoking is overrepresented in adults with ADHD, which may be related to its alleviation of attentional and cognitive symptoms. ADHD is associated with an increased risk and an earlier age of onset of cigarette smoking (Pomerleau et al., 1995). Maternal smoking during pregnancy increases the risk for ADHD in the offspring, and in utero exposure to nicotine in animals confers a heightened risk for an ADHD-like syndrome in the newborn.

In recent years evidence has emerged that nicotinic dysregulation may contribute to the pathophysiology of ADHD. This relationship is not surprising considering that nicotinic receptor activation enhances dopaminergic neurotransmission, mediated through the cholinergic pathway (Mereu et al., 1987). Acetylcholine acts as an agonist at a presynaptic heteroreceptor on dopamine nerve terminals, increasing the release of dopamine. In non-ADHD subjects, central nicotinic activation has been shown to improve attention, cognitive vigilance, and executive function (Levin, 1992). Because dopamine agonism is thought to be partially responsible for the therapeutic effects of anti-ADHD medications, this has led to the hypothesis that cholinergic agonists may be of value in the treatment of ADHD (Pliszka, 2001).

Support for a nicotinic hypothesis of ADHD can be derived from a recent study that evaluated the ther-

apeutic effects of nicotine in the treatment of ADHD. Although this controlled clinical trial documented that wearing a transdermal nicotine patch resulted in significant improvement of ADHD symptoms, working memory, and cognitive functioning, the trial was very short and included only a handful of patients (Levin et al., 1996).

The alpha-4 beta-2 nicotinic receptor agonist, ABT-418, resulted in preferential improvements in the inattentive cluster of symptoms relative to the behavioral symptoms, as well as improvements in higher level executive functioning, which are of great importance given findings of prominent executive dysfunction in adults with ADHD (Wilens et al., 1999). Doubts about clinical efficacy include the slow onset of action and an uncertain effect size. Preliminary results of a double-blind, randomized, 12-week, parallel-design pilot of galantamine vs. placebo did not support the clinical utility of this reversible acetylcholinestrase inhibitor (Biederman et al., 2006).

In a small randomized, double-blind, placebo-controlled, crossover proof-of-concept pilot of 11 adults with ADHD, treatment with ABT-089 was well tolerated. The clinical improvements were seen at the lower doses on both primary and secondary outcome measures (Wilens et al., 2006).

A small preliminary study examined the effects of nicotine with and without stimulant medication on ADHD symptoms, mood, and arousal in the everyday lives of smokers with ADHD. Participants, who were asked to abstain from smoking, underwent four conditions in randomized order: (1) nicotine patch + stimulant medication, (2) nicotine patch only, (3) placebo patch + stimulant medication, and (4) placebo patch only. Each condition continued for 2 days, during which self-reports of ADHD symptoms and mood were obtained using electronic diaries. Results revealed that nicotine patch and stimulant medication alone and in combination enhanced attentional processes and self-defined core symptoms in adults with ADHD (Gehricke et al., 2006).

A placebo-controlled study evaluating the effects of transdermal nicotine on attention in adult nonsmokers with and without attentional deficits supported the hypothesis that nicotine has differential effects on individuals varying in attentiveness. The results showed nicotine-induced improvement on some measures of sustained attention in the low-attention group and some decrement in working memory in the high-attention group, suggesting that nicotine may be more effective in optimizing attention than in improving optimal performance (Poltavski & Petros, 2006).

Donepezil, a cholinesterase inhibitor, may improve executive functioning in ADHD, but preliminary clinical impressions from a small open trial do not suggest efficacy.

In a small randomized, double-blind, placebo-controlled trial on the effect of chronic nicotine treatment for nonsmoking adults with ADHD, 40 participants were each enrolled in one of the following treatment combinations: control, nicotine only, methylphenidate only, or nicotine + methylphenidate (Wilens et al., 2005). Nicotine was administered via transdermal patches. The CGI scale was not significantly affected by either nicotine or methylphenidate during the chronic phase. On the Profile of Mood States (POMS), there was a significant improvement in the group given nicotine alone and in the nicotine + methylphenidate group ($p < 0.005$) on day 15. There was a very robust nicotine-induced attenuation of the rise in continuous performance test (CPT) hit reaction time standard error over session blocks on the Connors CPT, suggesting improved attentional consistency (Levin et al., 2001).

Nicotine potentiates the release of dopamine and norepinephrine as well as other neurotransmitters, such as serotonin and acetylcholine. The net increase in catecholaminergic stimulation resembles the actions of stimulants and may be critical for nicotine effects on attention. Interestingly, nicotine-induced attentional improvements are not blocked by haloperidol, so other pharmacological effects of nicotine may be important for its effects on attention. Results of studies provide evidence concerning the possible efficacy of nicotine treatment for ADHD, but additional research is needed on the possible use of nicotine for adults with ADHD.

Alpha-2 agonists

Clonidine, which at low dosages stimulates the presynaptic alpha-2 adrenergic autoreceptors, has been largely abandoned in the treatment of core symptoms of ADHD. Controversy has existed as to whether clonidine exerts its therapeutic effect via improvement in cognition or whether it simply has a nonspecific sedative effect. Increasingly, clonidine has been used more in conjunction with stimulants for the treatment of insomnia, aggression, and tics than as monotherapy for ADHD (Pliszka, 2003).

This antihypertensive agent may compromise cardiovascular status (producing bradycardia and hypotension) and prefrontal executive functions. An important clinical concern is the possibility of a sudden dose decrease – for example, by running out of pills – which is likely to happen in individuals with deficits in executive functions. Abrupt discontinuation can induce significant tachycardia and hypertension and has been associated with severe ventricular tachyarrhythmias (Popper, 2000).

By capitalizing on clonidine's sedative propensity, it can be employed to treat stimulant-induced insomnia and insomnia associated with ADHD. Yet, when clonidine is administered at nighttime in combination with daytime psychostimulants, significant rebound hypertension in the morning and bedtime hypotension may become potential hazards (Wilens et al., 1994).

Guanfacine, an alpha-2A agonist, was found to be 25 times more potent than clonidine in enhancing delayed response performance, 10 times less potent in lowering blood pressure, and much less likely to cause sedation (Arnsten et al., 1988). This differential response profile produced by these two alpha-2 agonists is attributed to the existence of three alpha-2 receptor subtypes. Guanfacine preferentially binds alpha-2A receptors, compared to the more general affinity of clonidine for alpha-2A, B, and C receptors (Lomasney et al., 1990). Studies have indicated that norepinephrine's beneficial actions in the prefrontal cortex (PFC) result from stimulation of postjunctional alpha-2A receptors (Friedman et al., 2004). Therefore, the adverse effects of alpha-2 agonists may be dissociated from their beneficial effects, according to their relative affinities for each receptor subtype. The ability of guanfacine to improve PFC function without significant adverse effects corresponds with its selectivity for the alpha-2A site (Friedman et al., 2004). Comparisons between guanfacine and clonidine, which lacks receptor specificity, support the superiority of guanfacine as a cognitive enhancer (Jakala et al., 1999). In comparison to clonidine, guanfacine produces less of an effect on blood pressure because of its weaker binding affinity for imidazoline receptors.

A preliminary study, in which 17 adult patients who met *DSM-IV* criteria for ADHD were randomized, used a double-blind, placebo-controlled, crossover design to compare the effects of guanfacine with that of d-amphetamine for the treatment of ADHD. The degree of efficacy of guanfacine, according to the *DSM-IV* Behavioral Checklist for Adults, and a subscale of the Controlled Oral Word Association Test COWAT, was similar to that of d-amphetamine. Methodological flaws include the short duration of each medication trial, the small sample size, and the fact that only a single morning dose was administered (Taylor & Russo, 2001).

Monoamine oxidase (MAO) inhibitors

There are two types of MAOs: MAO-A and MAO-B. MAO-A preferentially deaminates serotonin and norepinephrine, whereas MAO-B preferentially deaminates phenylethylamine. Both MAO-A and MAO-B metabolize dopamine and tyramine.

An open-label study with pargyline, a relatively selective irreversible MAO-B inhibitor, showed moderate improvement in adult ADHD (Wender et al., 1983).

Selegeline is a partial but relative selective inhibitor of MAO-B. At low doses, it is a selective inhibitor of MAO-B, and at higher doses, it inhibits both isoforms (Ernst et al., 1996). This agent undergoes an extensive first-pass effect, and its major plasma metabolites include L-amphetamine and L-metamphetamine, which may account for its apparent procognitive effects in some individuals with ADHD (Ernst et al., 1997). In comorbid Tourette disorder and ADHD, selegeline has been evaluated in a placebo-controlled, double-blind, crossover study of 24 children and adults. ADHD symptoms reportedly improved on selegeline without substantially increasing tics in most patients (Popper, 2000).

Ernst et al. (1996) reported dose-dependent improvements in ADHD symptoms with selegeline, but because of the high placebo response these improvements were not significantly different from that of placebo. The study design and selection bias may have contributed to the magnitude of the placebo response. Yet, as all subjects improved significantly with treatment, these results did not prove an absence of clinical efficacy.

Because of its selectivity and reversibility, moclobemide – a MAO-A inhibitor – has fewer side effects than conventional MAO inhibitors and requires less stringent dietary restrictions. Unfortunately controlled data on the efficacy of moclobemide in ADHD are not available.

In our opinion, the use of nonspecific irreversible MAO inhibitors such as tranylcipramine should be discouraged. Even when treatment is stopped, enzyme inhibition will continue until MAO levels return to normal as new enzyme is being synthesized. Therefore, although the elimination half-life of an MAO inhibitor is short, the half-life of enzyme inhibition is about 2 weeks. This means that, up to 2 weeks after the drug is stopped, transgressions of dietary restrictions or incorrect ingestion of stimulants could precipitate a serotonin syndrome or a hypertensive crisis. As patients with ADHD are characterized by impulsivity and disorganization, the prescription of these compounds may have detrimental effects.

Norepinephrine and dopamine reuptake inhibitors: Bupropion

Bupropion is an atypical catecholaminergic agent that has an indirect mixed agonist effect on dopamine and norepinephrine neurotransmission (Gobbi et al., 2003). It is approved for the treatment of depression and smoking cessation in adults and has been used off-label to treat adults with ADHD. It is rapidly absorbed, with peak plasma levels after 2 hours, and has an average elimination half-life of 14 hours. It has been formulated into a sustained-release (SR) preparation and a long-acting (XL) formulation, which can be administered twice and once daily, respectively. There is a slight increased risk for drug-induced seizures, and exacerbation of tic disorders has been reported. On the other hand, weight gain and sexual dysfunction have been minimal.

We identified five randomized controlled studies of bupropion. A controlled clinical trial with the SR preparation of bupropion was conducted in 40 subjects (bupropion, n = 21) from an outpatient clinic, recruited via advertisements and referrals (Wilens, Spencer, et al., 2001). The mean daily dose was 362 mg. Therapeutic benefits were delayed and were not observed until weeks 5 and 6. Ratings of "much" or "very much" improved using the CGI-I were attained in 52% of the patients taking bupropion SR versus 11% taking placebo. The improvements on the ADHD-RS were 76% for those taking bupropion and 37% for those taking placebo. The relatively short treatment time may not have allowed adequate time for the full therapeutic effect to take place (Wilens, Spencer, et al., 2001).

Another study compared bupropion SR with methylphenidate in 30 patients (bupropion, n = 11; methylphenidate, n = 8; placebo, n = 11) recruited by advertisements (Kuperman et al., 2001). The maximum daily dose was 300 mg for buproprion SR and 0.9 mg/kg for methylphenidate. Efficacy was measured with the CGI-I and the ADHD-RS. Although the response was better in both active treatment groups compared to placebo, the differences were not statistically significant. The large placebo response rate was explained by the fact that patients were mild to moderately ill (Kuperman et al., 2001). Most probably the study lacked power.

In a recent multicenter, randomized, double-blind, placebo-controlled study of 162 patients (bupropion, n = 81), once-daily bupropion XL was significantly more efficacious than placebo in treating core symptoms of ADHD, when measured by the ADHD-RS (53% vs. 31%, respectively). The study was completed by 133 patients. On the CGI-I, 38% were "much" or "very much" improved with bupropion XL versus 18% with placebo. The XL formulation of bupropion uses a diffusion-controlled vehicle, providing sustained benefit throughout the day, as shown by total CAARS-S:S scores at 10.00 am, 4.00 pm, and 10.00 pm. The improvement emerged as early as 2 weeks and continued throughout the 8-week study. At a mean final dose of bupropion XL of 393 mg/day, there were no significant differences from placebo in the most common adverse events (Wilens et al., 2005).

Bupropion SR was used in a 6-week controlled trial in 59 outpatients (bupropion, n = 35; Reimherr et al., 2005). The mean daily dose was 298 mg, and the effect was measured with the WRAADDS and the CGI-I. The response criterion was a reduction of 50% or more in the total WRAADDS score and a rating of "much" or "very much" improved on the CGI-I. The results showed a nonsignificant numerical trend favoring bupropion SR (Reimherr et al., 2005).

A double-blind, three-arm, 12-week trial comparing methylphenidate SR or bupropion SR with placebo showed that the active agents did not provide a clear advantage over placebo in reducing ADHD symptoms or additional cocaine use in methadone-maintained patients (Levin et al., 2006). Patients were recruited from several community-based methadone programs. A total of 98 patients were enrolled (placebo, n = 33; methylphenidate, n = 32; bupropion, n = 33). The daily doses were up to 400 mg of bupropion SR and up to 80 mg of methylphenidate.

Based on these data, a random-effects meta-analysis calculated a pooled odds ratio of 2.42, indicating that individuals who used bupropion were 2.4 times more likely to have improved on the CGI-I scale compared with patients on placebo (Verbeeck et al., 2009).

In addition to these controlled studies, several open-label studies of bupropion for adult ADHD have been published. In a 6- to 8-week open study of ADHD adults, sustained improvements were documented among 10 of 19 patients at 1 year, at an average dose of 360 mg/day (Wender & Reimherr, 1990). Two open-label studies in ADHD adults with comorbid substance abuse disorders suggested that bupropion is effective in treating ADHD symptoms and has mild anticraving effects with regard to cocaine use (Levin et al., 2002; Wilens, Spencer, et al., 2001). A 6-week open-label study, including 35 patients with ADHD plus a history of bipolar disorder (predominantly Type II), found that bupropion SR (mean dose, 362 mg/day) was useful in relieving ADHD symptoms in 30 of 35 patients, without significantly activating mania (Wilens et al., 2003).

In addition to being a second-line agent in uncomplicated ADHD, bupropion might be considered preferentially when ADHD presents comorbidly with uni- or bipolar depression, substance use disorder, or unwanted smoking.

Lithium

One small preliminary study using a randomized, double-blind, crossover design examined the efficacy of MPH and lithium in treating ADHD in adults. In this study, 32 patients received 8 weeks of MPH and 8 weeks of lithium treatment. Both agents produced similar improvements on the CAARS and on measures of behavioral domains that are often disturbed in patients with ADHD, such as irritability, aggressive outbursts, antisocial behavior, anxiety, and depression. The methodology was limited by the possibility of carryover effects inherent to crossover studies, the absence of a placebo arm, a slow drug titration regimen, and possibly suboptimal dosing (Dorrego et al., 2002).

Miscellaneous compounds

The efficacy of most of the agents in the treatment of ADHD discussed in this section remains to be established.

One small open study indicated improvements in both ADHD symptoms and temper outbursts in adults receiving propranolol up to 640 mg a day

(Mattes, 1986), but studies under controlled conditions are lacking. In addition, this beta-adrenoreceptor antagonist has been used as a supplement to mitigate psychostimulant-induced adverse effects such as tremor, anxiety, or palpitations.

Selective serotonin reuptake inhibitors (SSRIs) do not appear to be effective for attenuating core ADHD symptoms. In a double-blind trial of paroxetine and/or dextro-amphetamine in adults with ADHD, intermediate term outcome measures showed paroxetine to have no effect on ADHD (Weiss & Hechtman, 2006).

Complex changes of dopaminergic neurotransmission, mostly antidopaminergic effects, have been described with SSRIs. Several authors demonstrated that a serotonergically mediated reduction of dopamine activity plays an important role in the reduction of human vigilance after SSRI administration (Damsa et al., 2004). One exception is sertraline, which does not produce a significant decline in vigilance performance, presumably because of its concomitant effects on dopamine activity, which counteracts the negative effects of serotonin on dopamine transmission (Schmitt et al., 2002).

An SSRI-induced amotivational syndrome may emerge after several weeks or months of SSRI treatment of obsessive compulsive disorder (OCD) and probably depression, both in adults and children (Hoehn-Saric et al. 1990, 1991). The apathy or amotivational syndrome is associated with other subtle cognitive effects and may aggravate the hypofrontal dysfunction that characterizes a large proportion of patients with ADHD. Combining an SSRI with either a psychostimulant or an antidepressant that has significant noradrenergic properties appears to provide sufficient improvement in frontal symptoms to allow continued SSRI treatment (Popper, 1997).

Venlafaxine is a phenylethylamine with a structure similar to amphetamine. As it blocks the reuptake of serotonin, norepinephrine, and dopamine at increasing dosages, its use at higher dosages could be conceptualized as intramolecular co-pharmacy. Venlafaxine appears to have a lower risk of inducing frontal apathy than the SSRIs, probably because of its adrenergic and dopaminergic properties, which may buffer the serotonin-induced "DA-dependent" side effects. A high response rate was reported in five open studies of ADHD adults, but high dropout rates and small numbers temper these preliminary results (Berigan, 2003). As the current data are uncontrolled, further prospective trials are needed to determine the effective dosage and time course of the effects of venlafaxine.

Numerous dopaminergic agonists including carbi/levodopa, piribedil, and amantadine failed to show any effect on ADHD symptoms. Controlled clinical studies on the effects of selective dopamine agonists such as ropinirole are lacking.

Neuroleptic medications, which block DA receptors, are reported not to worsen ADHD symptoms in naturalistic settings and may have modest efficacy in the treatment of ADHD (Pliszka. 2001). However, we consider their use to be undesirable because iatrogenic akathisia and mental dulling can mimic ADHD symptoms. There is preliminary evidence that the novel antipsychotics may exert a positive effect on executive functioning, possibly mediated by cholinergic transmission in the medial prefrontal cortex (Ichikawa et al., 2002) or stimulation of D1 receptors.

Combined pharmacotherapy

Combination treatment, in which nonstimulants usually function as an adjuvant, is indicated in a variety of clinical situations, including partial or inadequate response to monotherapy, treatment refractoriness, patients manifesting with comorbidity, stimulant-induced side effects, or the emergence of psychiatric symptoms during stimulant treatment. Practical guidelines pertaining to these issues are beyond the scope of this chapter and are discussed in depth elsewhere (Pliszka, 2003; Wilens & Spencer, 2000). Although combinations of stimulants and nonstimulants are often clinically necessary, studies regarding the safety and efficacy of using multiple agents simultaneously remain virtually nonexistent.

Conclusions

Thirty-one controlled trials with nonstimulant medications have so far been published. Effects seen in uncontrolled studies are in general better than in controlled trials (Wilens, 2003), so well-designed RCTs must be taken as references for the evaluation of the real benefits of medications for ADHD, as they are for other psychiatric disorders. Nonpatented drugs are also underinvestigated. Apart from trials with atomoxetine and bupropion XR, the sample sizes are rather small. Comorbid disorders are estimated to occur for approximately two-thirds of adult patients with ADHD. As most studies exclude patients with active comorbid disorders, the generalizability of findings in research populations will always be in question.

Some of the studies report improvement on a variety of neuropsychological batteries measuring executive functioning. Because of the structured settings in which these evaluations take place and the ability of ADHD patients to hyperfocus, we cannot assume that such "in vitro" improvements can be generalized to better daily functioning. Most studies are of relatively short duration, and except for studies with atomoxetine, few studies have evaluated the effects on real-life outcomes, such as social, occupational, and academic functioning. Methodological differences, such as low drug dosages, different equivalencies in dosing strategies, diversity in assessment tools measuring ADHD symptoms, and small sample sizes, may explain some of the discrepancies in these studies' outcomes. Studies of ADHD adults should use measures of functional impairment that are specific to adult roles and sensitive to drug effects. Symptomatic reduction does not suffice, as effectiveness is ultimately determined by improvements in functional outcomes. Because the residual symptoms that persist into adulthood gravitate from the behavioral toward the cognitive domain, future studies have to implement "real-life" outcome measures that reflect such a shift in symptomatology

There is sufficient empirical evidence that compounds such as atomoxetine and bupropion complement the therapeutic armamentarium of psychostimulants. First, they may be viable treatment alternatives in cases where stimulants are ineffective or cause intolerable side effects. Second, there is an overrepresentation of comorbid disorders in ADHD, manifesting as uni- or bipolar depression, anxiety disorders, and substance use disorders. All of these disorders are targets for nonstimulant drugs. Bupropion and atomoxetine should be considered when there are concerns about abuse or diversion of psychostimulants. Other advantages of nonstimulants include the fact that they are nonscheduled agents and thus refills are permissible (Horrigan, 2001). In addition to having a preferential role in the treatment of concurrent psychiatric pathology, they may be used as adjuvant to psychostimulants in refractory ADHD. Several emerging and investigational nonstimulants, such as modafinil, nicotine, and guanfacine, may augment the therapeutic choices, but larger and more long-term studies of these experimental findings are warranted.

To establish the exact niche for nonstimulants, additional data assessing long-term efficacy and safety of single and combination agents are required. High-quality head-to-head trials are needed and provide the best assessment of comparative effectiveness and safety among these agents. The likelihood that there is a differential response to stimulants and nonstimulants in specific treatment domains (ADHD subtype, emotional dysregulation) requires further exploration.

In the quest for alternative interventions for the treatment of ADHD, new agents will face several challenges to match the advantages that are the hallmark of the use of psychostimulants. Psychostimulants have a formidable effect size, are safe, and, because of the immediacy of their clinical impact, can be given according to dosing strategies, including drug holidays, that are tailored to individual needs. Furthermore, because patients with ADHD are notorious for being disorganized, forgetful, and impulsive, simplicity and convenience are paramount to any pharmacological intervention (Biederman et al., 2004). So far the nonstimulants are hampered by their inferior effect size to that of stimulants, the need for daily dosing to maintain their clinical efficacy, and a delay in onset of clinical effects. Therefore, they serve predominantly as second-line treatments with regard to the treatment of core symptomatology in uncomplicated ADHD.

It has been suggested that at least three different psychostimulants be considered before exploring nonstimulant alternatives for children and adolescents with ADHD. Unfortunately, comparable guidelines for adults with ADHD have yet to be developed (Pliszka et al., 2000). Moreover, treatment recommendations for prescribing hierarchies for adult ADHD vary among different guideline committees (Peterson et al., 2008). In view of these disagreements, uncertainty remains regarding optimal treatment selection.

The literature supports the notion that compounds that are ultimately effective in the treatment of this disorder influence the bioavailability of dopamine and norepinephrine, either directly or indirectly, in regions of the brain implicated in ADHD. However, because the involvement of other transmitters or modulators has been suggested in the complex pathophysiology of ADHD, avenues beyond those of catecholaminergic involvement are being investigated. The potential reservoir of "dysexecutive antidotes" includes agents that antagonize histamine-3 receptors, GABA-B antagonists, and ampakines, which operate via the glutamatergic receptors.

References

Adler L, Dietrich A, et al. (2006). Safety and tolerability of once versus twice daily atomoxetine in adults with ADHD. *Ann Clin Psychiatry* 18(2):107–13.

Adler LA, Liebowitz M, et al. (2009). Atomoxetine treatment in adults with attention-deficit/hyperactivity disorder and comorbid social anxiety disorder. *Depress Anxiety* 26(3):212–21.

Adler LA, Spencer TJ, Levine LR, et al. (2008). Functional outcomes in the treatment of adults with ADHD. *J Atten Disord* 11(6):720–7.

Adler LA, Spencer TJ, Williams DW, et al. (2008). Long-term, open-label safety and efficacy of atomoxetine in adults with ADHD: final report of a 4-year study. *J Atten Disord* 12(3):248–53.

Adler LA, Spencer TJ, et al. (2009). Once-daily atomoxetine for adult attention-deficit/hyperactivity disorder: a 6-month, double-blind trial. *J Clin Psychopharmacol* 29(1):44–50.

Adler LA, Sutton VK, et al. (2006). Quality of life assessment in adult patients with attention-deficit/hyperactivity disorder treated with atomoxetine. *J Clin Psychopharmacol* 26(6):648–52.

Arnsten AF, Cai JX, et al. (1988). The alpha-2 adrenergic agonist guanfacine improves memory in aged monkeys without sedative or hypotensive side effects: evidence for alpha-2 receptor subtypes. *J Neurosci* 8(11):4287–98.

Bangs ME, Jin L, et al. (2008). Hepatic events associated with atomoxetine treatment for attention-deficit hyperactivity disorder. *Drug Saf* 31(4):345–54.

Bangs ME, Tauscher-Wisniewski S, et al. (2008). Meta-analysis of suicide-related behavior events in patients treated with atomoxetine. *J Am Acad Child Adolesc Psychiatry* 47(2):209–18.

Berigan T. (2003). Off-label use of venlafaxine in psychiatric and non-psychiatric conditions. *Prim Psychiatry* 10:82–116.

Biederman J, Mick E, et al. (2006). A double-blind comparison of galantamine hydrogen bromide and placebo in adults with attention-deficit/hyperactivity disorder: a pilot study. *J Clin Psychopharmacol* 26(2):163–6.

Biederman J, Spencer T, Wilens T. (2004). Evidence-based pharmacotherapy for attention-deficit hyperactivity disorder. *Int J Neuropsychopharmacol* 7(1):77–97.

Bymaster FP, Katner JS, et al. (2002). Atomoxetine increases extracellular levels of norepinephrine and dopamine in prefrontal cortex of rat: a potential mechanism for efficacy in attention deficit/hyperactivity disorder. *Neuropsychopharmacology* 27(5):699–711.

Damsa C, Bumb A, et al. (2004). "Dopamine-dependent" side effects of selective serotonin reuptake inhibitors: a clinical review. *J Clin Psychiatry* 65(8):1064–8.

Deroche-Gamonet V, Darnaudery M, et al. (2002). Study of the addictive potential of modafinil in naive and cocaine-experienced rats. *Psychopharmacology (Berl)* 161(4):387–95.

Dorrego MF, Canevaro L, et al. (2002). A randomized, double-blind, crossover study of methylphenidate and lithium in adults with attention-deficit/hyperactivity disorder: preliminary findings. *J Neuropsychiatry Clin Neurosci* 14(3):289–95.

Ernst M, Liebenauer LL, et al. (1996). Selegiline in adults with attention deficit hyperactivity disorder: clinical efficacy and safety. *Psychopharmacol Bull* 32(3):327–34.

Ernst M, Liebenauer LL, et al. (1997). Selegiline in ADHD adults: plasma monoamines and monoamine metabolites. *Neuropsychopharmacology* 16(4):276–84.

Faraone SV, Biederman J, et al. (2005). Atomoxetine and Stroop task performance in adult attention-deficit/hyperactivity disorder. *J Child Adolesc Psychopharmacol* 15(4):664–70.

Faraone SV, Spencer T, et al. (2004). Meta-analysis of the efficacy of methylphenidate for treating adult attention-deficit/hyperactivity disorder. *J Clin Psychopharmacol* 24(1):24–9.

Friedman JI, Stewart DG, et al. (2004). Potential noradrenergic targets for cognitive enhancement in schizophrenia. *CNS Spectr* 9(5):350–5.

Gehricke JG, Whalen CK, et al. (2006). The reinforcing effects of nicotine and stimulant medication in the everyday lives of adult smokers with ADHD: a preliminary examination. *Nicotine Tob Res* 8(1):37–47.

Gobbi G, Slater S, et al. (2003). Neurochemical and psychotropic effects of bupropion in healthy male subjects. *J Clin Psychopharmacol* 23(3):233–9.

Greenhill LL, Pliszka S, et al. (2002). Practice parameter for the use of stimulant medications in the treatment of children, adolescents, and adults. *J Am Acad Child Adolesc Psychiatry* 41(2 suppl):26S–49S.

Hoehn-Saric R, Harris GJ, et al. (1991). A fluoxetine-induced frontal lobe syndrome in an obsessive compulsive patient. *J Clin Psychiatry* 52(3):131–3.

Hoehn-Saric R, Lipsey JR, et al. (1990). Apathy and indifference in patients on fluvoxamine and fluoxetine. *J Clin Psychopharmacol* 10(5):343–5.

Horrigan JP. (2001). Present and future pharmacotherapeutic options for adult attention deficit/hyperactivity disorder. *Expert Opin Pharmacother* 2(4):573–86.

Ichikawa J, Dai J, et al. (2002). Atypical, but not typical, antipsychotic drugs increase cortical acetylcholine release without an effect in the nucleus accumbens or striatum. *Neuropsychopharmacology* **26**(3): 325–39.

Ishizuka T, Sakamoto Y, et al. (2003). Modafinil increases histamine release in the anterior hypothalamus of rats. *Neurosci Lett* **339**(2):143–6.

Jakala P, Riekkinen M, et al. (1999). Guanfacine, but not clonidine, improves planning and working memory performance in humans. *Neuropsychopharmacology* **20**(5):460–70.

Kollins SH, MacDonald EK, et al. (2001). Assessing the abuse potential of methylphenidate in nonhuman and human subjects: a review. *Pharmacol Biochem Behav* **68**(3):611–27.

Kumar R. (2008). Approved and investigational uses of modafinil : an evidence-based review. *Drugs* **68**(13):1803–39.

Kuperman S, Perry PJ, et al. (2001). Bupropion SR vs. methylphenidate vs. placebo for attention deficit hyperactivity disorder in adults. *Ann Clin Psychiatry* **13**(3):129–34.

Leonard BE, McCartan D, et al. (2004). Methylphenidate: a review of its neuropharmacological, neuropsychological and adverse clinical effects. *Hum Psychopharmacol* **19**(3):151–80.

Levin ED. (1992). Nicotinic systems and cognitive function. *Psychopharmacology (Berl)* **108**(4):417–31.

Levin ED, Conners CK, et al. (1996). Nicotine effects on adults with attention-deficit/hyperactivity disorder. *Psychopharmacology (Berl)* **123**(1):55–63.

Levin ED, Conners CK, et al. (2001). Effects of chronic nicotine and methylphenidate in adults with attention deficit/hyperactivity disorder. *Exp Clin Psychopharmacol* **9**(1):83–90.

Levin FR, Evans SM, et al. (2002). Bupropion treatment for cocaine abuse and adult attention-deficit/hyperactivity disorder. *J Addict Dis* **21**(2):1–16.

Levin FR, Evans SM, et al. (2006). Treatment of methadone-maintained patients with adult ADHD: double-blind comparison of methylphenidate, bupropion and placebo. *Drug Alcohol Depend* **81**(2):137–48.

Lomasney JW, Lorenz W, et al. (1990). Expansion of the alpha 2-adrenergic receptor family: cloning and characterization of a human alpha 2-adrenergic receptor subtype, the gene for which is located on chromosome 2. *Proc Natl Acad Sci USA* **87**(13):5094–8.

Mattes JA. (1986). Propranolol for adults with temper outbursts and residual attention deficit disorder. *J Clin Psychopharmacol* **6**(5):299–302.

Mereu G, Yoon KW, et al. (1987). Preferential stimulation of ventral tegmental area dopaminergic neurons by nicotine. *Eur J Pharmacol* **141**(3):395–9.

Michelson D, Adler L, et al. (2003). Atomoxetine in adults with ADHD: two randomized, placebo-controlled studies. *Biol Psychiatry* **53**(2):112–20.

No benefit noted from Provigil (modafinil) in ADHD disorder [press release]. (2000, Jul. 31). West Chester, PA: Cephalon, Inc.

Peterson K, McDonagh MS, et al. (2008). Comparative benefits and harms of competing medications for adults with attention-deficit hyperactivity disorder: a systematic review and indirect comparison meta-analysis. *Psychopharmacology (Berl)* **197**(1):1–11.

Pliszka SR. (2001a). Comparing the effects of stimulant and non-stimulant agents on catecholamine function: implications for theories of attention deficit hyperactivity disorder. In: Solanto MV, Arnsten AFT, Castellanos FX, eds. *Stimulant Drugs and ADHD: Basic and Clinical Neurosciences*. Oxford: Oxford University Press: 332–52.

Pliszka SR. (2001b). New developments in psychopharmacology of attention deficit hyperactivity disorder. *Expert Opin Investig Drugs* **10**(10):1797–807.

Pliszka SR. (2003). Non-stimulant treatment of attention-deficit/hyperactivity disorder. *CNS Spectr* **8**(4):253–8.

Pliszka SR, Greenhill LL, et al. (2000). The Texas Children's Medication Algorithm Project: Report of the Texas Consensus Conference Panel on Medication Treatment of Childhood Attention-Deficit/Hyperactivity Disorder. Part II: Tactics. Attention-Deficit/Hyperactivity Disorder. *J Am Acad Child Adolesc Psychiatry* **39**(7):920–7.

Poltavski DV, Petros T. (2006). Effects of transdermal nicotine on attention in adult non-smokers with and without attentional deficits. *Physiol Behav* **87**(3): 614–24.

Pomerleau OF, Downey KK, et al. (1995). Cigarette smoking in adult patients diagnosed with attention deficit hyperactivity disorder. *J Subst Abuse* **7**(3): 373–8.

Popper CW. (1997). Antidepressants in the treatment of attention-deficit/hyperactivity disorder. *J Clin Psychiatry* **58**(suppl 14):14–29; discussion 30–1.

Popper CW. (2000). Pharmacologic alternatives to psychostimulants for the treatment of attention-deficit/hyperactivity disorder. *Child Adolesc Psychiatr Clin North Am* **9**(3):605–46, viii.

Reimherr FW, Hedges DW, et al. (2005). Bupropion SR in adults with ADHD: a short-term, placebo-controlled trial. *Neuropsychiatr Dis Treat* **1**(3):245–51.

Reimherr FW, Marchant BJ, et al. (2005). Emotional dysregulation in adult ADHD and response to atomoxetine. *Biol Psychiatry* **58**(2):125–31.

Scammell TE, Estabrooke IV, et al. (2000). Hypothalamic arousal regions are activated during modafinil-induced wakefulness. *J Neurosci* **20**(22):8620–8.

Schmitt JA, Ramaekers JG, et al. (2002). Additional dopamine reuptake inhibition attenuates vigilance impairment induced by serotonin reuptake inhibition in man. *J Psychopharmacol* **16**(3):207–14.

Simpson D, Plosker GL. (2004). Atomoxetine: a review of its use in adults with attention deficit hyperactivity disorder. *Drugs* **64**(2):205–22.

Spencer, T., J. Biederman, et al. (1998). Adults with attention-deficit/hyperactivity disorder: a controversial diagnosis. *J Clin Psychiatry* **59**(suppl 7):59–68.

Spencer T, Biederman J, et al. (2002). A double-blind comparison of desipramine and placebo in children and adolescents with chronic tic disorder and comorbid attention-deficit/hyperactivity disorder. *Arch Gen Psychiatry* **59**(7):649–56.

Spencer T, Biederman J, et al. (2004). Stimulant treatment of adult attention-deficit/hyperactivity disorder. *Psychiatr Clin North Am* **27**(2):361–72.

Stahl SM. (2002). Awakening to the psychopharmacology of sleep and arousal: novel neurotransmitters and wake-promoting drugs. *J Clin Psychiatry* **63**(6): 467–8.

Swanson JM. (2003). Role of executive function in ADHD. *J Clin Psychopharmacol* **64**(suppl 14):35–9.

Taylor FB, Russo J. (2000). Efficacy of modafinil compared to dextroamphetamine for the treatment of attention deficit hyperactivity disorder in adults. *J Child Adolesc Psychopharmacol* **10**(4):311–20.

Taylor FB, Russo J. (2001). Comparing guanfacine and dextroamphetamine for the treatment of adult attention-deficit/hyperactivity disorder. *J Clin Psychopharmacol* **21**(2):223–8.

Turner DC, Clark L, et al. (2004). Modafinil improves cognition and response inhibition in adult attention-deficit/hyperactivity disorder. *Biol Psychiatry* **55**(10):1031–40.

Verbeeck W, Tuinier S, et al. (2009). Antidepressants in the treatment of adult attention-deficit hyperactivity disorder: a systematic review. *Adv Ther* **26**(2): 170–84.

Weiss M, Hechtman L. (2006). A randomized double-blind trial of paroxetine and/or dextroamphetamine and problem-focused therapy for attention-deficit/hyperactivity disorder in adults. *J Clin Psychiatry* **67**(4): 611–9.

Wender PH, Reimherr FW. (1990). Bupropion treatment of attention-deficit hyperactivity disorder in adults. *Am J Psychiatry* **147**(8):1018–20.

Wender PH, Wood DR, et al. (1983). An open trial of pargyline in the treatment of attention deficit disorder, residual type. *Psychiatry Res* **9**(4):329–36.

Wernicke JF, Adler L, et al. (2004). Changes in symptoms and adverse events after discontinuation of atomoxetine in children and adults with attention deficit/hyperactivity disorder: a prospective, placebo-controlled assessment. *J Clin Psychopharmacol* **24**(1):30–5.

Wernicke JF, Faries D, et al. (2003). Cardiovascular effects of atomoxetine in children, adolescents, and adults. *Drug Saf* **26**(10):729–40.

Wilens TE. (2003). Drug therapy for adults with attention-deficit hyperactivity disorder. *Drugs* **63**(22):2395–411.

Wilens TE, Adler LA, et al. (2008). Atomoxetine treatment of adults with ADHD and comorbid alcohol use disorders. *Drug Alcohol Depend* **96**(1–2):145–54.

Wilens TE, Biederman J, et al. (1994). Clonidine for sleep disturbances associated with attention-deficit hyperactivity disorder. *J Am Acad Child Adolesc Psychiatry* **33**(3):424–6.

Wilens TE, Biederman J, et al. (1995). A systematic assessment of tricyclic antidepressants in the treatment of adult attention-deficit hyperactivity disorder. *J Nerv Ment Dis* **183**(1):48–50.

Wilens TE, Biederman J, et al. (1996). Six-week, double-blind, placebo-controlled study of desipramine for adult attention deficit hyperactivity disorder. *Am J Psychiatry* **153**(9):1147–53.

Wilens TE, Biederman J, et al. (1999). A pilot controlled clinical trial of ABT-418, a cholinergic agonist, in the treatment of adults with attention deficit hyperactivity disorder. *Am J Psychiatry* **156**(12):1931–7.

Wilens TE, Biederman J, et al. (2001). An open study of sustained release bupropion in adults with attention-deficit/hyperactivity disorder and substance use disorders. Paper presented at: 48th Annual Meeting of the Academy of Child and Adolescent Psychiatry; October 23–28; Honolulu.

Wilens TE, Haight BR, et al. (2005). Bupropion XL in adults with attention-deficit/hyperactivity disorder: a randomized, placebo-controlled study. *Biol Psychiatry* **57**(7):793–801.

Wilens TE, Prince JB, et al. (2003). An open trial of bupropion for the treatment of adults with attention-deficit/hyperactivity disorder and bipolar disorder. *Biol Psychiatry* **54**(1):9–16.

Wilens TE, Spencer TJ. (2000). The stimulants revisited. *Child Adolesc Psychiatr Clin North Am* **9**(3):573–603, viii.

Wilens TE, Spencer TJ, et al. (2001). A controlled clinical trial of bupropion for attention deficit hyperactivity disorder in adults. *Am J Psychiatry* **158**(2):282–8.

Wilens TE, Spencer TJ, et al. (2002). A review of the pharmacotherapy of adults with attention-deficit/hyperactivity disorder. *J Atten Disord* **5**(4):189–202.

Wilens TE, Verlinden MH, et al. (2006). ABT-089, a neuronal nicotinic receptor partial agonist, for the treatment of attention-deficit/hyperactivity disorder in adults: results of a pilot study. *Biol Psychiatry* **59**(11):1065–70.

Wilens TE, Waxmonsky J, Scott M, et al. (2005). An open trial of adjunctive donepezil in attention-deficit hyperactivity disorder. *J Child Adolesc Psychopharmacol* **15**(6):947–55.

Zerbe RL, Rowe H, et al. (1985). Clinical pharmacology of tomoxetine, a potential antidepressant. *J Pharmacol Exp Ther* **232**(1):139–43.

Medication management in adult ADHD

J. J. Sandra Kooij

Introduction

Once the diagnosis has been established, ADHD in adults is treated most effectively with a combined approach consisting of psychoeducation, medication, coaching, and cognitive behavioral therapy (Kooij, 2003; Safren et al., 2005; Solanto et al., 2007; Weiss et al., 2001). This chapter offers a practical guide to the medication management of ADHD in adults from a clinical point of view. It presents the following topics: opinions and fears about medication, the impact of not treating ADHD with medication, psychoeducation and the motivational approach, the order of treatment, available medications, combining stimulants and other medications, set-up with stimulants and other medications, appropriate dosing, measuring efficacy and the frequency of control visits, and dealing with noncompliance.

Opinions and fears about medication

The general public, as well as every patient and family member, may have an opinion about medication in general and about the use of medications for psychiatric disorders in particular. As the general public has not yet been very well informed about lifetime symptoms and impairment of ADHD in adulthood, family members and patients may be understandably hesitant about diagnosis and treatment (Corkum et al., 1999; Safer, 2000). To be able to address specific fears or misconceptions it is important to get to know each patient's attitude toward medication (Buitelaar, 2001; Hawthorne, 2007; McLeod et al., 2007). Patients may be very reluctant to use medications, and eagerness to get a prescription for stimulant medication has been seen very rarely in outpatient psychiatric clinics so far, although this may be different in substance use disorder clinics. When physicians or psychiatrists pro-

pose that patients use medication for their disorder(s), patients usually voice some of the following concerns: a fear of side effects, of losing control, or of being "poisoned" by chemical substances that will change their personal behavior; misinformation about the chance of addiction; being reminded that they have a disorder on a daily basis by taking medication; and moral skepticism and disapproval of having to take a pill for symptoms of inattention like laziness or being late. It may be useful to offer information about facts and myths regarding medication not only to the patient but also to his or her family.

Although stimulants are the most studied and most effective treatment for ADHD, their use, particularly in adults, remains controversial among mental health care professionals. With no standard education provided on ADHD in adults in medical training, reluctance and uncertainty about using drugs that are classified as control drugs, that are not licensed for use in adults, and that are related to substances of abuse are understandable. For a long time ADHD was considered to be a disorder limited to childhood, and doctors treating adult ADHD patients are generally resistant to the use of stimulants because they are not used to prescribing these medications in adults and because of unsubstantiated concerns over their abuse potential. This high level of resistance is not shared by child and adolescent mental health services that are aware of the potential benefits and relative safety of stimulants in children, although there was initial resistance to the use of stimulants in children when they were first introduced. It is an unusual scenario that a treatment considered suitable in children is not generally accepted for use in adults, and it creates a particular problem for individuals making the transition from child to adult psychiatric services. Continued research into the safety and efficacy of stimulants in

ADHD in Adults: Characterization, Diagnosis and Treatment, ed. Jan Buitelaar, Cornelis Kan and Philip Asherson.
Published by Cambridge University Press. © Cambridge University Press 2011.

adult patients and more effort to incorporate knowledge about adult ADHD into professional training and education are clearly of high priority.

Impact of not treating ADHD with medication

In clinical practice, one of the most frequently asked questions about medication is whether ADHD can be treated without it. The honest answer is "not really." After more than a decade of experience treating several hundred patients, positive results using psychoeducation, coaching, and psychotherapy without medication have been scarce. Clinical experience indicates that most patients forget appointments with their therapist if they are not being treated with medication, thereby interrupting their treatment. Patients may also be easily distracted from the treatment goals once another therapy comes along that seems more appealing. A substantial group of those patients who do not want to use medication for ADHD do not show up any more after 3 months. Others resist appropriate medication for years, during which they do not make any real progress. By letting the patient decide whether or not to take medication, the therapist may be suggesting that treatment options have equal outcome, which they do not. Leaving the decision to take medication to the patient alone may thus lead to a less favorable outcome. Not trying the most effective treatment for ADHD also cannot be defended when taking into account the scarcity of mental health services, the waiting lists of patients in need for treatment, and the inefficacy and costs associated with failed treatments.

In other words, the inattention symptoms of ADHD, if not addressed by medication, hinder appropriate treatment by causing the patient to fail to stick to an appointment schedule, remember or plan activities, or pay attention to the instructions of the therapist. At the same time, ADHD in adulthood usually has a great impact on several areas of daily functioning such as work performance, driving skills, relationships with friends and family, alcohol and drug abuse, self-esteem, handling of finances, sexuality, weight, sleep, and health in general. The lifetime symptoms and impairment of ADHD therefore justify the best treatment available, which many adults receive for the first time in their life.

Psychoeducation and a motivational approach

Mental health care professionals should explain to patients and family that the symptoms and impairment of ADHD can be treated effectively by medications and that the least they can do is let the patient try a course to see if it would be helpful. To help patients make up minds to take medication, professionals can share their experiences with treating patients who did not use medication and therefore failed to make progress. In addition, it may be very helpful for experienced patients who have benefited from using medication to explain to new patients the pros and cons of trying medication (Schuijers & Kooij, 2007). Patients may accept advice from fellow ADHD patients much easier than from their doctors. They can be reassured by knowing that they will always make the final decision whether to continue the medication, thereby increasing their experience of personal control. Information, provided both verbally and in a written handout, should be offered on these topics: the efficacy and safety of stimulants and other medications for ADHD, the order of treatment in case of comorbidity, dosing and timing, side effects, rebound symptoms after the medication wears off, dealing with sleep problems, the drawbacks of the concurrent use of alcohol or drugs, legal regulations regarding driving while using stimulants, the need for a statement from a physician when taking medication abroad, the need to stop the use of stimulants in case of pregnancy, and the responsible use of the prescribed medication; that is, the risk of abuse of stimulants by others or by injecting or snorting the (short-acting) medication (Weiss et al., 2001).

Order of treatment in comorbid ADHD

In epidemiological as well as clinical populations, ADHD in adults is highly comorbid. The most frequently diagnosed comorbid disorders are anxiety, mood, sleep, substance use, and personality disorders (Biederman et al. 1993; Fayyad et al., 2007; Kooij, Aeckerlin, et al., 2001; Kooij et al., 2004; McGough et al., 2005).

Anxiety, mood, and substance use disorders are generally treated first, because their symptoms are often more disabling and may interfere with a proper evaluation of the efficacy of the ADHD medications. However, where ADHD and personality disorder occur together, treatment of ADHD can effectively diminish problems of inattention, impulsivity, mood swings, and associated aggressive behavior and may lead to increased adherence to other treatment programs, such as psychotherapy for personality disorders. Therefore, treatment of ADHD is usually advised before starting treatment of personality disorders.

The order of treatment is important in anxiety patients. Comorbid anxiety disorders must be treated first, as the tachycardia that may accompany stimulant treatment may increase symptoms of anxiety. Anxious patients may easily become fearful of a slightly higher pulse rate, thereby increasing their feelings of panic. After such an experience, these patients will be very reluctant to try stimulants again. Once the anxiety disorder is successfully treated with an antidepressant, these phenomena usually do not occur or to a much lesser extent. To our knowledge, the effects of cognitive behavioral therapy on the experience of anxiety while using stimulants have never been studied. According to clinical experience, antidepressants can be well combined with stimulants. Atomoxetine may be another option for ADHD treatment in patients with anxiety (Turgay, 2006).

An irritable mood, changing four to five times a day, is seen in 90% of adults with ADHD and is not usually the consequence of comorbid depression or bipolar disorder (Kooij, Middelkoop, et al., 2001). In this case treatment should be targeted at the ADHD. In contrast, depression and chronic dysthymia frequently accompany ADHD and deserve treatment priority as they are usually prominent and cause severe impairment. In addition, a depressed patient may have a negative attitude in general, and therefore it may be difficult to observe positive effects of the ADHD medication. After remission of the depressive episode, stimulants may be added to the antidepressant medication.

Bipolar patients with ADHD should be treated first with a mood stabilizer as their (hypo)manic symptoms may exacerbate while using antidepressants, stimulants, or the combination of both. Mood stabilizers may protect against this unwanted effect. Psychotic symptoms should be diagnosed and treated first using conventional antipsychotic medication.

In most cases substance use disorders should be treated first because of the known risks and impairments associated with them. Ongoing substance abuse will interfere with evaluation of ADHD treatment response, interactions will emerge, and side effects can be intensified. Therefore all substance use should be minimized before the start of medication for ADHD. Patients are instructed to reduce their intake of alcohol and drugs to a certain level, and only after they do so can they start the ADHD medication; after that, intake is further reduced. Because many people with ADHD used alcohol or drugs to reduce ADHD symptoms such as restlessness, inattention, or irritability, it may be easier for them to reach the ultimate goal of stopping alcohol/drug use when using ADHD medication. Many patients report they can refrain from substance use with the use of ADHD medication.

Patients have to record their intake of substances before the start of and during medication treatment, until the physician and the patient agree on the data. Generally, patients who indicate they cannot limit their alcohol beverages should drink no more. Others who can stop after one or two drinks may use this limited amount of alcohol only on the weekends or at social occasions, thereby inducing a pattern of intermittent alcohol intake. Although there are no data to support the exact number of beverages allowed, this rule may offer some practical guidance to patients and doctors as how to deal with drinking alcohol while on medication.

Likewise, cannabis use is widespread among ADHD adults and, according to clinical experience, one of the most difficult addictions to deal with. Patients may smoke many cannabis cigarettes per day, usually to treat their restlessness and sleep problems, but doing so may lead to a reversed day-and-night rhythm. They should be instructed about the detrimental effects of cannabis on their attention and daily rhythm and encouraged to reduce the number of cannabis cigarettes smoked and to record them daily. When the lowest level the patient can handle has been reached, the ADHD medication is started and then the number of cigarettes is cut back further. Usually patients keep on using one cannabis cigarette to get to sleep, although this is not preferable. Melatonin may be more appropriate for the delayed sleep phase disorder with which many adults with ADHD seem to be afflicted. However, more research in this field is needed before clinical guidelines can be given on dosage and timing of melatonin for sleep-onset problems in adults with ADHD (Rybak et al. 2006, 2007; Van der Heijden et al., 2007).

Hard drugs must be stopped completely before ADHD medication is started. However, patients do not need to be clean for a long time before they can start, as this requirement would reduce the chances of their getting effective treatment for ADHD.

Clinical experience supports the view that treatment of ADHD with stimulants may diminish the need for substance use in adults. A recent study and meta-analysis of previous studies confirmed reports that treatment of ADHD with stimulants does indeed reduce the risk of substance abuse in adolescents (Wilens, Faraone, et al., 2003). The concerns of some professionals that use of stimulants in ADHD may lead to drug abuse (a gateway hypothesis) are not supported by available evidence, but more research on the effects of medication on ADHD and possible abstinence of substance abuse is needed in adults.

Available medications

ADHD symptoms in adults as well as in children can be treated effectively with medications. The stimulants (methylphenidate or dexamphetamine) are dopaminergic and noradrenergic agonists and are the first-choice treatments for ADHD in both children and adults. Numerous studies have shown the beneficial effects of stimulant medication on the core symptoms of ADHD in children and adolescents (Prince, 2006; Wilens, Biederman, et al., 1995). The number of drug trials in adults is far lower than that for childhood ADHD, but they consistently demonstrate similar response rates up to 78% (Biederman et al., 2006; Conners, 2002; Kooij et al., 2004; Paterson et al., 1999; Prince & Wilens, 2002; Spencer et al., 2001, 2005). Several short- and long-acting formulations of methylphenidate and dexamphetamine are available, as well as nonstimulants like atomoxetine, a long-acting noradrenergic reuptake inhibitor proven effective and licensed for ADHD symptoms in children but only in adults when treatment was initiated in childhood or adolescence (Michelson et al., 2003; Turgay, 2006). Nevertheless, because both stimulants and atomoxetine are effective in adults with ADHD, experts in the management of adult ADHD recommend their clinical use, both for individuals who started treatment in childhood/adolescence and for those receiving a first-time diagnosis of ADHD in adulthood (Banaschewski et al., 2006).

The long-acting antidepressant and dopaminergic agonist, bupropion hydrochloride XL, has been licensed for smoking cessation and depression and, although not licensed for ADHD, has shown efficacy for ADHD in controlled trials in children,

adolescents, and adults (Cantwell, 1998; Reimherr et al., 2005; Solhkhah et al., 2005; Waxmonsky, 2005; Wilens, Haight, et al., 2005; Wilens, Spencer, et al., 2001). Other options may be modafinil, licensed for narcolepsy; tricyclic antidepressants; reboxetine, a selective norepinephrine reuptake inhibitor (SNRI); and the alpha-2-agonists, guanfacine and clonidine, although they have been less studied and have shown less efficacy in ADHD than the medications mentioned earlier (Biederman et al., 2004; Ratner et al., 2005). There are some preliminary studies indicating efficacy of nicotinic receptor agonists for the cognitive dysfunction in ADHD (Wilens & Decker, 2007).

All of these medications are available in the United States, although those in the rest of the world may have fewer options. Most medications are still only licensed for use in children and adolescents, but this may change in the future. Medication studies in adults with ADHD for the purpose of registration are ongoing, leading to more treatment options for adults with ADHD in other countries around the world.

Combining stimulants and other medications

Recently, there has been increasing interest in combining nonstimulant therapies with stimulants to further enhance treatment effects (Waxmonsky, 2005). Data on the combined use of antidepressants or mood stabilizers and stimulants are still scarce, but clinical experience suggests that the combinations are effective and safe (Kafka & Hennen, 2000; Weiss et al., 2001). Although it is possible to introduce two medications at the same time, it is usually advisable to introduce one at a time. Doing so facilitates evaluation of each medication and helps the patient understand for which disorder he or she is taking the medication.

Serotonergic reuptake inhibitors (SSRIs) and tricyclic antidepressants (TCAs) for anxiety or depression may be combined with stimulants for ADHD. Because stimulants may increase the blood concentration of TCAs, the level of TCAs should be established and the dose adjusted if necessary (Weiss & Hechtman, 1993). After a depressive episode is remitted, the hyperactive symptoms of ADHD may return and become more prominent, sometimes suggesting even a hypomanic episode. However, if this reflects normal hyperactive behavior, the patient will be able to tell that it is the normal state, just as he or she felt before the depressive episode began. Obviously, a hypomanic episode is a possibility in patients susceptible to bipolar disorder, and careful evaluation is needed in such cases.

Mood stabilizers can be combined with stimulants or atomoxetine according to some studies of treatment-refractory bipolar depression treated with stimulants, as well as clinical experience in ADHD children and adults with bipolar disorder (Carlson et al., 2004; Hah & Chang, 2005; Lydon & El-Mallakh, 2006; Scheffer et al., 2005; Wilens, Spencer, et al., 1995). Data on the combined use of atomoxetine and stimulants or antidepressants are still lacking (Adler et al., 2006).

In general the use of stimulants (dopamine agonists) is not advised for treatment of ADHD with comorbid psychotic symptoms, and in a few cases stimulants may trigger a relapse (or first episode) of a psychotic illness. Nonstimulant treatments for ADHD, like noradrenaline reuptake inhibitors (atomoxetine, reboxetine) or the tricyclic antidepressants, could be considered in such cases. In some cases stimulants have been used alongside traditional antipsychotics and, despite the apparent contradiction in such a regime, have been successful in controlling both conditions. For this reason it may be reasonable to maintain such a combination where it has already been initiated and appears to be successful.

Set-up with stimulants, atomoxetine, and bupropion XL

Before starting the use of stimulants, the presence of contraindications like pregnancy and (a history of) psychosis must be verified. In pregnant women the use of hard drugs like heroin or amphetamines results in an increased incidence of prematurity, low birthweight, intrauterine growth retardation, and microcephaly. Congenital anomalies were found in 2.8% of amphetamine-exposed infants (Thaithumyanon et al., 2005). The risk of congenital birth defects using stimulants for ADHD during pregnancy in adult women is not known, as no studies have been performed in this group (Rayburn & Bogenschutz, 2004). In general, there are insufficient data about the effects of stimulants on the fetus during pregnancy; this knowledge will only increase through the publication of case reports of individual patients who have used stimulants during pregnancy (2005). Trying to get pregnant may not be regarded as a contraindication to stimulant treatment, as a stimulant can easily be discontinued immediately after an early pregnancy test turns out positive. In that situation, exposure to the stimulant will thus be limited to the first 2 weeks of pregnancy. This risk of exposure has to be weighed against the risk of not treating the ADHD, which may lead to conflicts in relationships, including the relationship with the partner. These risks must be discussed with the patient and partner in advance.

As mentioned earlier, a (history of) psychosis limits the use of stimulants as they may induce a relapse of a psychotic episode. However, careful evaluation of the nature of the psychotic episode may be helpful because there are different treatment options for a bipolar versus a schizophrenic psychotic episode. In patients with a bipolar disorder, stimulants may be combined with mood stabilizers, whereas in patients with schizophrenia, antipsychotics are the first choice and may be more appropriately used with atomoxetine, bupropion XL, or a TCA. However, sometimes patients do improve with a combination of an antipsychotic and a stimulant, and in such cases treatment may be continued.

Relative contraindications for stimulants are hyperthyroidism, high blood pressure, cardiac rhythm abnormalities, glaucoma, seizures or epilepsy, and tics. These disorders must be treated first, and after consultation with the attending physician, stimulant treatment may be added.

As stated earlier, comorbid anxiety, mood, and substance use disorders have to be treated first as well. As soon as the comorbid disorder is in remission, the stimulant for ADHD is added, usually to an SSRI or TCA. A short physical exam including blood pressure, pulse, and weight is required before starting the medication, and these parameters are repeated during treatment. An electrocardiogram is only performed in case of a history of or existing cardiac disease. During treatment the pulse will increase; blood pressure may remain unchanged, decrease, or increase; and weight usually decreases (without additional caloric intake, mean weight loss is 1–2 kg in the first few weeks; Kooij et al., 2004; Wilens, Hammerness, et al., 2005).

It is important to discuss the most common side effects with the patient, such as headache in the first few days, loss of appetite and weight, nervousness, palpitations or tachycardia, sleeping problems, and dry mouth. If the patient loses more weight than is considered appropriate, he or she may be instructed to eat regularly even in the absence of appetite; otherwise the medication may have to be discontinued. If blood pressure increases while using a stimulant but the stimulant is needed because it is effective for ADHD, the blood pressure may need to be treated as well. Patients developing higher blood pressure while using stimulants, who often have a family history of hypertension and cardiac disease, may in fact be detected earlier than they otherwise would have been. Patients complaining of nervousness or edginess may benefit from a lower dose of the stimulant, whereas patients who get anxious or panicky may be those with a previously undiagnosed comorbid anxiety disorder. The anxiety disorder can be treated effectively by stopping the stimulant, starting an SSRI, and then adding the stimulant again. Persistent tachycardia that is not accompanied by anxiety symptoms may be well treated by a low dose of propanolol or another beta blocker.

According to clinical experience in an outpatient population of more than one thousand adult patients with ADHD, stimulants are seldom abused. However, in the case of abuse, the prescription should be stopped. Long-acting methylphenidate formulations that protect against possible abuse may be preferred, or atomoxetine or bupropion XL may be used.

Sleep onset may be more difficult when using a stimulant, although most patients report they sleep better using this medication (Boonstra et al., 2007; Kooij, Middelkoop, et al., 2001). Moreover, the majority of adult patients, like children with ADHD, may have suffered from chronic sleep-onset problems before starting the medication. Because these problems usually are of the delayed sleep phase type, careful assessment of sleeping patterns and problems may be useful beforehand (Van der Heijden et al., 2005).

However, the most important side effect to inform the patient about is the emergence of so-called rebound symptoms after the medication wears off. During this period of 1 to 2 hours, the symptoms of ADHD may increase temporarily, leading to tiredness, irritability, restlessness, impulsivity, and a drop in concentration. After this short period, the symptoms of ADHD return to their usual level of severity. These rebound symptoms are not only unwanted but also may be even more severe than the disorder for which the medication was taken. Likely, rebound symptoms are the side effects that are discussed most among patients and that may have generated negative press about stimulants. Patients need to understand in advance the difference between effects during the time the medication is working and after it wears off. Therefore the duration of effectiveness of every stimulant

preparation has to be explained to patients so they can distinguish side effects from rebound symptoms.

Rebound symptoms can be treated effectively by taking another dose of the stimulant until bedtime, when the medication is supposed to wear off. Stimulant preparations that are effective during an adult 16-hour day are lacking, so it may be an art to titrate for every individual patient the proper dosage and timing of the stimulant needed to treat symptoms in an optimal way during the day and evening, with little or no side effects, no negative impact on sleep, and no rebound.

The problem is caused by the short time in which most stimulants have an effect, varying from 2–4 hours per dose of short-acting methylphenidate, to 5–8 hours per dose of other longer acting methylphenidate preparations, to 8–12 hours per tablet of long-acting osmotic-release oral system (OROS) methylphenidate. Adults usually want to be active during a 16-hour day, and we currently lack appropriate stimulant preparations for this length of time. Matching stimulant preparations with different pharmacokinetic profiles, resulting in different periods of effectiveness, with the individual metabolism of the patient may enable optimal dosing for adults.

The nonstimulant atomoxetine, which works for 24 hours, does not produce the side effect of rebound symptoms and may be considered in those patients who cannot comply with the dosing regime of the stimulants. Atomoxetine may also be prescribed to patients with comorbid anxiety, substance use disorders, or a history of psychosis (Turgay, 2006). Its most common side effects, which should be discussed with the patient, are the suppression of appetite, nausea, headache, lowered sexual drive and performance, and somnolence. Because 2D6 inhibitors (e.g. paroxetine and fluoxetine) may increase atomoxetine plasma levels, caution should be used when they are co-administered. Atomoxetine is contraindicated in patients who have taken MAO inhibitors within 15 days and in those with narrow-angle glaucoma; the drug should be used with caution in patients with hypertension, hypotension, tachycardia, cardiovascular or cerebrovascular disease, or urinary retention. In patients with impaired autonomic function, atomoxetine, which is a norepinephrine transporter blocker, was shown to induce dramatic increases in blood pressure (Shibao et al., 2007).

Another nonstimulant with proven efficacy for ADHD is long-acting bupropion XL. This medication also has a 24-hour profile and may be indicated in ADHD and comorbid depression, bipolar disorder, or substance use disorders (Solhkhah et al., 2005; Wilens, Haight, et al., 2005; Wilens, Spencer, et al., 2001). Bupropion XL is licensed for smoking cessation and depression and has shown efficacy for ADHD in children as well as adults in randomized controlled trials. Another advantage of bupropion XL is that it has been associated with fewer sexual side effects and less induction of (hypo)manic episodes than SSRIs (Wilens, Prince, et al., 2003). Side effects are weight loss, dry mouth, nausea, difficulty sleeping, dizziness, sore throat, constipation, and a dose-dependent increased risk of epileptic seizures. Using 300 mg bupropion XL the chance of seizures is 0.1%; using a dose above 400 mg increases the chance to 0.4%. Therefore, it is advised not to prescribe this medication to patients with a history of seizures without consultation with a neurologist. Bupropion XL is a moderate 2D6 inhibitor, leading to higher concentrations of concomitant medications that are metabolized by 2D6, such as venlafaxine, nortriptyline, and desipramine.

Appropriate dosing

The usual initial dose of short-acting methylphenidate is given six times a day, or a 10-mg tablet every 2–4 hours: at 8:00 am, 12:00 pm, 4:00 pm, and 8:00 pm. Short-acting dexamphetamine tablets of 5 mg are given three to four times a day, every 4–5 hours: at 8:00 am, 12:00 pm, 4:00 pm, and 8:00 pm. After one week the dose and frequency of dosing may be adjusted according to effects and side effects. Most patients need sustained medication treatment until bedtime to prevent rebound symptoms in the evening or just before going to bed. The effects of short-acting stimulants start within 30 minutes and continue (depending on dose and individual pharmacokinetic profiles) for around 2–4 hours for short-acting methylphenidate and a little longer for dexamphetamine. Titration to an effective dose is important (Faraone et al., 2004). Doses are titrated in 3 weeks, from 0.5 mg up to 1.0 mg/k/day for methylphenidate and from 0.25 mg up to 0.5mg/k/day for dexamphetamine, to ensure adequate coverage for adults (Kooij et al., 2004; Spencer, Biederman, et al., 2005). The dose of dexamphetamine is usually half of the dose of methylphenidate, as the strength of dexamphetamine is twice that of methylphenidate (Elia et al., 1991). The most common dose range

used in European adult ADHD clinics is 10–20 mg of immediate-release methylphenidate, taken four to six times daily, or dexamphetamine 10–15 mg, three to four times a day, with both higher and lower dosing required in individual cases. It is thus necessary to take a dose every 2–4 hours throughout the day to obtain a sustained effect.

Because patients need to take medication on time at least four to six times per day between 8:00 am and 11:00 pm, they should use a timer. Forgetting a dose or taking it too late usually results in a temporary increase in ADHD symptoms due to rebound. This unwanted effect may lead to a roller coaster of ADHD symptoms, which decrease and increase throughout the day. The need to take a dose so often and on time in adults whose main complaints are forgetfulness and distractibility has been the greatest obstacle for compliance to treatment (Kooij et al., 2004; Perwien et al., 2004; Steinhoff, 2004). Compliance problems are therefore the main limitation to the effectiveness of short-acting stimulants in adult patients.

To increase the ease of taking stimulants, improve compliance, and smooth out medication effects, long-acting preparations are now available and need to be taken only once or twice a day. This is particularly useful for adults with ADHD who, in contrast to children, are supposed to organize their own medication management.

The use of sustained-release stimulants has been less extensively investigated in the adult ADHD population, but their similar effect sizes to immediate-release methylphenidate suggest that the guidelines for their use in older children and adolescents may be followed for adults. As with immediate-release preparations, titration to a clinically effective dose is required. In a large placebo-controlled trial of OROS methylphenidate in 141 adult patients with *DSM-IV* ADHD, dosage could be titrated up to 1.3 mg/k/day. The average daily dose used in this study was 72 mg, and the maximum was 108 mg per day (Biederman et al., 2006). This dose range is in accordance with clinical experience in adults.

With the availability of several longer acting formulations of methylphenidate, new combinations can be tried to cover the full 16-hour day of an adult patient. Although these formulations have not all been studied in adults and they contain different percentages of both immediate- and sustained-release forms of the medication designed for use in the morning, early clinical experience indicates that OROS methylphenidate and methylphenidate formulations that work for 5–8 hours may be combined effectively. For fast metabolizers who experience rebound symptoms at 3:00 pm after taking OROS methylphenidate in the early morning, another dose of OROS methylphenidate may be appropriate without inducing sleep problems or rebound symptoms around bedtime. When OROS methylphenidate wears off at 5:00 pm, adding another longer acting methylphenidate formulation that works for around 5–6 hours is advised. When combining different methylphenidate formulations to cover an adult day and evening, higher dosages per day may be reached than in the past. Therefore, careful monitoring of pulse, blood pressure, weight, efficacy, rebound symptoms, and side effects, as well as sleep, is necessary. The most important goal is to prevent rebound symptoms during the day and at bedtime. If needed a half-tablet of 10-mg short-acting methylphenidate just before bedtime may reduce rebound symptoms, after which the patient may be quiet enough to fall asleep.

Atomoxetine is started at 40 mg and, depending on side effects, increased in 1 to 2 weeks to 80–100 mg/day. The maximum dosage is 1.2–1.4 mg/kg/day. Efficacy evolves gradually, and it may take 6 weeks on the highest dose before clinical effects of atomoxetine emerge. Patients have to be informed in advance as this action is much slower than with the stimulants.

Bupropion XL is started once daily at 150 mg and increased weekly to 300 mg and then up to 450 mg if needed. Efficacy may evolve after 2 weeks on the highest dose.

Measuring efficacy and the frequency of control visits

Stimulants work within 30 minutes of intake, but may be evaluated with the patient after 1 week by telephone and after 2 weeks during a visit. The patient may need a bit more time to experience and to interpret the effects of the medication on his or her behavior in different settings. Typical patient reports of the initial effects of the stimulant medication include being able to read for a longer time, being more organized, finding it easier to make decisions and to clear a desktop or clean up a room, less impulsive and stressful driving, and reduced irritability. To monitor the effects of the medication, instruments like the self-report ADHD Rating Scale (DuPaul et al., 1998), the investigator-based Clinical Global Impressions CGI; (Kooij et al., 2004; NIMH,

1985), or other personalized lists of target symptoms and side effects may be used at baseline and after 1 and 2 weeks of medication use. After 1 week the dose may be increased if there is no or minimal effect and little side effects. After 2 weeks this dosage is evaluated, and side effects, blood pressure, weight, and pulse are checked. It is important to determine with the patient the time of the day when side effects occur to establish the difference between side effects that happen when the medication is actually working and rebound symptoms that may emerge after the medication wears off. Side effects that usually occur are appetite suppression, 1–2 kg weight loss, tachycardia and nervousness, and difficulty falling asleep (either caused by preexisting sleep-onset problems, the medication still working, or the medication wearing off at that time). Some patients have an increased feeling of depression because they have more insight into their situation since using the medication, or the improved cognitive functioning brought about by medication use may enable them to see the chaos that lays behind and ahead. This may lead to demoralization that has to be addressed and explained. Another possibility may be a subsyndromal depression becoming more obvious during stimulant treatment. Depressive episodes should be treated with a antidepressant.

Sometimes hypomanic symptoms emerge, especially during combined treatment of a stimulant with venlafaxine in patients susceptible for bipolar disorder. In that case the antidepressant and sometimes also the stimulant may be discontinued, and a mood stabilizer has to be started. After stabilization of the hypomanic episode, depending on the need for antidepressant or stimulant treatment, both may be reconsidered while continuing the mood stabilizer.

When anxiety emerges or increases using a stimulant, adding an SSRI is safe according to clinical experience and usually effective. In case of persistent tachycardia without anxiety, a low dose of propanolol may be helpful.

A patient who feels like "a zombie" using methylphenidate may be a nonresponder, as the stimulant should increase alertness and not induce sleepiness or lethargy. In that case dexamphetamine may be tried, as these stimulants have a different way of action in the brain. Methylphenidate is a reuptake inhibitor of dopamine and noradrenaline, whereas dexamphetamine increases the release of both neurotransmitters. In a patient, one or both can be effective (Elia et al., 1991).

As soon as the patient and physician agree on the proper dosage for optimal effect and minimal side effects, the timing of the medication is appropriate during an adult 16-hour day, and the patient has no further questions regarding the medication, the frequency of control visits can be reduced to every 1 to 3 months. Periodic control of blood pressure, pulse, and weight is useful (Wilens, Hammerness, et al., 2005). In case of relapse or lack of treatment progress, the possibility of alcohol or drug abuse should be discussed with the patient. Ongoing alcohol and drug abuse are frequent reasons for noncompliance and treatment dropout. However, when the patient benefits from the medication, the psychological treatment usually becomes more important and effective, addressing acceptance of the disorder and treatment and learning skills to organize oneself more successfully.

Patients may ask whether it is necessary to take the medication everyday. To keep up their motivation for continued medication use, some patients at times like to feel the difference between being on and off the medication. Others want to stop the medication on the weekends so they can use alcohol or drugs. This may not be a good exchange. It is important to explain to the patient that ADHD is a chronic disabling disorder that affects not only the work or school setting but that also influences cognition, memory, mood, vitality, and initiative every day. Maintaining social contacts, keeping appointments, doing long-range planning, driving, being able to organize oneself while running the household, handling the finances, shopping, and the like are all usually performed less well without medication. Medication for ADHD should therefore be taken every day and not on demand.

Driving and stimulant use

Driving while using a stimulant is a relatively new phenomenon for adult psychiatry and for the driving license agency. Although clinical experience indicates that patients with ADHD drive better while using a stimulant and several controlled studies point in the same direction, the final study on this subject has not yet been published (Cox, Humphrey, et al., 2004; Cox, Merkel, et al., 2004; Barkley & Cox, 2007; Barkley et al., 2005). Therefore, depending on the legal regulations in different countries, driving may be allowed under certain conditions. In the Netherlands, for instance, stimulants for ADHD are allowed if an experienced psy-

chiatrist has examined the patient regarding compliance, dosing, and timing of the medication and eventual rebound symptoms. The recommendation of the psychiatrist is sent to the driving license agency, who decides whether the patient can drive. Sometimes an additional driving test is required. As rebound symptoms while driving are considered dangerous for road safety in general, inadequate dosing should be avoided. If dosing or timing is not appropriate, the patient is declared unfit and is advised to use long-acting methylphenidate or atomoxetine. He or she may return for a second examination after following the revised treatment plan.

Dealing with noncompliance

Noncompliance to medication usually occurs when the patient uses a short-acting stimulant that has to be taken several times a day and forgets to take it because of the cognitive disabilities that accompany ADHD. Long-acting medication may therefore be a relief to the patient as well as the physician, who can discuss other topics during consultation than forgetfulness and the resulting noncompliance. Treatment is more successful and the patient makes more and faster progress when the medication is taken. Another problem resulting in noncompliance is when the patient has difficulty accepting the disorder and the need for medication. The perceptions of the patient (and partner or family) regarding what it means to have ADHD, to have to take medication on a daily basis for years, and not to be able to function well without it have to be addressed. Some patients never comply before this subject has been really discussed and they have had the opportunity to mourn what may be called "the loss of (the illusion of) the normal self."

Patients often ask how long they will have to take medication for ADHD. Pharmacological treatment of ADHD does not cure the disorder as symptoms return immediately after discontinuation of the medication. Therefore lifetime medication is a possibility in many cases and needs to be reviewed at regular intervals. Regular follow-up of the need for stimulant medication should be done at least once every few years. If the medication is discontinued, evaluation of the level of symptoms and of psychosocial functioning off medication for a few months should facilitate the decision how to proceed. If symptoms return and lead to impairment in work and/or social relationships, continued prescription of medication is advised.

References

Adler LA, Reingold LS, et al. (2006). Combination pharmacotherapy for adult ADHD. *Curr Psychiatry Rep* 8(5):409–15.

Banaschewski T, Coghill D, et al. (2006). Long-acting medications for the hyperkinetic disorders. A systematic review and European treatment guideline. *Eur Child Adolesc Psychiatry* 15(8):476–95.

Barkley RA, Cox D. (2007). A review of driving risks and impairments associated with attention-deficit/hyperactivity disorder and the effects of stimulant medication on driving performance. *J Safety Res* 38(1):113–28.

Barkley RA, Murphy KR, et al. (2005). Effects of two doses of methylphenidate on simulator driving performance in adults with attention deficit hyperactivity disorder. *J Safety Res* 36(2):121–31.

Biederman J, Faraone SV, et al. (1993). Patterns of psychiatric comorbidity, cognition, and psychosocial functioning in adults with attention deficit hyperactivity disorder. *Am J Psychiatry* 150(12):1792–8.

Biederman J, Mick E, et al. (2006). A randomized, placebo-controlled trial of OROS methylphenidate in adults with attention-deficit/hyperactivity disorder. *Biol Psychiatry* 59(9):829–35.

Biederman J, Spencer T, et al. (2004). Evidence-based pharmacotherapy for attention-deficit hyperactivity disorder. *Int J Neuropsychopharmacol* 7(1): 77–97.

Boonstra AM, Kooij JJS, et al. (2007). Hyperactive night and day? Actigraphy studies in adult ADHD: baseline comparison and the effect of methylphenidate. *Sleep* 30(4):433–42.

Buitelaar JK. (2001). Discussion of attention deficit-hyperactivity disorder (ADHD): facts, opinions and emotions. *Ned Tijdschr Geneeskd* 145(31):1485–9 [in Dutch].

Cantwell DP. (1998). ADHD through the life span: the role of bupropion in treatment. *J Clin Psychiatry* 59(suppl 4): 92–4.

Carlson PJ, Merlock MC, et al. (2004). Adjunctive stimulant use in patients with bipolar disorder: treatment of residual depression and sedation. *Bipolar Disord* 6(5):416–20.

Conners CK. (2002). Forty years of methylphenidate treatment in Attention-Deficit/Hyperactivity Disorder. *J Atten Disord* 6(suppl 1): S17–30.

Corkum P, Rimer P, et al. (1999). Parental knowledge of attention-deficit hyperactivity disorder and opinions of treatment options: impact on enrollment and adherence to a 12-month treatment trial. *Can J Psychiatry* 44(10):1043–8.

Cox DJ, Humphrey JW, et al. (2004). Controlled-release methylphenidate improves attention during on-road driving by adolescents with attention-deficit/hyperactivity disorder." *J Am Board Fam Pract* 17(4):235–9.

Cox DJ, Merkel RL, et al. (2004). Impact of methylphenidate delivery profiles on driving performance of adolescents with attention-deficit/hyperactivity disorder: a pilot study. *J Am Acad Child Adolesc Psychiatry* 43(3):269–75.

DuPaul GJ, Power TJ, et al. (1998). *ADHD Rating Scale-IV. Checklists, Norms and Clinical Interpretation.* New York: Guilford Press.

Elia J, Borcherding BG, et al. (1991). Methylphenidate and dextroamphetamine treatments of hyperactivity: are there true nonresponders? *Psychiatry Res* 36(2): 141–55.

Faraone SV, Spencer T, et al. (2004). Meta-analysis of the efficacy of methylphenidate for treating adult attention-deficit/hyperactivity disorder. *J Clin Psychopharmacol* 24(1):24–9.

Fayyad J, de Graaf R, et al. (2007). Cross-national prevalence and correlates of adult attention-deficit hyperactivity disorder. *Br J Psychiatry* 190:402–9.

Hah M, Chang K. (2005). Atomoxetine for the treatment of attention-deficit/hyperactivity disorder in children and adolescents with bipolar disorders. *J Child Adolesc Psychopharmacol* 15(6):996–1004.

Hawthorne S. (2007). ADHD drugs: values that drive the debates and decisions. *Med Health Care Philos* 10(2):129–40.

Kafka MP, Hennen J. (2000). Psychostimulant augmentation during treatment with selective serotonin reuptake inhibitors in men with paraphilias and paraphilia-related disorders: a case series. *J Clin Psychiatry* 61(9):664–70.

Kooij JJS. (2003). *ADHD in Adults. Introduction to Diagnosis and Treatment* [in Dutch]. Lisse: Harcourt.

Kooij JJS, Aeckerlin LP, et al. (2001). Functioning, comorbidity and treatment of 141 adults with attention deficit hyperactivity disorder (ADHD) at a Psychiatric Outpatients' Department. *Nederlands Tijdschrift voor Geneeskunde* 145(31):1498–1501 [in Dutch].

Kooij JJS, Buitelaar JK, et al. (2004). Internal and external validity of Attention-Deficit Hyperactivity Disorder in a population-based sample of adults. *Psychological Medicine*, 2004, 34, 1–11.

Kooij JJS, Burger H, et al. (2004). Efficacy and safety of methylphenidate in 45 adults with attention-deficit/hyperactivity disorder. A randomized placebo-controlled double-blind cross-over trial. *Psychol Med* 34(6):973–82.

Kooij JJS, Middelkoop HAM, et al. (2001). The effect of stimulants on nocturnal motor activity and sleep quality in adults with ADHD: an open-label case-control study. *J Clin Psychiatry* 62(12):952–6.

Lydon E, El-Mallakh RS. (2006). Naturalistic long-term use of methylphenidate in bipolar disorder. *J Clin Psychopharmacol* 26(5):516–8.

McGough JJ, Smalley SL, et al. (2005). Psychiatric comorbidity in adult attention deficit hyperactivity disorder: findings from multiplex families. *Am J Psychiatry* 162(9):1621–7.

McLeod JD, Fettes DL, et al. (2007). Public knowledge, beliefs, and treatment preferences concerning attention-deficit hyperactivity disorder. *Psychiatr Serv* 58(5):626–31.

Michelson D, Adler L, et al. (2003). Atomoxetine in adults with ADHD: two randomized, placebo-controlled studies. *Biol Psychiatry* 53(2):112–20.

NIMH. (1985). CGI (Clinical Global Impression) Scale. *Psychopharmacol Bull* 21:839–44.

NTP-CERHR. (2005). Monograph on the potential human reproductive and developmental effects of methylphenidate. *Ntp Cerhr Mon* 16: vii–III1.

Paterson R, Douglas C, et al. (1999). A randomised, double-blind, placebo-controlled trial of dexamphetamine in adults with attention deficit hyperactivity disorder. *Aust N Z J Psychiatry* 33(4):494–502.

Perwien A, Hall J, et al. (2004). Stimulant treatment patterns and compliance in children and adults with newly treated attention-deficit/hyperactivity disorder. *J Manag Care Pharm* 10(2):122–9.

Prince JB. (2006). Pharmacotherapy of attention-deficit hyperactivity disorder in children and adolescents: update on new stimulant preparations, atomoxetine, and novel treatments. *Child Adolesc Psychiatr Clin North Am* 15(1):13–50.

Prince JB, Wilens TE. (2002). Pharmacotherapy of adult ADHD. In: Goldstein S, Ellison AT, eds. *Clinicians' Guide to Adult ADHD: Assessment and Intervention*. San Diego: Academic Press: 165–86.

Ratner S, Laor N, et al. (2005). Six-week open-label reboxetine treatment in children and adolescents with attention-deficit/hyperactivity disorder. *J Am Acad Child Adolesc Psychiatry* 44(5):428–33.

Rayburn WF, Bogenschutz MP. (2004). Pharmacotherapy for pregnant women with addictions. *Am J Obstet Gynecol* 191(6):1885–97.

Reimherr FW, Hedges DW, et al. (2005). Bupropion SR in adults with ADHD: a short-term, placebo-controlled trial. *Neuropsychiatr Dis Treatment* 1(3):245–51.

Rybak YE, McNeely HE, et al. (2006). An open trial of light therapy in adult attention-deficit/hyperactivity disorder. *J Clin Psychiatry* 67(10):1527–35.

Rybak YE, McNeely HE, et al. (2007). Seasonality and circadian preference in adult attention-deficit/hyperactivity disorder: clinical and neuropsychological correlates. *Compr Psychiatry* 48(6):562–71.

Safer DJ. (2000). Are stimulants overprescribed for youths with ADHD? *Ann Clin Psychiatry* 12(1):55–62.

Safren SA, Otto MW, et al. (2005). Cognitive-behavioral therapy for ADHD in medication-treated adults with continued symptoms. *Behav Res Ther* 43(7):831–42.

Scheffer RE, Kowatch RA, et al. (2005). Randomized, placebo-controlled trial of mixed amphetamine salts for symptoms of comorbid ADHD in pediatric bipolar disorder after mood stabilization with divalproex sodium. *Am J Psychiatry* 162(1):58–64.

Schuijers F, Kooij JJS. (2007). *ADHD' ers voor elkaar. Lotgenotenproject*. Bilthoven: Vereniging Impuls [in Dutch].

Shibao C, Raj SR, et al. (2007). Norepinephrine transporter blockade with atomoxetine induces hypertension in patients with impaired autonomic function. *Hypertension* 50(1):47–53.

Solanto MV, Marks DJ, et al. (2008). Development of a new psychosocial treatment for adult ADHD. *J Atten Disord* 11(6):728–36.

Solhkhah R, Wilens TE, et al. (2005). Bupropion SR for the treatment of substance-abusing outpatient adolescents with attention-deficit/hyperactivity disorder and mood disorders. *J Child Adolesc Psychopharmacol* 15(5):777–86.

Spencer T, Biederman J, et al. (2001). Efficacy of a mixed amphetamine salts compound in adults with attention-deficit/hyperactivity disorder. *Arch Gen Psychiatry* 58(8):775–82.

Spencer T, Biederman J, et al. (2005). A large, double-blind, randomized clinical trial of methylphenidate in the treatment of adults with attention-deficit/hyperactivity disorder. *Biol Psychiatry* 57(5):456–63.

Steinhoff KW. (2004). Attention-deficit/hyperactivity disorder: medication treatment-dosing and duration of action. *Am J Manag Care* 10(4 suppl): S99–106.

Thaithumyanon P, Limpongsanurak S, et al. (2005). Perinatal effects of amphetamine and heroin use during pregnancy on the mother and infant. *J Med Assoc Thai* 88(11):1506–13.

Turgay A. (2006). Atomoxetine in the treatment of children, adolescents and adults with attention deficit hyperactivity disorder. *Therapy* 3(1):19–38.

Van Der Heijden KB, Smits MG, et al. (2005). Idiopathic chronic sleep onset insomnia in attention-deficit/hyperactivity disorder: a circadian rhythm sleep disorder. *Chronobiol Int* **22**(3):559–70.

Van Der Heijden KB, Smits MG, et al. (2007). Effect of melatonin on sleep, behavior, and cognition in ADHD and chronic sleep-onset insomnia. *J Am Acad Child Adolesc Psychiatry* **46**(2):233–41.

Waxmonsky JG. (2005). Nonstimulant therapies for attention-deficit hyperactivity disorder (ADHD) in children and adults. *Essent Psychopharmacol* **6**(5):262–76.

Weiss G, Hechtman LT. (1993). *Hyperactive Children Grown Up: ADHD in Children, Adolescents, and Adults.* 2nd ed. New York: Guilford Press.

Weiss M, Hechtman LT, Weiss G. (2001). *ADHD in Adulthood. A Guide to Current Theory, Diagnosis, and Treatment.* Baltimore: Johns Hopkins University Press.

Wilens TE, Biederman J, et al. (1995). Pharmacotherapy of adult attention deficit/hyperactivity disorder: a review. *J Clin Psychopharmacol* **15**(4):270–9.

Wilens TE, Decker MW. (2007). Neuronal nicotinic receptor agonists for the treatment of attention-deficit/hyperactivity disorder: focus on cognition. *Biochem Pharmacol* 7:7.

Wilens TE, Faraone SV, et al. (2003). Does stimulant therapy of attention-deficit/hyperactivity disorder beget later substance abuse? A meta-analytic review of the literature. *Pediatrics* **111**(1):179–85.

Wilens TE, Haight BR, et al. (2005). Bupropion XL in adults with attention-deficit/hyperactivity disorder: a randomized, placebo-controlled study. *Biol Psychiatry* **57**(7):793–801.

Wilens TE, Hammerness PG, et al. (2005). Blood pressure changes associated with medication treatment of adults with attention-deficit/hyperactivity disorder. *J Clin Psychiatry* **66**(2):253–9.

Wilens TE, Prince JB, et al. (2003). An open trial of bupropion for the treatment of adults with attention-deficit/hyperactivity disorder and bipolar disorder. *Biol Psychiatry* **54**(1):9–16. 168–186

Wilens TE, Spencer TJ, et al. (1995). Pharmacotherapy of adult ADHD. In: Nadeau KG, ed. *A Comprehensive Guide to Attention Deficit Disorder in Adults: Research, Diagnosis, and Treatment.* Philadelphia: Brunner/Mazel: 168–86.

Wilens TE, Spencer TJ, et al. (2001). A controlled clinical trial of bupropion for attention deficit hyperactivity disorder in adults. *Am J Psychiatry* **158**(2): 282–8.

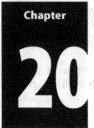

Chapter 20

Abuse potential of stimulant drugs used to treat ADHD

Scott H. Kollins

Introduction

The use of psychostimulants and, more recently, other classes of drugs for the treatment of attention-deficit hyperactivity disorder (ADHD) is widespread. Although it is generally agreed that use in the United States is higher than in other countries, evidence for increasing medication use for ADHD in other countries exists (Schmidt-Troschke et al., 2004). The medications used to treat ADHD have unequivocal support for their efficacy in managing the core symptoms of ADHD in both children and adults (Faraone & Biederman, 2002; Faraone, Biederman, & Roe, 2002; Faraone et al., 2004; Wolraich, 2003). However, significant controversy has arisen in recent years over the possibility that stimulant use may be associated with substance use and abuse (Greenhill, Halperin, & Abikoff, 1999), and a significant challenge confronting researchers, clinicians, and the public is to understand the myriad issues pertaining to stimulant drug use and ADHD. To this end, the purpose of this chapter is (1) to delineate several related questions pertaining to stimulant drug use and ADHD and (2) to review the relevant research that bears on these questions. Specifically, this chapter addresses the following questions:

- Does stimulant drug use for treating ADHD increase the risk for substance abuse later in life?
- Do ADHD medications have the potential for abuse?
- What is the distinction between drug abuse and misuse/diversion with respect to ADHD medications?

Does stimulant drug use for treating ADHD increase the risk for substance abuse later in life?

Animal models

In recent years, there has been considerable controversy over whether early treatment with stimulant medications may increase the risk for drug abuse later in life. This concern has been fueled by at least two observations: (1) individuals with ADHD are at increased risk for substance use disorders, even when controlling for other factors, such as conduct disorder (Biederman et al., 1997), and (2) a sizable literature in nonhuman species supports the notion that repeated exposure to stimulant drugs produces sensitization to subsequent effects of stimulant drugs (Robinson & Becker, 1986; Stewart & Badiani, 1993).

Regarding the latter observation, the relevance of the nonhuman stimulant sensitization literature to the practice of clinical psychopharmacology (Volkow & Insel, 2003) has been questioned, largely because traditional studies of stimulant sensitization have used doses and dosing regimens that are not analogous to those used in clinical practice. Recently, researchers have begun to explore the impact of repeated methylphenidate (MPH) exposure in animal studies under conditions that resemble clinical practice using endpoints that are relevant to understanding the onset of substance abuse. Exposure to comparatively low doses of MPH (2 mg/kg) early in life (preadolescence) has been shown to reduce sensitivity to the rewarding properties of cocaine and other natural reinforcers later in life (Andersen et al.,

ADHD in Adults: Characterization, Diagnosis and Treatment, ed. Jan Buitelaar, Cornelis Kan and Philip Asherson.
Published by Cambridge University Press. © Cambridge University Press 2011.

2002; Bolanos et al., 2003; Carlezon, Mague, & Andersen, 2003). When rats are exposed to similar doses of MPH later in life (i.e., during adolescence), however, the effects seem to be different. Exposure during this developmental stage has been shown to increase the acquisition of cocaine self-administration later in life and to alter the firing rates of dopamine neurons in the ventral tegmental area (Brandon et al., 2001; Brandon, Marinelli, & White, 2003; Brandon & Steiner, 2003). These findings are consistent with research showing that MPH exposure during adulthood facilitates cocaine self-administration (Schenk & Izenwasser, 2002). Finally, evidence exists that early exposure to 2 mg/kg MPH during adolescence results in significantly decreased striatal DAT density later in life (Moll et al., 2001).

Collectively, these nonhuman studies demonstrate that (1) exposure to relatively low doses of MPH can have persistent effects on endpoints associated with substance use; (2) the timing of exposure is critical in predicting the expression of effects and adolescent exposure may result in the highest risk for substance use outcomes (i.e., cocaine self-administration); and (3) the pattern of effects appears to be mediated by alterations in dopaminergic functioning. In short, the animal studies of MPH exposure provide converging evidence for enduring effects that may be relevant to substance use and abuse, especially when exposure occurs in adolescence.

Clinical/human evidence

Experimental and laboratory findings

To date, only a handful of studies have experimentally studied the phenomenon of stimulant sensitization in human participants using drugs relevant to ADHD treatment. Two studies demonstrated sensitization of eye blinking, activity ratings, and self-reported mood in healthy adults following repeated doses of amphetamine (AMP; 0.25 mg/kg p.o.) administered 48 hours apart (Strakowski & Sax, 1998; Strakowski et al., 1996), although other studies have failed to replicate the sensitization of subjective effects of AMP (Brauer, Andre, & de Wit, 1996; Kelly, Foltin, & Fischman, 1991; Wachtel & de Wit, 1999). Although not designed to directly assess behavioral sensitization, another study reported increased metabolism in the frontal, parietal, and occipital cortices, as well as the hippocampus, after repeated doses of MPH, as compared to a single administration (Volkow et al., 1998).

Experimental and descriptive studies of repeated stimulant administration in humans suggest that, under some conditions, changes in behavior (Strakowski & Sax, 1998; Strakowski et al., 1996) and brain function (Volkow et al., 1998) do occur. However, the relevance of these studies to the practice of clinical psychopharmacology remains limited. To date, no studies have examined repeated MPH or AMP effects on behavioral endpoints following dosing regimens that are comparable to those used in clinical practice. Moreover, no studies have examined clinical samples to whom stimulants are most likely to be prescribed.

Naturalistic clinical studies

Particularly in light of the previously reviewed animal research, a number of recent studies have examined data from longitudinally followed ADHD samples. These samples are informative because some of the patients in them have been treated with stimulants, whereas others have not. One of the first published studies to report on this issue found that individuals treated with stimulant medication were more likely to smoke cigarettes and have problems with cocaine use than individuals who had not received stimulant treatment (Lambert & Hartsough, 1998). Other studies have reported that, by contrast, individuals treated with stimulants are at lower risk for substance use problems (Biederman et al., 1999), and recent meta-analyses have supported the idea that treatment with stimulant medication serves a protective function against the development of substance use problems (Faraone & Wilens, 2003; Wilens et al., 2003). Two recent studies however were unable to find evidence for either a protective or a negative relationship between the duration or cumulative amount of stimulant treatment for ADHD and later SUD (Biederman et al., 2008; Molina et al., 2007). Another recent study however did find that early age at initiating stimulant treatment for ADHD was linked with a lower risk for later SUD (Mannuzza et al., 2008). This finding awaits replication.

Collectively, findings from naturalistic studies of longitudinally followed ADHD youth suggest that stimulant treatment early in life serves a protective function against the development of substance use disorders, although these findings should be regarded with some caution given the relatively small number of studies that have been conducted (i.e. the meta-analysis contained data from six studies).

Do ADHD medications have the potential for abuse?

Methods of abuse liability assessment

To meaningfully evaluate whether ADHD drugs have the potential for abuse, it is important to first consider the methods by which this liability is assessed. Abuse liability testing is an important component in the development, marketing, and ongoing clinical assessment of any psychoactive drug. Decisions regarding the eventual approval of a drug and the manner in which it is controlled and prescribed are guided, to a large extent, by research targeting a drug's potential for abuse. The history of such abuse potential testing has been concisely reviewed elsewhere (Balster & Bigelow, 2003; Jaffe & Jaffe, 1989).

Abuse liability assessments that use behavioral endpoints as dependent measures can be particularly informative with respect to the likelihood that, under a particular configuration of environmental conditions, a drug might be misused. Three behavioral paradigms have been used extensively to assess the abuse potential of a wide range of drugs: reinforcing, discriminative-stimulus, and subjective effects.

Reinforcing effects

The reinforcing effects of a drug may be the single most important determinant of its abuse potential because those drugs that function as reinforcers in laboratory animals are often abused by humans, and conversely, compounds not abused in humans are typically not self-administered in nonhuman species (Brady & Lukas, 1984; Fishman, 1973). Preclinical studies with laboratory animals typically assess a drug's reinforcing effects by determining whether it maintains self-administration (Brady, Hienz, & Ator, 1990; Yokel, 1987), wherein animals receive administrations (usually intravenous) of a drug or vehicle (i.e., placebo) contingent on some response (e.g., a lever press). Drugs that maintain rates of self-administration greater than those observed with vehicle are considered to be reinforcers and have a high potential for abuse (LeSage, Stafford, & Glowa, 1999).

Comparable procedures used with human participants have demonstrated that adult human subjects will emit responses at high rates for contingent administration of drugs such as cocaine (Ward et al., 1997). An alternative method for assessing the reinforcing effects of drugs commonly used with human participants involves a choice procedure in which subjects are exposed to a drug and placebo under double-blind conditions on separate days (usually administered orally) and are then given the opportunity to choose which drug they wish to administer on subsequent days (De Wit & Johanson, 1987). With this procedure, the reliable selection of the capsule containing the drug (e.g. *d*-amphetamine) illustrates how it functions to reinforce the choice selection and is believed to predict the abuse potential of the drug under investigation (Johanson & Uhlenhuth, 1980).

Discriminative-stimulus effects

The discriminative-stimulus effects of a drug help determine whether drugs share similar interoceptive effects, and as such, they represent a second paradigm for assessing a drug's abuse potential. Preclinical laboratory studies characterize a drug's interoceptive or discriminative-stimulus effects using drug-discrimination procedures, in which one response (e.g., right lever press) is reinforced following the administration of a drug and a different response (e.g., left lever press) is reinforced following the administration of vehicle/placebo. Following training, novel drugs are administered to determine if they share discriminative-stimulus effects with the training drug (i.e., produce similar response patterns). The drug-discrimination procedure has several advantages. First, drug discrimination is pharmacologically specific in that drugs from the same class as the training drug generally increase drug-appropriate responding as a function of dose, whereas drugs from different classes generally produce placebo-appropriate responding (Glennon, Jarbe, & Frankenheim, 1991). Second, results from drug-discrimination studies are generally concordant with drug action at the cellular level (Glennon & Young, 1987). Third, the discriminative-stimulus effects of drugs in laboratory animals are thought to be a model of the subjective effects of drugs in humans (Preston & Bigelow, 1991). Drugs that produce similar discriminative-stimulus effects in laboratory animals generally produce similar subjective effects in humans.

Subjective effects

A final paradigm for assessing the abuse potential of a drug is measuring its subjective effects in humans. A drug's subjective (or self-reported) effects are typically measured using standardized questionnaires and rating scales. The strength of these subjective effects s inferred from the difference between ratings before and after drug administration or after drug administration compared to placebo administration. The extent to which the drug effects are associated with subjective ratings of euphoria, drug liking, or similarity to other drugs of abuse is the extent to which the drug is believed to have abuse potential. Drug effects on subjective effects measures tend to be dose dependent and pharmacologically specific and, as such, are believed to be strongly correlated with a drug's abuse potential (Jaffe & Jaffe, 1989).

As noted previously, the extent to which a drug exerts reinforcing, discriminative-stimulus, and subjective effects consistent with abuse potential is not itself the sole determinant of whether a drug will be abused by humans in natural environments. The validity of these assays for predicting abuse potential has been debated previously (Fischman & Mello, 1984), and there are instances where drugs that predict abuse in laboratory evaluations are not abused; conversely, there are drugs (or combinations of drugs) that are abused in humans that have never been evaluated or whose evaluation would not predict significant abuse (Brady & Lukas, 1984). These discrepancies warrant caution when interpreting the validity of the behavioral assays used to assess abuse potential.

Abuse liability of stimulant drugs used to treat ADHD

The abuse liability of both MPH and AMP, which are the most commonly used drugs to treat ADHD, has been extensively evaluated. Studies in both non-humans and in human volunteers have repeatedly demonstrated that both drugs function as reinforcers, are reliably discriminated, and substitute fully for cocaine and other drugs of abuse. In addition, in humans, both drugs produce subjective effects suggestive of abuse potential (Kollins, 2003; Kollins, MacDonald, & Rush, 2001).

Reinforcing effects

A number of studies have reported that intravenously administered MPH and AMP reliably maintain self-administration in a range of species and that the only differences between these two compounds is their relative potency, with AMP exhibiting approximately twice the potency of MPH (Nielsen et al., 1984: Risner & Jones, 1975, 1976). Other studies in non-humans have shown that rates of self-administration

maintained by MPH are comparable to those seen with cocaine (Aigner & Balster, 199; Bergman et al., 1989; Collins et al., 1984; Wilson, Hitomi, & Schuster, 1971). There are fewer studies of the reinforcing effects of MPH and AMP in humans, but they have generally shown that oral administration of these drugs, even at dose levels comparable to those used in clinical practices, results in reinforcing effects of both drugs compared to placebo (Rush et al., 2001). Two studies have been conducted that assess the reinforcing effects of orally administered MPH using a choice procedure in patients with ADHD. These studies reported that MPH was reliably chosen over placebo and that this effect tended to be dose dependent (Fredericks & Kollins, 2004; MacDonald Fredericks & Kollins, 2005). Importantly, however, these studies also reported that, in spite of the observed reinforcing effects of MPH in ADHD patients, there was a marked lack of subjective effects indicative of abuse liability. The authors interpreted these findings as a demonstration of how the reinforcing effects of MPH in ADHD patients are associated with clinical efficacy rather than abuse liability.

Discriminative-stimulus effects

A number of studies have shown that intravenously or intraperitoneally administered MPH substitutes fully for both AMP and cocaine in rodents, pigeons, and nonhuman primates (de la Garza & Johnson, 1987; Evans & Johanson, 1987; McKenna & Ho, 1980; Wood & Emmett-Oglesby, 1988).

Four studies have examined the discriminative-stimulus effects of orally administered MPH in human studies. d-Amphetamine was used as a training drug in two of these studies, and fixed doses of 30 and 20 mg d-amphetamine, respectively, were shown to be reliably discriminated (Heishman & Henningfield, 1991; Rush, Kollins, & Pazzaglia, 1998). In these studies, 20- to 60-mg methylphenidate fully substituted for the d-amphetamine training stimulus. One other study demonstrated that, in cocaine abusers, 200-mg oral cocaine could be reliably discriminated from placebo and that 15- to 90-mg methylphenidate dose dependently increased cocaine-appropriate responding, with the highest doses (60–90 mg) fully substituting for the training stimulus (Rush & Baker, 2001).

Subjective effects

A number of studies have investigated the subjective effects of MPH in healthy adult volunteers and experienced drug users. These studies have shown that both MPH and AMP produce significant changes in subjective effects compared to placebo and that amphetamine is roughly twice as potent in producing these effects compared to MPH (Martin et al., 1971; Smith & Davis, 1977). Studies have also shown that MPH exhibits comparable effects as cocaine when administered orally. For example, one study directly compared the subjective effects of oral cocaine (50–300 mg) and MPH (15–90 mg) in human participants and reported that MPH and cocaine both dose dependently increased ratings of "drug liking" and that MPH was more potent (Rush & Baker, 2001).

Few studies have directly assessed the subjective effects of ADHD medications in the actual patients who are receiving them for clinical purposes. Generally, these studies have reported that MPH fails to produce reliable subjective effects compared to placebo (Fredericks & Kollins, 2004; Kollins et al., 1998; MacDonald Fredericks & Kollins, 2005). These findings are particularly striking because, in two of the studies, MPH was shown to exhibit reinforcing effects (Fredericks & Kollins, 2004; MacDonald Fredericks & Kollins, 2005). These findings highlight the importance of considering a range of behavioral endpoints in assessing the abuse potential of different drugs.

Collectively, studies with non-ADHD samples provide evidence that both AMP and MPH produce subjective effects that are indicative of abuse potential. However, in the ADHD patients themselves, there is preliminary evidence suggesting that they may not experience the same subjective effects of these drugs. This finding is consistent with clinical anecdotal evidence that ADHD patients do not take their medication because of dysphoric subjective effects, and it may be related to underlying dopaminergic differences between ADHD and non-ADHD individuals (Solanto, 2002).

Summary of abuse liability of stimulant drugs

The reviewed studies provide support for the assertion that both MPH and AMP exhibit profiles consistent with abuse liability. These drugs both produce reinforcing effects, substitute for cocaine in drug discrimination studies, and produce subjective effects indicative of abuse liability. Several important caveats should be noted, however. First, although only a few studies have reported on this, findings suggest that the abuse potential of ADHD medications may actually be lower in the patients themselves. Another important consideration pertains to the drug formulations used

in the reviewed studies. All of the studies reviewed included either injected or immediate-release oral stimulants. Since the late 1990s the proportion of children receiving extended-release formulations of MPH or alternative formulations of AMP (i.e., mixed-salt amphetamine products) has increased substantially. The abuse potential of these alternative formulations of MPH and AMP has not been extensively characterized. There is some evidence that longer acting formulations may have reduced abuse potential in non-ADHD samples (Kollins et al., 1998).

Abuse liability of nonstimulant drugs used to treat ADHD

Recently, nonstimulant drugs have been used more widely for treating ADHD in adults in children. In the US, the selective norepinephrine reuptake inhibitor atomoxetine was approved by the Food and Drug Administration (FDA) in November 2002. Another nonstimulant compound, modafinil, was approved by the FDA in 2006 for the treatment of ADHD. Consistent with FDA requirements, these compounds have also undergone abuse liability testing, though not as extensively as the stimulant drugs. In general, neither atomoxetine nor modafinil has demonstrated significant abuse potential. Studies in nonhumans have shown that atomoxetine fails to maintain self-administration, and studies in humans have shown that this drug fails to produce significant subjective effects compared to placebo (Gasior et al., 2005; Heil et al., 2002). Similarly, modafinil has failed to produce significant reinforcing or subjective effects in human and nonhuman studies (Jasinski, 2000; Jasinski & Kovacevic-Ristanovic, 2000; Myrick et al., 2004; Rush et al., 2002; Stoops et al., 2005).

What is the distinction between drug abuse and misuse/diversion?

To fully describe the abuse potential of medications used to treat ADHD, it is important to distinguish between substance abuse and misuse/diversion. Much of the controversy over the use of these medications centers on widespread reports of the drugs' misuse, which is often mistakenly referred to as abuse. By definition, substance abuse refers to the continued use of a drug that leads to significant impairment characterized by failure to fulfill important obligations, recurrent use under hazardous conditions, and legal and interpersonal problems (American Psychiatric Association, 1994). However, much of the popular press and anecdotal information regarding the nonmedical use of MPH and AMP center on their stimulant properties. For example, one review characterized this pattern of use by college students in an effort to stay up later and "party" longer or to sharpen mental skills and study harder (Weiner, 2000). As such, it may be possible that the perception of low abuse liability is generated by the fact that the drug rarely leads to significant impairment. In any case, researchers and policymakers alike need to pay close attention to the distinction between drug abuse and misuse/diversion and their respective consequences.

Evidence for abuse of ADHD medications

Despite the fact that both MPH and AMP have documented abuse potential, there is fairly limited evidence that these drugs, in the formulations used to treat ADHD, are abused in any widespread manner. A search of the medical literature results in a handful of case reports of MPH abuse, almost all of which described an intravenous route of administration with subsequent medical complications. Several other studies and reviews have reported methylphenidate abuse in specific groups of individuals (e.g. methadone maintenance patients; Raskind & Bradford, 1975) and in the general population (Crutchley & Temlett, 1999; Weiner, 2000). It is generally accepted, however, that the drugs used to treat ADHD are not abused to the same extent as other stimulants like cocaine and methamphetamine. Some empirical work suggests that the differences in actual rates of abuse between MPH and cocaine may be related to the pharmacodynamic actions of the drugs in the brain (Volkow et al., 1995), which may account for the more prevalent abuse of cocaine as compared to methylphenidate.

Evidence for misuse/diversion of ADHD medications

Considerable evidence points to widespread patterns of diversion and misuse of ADHD medications among young people. To reiterate, these studies do not assess clinically defined patterns of drug abuse or dependence, but rather highlight the fact that the stimulant drugs used to treat ADHD are commonly used by nondiagnosed individuals for other purposes. One

study that surveyed children and adolescents who had been prescribed methylphenidate found that nearly one in five had been approached to sell, give away, or trade their medication at least once in the past 5 years (Musser et al., 1998). More recent work has characterized the diversion and misuse of prescription stimulants as widespread on college campuses. These studies have consistently found demographic differences among those most likely reporting misuse of the drugs, with Caucasian males more likely to misuse prescription stimulants than females or other ethnic groups (McCabe, Teter, & Boyd, 2001, 2004; Teter et al., 2005). These studies have also found that individuals reporting illicit use of prescription ADHD medications are more likely to report other kinds of alcohol and drug use (McCabe, Teter, & Boyd, 2004). In a comprehensive, population-based survey of more than 50,000 individuals, an estimated 2.6% of individuals aged 12–17 and 5.9% of individuals aged 18–25 years of age reported ever having misused an ADHD medication (Kroutil et al., 2006).

Particular attention should be paid to actual rates of misuse and abuse in individuals to whom the drug is most likely to be medically prescribed. Several studies have shown that although children and college students with ADHD may learn to reliably discriminate their medication from placebo, and choose to take it more than placebo, the magnitude of their subjective effects is lower than might be expected (Fredericks & Kollins, 2004; Kollins et al., 1998; MacDonald Fredericks & Kollins, 2005). As noted, this discordance among indices of abuse liability may reflect underlying neurobiological differences in ADHD versus non-ADHD individuals.

Summary: Abuse and misuse/diversion of ADHD medications

Both the literature and clinical experience support the notion that clinically significant levels of abuse of or dependence on stimulant drugs prescribed for ADHD are comparatively rare. However, a much more widespread problem seems to be the misuse and diversion of these medications to individuals not diagnosed with ADHD. Anecdotally, this diversion is usually associated with efforts to increase concentration and attention, often in competitive academic environments. This observation is supported by at least one study that assessed the motives for illicit prescription stimulant use among college students and found that more individuals reported taking the medications to increase concentration than to "get high" per se (Teter et al., 2005). Also of interest is that there seems to be evidence that the ADHD patients who are most likely to receive the medications in question do not report the same magnitude of subjective effects as nondiagnosed individuals. This is an important finding in light of concerns about ADHD patients becoming addicted to their medication.

Conclusions/clinical implications

This chapter has delineated answers to several related but distinct questions pertaining to the abuse potential of stimulant drugs used to treat ADHD. First, the bulk of the clinical evidence suggests that treatment of ADHD with stimulant drugs reduces the risk for subsequent drug abuse, although more research is needed in this area. Second, a considerable literature in a number of species supports the abuse potential of the most commonly used medications to treat ADHD: MPH and AMP. This abuse potential is the primary reason these products are tightly regulated by the US FDA and other agencies. Third, alternatives to stimulant drugs, such as atomoxetine and modafinil, do not seem to share the same level of abuse liability as the stimulant drugs. Finally, although there are rare cases of actual abuse or dependence on MPH or AMP as formulated for the treatment of ADHD, a more salient concern is the extent to which these drugs are diverted and misused in non-ADHD individuals.

Several important clinical implications derive from this review. First, it is important for clinicians to provide as much information as possible to their patients regarding the abuse potential of these medications. Parents and adult patients are often reluctant to initiate effective treatment for ADHD because of concerns based on misinformation and myth. Second, clinicians should exercise caution when prescribing medications to potential high-risk groups. For example, adolescents and college students are the most likely to report misuse of ADHD medications, so when prescribing to patients in this age range, extra time should be taken to explain the importance of keeping their medication out of the hands of nonpatients. However, any caution in prescribing these medications for ADHD patients needs to be weighed against the incontrovertible support for their efficacy in reducing the requisite symptoms and accompanying impairment of ADHD.

References

Aigner TG, Balster RL. (1979). Rapid substitution procedure for intravenous drug self-administration studies in rhesus monkeys. *Pharmacol Biochem Behav* **10**(1):105–12.

American Psychiatric Association. (1994). *Diagnostic and statistical manual of mental disorders.* 4th ed. Washington, DC: American Psychiatric Association.

Andersen SL, Arvanitogiannis A, Pliakas AM, LeBlanc C, Carlezon WA, Jr. (2002). Altered responsiveness to cocaine in rats exposed to methylphenidate during development. *Nat Neurosci* **5**(1):13–14.

Balster RL, Bigelow GE. (2003). Guidelines and methodological reviews concerning drug abuse liability assessment. *Drug Alcohol Depend* **70**(3 suppl): S13–40.

Bergman J, Madras BK, Johnson SE, Spealman RD. (1989). Effects of cocaine and related drugs in nonhuman primates. III. Self-administration by squirrel monkeys. *J Pharmacol Exp Ther* **251**(1):150–5.

Biederman J, Wilens T, Mick E, Faraone SV, Weber W, Curtis S, et al. (1997). Is ADHD a risk factor for psychoactive substance use disorders? Findings from a four-year prospective follow-up study. *J Am Acad Child Adolesc Psychiatry* **36**(1):21–9.

Biederman J, Wilens T, Mick E, Spencer T, Faraone SV. (1999). Pharmacotherapy of attention-deficit/ hyperactivity disorder reduces risk for substance use disorder. *Pediatrics* **104**(2):e20.

Biederman J, Monuteaux MC, Spencer T, Wilens TE, Macpherson HA, Faraone SV. (2008). Stimulant therapy and risk for subsequent substance use disorders in male adults with ADHD: a naturalistic controlled 10-year follow-up study. *Am. J Psychiatry* **165**:597–603.

Bolanos CA, Barrot M, Berton O, Wallace-Black D, Nestler EJ. (2003). Methylphenidate treatment during pre- and periadolescence alters behavioral responses to emotional stimuli at adulthood. *Biol Psychiatry* **54**(12):1317–29.

Brady JV, Hienz RD, Ator NA. (1990). Stimulus functions of drugs and the assessment of abuse liability. *Drug Dev Res* **20**:231–49.

Brady JV, Lukas SE. (1984). *Testing Drugs for Physical Dependence Potential and Abuse Liability.* National Institute on Drug Abuse Monograph No. 52 (ADM)90–1332. Washington, DC: Department of Health and Human Services.

Brandon CL, Marinelli M, Baker LK, White FJ. (2001). Enhanced reactivity and vulnerability to cocaine following methylphenidate treatment in adolescent rats. *Neuropsychopharmacology* **25**(5):651–61.

Brandon CL, Marinelli M, White FJ. (2003). Adolescent exposure to methylphenidate alters the activity of rat midbrain dopamine neurons. *Biol Psychiatry* 54(12):1338–44.

Brandon CL, Steiner H. (2003). Repeated methylphenidate treatment in adolescent rats alters gene regulation in the striatum. *Eur J Neurosci* 18(6):1584–92.

Brauer LH, Ambre J, de Wit H. (1996). Acute tolerance to subjective but not cardiovascular effects of d-amphetamine in normal, healthy men. *J Clin Psychopharmacol* 16(1):72–6.

Carlezon WA, Jr., Mague SD, Andersen SL. (2003). Enduring behavioral effects of early exposure to methylphenidate in rats. *Biol Psychiatry* 54(12): 1330–7.

Collins RJ, Weeks JR, Cooper MM, Good PI, Russell RR. (1984). Prediction of abuse liability of drugs using IV self-administration by rats. *Psychopharmacology (Berl)* 82(1–2):6–13.

Crutchley A, Temlett JA. (1999). Methylphenidate (Ritalin) use and abuse. *S Afr Med* 89(10):1076–9.

de la Garza R, Johanson CE. (1987). Discriminative stimulus properties of intragastrically administered d-amphetamine and pentobarbital in rhesus monkeys. *J Pharmacol Exp Ther* 243(3):955–62.

De Wit H, Johanson CE. (1987). A drug preference procedure for use with human volunteers. In: Bozarth MA, ed. *Methods of Assessing the Reinforcing Properties of Abused Drugs.* New York: Springer-Verlag: 559–72.

Evans SM, Johanson CE. (1987). Amphetamine-like effects of anorectics and related compounds in pigeons. *J Pharmacol Exp Ther* 241(3):817–25.

Faraone SV, Biederman J. (2002). Efficacy of Adderall for Attention-Deficit/Hyperactivity Disorder: a meta-analysis. *J Atten Disord* 6(2):69–75.

Faraone SV, Biederman J, Roe C. (2002). Comparative efficacy of Adderall and methylphenidate in attention-deficit/hyperactivity disorder: a meta-analysis. *J Clin Psychopharmacol* 22(5):468–73.

Faraone SV, Spencer T, Aleardi M, Pagano C, Biederman J. (2004). Meta-analysis of the efficacy of methylphenidate for treating adult attention-deficit/ hyperactivity disorder. *J Clin Psychopharmacol* 24(1):24–9.

Faraone SV, Wilens T. (2003). Does stimulant treatment lead to substance use disorders? *J Clin Psychiatry* 64(suppl 11):9–13.

Fischman MW, Mello NK. (1989). *Testing Drugs for Physical Dependence Potential and Abuse Liability.* National Institute on Drug Abuse Monograph No. 92, No. (ADM)90–1332. Washington, DC: Department of Health and Human Services Publication.

Fishman DB. (1973). Holt's Rorschach measure of adaptive regression, mathematical artifact, and prediction of psychotherapy outcome. *J Pers Assess* 37(4):328–33.

Fredericks EM, Kollins SH. (2004). Assessing methylphenidate preference in ADHD patients using a choice procedure. *Psychopharmacology (Berl)* 175(4):391–8.

Gasior M, Bergman J, Kallman MJ, Paronis CA. (2005). Evaluation of the reinforcing effects of monoamine reuptake inhibitors under a concurrent schedule of food and i.v. drug delivery in rhesus monkeys. *Neuropsychopharmacology* 30(4):758–64.

Glennon RA, Jarbe TUC, Frankenheim J. (1991). *Drug Discrimination: Applications to Drug Abuse Research.* Rockville, MD: US Department of Health and Human Services.

Glennon RA, Young R. (1987). The study of structure activity relationships using drug discrimination methodology. In: Bozarth MA, ed. *Methods of Assessing the Reinforcing Properties of Abused Drugs.* New York: Springer-Verlag: 373–90.

Greenhill LL, Halperin JM, Abikoff H. Stimulant medications. (1999). *J Am Acad Child Adolesc Psychiatry* 38(5):503–12.

Heil SH, Holmes HW, Bickel WK, Higgins ST, Badger GJ, Laws HF, et al. (2002). Comparison of the subjective, physiological, and psychomotor effects of atomoxetine and methylphenidate in light drug users. *Drug Alcohol Depend* 67(2):149–56.

Heishman SJ, Henningfield JE. (1991). Discriminative stimulus effects of d-amphetamine, methylphenidate, and diazepam in humans. *Psychopharmacology (Berl)* 103(4):436–42.

Jaffe JH, Jaffe SK. (1989). Historical perspectives on the use of subjective effects measures in assessing the abuse potential of drugs. In: Fishman MW, Mello NK, eds. *Testing for Abuse Liability of Drugs in Humans.* National Institute on Drug Abuse Monograph No. 92 (ADM)89–1613. Washington, DC: Department of Health and Human Services: 43–72.

Jasinski DR. (2000). An evaluation of the abuse potential of modafinil using methylphenidate as a reference. *J Psychopharmacol* 14(1):53–60.

Jasinski DR, Kovacevic-Ristanovic R. (2000). Evaluation of the abuse liability of modafinil and other drugs for excessive daytime sleepiness associated with narcolepsy. *Clin Neuropharmacol* 23(3):149–56.

Johanson CE, Uhlenhuth EH. (1980). Drug preference and mood in humans: d-amphetamine. *Psychopharmacology (Berl)* 71(3):275–9.

Kelly TH, Foltin RW, Fischman MW. (1991). The effects of repeated amphetamine exposure on multiple measures of human behavior. *Pharmacol Biochem Behav* **38**(2):417–26.

Kollins SH. (2003). Comparing the abuse potential of methylphenidate versus other stimulants: a review of available evidence and relevance to the ADHD patient. *J Clin Psychiatry* **64**(suppl 11):14–18.

Kollins SH, MacDonald EK, Rush CR. (2001). Assessing the abuse potential of methylphenidate in nonhuman and human subjects: a review. *Pharmacol Biochem Behav* **68**(3):611–27.

Kollins SH, Rush CR, Pazzaglia PJ, Ali JA. (1998). Comparison of acute behavioral effects of sustained-release and immediate-release methylphenidate. *Exp Clin Psychopharmacol* **6**(4):367–74.

Kollins SH, Shapiro SK, Newland MC, Abramowitz A. (1998). Discriminative and participant-rated effects of methylphenidate in children diagnosed with attention deficit hyperactivity disorder (ADHD). *Exp Clin Psychopharmacol* **6**(4):375–89.

Kroutil LA, Van Brunt DL, Herman-Stahl MA, Heller DC, Bray RM, Penne MA. (2006). Nonmedical use of prescription stimulants in the United States. *Drug Alcohol Depend* **84**(2):135–43.

Lambert NM, Hartsough CS. (1998). Prospective study of tobacco smoking and substance dependencies among samples of ADHD and non-ADHD participants. *J Learn Disabil* **31**(6):533–44.

LeSage MG, Stafford D, Glowa JR. (1999). Preclinical research on cocaine self-administration: environmental determinants and their interaction with pharmacological treatment. *Neurosci Biobehav Rev* **23**(5):717–41.

MacDonald Fredericks E, Kollins SH. (2005). A pilot study of methylphenidate preference assessment in children diagnosed with attention-deficit/hyperactivity disorder. *J Child Adolesc Psychopharmacol* **15**(5):729–41.

Mannuzza S, Klein RG, Truong NL, Moulton JL 3rd, Roizen ER, Howell KH, Castellanos FX (2008). Age of methylphenidate treatment initiation in children with ADHD and later substance abuse: prospective follow-up into adulthood. *Am.J Psychiatry* **165**:604–9.

Martin WR, Sloan JW, Sapira JD, Jasinski DR. (1971). Physiologic, subjective, and behavioral effects of amphetamine, methamphetamine, ephedrine, phenmetrazine, and methylphenidate in man. *Clin Pharmacol Ther* **12**(2):245–58.

McCabe SE, Teter CJ, Boyd CJ. (2004). The use, misuse and diversion of prescription stimulants among middle and high school students. *Subst Use Misuse* **39**(7):1095–116.

McCabe SE, Teter CJ, Boyd CJ, Guthrie SK. (2004). Prevalence and correlates of illicit methylphenidate use among 8th, 10th, and 12th grade students in the United States, 2001. *J Adolesc Health* **35**(6):501–4.

McKenna ML, Ho BT. (1980). The role of dopamine in the discriminative stimulus properties of cocaine. *Neuropharmacology* **19**(3):297–303.

Molina BS, Flory K, Hinshaw SP, Greiner AR, Arnold LE, Swanson JM, Hechtman L, Jensen PS, Vitiello B, Hoza B, Pelham WE, Elliott GR, Wells KC, Abikoff HB, Gibbons RD, Marcus S, Conners CK, Epstein JN, Greenhill LL, March JS, Newcorn JH, Severe JB, Wigal T (2007). Delinquent behavior and emerging substance use in the MTA at 36 months: prevalence, course, and treatment effects. *J Am. Acad. Child Adolesc. Psychiatry* **46**:1028–40.

Moll GH, Hause S, Ruther E, Rothenberger A, Huether G. (2001). Early methylphenidate administration to young rats causes a persistent reduction in the density of striatal dopamine transporters. *J Child Adolesc Psychopharmacol* **11**(1):15–24.

Musser CJ, Ahmann PA, Theye FW, Mundt P, Broste SK, Mueller-Rizner N. (1998). Stimulant use and the potential for abuse in Wisconsin as reported by school administrators and longitudinally followed children. *J Dev Behav Pediatr* **19**(3):187–92.

Myrick H, Malcolm R, Taylor B, LaRowe S. (2004). Modafinil: preclinical, clinical, and post-marketing surveillance – a review of abuse liability issues. *Ann Clin Psychiatry* **16**(2):101–9.

Nielsen JA, Duda NJ, Mokler DJ, Moore KE. (1984). Self-administration of central stimulants by rats: a comparison of the effects of d-amphetamine, methylphenidate and McNeil 4612. *Pharmacol Biochem Behav* **20**(2):227–32.

Preston KL, Bigelow GE. (1991). Subjective and discriminative effects of drugs. *Behav Pharmacol* **2**(4 and 5):293–313.

Raskind M, Bradford T. (1975). Methylphenidate (ritalin) abuse and methadone maintenance. *Dis Nerv Syst* **36**(1):9–12.

Risner ME, Jones BE. (1975). Self-administration of CNS stimulants by dog. *Psychopharmacologia* **43**(3):207–13.

Risner ME, Jones BE. (1976). Characteristics of unlimited access to self-administered stimulant infusions in dogs. *Biol Psychiatry* **11**(5):625–34.

Robinson TE, Becker JB. (1986). Enduring changes in brain and behavior produced by chronic amphetamine administration: a review and evaluation of animal models of amphetamine psychosis. *Brain Res* **396**(2):157–98.

Rush CR, Baker RW. (2001). Behavioral pharmacological similarities between methylphenidate and cocaine in cocaine abusers. *Exp Clin Psychopharmacol* **9**(1):59–73.

Rush CR, Essman WD, Simpson CA, Baker RW. (2001). Reinforcing and subject-rated effects of methylphenidate and d-amphetamine in non-drug-abusing humans. *J Clin Psychopharmacol* **21**(3):273–86.

Rush CR, Kelly TH, Hays LR, Baker RW, Wooten AF. (2002). Acute behavioral and physiological effects of modafinil in drug abusers. *Behav Pharmacol* **13**(2):105–15.

Rush CR, Kollins SH, Pazzaglia PJ. (1998). Discriminative-stimulus and participant-rated effects of methylphenidate, bupropion, and triazolam in d-amphetamine-trained humans. *Exp Clin Psychopharmacol* **6**(1):32–44.

Schenk S, Izenwasser S. (2002). Pretreatment with methylphenidate sensitizes rats to the reinforcing effects of cocaine. *Pharmacol Biochem Behav* **72**(3):651–7.

Schmidt-Troschke SO, Ostermann T, Melcher D, Schuster R, Erben CM, Matthiessen PF. (2004). The use of methylphenidate in children: analysis of prescription usage based in routine data of the statutory health insurance bodies concerning drug prescriptions. *Gesundheitswesen* **66**(6):387–92.

Smith RC, Davis JM. (1977). Comparative effects of d-amphetamine, l-amphetamine, and methylphenidate on mood in man. *Psychopharmacology (Berl)* **53**(1):1–12.

Solanto MV. (2002). Dopamine dysfunction in AD/HD: integrating clinical and basic neuroscience research. *Behav Brain Res* **130**(1–2):65–71.

Stewart J, Badiani A. (1993). Tolerance and sensitization to the behavioral effects of drugs. *Behav Pharmacol* **4**(4):289–312.

Stoops WW, Lile JA, Fillmore MT, Glaser PE, Rush CR. (2005). Reinforcing effects of modafinil: influence of dose and behavioral demands following drug administration. *Psychopharmacology (Berl)* **182**(1):186–93.

Strakowski SM, Sax KW. (1998). Progressive behavioral response to repeated d-amphetamine challenge: further evidence for sensitization in humans. *Biol Psychiatry* **44**(11):1171–7.

Strakowski SM, Sax KW, Setters MJ, Keck PE, Jr. (1996). Enhanced response to repeated d-amphetamine challenge: evidence for behavioral sensitization in humans. *Biol Psychiatry* **40**(9):872–80.

Teter CJ, McCabe SE, Cranford JA, Boyd CJ, Guthrie SK. (2005). Prevalence and motives for illicit use of prescription stimulants in an undergraduate student sample. *J Am Coll Health* **53**(6):253–62.

Volkow ND, Ding YS, Fowler JS, Wang GJ, Logan J, Gatley JS, et al. (1995). Is methylphenidate like cocaine? Studies on their pharmacokinetics and distribution in the human brain. *Arch Gen Psychiatry* **52**(6):456–63.

Volkow ND, Insel TR. (2003). What are the long-term effects of methylphenidate treatment? *Biol Psychiatry* **54**(12):1307–9.

Volkow ND, Wang GJ, Fowler JS, Hitzemann R, Gatley J, Ding YS, et al. (1998). Differences in regional brain metabolic responses between single and repeated doses of methylphenidate. *Psychiatry Res* **83**(1):29–36.

Wachtel SR, de Wit H. (1999). Subjective and behavioral effects of repeated d-amphetamine in humans. *Behav Pharmacol* **10**(3):271–81.

Ward AS, Haney M, Fischman MW, Foltin RW. (1997). Binge cocaine self-administration in humans: intravenous cocaine. *Psychopharmacology (Berl)* **132**(4):375–81.

Wee S, Woolverton WL. (2004). Evaluation of the reinforcing effects of atomoxetine in monkeys: comparison to methylphenidate and desipramine. *Drug Alcohol Depend* **75**(3):271–6.

Weiner AL. (2000). Emerging drugs of abuse in Connecticut. *Conn Med* **64**(1):19–23.

Wilens TE, Faraone SV, Biederman J, Gunawardene S. (2003). Does stimulant therapy of attention-deficit/hyperactivity disorder beget later substance abuse? A meta-analytic review of the literature. *Pediatrics* **111**(1):179–85.

Wilson MC, Hitomi M, Schuster CR. (1971). Psychomotor stimulant self administration as a function of dosage per injection in the rhesus monkey. *Psychopharmacologia* **22**(3):271–81.

Wolraich ML. (2003). Annotation: the use of psychotropic medications in children: an American view. *J Child Psychol Psychiatry* **44**(2):159–68.

Wood DM, Emmett-Oglesby MW. (1988). Substitution and cross-tolerance profiles of anorectic drugs in rats trained to detect the discriminative stimulus properties of cocaine. *Psychopharmacology (Berl)* **95**(3):364–8.

Yokel RA. (1987). Intravenous self administration: Response rates, the effects of pharmacological challenges, and drug preferences. In: Bozarth MA, ed. *Methods of Assessing the Reinforcing Properties of Abused Drugs.* New York: Springer-Verlag: 1–34.

Chapter

21

Psychoeducation for adults with ADHD
Impressions from the field

Anne M. D. N. van Lammeren and Richard Bruggeman

Introduction

Broadly speaking, psychoeducation for adults with attention-deficit/hyperactivity disorder (AHDH) provides adequate educational information about the disorder, its causes, as well as symptoms, and about available treatment options. It relies not only on traditional medical models but also on the more competence-based approaches such as empowering patients and teaching them how to cope.

Making sure ADHD patients, their partners, and family have access to adequate information is an important first step because, in spite of the exposure ADHD has received, not many people know exactly what it is: misconceptions and myths about the disorder abound (Sonagu & Balding, 1993). Just by giving people a better understanding of the nature of ADHD, psychoeducation proves a useful starting point for dealing with the symptoms and the dysfunction related to it.

It is still largely unusual to involve partners, family members, or even close friends or colleagues in the treatment of adult patients, but provided that patients agree, the advantages of letting them take part in psychoeducation sessions are many. Once patients, partners, and family begin to understand the basic facts about ADHD and the consequences it has for the way adults with ADHD tend to function, and once they develop a growing awareness of the symptoms, impairments, and strengths that come with ADHD and its comorbid disorders, they will all come to play a more active and beneficial role in its treatment. Furthermore, greater respect and deeper understanding between patients, partners, and family will generate a more constructive way of talking with each other and with the professionals involved. The more knowledgeable patients and their relatives and caregivers are, the

more positive health-related outcomes will be achieved for all (Lukens & McFarlane, 2004).

A beneficial recent development is that providing adequate information to patients has become a prerequisite for good clinical practice for health workers. Recent requirements on federal and international levels mandate that professionals provide psychoeducation as part of treatment (Lukens & McFarlane, 2004). For example, Dutch law (Law on Medical Treatment Agreement [WGBO] Civil Code) requires all physicians to give patients the information they need about their disease and to outline the available treatment options open to them. In the United States, special education programs are geared to children with ADHD in the Education Act for Individuals with Disabilities of the Civil Rights Act (1990).

However, there is as yet no evidence-based research supporting the effectiveness of psychoeducation for adults with ADHD in alleviating their symptoms and improving their quality of life. Looking at family or group psychoeducation in adult psychiatry for which there is evidence-based research (Dixon et al., 2001), there is a major focus on work with consumers and families with relatives suffering from schizophrenia or schizoaffective disorders; in addition, a good deal of attention is paid to other psychiatric disorders such as bipolar disorder, major depression, obsessive-compulsive disorder, anorexia nervosa, and borderline personality disorder, as well as to somatic disease such as cancer (Lukens & McFarlane, 2004).

Because they incorporate illness-specific information and tools for managing related problems, psychoeducational programs are inherently flexible, which makes them likely to be effective for adult patients with ADHD.

This chapter is based on our clinical experience in leading psychoeducational groups in which ADHD

ADHD in Adults: Characterization, Diagnosis and Treatment, ed. Jan Buitelaar, Cornelis Kan and Philip Asherson.
Published by Cambridge University Press. © Cambridge University Press 2011.

patients participated at the Outpatients Clinic of the University Medical Centre, Groningen, the Netherlands. Our impressions are highly encouraging for the way they show that, together with other psychosocial interventions for AHDH, psychoeducation for adults can play a significantly beneficial role. In this chapter we first give an update of existing research on psychoeducation for adults with ADHD. We then highlight some of the arguments in favor of psychoeducation and finally make some clinical suggestions on how to provide psychoeducation to adult patients with ADHD and their partners and family.

Literature about psychoeducation for adults with ADHD

In a review article, "Psychosocial treatments for ADHD in teens and adults," Murphy (2005) highlighted the importance of psychoeducation about ADHD to both patients and people in their environment, such as partners, friends, and associates. Brown (2000), in a chapter on psychosocial interventions, argued that psychoeducation should be given to patients and family members together because it gives them hope and helps motivate them to participate in treatment. These authors provided general information on how psychoeducation should be given. As already mentioned, there are no evidence-based guidelines for psychoeducation for adults with ADHD. In searching electronic databases such as MEDLINE (1966–July 2005), PsycINFO (1872–July 2005), EMBASE (1993–July 2005), ERIC (1991–June 2004), and Psydexplus (1977–June 2005), we found not one single article on psychoeducation for adults with ADHD. Thus, the programs that are given today are largely based on common sense and clinical experience, and guidelines are extrapolated from the literature about children with ADHD.

Indeed, the literature on children with ADHD contains some research on the effects of nonmedical treatments, including psychoeducation for children, parents, and teachers. Yet even in that literature, the effect of psychoeducation, especially as treatment for ADHD by itself, has not been investigated, but always as part of a broader psychosocial intervention scheme, such as behavior therapy and parent training, or in combination with medication. McCleary and Ridley (1999) described an evaluation of a psychoeducation group for parents of adolescents with ADHD in which the parents reported that they found this approach

effective, especially because of the information they received about ADHD and what they learned about other families' experiences. After 10 weeks of 2-hour sessions, parents felt more competent. Although this study had its limitations – there was no control group – it supports our hypothesis that psychoeducation for family members of adults with ADHD will prove beneficial.

ADHD psychoeducation groups

Procedure and structure

The following suggestions on how to perform psychoeducation with adults with ADHD are based on extrapolations from the literature and on our clinical experience gained from running psychoeducational groups over a 5-year period at the University Medical Center in Groningen. Adults with ADHD often tend to know quite a lot already about ADHD. Most will have surfed the Internet and made themselves familiar with sites of advocacy groups, will have read a few books on the subject, and will have discussed aspects of the disorder with others. Sometimes they are so well informed that they seem to know more about ADHD than their mental health worker as not every psychiatrist/psychologist is necessarily familiar with the disorder. We therefore recommend strongly that psychoeducation for adults with ADHD be given by a psychiatrist or a psychologist who has specialized in ADHD.

Usually information about a mental disorder is given on a one-to-one basis, but the advantages of group psychoeducation for ADHD as part of a formal treatment plan are obvious. First, sharing experiences and knowledge with others reduces the feeling people tend to have of being the only one with their kind of problem. Second, the group helps patients recognize and normalize their experiences (Lukens & McFarlane, 2004). In addition to receiving information from the clinician (so-called expert power), patients also learn from each other, a process known as "referent power."

In addition, it is of paramount importance to involve partners and family or close friends at some later stage in the group process. In the groups we led, patients were allowed to invite partners, children, family, and also close friends to the fifth and sixth sessions. This invitation can be extended to primary caregivers, study advisers, colleagues, etc. To involve colleagues may at first seem a bit unusual, but then adults with ADHD have problems not just in personal relationships but also at work and in keeping track of their finances, driving their car, and participating in community institutions. Another possibility is to have separate psychoeducation programs for partners and for family and close friends.

Patients may join a psychoeducation group on their own, or they may be referred to one by their health care workers. The professional leading the psychoeducation sessions may want to do an intake to pinpoint a patient's specific problems and needs.

Ideally, a group should be made up of at least 6 but not more than 10 adults with ADHD. If every member decides to involve his or her partner, the group will have a maximum of 20 participants in the fifth and sixth sessions. For these later sessions we usually ask patients to keep the number of invited family members down to no more than three. Theoretically, this means there could be groups of 40, but practically this is unlikely to happen. In our experience, participants initially appear enthusiastic about inviting partners and family, but many then retract the invitation or prove unable to ensure that people do come with them. One reason may be that adult patients are ashamed to involve partners and family or that family members still feel stigmatized by previous experiences (Harborne, Wolpert, & Clare, 2004). Of course, practical problems, such as an inconvenient time of the group session, finding someone to take care of the children, and the like, may limit participation of family members and friends.

One obvious problem – common in people with ADHD, as it directly relates to their attention and time management problems – is that they simply forget the meeting time. One can try to solve this problem by sending the patients a reminder the week before and having the clinic's secretary phone them on the day of the meeting. This proves partly effective, and we still are looking for ways of helping the patients to come in time.

In the literature the duration of the group – which normally meets in one 90-minute session per week – has varied from a few weeks to one year. We believe a limited duration is the most effective, as the aim is to provide education, not therapy. Therefore, at our clinic we offer a general program of four sessions for individuals with ADHD alone, and then in the fifth and sixth sessions they can invite partners and family members. Topics for the first two sessions are fixed, but in the third and the fourth session participants choose topics from a list they have been given in the first session. Patient with ADHD need to be given information piecemeal, and key concepts should be mentioned repeatedly. In addition, as patients with ADHD across the life span will need periodic interventions, they should be able to attend a psychoeducation group cycle more than once.

The length of each session may vary. We started out with sessions of 1 hour, because we thought patients with ADHD would find this time already long enough for them to try and sit still and concentrate. Yet participants protested almost from the start that 1 hour was too short to allow topics to be adequately discussed and also for them to have time to share their experiences, something they proved very keen on doing. Therefore, in consultation with the participants themselves, we decided to extend sessions to 90 minutes, with a break of 15 minutes in the middle; this timing turned out to satisfy all sides involved. Even then, after the 90-minute meetings end, the participants often spend additional time socializing because of their need to share their experiences. We provide the opportunity for them to remain in the meeting room and have coffee and tea for an additional half-hour after the main session. Those who find sharing experiences particularly effective are strongly advised to contact an ADHD advocacy organization that organizes self-help groups.

The role of the professional

Patients with ADHD have been criticized throughout their lives for their behavior, and they feel frustrated, often blame themselves, and show low levels of self-esteem. The professional's positive attitude, with every so often a bit of humor, can be the beginning of a constructive interaction with participants. Needless to say, it is most important for professionals to show respect and empathy toward the participants.

The professional, usually a psychiatrist or psychologist, should have a fair amount of experience in working with adults with ADHD and be able to differentiate between ADHD problems and those due to comorbid disorders. He or she has to highlight that what the group is doing is education and not group psychotherapy. The professional who notices that a participant has psychological problems can provide feedback and advise that individual to talk the problem over with his or her caregiver.

The professional leads the group and monitors the time. As patients with ADHD suffer from attention problems, difficulties with organization and with time awareness, restlessness, and impulsivity in speaking – all of which will come out in the psychoeducation sessions – the information given should be accurate and easy to understand, again with key concepts repeatedly emphasized. The overall program should be well structured, and the professional has to be decisive, though always respectful, in dealing with the impulsive behavior of the participants. Because some adults with ADHD talk excessively, whereas others have inattention problems and are very quiet, the professional also has to make sure that each participant is given the opportunity to participate.

Three rules have to be clear from the start to all participants: (1) do not talk about other group members to people not involved in this group, (2) do not miss sessions, and (3) be on time. The second and third rules can pose a problem for patients with ADHD as explained earlier.

Most participants are eager to understand their symptoms and are on the whole highly motivated to learn skills that help them cope with their problems; they start to externalize less as the sessions go on and are usually very willing to work on themselves. Despite the distress, sessions often include moments of joyfulness. Because groups of ADHD patients are generally highly motivated and actively involved, working with them is a gratifying experience.

Finally, before the sessions begin, we recommend giving participants a manual containing an outline of the program, handouts with information about the topics to be addressed, and references for literature and useful internet sites; for example, of advocacy groups. The manual should be written in concise, clear language, using short and simple sentences, and with a good deal of pictorial information.

Outline of a six-session program

In this section we outline a six-session program for individuals with ADHD that incorporates the elements of psychoeducation (see Table 21.1).

In their study of a psychoeducational program for families with children with ADHD and depression, the Patient and Family Education Program (PFEP), Lopez et al. (2005) noted that the amount of education they provided proved too much for some parents, who said they felt overwhelmed by it. This tallies with our own clinical experience. In our initial groups, adult ADHD participants claimed we told them too much about

Table 21.1 Key concepts of psychoeducation

Recognition of the symptoms belonging to ADHD for each individual

Recognition of the positive aspects of ADHD for each individual

Becoming aware of the functional disabilities due to ADHD

Consequences of having ADHD on different areas of life (work, social life, relationship, parenting)

Learning how to find reliable information on ADHD

Learning to think in a constructive way how to deal with the problems related to ADHD

comorbid disorders, that this information was confusing, and that they were unable to absorb it. We learned that we not only had to keep track of how much time we dedicated to each topic but also had to estimate the relevance of the topic and the content of the information we were providing.

Providing education about the nature, causes, and the course of ADHD symptoms through the life span involves giving alternative explanations for their behaviors – for example, their failure to complete their homework is not due to laziness but to the symptoms of ADHD – and clarifying the problems participants confront. Participants often experience feelings of relief but also of grief. We always end sessions with a review of the participants' strengths, so as to give them a sense of hope and also to emphasize their self-reliance and efficacy (Bandura, 1986), so they can gain confidence in their ability to perform specific behaviors adequately or to change certain conditions successfully.

First session

The first session starts with an introduction about the program itself and sets out the group rules. The participants then introduce themselves and briefly tell the other group members about their expectations for the group.

Next, the professional assesses the knowledge that participants already have and their needs, interests, and strengths so he or she can tailor the information accordingly. The professional writes key words on a blackboard so they can easily be referred to again in the discussion. Lopez et al. (2005) suggested that participants be asked to choose the topics for discussion from a list of relevant concerns and questions prepared by staff members. Examples include "What does it mean to have ADHD? What are psychiatric comorbid disorders? How does the disorder affect my leisure time?"

For some topics one may want to invite guest speakers or, in sessions three and four, ask one of the participants to give an introduction to the discussion.

In Session One, information is provided about the signs and symptoms of ADHD, hereditary and environmental causes, comorbid disorders, its lifetime course, impairments, and myths and misconceptions. We illustrate how a professional diagnosis of ADHD is made and which diagnostic tools are used, briefly summarizing the usefulness and limitations of the DSM-IV classification system (American Psychiatric Association, 1994) and the history of the concept of ADHD.

Because people with ADHD display a considerable variety of behaviors (Barkley, 1991), not all participants know how pervasive the handicaps of ADHD can be in their own lives. They may hear their partners or family members talk about behavioral problems that they themselves are unaware of having. That is why we ask all participants to describe the handicaps they are aware of that they suffer because of ADHD. We write their responses on the blackboard and then explain which of them are due to ADHD and which are symptoms of a comorbid disorder or can be considered as personality traits. We then concentrate on the symptoms of ADHD.

After making a list of what patients already know, we ask each of them about the misconceptions and myths of ADHD they have encountered. An example of a still widely held misconception is that ADHD is the result of a poor diet (Sonuga & Balding, 1993). As beliefs about causation influence the kind of treatment a patient chooses, it is important to address this issue (Bussing et al., 2003).

Another misconception is that being diagnosed with ADHD gives an individual a license to behave irresponsibly or an excuse to be lazy and maladaptive. Not surprisingly, in the last two psychoeducation sessions in which partners participate, this misconception in particular elicits strong emotions.

Second session

In the second session patients learn about treatment options and recommendations, including medication, psychosocial treatments, and alternative treatments. Treatment is an important topic in psychoeducation, and patients and partners tend to ask a lot of questions about medication. It is often necessary to reiterate that ADHD is not a disorder of motivation or will and that medication can have an effect on the neurobiological

factors involved. Some patients are apprehensive about psychostimulants and feel strongly that they should be avoided. Others expect medication to take care of all their problems. Patients and partners need unbiased information about scientific research, the value but also the limitation of medications, their effects and side effects, and alternatives to medication – all of which the professional preferably provides in a dispassionate tone of voice.

Education about psychosocial treatments includes information about behavior management techniques, family therapy, coaching, or developing self-management techniques, which are interventions that teach an adult to manage more effectively in their work, social, and family relationships. We explain that these interventions can be all the more effective when given by a professional familiar with comorbid disorders and their symptoms, which can interfere with the treatment.

Many patients are seeking alternative treatments, and in the groups we have led, they often ask our opinion about them. It is important to provide relevant scientific information about the advantages and disadvantages of specific alternative treatments, such as neurofeedback, the few-food diet, and fatty acids treatment, and how promising they can be for the treatment of ADHD (Arnold, 2001).

Third and fourth sessions

Topics that participants selected from the list they were given in Session One are discussed in the third and the fourth sessions. In our groups, the most common topics have been career and work problems, leisure time, marital problems, friendships, finances, lifetime management of behaviors, the use of drugs and alcohol, and comorbid disorders, such as personality and anxiety disorders. Additional educational materials are provided that are relevant for the subject and are not included in the manual.

One or two participants prepare a short introduction to each topic. This task engages them in the group, and patients often comment on the final evaluation form that at first they were afraid to give an introduction, but that in the end it proved instructive and raised their self-esteem.

Fifth and sixth sessions

In the last two sessions participants invite their partners, family, children (older than age 12), and close friends to participate. Psychoeducation emphasizes the importance of working with the partners and family, both as a way of obtaining further relevant information and of providing information and support to the relatives (Falloon, Boyd, & McGill, 1984, Weiss et al., 1999). As they often have limited access to resources, partners may well be exhausted and feel helpless, disappointed, and frustrated. We start the fifth session in the same way as the first – with an introduction of the participants and assessment of existing knowledge and misconceptions. What often occurs is that, as soon as the professional starts providing information, the participants with ADHD, who already had heard most of it, will take over and begin explaining to their partners and family members what they had learned about ADHD in the previous sessions. We are often amazed by how much information they retain and how clearly they are able to explain symptoms, treatment, and other aspects of ADHD, often with a good deal of humor in the bargain. This always works to break the ice, and partners and family members soon begin to feel more comfortable in and with the group. Issues that often come up for discussion are the role of heredity, raising the children, housekeeping, intimacy, and how to live with a person with ADHD.

Many parents continue to feel stigmatized when they talk about the past and the problems they have had with their ADHD children. A study by Harborne et al. (2004) of parents' views of the etiology of ADHD in their children found that parents often felt blamed for their children's difficulties and that they had to fight professionals, teachers, families, and friends to gain recognition and respect for their children while they themselves experienced a good deal of distress. In these sessions blame is an important issue, and we provide information on how to cope with it. If this proves insufficient, we suggest they talk about it in a family session or refer them to a family therapist. In general, we do not deal with blame in the psychoeducation group as we are keen not to let the group develop into a therapy session.

Overview and recommendations

Psychoeducation for adults with ADHD is an important psychosocial intervention and should be incorporated into all treatment plans.

We were unable to find evidence-based guidelines on how to provide psychoeducation for ADHD adults. Extrapolating information from psychoeduca-

tion groups for parents with children with ADHD and for adults with other psychiatric disorders and consulting with patients with ADHD, we put together a psychoeducation program that also fully takes into consideration our own clinical experience.

Many questions remain as yet unanswered. For example, how much information should be given, do partners need their own education program, how can we successfully motivate partners to become actively involved, who will benefit most from psychoeducation, and, conversely, who is likely to drop out? Further research is also needed to identify active ingredients of psychoeducation for adult patients with ADHD and to explore to what extent participation helps improve the overall treatment.

Acknowledgement

The authors wish to thank Dick Bruggeman for his comments on an earlier version of the manuscript.

References

American Psychiatric Association. (1994). *Diagnostic and Statistical Manual of Mental Disorders*. 4th ed. Washington, DC: American Psychiatric Association.

Arnold LE. (2001). Alternative treatments for adults with attention-deficit hyperactivity disorder (ADHD). *Ann N Y Acad Sci* **931**:310–41.

Bandura A. (1986). *Social Foundations of Thought and Action: A Social Cognitive Theory*. Englewood Cliffs, NJ: Prentice-Hall.

Barkley RA. (1991). *Attention Deficit Hyperactivity Disorder: A Clinical Workbook*. New York. Guilford Press.

Brown TE. (2000). Psychosocial interventions for attention-deficit disorders and comorbid conditions. In: **Brown TE,** ed. *Attention-Deficit Disorders and Comorbidities in Children, Adolescents, and Adults* (pp. 537–569). Washington, DC: American Psychiatric Press: 537–69.

Bussing R, Gary FA, Mills TL, Garvan CW. (2003). Parental explanatory models of ADHD. Gender and cultural variations. *Soc Psychiatry Psychiatr Epidemiol* **38**:563–75.

Dixon L, McFarlane WR, Lefley H, et al. (2001). Evidence-based practices for services to families of people with psychiatric disabilities. *Psychiatr Serv* **52**:903–910.

Falloon IR, Boyd JL, McGill CW. (1984). *Family Care of Schizophrenia*. New York: Guilford Press.

Harborne A, Wolpert M, Clare L. (2004). Making sense of ADHD: a battle for understanding? Parents' view of their children being diagnosed with ADHD. *Clin Child Psychol Psychiatry* **9**(3):327–39.

Lopez MA, Toprac MG, Crismon ML, et al. (2005). A psychoeducational program for children with ADHD or depression and their families: results from the CMAP feasibility study. *Comm Ment Health J* **41**(1):51–66.

Lukens EP, McFarlane WR. (2004). Psychoeducation as evidence-based practice: considerations for practice, research and policy. In: Roberts AR, Yeager KR, eds. *Foundations of Evidence-Based Social Work Practice*. New York: Oxford University Press: 214–319.

McCleary L, Ridley T. (1999). Parenting adolescents with ADHD: evaluation of a psychoeducation group. *Patient Educ Couns* **38**:3–10.

Murphy K. (2005). Psychosocial treatments for ADHD in teens and adults: a practice-friendly review. *J Clin Psychiatry* **61**(5):607–19.

Sonuga BE, Balding J. (1993). British parents' beliefs about the causes of three forms of childhood psychological disturbances. *J Abnorm Child Psychol*: **21**: 367–76.

Weiss M, Hechtman L, Weiss G. (1999). *ADHD in Adulthood: A Guide to Current Theory, Diagnosis, and Treatment*. Baltimore: Johns Hopkins University Press.

Website with materials from the CMAP patient and family education program are available at http://www.dshs. state.tx.us/mhprograms/cmap.shtm.

Chapter

22

Coaching in ADHD

Doris Ryffel

Introduction

Our current understanding of ADHD is based on the assumption of the bio-psycho-social nature of this condition throughout the life span. On this premise experience proves that a multimodal treatment is the most promising approach to overcome the impairing traits of ADHD.

Medication, psychotherapy, and coaching are the three pillars in the ADHD treatment plan. ADHD is a lifelong disability that requires ongoing management, reinforcement, and support. Without adequate identification and proper treatment ADHD may have serious consequences: problems with relationships, academic and professional failure, and the possible development of other psychiatric disorders.

To overcome these difficulties a person has to be capable of taking control of his or her life. Through specific ADHD coaching the individual learns to cope with the daily challenges of life and gains control. The coaching process usually begins once the medication regimen is effective and psychotherapy has been successful.

What is ADHD coaching?

The concept of ADHD coaching appears for the first time in the 1994 book, *Driven to Distraction* by E. M. Hallowell and John J. Ratey.

Coaching builds on a partnership between the therapist and patient with the aim of designing an effective plan of action to improve performance in everyday life. Two steps are needed to achieve this aim. First, the individual has to gain insight and understand why and how ADHD gets in the way of effective functioning. The next step is acceptance of the condition while at the same time viewing it as the chance for a new start: knowledge is power.

With the help of a coach new plans are set in place, and achievable goals and realistic expectations are identified to terminate the pattern of never finishing ongoing projects. Strategies for improvement, such as developing social skills (Novotni, 1999), acquiring learning skills, planning environmental structuring techniques, coping with forgetfulness and disorganization, and gaining time and money management skills, are target areas. Positive results will be within reach only through a commitment to work together in a scheduled time frame.

Comorbid conditions can be a serious impediment for coaching. If the individual with ADHD also suffers from depression, anxiety disorder, or substance abuse, these psychiatric conditions have to be treated adequately before coaching can take place.

Life circumstances such as troublesome relationships and financial problems but also highlights such as childbirth can make it difficult to carry out a consistent coaching process.

Is coaching therapy?

Cognitive-behavioral therapy (CBT), the psychotherapeutic method used for treating ADHD, and coaching can flow into one another when the psychotherapist and coach are one and the same person, but coaching in itself cannot be defined as therapy. A coach deals with practical issues in everyday life: planning, organization, setting priorities, and managing time. One could simply say that coaching is about the questions – what, when, and how – and CBT is about the why. CBT and coaching should work together because they share the aim of helping the individual with ADHD develop a healthy self-esteem. This aim goes along with the acceptance of strengths and limitations and the ability to have self-control, tolerate frustrations, achieve a degree of self-discipline, be able to manage

ADHD in Adults: Characterization, Diagnosis and Treatment, ed. Jan Buitelaar, Cornelis Kan and Philip Asherson.
Published by Cambridge University Press. © Cambridge University Press 2011.

different situations, and find those hidden capabilities and talents that may compensate for other shortcomings. Therapist and coach both have the crucial task of increasing the self-awareness and strengthening the self-control of the individual with ADHD so he or she can develop a healthy self-esteem.

The coaching process

Because coaching is about understanding ADHD sufferers and paying attention to their individual difficulties, there are different kinds of coaching. Aims are formulated and strategies are developed together with the individual that allow these aims to become reality. Depending on the individual's need for therapy, situation in life, and educational level, the coach makes a plan and offers corresponding support.

ADHD involves a more or less pronounced impairment in the executive functions (Brown, 2005). Individuals with ADHD report chronic deficits in six areas:

1. Impaired faculty to organize and prioritize and a lack of motivation
2. Difficulty in focusing and maintaining attention
3. Reduced concentration, marked distractibility, and difficulty in maintaining a sustained effort
4. Impaired self-control of emotions and diminished tolerance of frustration
5. Impaired verbal working memory and as a consequence little self-monitoring, self-control, and self-questioning
6. Impaired capacity to inhibit behavior

To address these difficulties, the coaching process should incorporate these six elements (Ratey et al., 2001):

1. *Identification* of difficulties and problems in the individual's current situation
2. *Formulation* of new plans and aims, considering the individual's capabilities, desires, possibilities, and limitations
3. *Structuring and planning*: Discussion of potential solutions to problems so that the formulated aims can be put into practice
4. *Management of time*: Fixing of time frames with the aid of hourly, daily, and weekly time tables and the use of diaries, bulletin boards, organizers, and special watches
5. *Checks*: To support self-monitoring, self-control, and self-regulation, the coach regularly checks the progress made by the individual

6. *Emotional support*: Last but not least, coaching imparts encouragement and positive feedback; in the case of a setback the coach is empathetic and tries to continue the work with the individual, always based on the principle of hope

ADHD individuals often have a tendency to understand only part of the information given to them. Asking for confirmation is helpful and shows whether the directives have been understood, so that misunderstandings can be avoided. Clarity, good timing, and not demanding too much will help. Small steps lead to goal achievement in the long run and are implemented more consistently.

No value judgments should be made in the case of setbacks. On the contrary, praise is more productive. A lesson can also be drawn from a mishap. The so-called sandwich method has stood the test: praise, critical remark, and praise. In this way, the individual's attention is aroused, and he or she keeps at the task and does not indulge in self-pity. Of course, the coach should offer praise and positive reinforcement for success.

Assigning homework tailored to adults is a good way to assess progress in the coaching process. Although adults with ADHD often associate homework with negative school memories, when the coach points out that it is a different kind of homework, most adults are willing to accomplish the assigned task. The assignment should reflect current issues and provide a way for problem solving, as the individual formulates possible solutions. The coach should give clear, explicit guidelines taking into account the individual's situation, lifestyle, and domestic difficulties.

We know how capable of enthusiasm ADHD individuals are and what a wealth of original ideas they have. By working with the individual resources of each patient, it is not unusual to discover creative potential that had previously lain dormant. The coach should formulate short-, medium-, and long-term goals together with the individual and then help him or her sort things out and reformulate unattainable hopes and expectations into attainable goals. All agreements should be set down in writing, but flexibility is nevertheless mandatory.

The ability to carry out a complex activity in a targeted and consistent manner and to achieve a successful result requires attention. Deficits of attention result in compromised actions in the areas of perceptive functions, organization of activities, and the directed execution of actions. To apply an attentive behavior effectively, the following five conditions must be met:

1. The task must be understood.
2. The aim of the assignment must be kept in focus throughout.
3. A strategy for solutions must be developed.
4. Internal and external disturbing factors should be filtered out as far as possible.
5. The coach should work with the individual and monitor the activity leading to the solution.

This approach promotes the individual's self-awareness, self-confidence, self-motivation, and self-management.

The ADHD coach

ADHD coaches may come from a variety of professional backgrounds, but should have the following knowledge and skills:

- Have knowledge of the disorder and the characteristic symptoms of ADHD, and the knowledge should be continuously updated
- Be capable of listening patiently to the affected person
- Be future-oriented and able to formulate new goals with the patient
- Be able to work in a structured manner and communicate this structure to the patient – in this way, goals become reality!
- Be aware that successful coaching requires time and should therefore be prepared to invest this time
- Talk with experts, schools, and employers; networking is frequently the only way to sort out a situation that is seemingly beyond remedy
- Not take over the patient's responsibility but always support him or her in all endeavors and realistic plans
- Be flexible; coaching may take place via face-to-face dialogue, telephone, or e-mail, depending on the patient's particular situation and issues
- Be characterized by personal integrity, neither benefiting from nor abusing the patient's situation, and be able to handle confidential information with discretion as would a physician or a psychologist

- Have empathy and understanding, offering encouraging and positive feedback whenever possible

A good coach is characterized by empathy, compassion, and a motivating attitude. However, one important point should be heeded: although it is natural to be happy about the successes of patients, the coach should still strive to remain as emotionally neutral as possible. He or she should show joy at the individual's success but within limits; otherwise pressure is put on the patient who does not want to disappoint the coach. The coach should always remember that the achievement of goals requires time.

Case vignette 1

Marlene, a 20-year-old patient, came to my practice 2 years ago when she was 18 years old. From childhood she had experienced difficulty in school, suffering from poor concentration, increased distractibility, and insufficient strategies to cope with stress. Furthermore she showed emotional instability characterized by the switch within a short time from a feeling of anger and despair into feeling happy. Inner restlessness and low self-esteem finally led to a social phobia, with withdrawal and depressive symptoms. A precise evaluation revealed that deficits from the ADHD diagnosed in childhood continued to be present.

Because the primary target of therapy was mood stabilization, an antidepressant medication was started. Once she was emotionally stabilized, stimulants were prescribed in addition to the antidepressant medication. Psychotherapy with weekly sessions was conducted at the same time; it focused on the social phobia that caused her to shy away from contacts. Then coaching was started to address her ADHD-specific symptoms.

At the start of therapy Marlene offered the following self-observations as being particularly troubling:

- Sometimes I get lost when writing or reading a text and have to start all over again. I lose the thread of what it is all about. I lose the context or the relationship to what I have been thinking a moment ago. I also am afraid of forgetting my ideas instantly when I am together with others; therefore, I cannot communicate effectively.
- Quite often I have the feeling of being looked at as if I am stupid. I'm afraid that the other person is

angry or upset with me. I simply don't want to expose myself, don't want to attract attention. I worry very much whether the people with whom I deal reject me. I fear they believe that I cause my mishaps intentionally.

- My father says, "Why do you just talk without thinking first?" I have the impression that my father considers me to be stupid and I don't believe him if he denies this.
- Frequently I have the feeling of having to lean on others as if I need their attention and support in order to remain focused.
- I feel that time is running out and when I am aware that time is limited I become fussy. Therefore group work means trouble for me.
- Sometimes I have great difficulty not to lose the thread and on other occasions I can stay focused for hours without problem.

My first goal was to explore Marlene's resources (Kolberg & Nadeau, 2002). The purpose was to make the patient see her positive sides, capabilities, and strengths and not only her deficits, which she knew sufficiently well, for which she reproached herself and which made her despair. The result was discovery of a whole range of positive properties: her sensitivity, her talent in writing good texts full of fantasy, her varied interests, and her helpfulness. These properties became a valid "trump card" that I reactivated in the course of the coaching when her negative view of things prevailed. A comprehensive and detailed identification of problems followed.

A plan for the week was established, incorporating the following elements:

- To arrange the workplace in her room so that there would be enough space to open her books and files and she would not be distracted by a thousand other things
- To ask somebody from the school class to study with her; she is able to memorize subject matter better when discussing it with others.
- To take notes during school lessons, in particular if the teacher presents an uninteresting subject in a monotonous voice. Taking notes facilitates her focusing and keeps her from losing the thread. She finds it easier to retain a visual impression than to listen for a long time.
- To reserve in her diary a fixed time for learning and to keep herself free exclusively for this time

(e.g., a half-hour each school night or 2 hours on Sunday)
- To first gain an overview of the subject material being studied. What precisely is the content, and how is the topic treated? In this way what she reads makes sense, can be classified, and is easier to link to already acquired knowledge and experience.

It is imperative for Marlene to receive repeated feedback and encouragement, although she is highly motivated to implement the proposals that we elaborated together. She herself asked to summarize and write down at the end of each coaching session what we had discussed.

It is human nature to want to solve our problems independently. This means that, even when help is requested, the coach should make sure that the patient is serious about wanting it. The coach will inevitably feel frustrated and annoyed if appointments and agreements are not kept.

As a coach one should be flexible and ask questions time and again to ensure that the chosen strategy is the appropriate one; otherwise it must be changed.

Case vignette 2

Is there a relationship between ADHD and a person's intelligence? Research over the past several decades has shown that the chronic nature of ADHD is independent of intelligence, despite a marked impairment in coping with life caused by ADHD-typical symptoms.

The 44-year-old patient is a physician, married, and the father of a 15-year-old son with ADHD. Here are catch words from the life story written by the patient himself:

- I could read by the age of 5 and played the piano before going to school.
- I had difficulty learning something new at school and could not overcome obstacles step by step.
- It seemed totally unthinkable for me to choose a profession. Already in adolescence I had no idea of "real life" and lived many hours of the day in an internal pseudo-world in which I was the greatest and did not need to prove myself.
- As time went by I felt my depressive traits reinforced by the increasing awareness of my learning disability: poor concentration already

after a few minutes with extreme flight of thoughts.

- I experienced difficulty doing my homework; my room was disorganized.
- Occasionally I was able to overcome my procrastinating nature, when I had to accomplish under pressure, although typically "in a hurry, and therefore not perfect."
- It was by mere chance that I started to study medicine.
- My marriage was difficult. I didn't know that I have ADHD. My wife could never really count on me. I could never make final decisions. The personified ambivalence: I stand at a crossroads, not by choice but because I cannot make up my mind which way to take.
- Like everything important in my life, I forgot the details of my son's child-psychiatric consultation or maybe I didn't understand them to start with, owing to my massive problem of perception.

He had undergone several psychotherapies that, however, did not bear fruit. He reported that he had difficulty in concentrating and was unable to read a book to the end because he would lose the thread. He also said, "I am unable to make decisions, have no friends, and I am dominated by my feelings. I also cannot handle money, am an impulsive shopper but fortunately it is my wife who manages our financial matters."

He continued, "In my profession I am under great pressure. I constantly feel that I am not up to it. It is above all the organization and the telephone that cause me headaches." However, his contact with patients is good and in principle he enjoys the medical profession. Because of his subjective impression of being overworked he finds neither time nor leisure for his wife and children.

After a thorough ADHD assessment, therapy was started. It was obvious from the beginning that in addition to medication this patient required coaching. Coaching covered the following topics:

Organization: We discussed the concrete details of organizing his practice, above all how to better organize administrative tasks such as writing reports, answering written queries, and billing. The doctor's receptionist is involved as well, helping prioritize tasks according to their importance and urgency.

Time management: He is virtually eaten up by his patients; he is good-natured and can never say "no." Because of this trait he is, of course, loved by his patients – but at the cost of his own health and his family. He must learn to draw limits, limiting the number of patients and setting a fixed time for consultations by phone.

Marital relationship: As the daily professional demands overwhelm him, his marital relationship is under pressure. Having dinner once a week just with his wife is imperative.

Up to now little progress has been made. There is no correlation between ADHD and intelligence. Despite his strong willingness to change, this highly gifted physician is unable, due to his marked ADHD, to adhere to clear agreements.

Case vignette 3

The 42-year-old patient is married and the mother of four children. She is a nurse by profession but does not work as such, having to help on her husband's farm. The patient was diagnosed with ADHD, inattentive type, and depression.

The burden of reconciling the demands of family, household, and farm was increasingly too much for her. The patient first received an antidepressant treatment, and after mood stabilization was achieved, she was prescribed a stimulant. Although there was considerable improvement, marked symptoms persisted with regard to her short-term memory – working memory – which made it difficult for her to cope with everyday life.

She reported the following problems:

- I can't remember names. This leads to embarrassing situations when I meet acquaintances and I am unable to greet them by name.
- It is still difficult for me to keep an appointment. It often occurs that I mix up dates and days, thereby missing the parents' evening at school, for example.
- I am looking for my keys and purse all the time.
- Although I can concentrate better with Ritalin when reading, I am still unable to retain what I have read. I have therefore developed over the years an actual defensive attitude toward reading which I have to actively fight against now.
- I am now better able to organize household chores but the routine bores me. Often I am overcome by lethargy so that much is left undone.

The following coaching strategies were used to address these problems:

Impaired memory, disturbed short-term memory, and forgetting names: Visualize the person concerned and at the same time name the person. Through the visual and acoustic stimulus and with constant exercise the patient will be able, in the course of time, to memorize names better.

Keeping appointments: It is typical that this patient kept three diaries at the same time. As a result, she entered some of her appointments in one or the other diaries. It is hardly surprising she could not remember important dates.

Coaching strategy: keep only one diary in which every appointment is entered in detail. In addition, open the diary each morning.

Losing and misplacing objects: Place keys, purse, and diary always in the same place and urge her family members to do the same.

Reading and retaining information: External and internal distraction (her own thoughts) lead to her feeling overwhelmed by input so that she could not process what she read. Shakespeare's words in *Hamlet* (Act III, scene 3) could not illustrate this condition better:

My words fly up, my thoughts remain below:
Words without thoughts never to heaven go.

Coaching strategy: Read for short periods with breaks in between. Being a housewife, she was advised to turn to light physical activity during the short breaks (fold the laundry, empty the dishwasher). During these breaks she can reflect on what she has read and transfer it from short-term into long-term memory so that she would later be able to recall it.

Feeling bored: Patients frequently report that they are unable to fulfill their duties without a "kick." Household chores are monotonous and boring because they are repetitive. No sooner is the clean and ironed laundry neatly stacked away in the closet than the laundry basket is full again, and the individual experiences the frustration of having to begin the Sisyphean task all over again.

Coaching strategy: This patient developed her own strategy to escape from feelings of boredom, lethargy, and frustration. With increasing frequency she invited a friend of hers for afternoon tea. This stimulated and motivated her to keep her home tidy, bake cakes and biscuits, and try out new recipes. She had set herself a target and could then work more efficiently. Thanks to the increased contact with other women she gained greater enjoyment out of her life.

Conclusion

Once the diagnosis of ADHD has been made in a patient, the following five-pronged multimodal therapeutic approach has proven successful:

1. *Information* about the nature of the ADHD disorder and its impact on coping with life. With the patient's consent, the partner, family members, and if necessary the employer should also be informed as far as possible.
2. *Medication* to attain emotional stabilization and to regulate the ADHD symptoms. It will frequently be necessary to combine basic stimulant therapy with antidepressant medication.
3. *Psychotherapy, specially cognitive behavior therapy*, adapted and modified with regard to the patient's ADHD
4. *Coaching* to restructure everyday life, formulate goals, and make it possible to put these goals into practice
5. *Activation* of all existing resources

Although to this day there is no published research evaluating the effectiveness of coaching, empirical reports find that it is very helping for ADHD-affected individuals because it is a psychoeducational approach designed to help them practice adaptive and coping behaviors. Its benefits are the development of specific skills and strategies that are applicable on a daily basis and lead to the attainment of goals. To a certain degree, coaching enables ADHD-specific challenges to be mastered and overcome.

For the past 12 years I have evaluated and treated adults with ADHD, and it is my opinion that ADHD adults receiving both medications and behavioral treatments, including coaching, have the best opportunity to improve their well-being. However, more research is needed to demonstrate this fact. I hope that in the near future encouraging findings will emerge that support the effectiveness of coaching in adults with ADHD.

References

Brown TE. (2005). *Attention Deficit Disorder: The Unfocused Mind in Children and Adults*. New Haven: Yale University Press.

Hallowell EM, Ratey JJ. (1994). *Driven to Distraction*. New York: Touchstone.

Kolberg J, **Nadeau K.** (2002). *ADD-Friendly Ways to Organize Your Life*. New York: Brunner-Rutledge.

Novotni M. (1999). *What Does Everybody Else Know That I Don't?* Plantation, FL: Specialty Press.

Ratey N, et al. (2001). *The Guiding Principles for Coaching Individuals with Attention Deficit Disorders*. Wilmington, DE: ADDA.

Further reading

Ryffel D. (2001). *ADS bei Erwachsenen*. Bern: H. Huber.

Ryffel D. (2003). *ADS/ADHS: Wir flen uns anders*. Bern: H. Huber.

Ryffel D. (2004). *ADHS bei Frauen- den Geflen ausgeliefert*. Bern: H. Huber.

Chapter 23

Clinical application of research on cognitive-behavioral therapies for adults with ADHD

Stephen P. McDermott

Introduction

Attention-deficit hyperactivity disorder (ADHD) is a prevalent disorder estimated to affect 2–9% of school-aged children (the term "ADHD" used in this chapter also refers to previous definitions of the disorder; Anderson et al., 1987; Bauermeister, Canino, & Bird, 1994; Safer & Krager, 1988). Prospective, long-term follow-up studies have shown the persistence of the syndrome in approximately 50% of young adults diagnosed as having ADHD in childhood (Mannuzza et al., 1991, 1993; Weiss, et al., 2008). Epidemiological data suggest that as many as 5% of adults may have ADHD (Murphy & Barkley, 1996).

Studies of adults with ADHD have demonstrated high rates of comorbidity with depression, anxiety, substance use, and conduct/antisocial disorders (Biederman et al., 1993; Shekim et al., 1990). It is not surprising that studies indicate that 20–25% of adult outpatients with depression or substance abuse also have ADHD (Alpert et al., 1996; T. Wilens et al., 1994).

Further, many authors describe obstacles associated with ADHD in adults that are neither the core symptoms of ADHD nor of distinct comorbid disorders. ADHD adults are often described as having problems with procrastination, boredom intolerance, frustration intolerance, and disorganization. They have also been shown to have more relationship difficulties as well as academic and occupational underachievement despite adequate intellectual abilities (Biederman et al., 1993; Mannuzza et al., 1993). Ratey and associates (1992) noted that "associated problems" and comorbid disorders often cause more distress and dysfunction for ADHD adults than the core symptoms and are often the reasons these patients seek treatment.

Before 1999, little information existed in the published literature on the use of psychotherapies for ADHD adults (Bemporad & Zambenedetti, 1996;

Hallowell, 1995; McDermott, 2000; Weiss & Murray, 2003; Wilens et al., 1999). Although not tested under controlled conditions, traditional psychotherapies were reported to be generally ineffective in treating ADHD adults (Bemporad, 2001; Ratey et al., 1992; Weiss & Murray, 2003). In a retrospective assessment of the histories of 60 adults with ADHD, Ratey and associates (1992) reported that the majority of patients did not respond favorably to adequate psychotherapeutic treatment delivered by experienced psychotherapists using both short-term focused and long-term unstructured psychotherapies. However, these retrospective patient accounts were limited to descriptions of diverse, broadly defined psychotherapeutic interventions. Moreover, these adults were not diagnosed or treated for their ADHD at the time of their psychotherapeutic involvement. Two researchers (Weiss & Murray, 2003) summarized this period of time before 2000 as follows:

> There is a scarcity of controlled studies on the efficacy of psychosocial treatments for adults with ADHD. Clinicians with experience in treating adults with ADHD have used a variety of psychological interventions, including education about the disorder, involvement in a support group, skills training (e.g., vocational, organizational, time management, financial) and coaching. ... Cognitive behaviour therapy, training of parenting skills for adult parents with ADHD, vocational counseling and educational remediation may be helpful interventions, but controlled studies are needed to investigate their usefulness (p. 719).

Pharmacological therapies have generally been the mainstay of treatment of adults with ADHD (Davidson, 2008; Dodson, 2005; Wilens, Biederman, & Spencer, 2002). Although numerous studies have shown medications (primarily stimulants) to be effective treatments for a given research sample of adults with ADHD (for a review, see Wilens, Spencer, &

ADHD in Adults: Characterization, Diagnosis and Treatment, ed. Jan Buitelaar, Cornelis Kan and Philip Asherson.
Published by Cambridge University Press. © Cambridge University Press 2011.

Biederman, 2001), approximately 30% of adults in ADHD psychopharmacological outcome studies do not respond to medications alone. Moreover, adults in these treatment trials who are considered responders typically show a reduction in only 50% or less of the core symptoms of ADHD (Safren et al., 2005), even though in most studies, a successful response is considered a 50% or greater reduction of symptoms (Spencer et al., 1996). Recent evidence suggests that these residual symptoms can have a significant impact on an adult's ability to function in an effective way. Young and Gudjonsson (2008) examined adults who met full criteria for ADHD in childhood. They compared those adults who had "partial remission" of their ADHD (i.e., loss of some, but not all, of their ADHD symptoms) with adults with childhood ADHD who were in "full remission" (i.e., no longer had sufficient symptoms to meet criteria for ADHD). Adults with ADHD with partial remission had significantly more depression, anxiety, problems with friendships, antisocial activities and police contact, and drug and alcohol abuse than normal controls, whereas adults in full remission showed no significant differences in these criteria compared with normal controls. Young and Gudjonsson (2008, p. 162) noted that "symptom remission is associated with improvement in neuropsychological, clinical, and psychosocial problems," but also found that, even among adults with full remission of their ADHD symptoms, neuropsychological problems continued to exist (in comparison to the normal controls). These issues, among others, led clinicians and researchers to pursue the development of a psychotherapeutic approach to the treatment of adults with ADHD.

Cognitive-behavioral interventions have emerged as one of the best studied and most efficacious psychotherapeutic interventions in ADHD children and adolescents (Barkley, 1990, 2002; Hinshaw & Erhardt, 1991; Swanson et al., 2002) although outcome studies have shown mixed results (Safren et al., 2005). Cognitive-behavioral therapy (CBT) for adults shares many characteristics with psychotherapies used in pediatric ADHD groups, namely training in self-evaluation, social skills, anger and impulse management, as well as self-instruction relating to coping skills and problem solving (Barkley, 1990); hence there was an interest in examining the use of CBT for adults with ADHD. The proactive, focused, structured, and goal-directed nature of CBT is compelling given the nature of the disturbances in ADHD (Bemporad &

Zambenedetti, 1996; Hallowell, 1995). Yet, the child CBT protocols were not directly adaptable to ADHD adults, given their reliance on parental involvement for structure and motivation (Ramsay & Rostain, 2005; Safren et al., 2005).

Further, it is estimated that about 70% of adults with ADHD have at least one comorbid disorder, and many have several (Wilens et al., 2002). These disorders often compound the functional impairment of ADHD in adults and may interfere with their treatment; for example, the use of stimulants in patients with severe anxiety disorders or histories of stimulant dependence. CBT has demonstrated efficacy for major depression (Bockting et al., 2006; DeRubeis et al., 1999) and anxiety (Siev & Chambless, 2007; van Apeldoorn et al., 2008) and shows promise in substance abuse (Kadden et al., 1989, 2007; Najavits & Weiss, 1994), all disorders that are highly comorbid with ADHD in adults.

The theoretical construct of CBT addresses the interaction of cognition, behavior, and affect (McDermott & Wright, 1992) – areas that are speculated to be dysregulated in ADHD (Hinshaw & Erhardt, 1991). Yet the nature of the dysfunction in adults with ADHD can interfere with the process of therapy, including CBT. As Ramsey and Rostain (2005, p. 74) noted,

Adults with ADHD often present with two major therapy goals: (a) developing coping strategies with which to manage their symptoms of ADHD and (b) dealing with the pervasive emotional and functional effects that living with ADHD has had on their lives (including the presence of comorbid disorders; (Brown, 2000; Hallowell, 1995; McDermott, 2000; Ramsay & Rostain, 2003).

Yet, the very problems faced by these adults in their lives, which stem from the characteristic executive function problems of ADHD, pose challenges to their getting the most out of psychotherapy. These challenges include problems such as being unable to concentrate on a theme during a session, having difficulty remembering and generalizing insights developed during sessions to one's life, and poor follow through on therapeutic homework, to name a few. At their worst, these difficulties could lead to premature termination and/or a negative therapy experience that would replicate and perpetuate the sense of frustration and failure that the patient likely experienced throughout his or her life as a consequence of living with ADHD.

This chapter examines the design and results of six studies of psychosocial treatments for adults with ADHD. A summary, examining the similarities and differences among the therapies, discusses general clinical guidelines that can be deduced from the group of studies as a whole.

The studies

Research into the development of effective psychosocial treatments for adults with ADHD has expanded dramatically over the past decade or so (Table 23.1). The six major psychosocial research studies since 1999 are Wilens et al. (1999); Hesslinger et al. (2002), which is a modification of Linehan's dialectical behavior therapy (Linehan, 1993a, 1993b); Stevenson et al. (2002), based on cognitive remediation and CBT (Stevenson, personal communication, July 19, 2006), and Stevenson et al. (2003), which was a modification of the 2002 protocol requiring less direct therapist involvement; and Safren et al. (2004), an adaptation of standard CBT techniques and the treatment guidelines in McDermott (2000)).

Wilens et al. (1999)

The first report of a psychotherapy specifically developed for adults with ADHD was a case series, published by Wilens and co-workers in 1999, of 26 patients who were treated with a modified form of Beck's cognitive therapy (CT; McDermott, 1995, 2000). In 1999, Weiss, Hechtman, and Weiss noted, "Cognitive therapy is the only form of psychotherapy that has been systematically adapted specifically for adult ADHD and then tested empirically" (p. 196). McDermott's modifications of CT addressed, in part, the impediments created by ADHD to standard cognitive therapy in adults. In particular, the modified treatment emphasizes the role of beliefs as determinants of which components adults attend to in a specific situation, how this belief/attention interaction affects their perception of the situation and any necessary problem solving, and how emotional lability sidetracks ADHD treatments in adults. Weiss et al. (1999, p. 198) described this modification as follows: "What is unique to this adaptation of cognitive therapy to those with ADHD is the emphasis on capturing attention away from emotionally charged immediate events and redirecting it into a more neutral but productive problem-solving mode."

All but 2 of the 26 patients in the case series were treated with medications. Patients generally had their medications stabilized early in treatment. Both retrospective and prospective measures were obtained for ADHD, depression, and anxiety. Clinically significant improvement was found in all three domains

for medication treatment, and CT produced improvement beyond that seen from medications. However, Weiss et al. (1999, p. 198) noted, "Although McDermott (1995) ascribed this post-medication improvement to the cognitive therapy itself, the design of the study does not rule out that this continued improvement might represent long-term medication impact on functioning."

This report of Wilens et al. (1999) was limited in scope because it was a retrospective though independent chart review of cases with only one therapist. Many assessments were made by prospective patient self-report, but there were no independent patient evaluators. Weiss et al. (1999, p. 198) summarized their interpretation of this study: "These findings, based on an open trial that did not control for the effect of delayed improvements from medication alone, are difficult to interpret until more rigorously controlled studies are done. However, they challenge assumptions that therapy cannot address the core symptoms of ADHD."

Hesslinger et al. (2002)

More recent studies have attempted to test more directly the effectiveness of CBT for adults with ADHD. Hesslinger and associates (2002) noted similarities between adults with ADHD and adults with borderline personality disorder (BPD), including "deficits in affect regulation, impulse control, substance abuse, low self esteem and disturbed interpersonal relationships (which) are common in both conditions" (p. 178) while acknowledging important differences. In their controlled, open "exploratory pilot study" (p. 183) of eight patients, they used a structured skills training program based on dialectic behavior therapy (DBT), a form of cognitive-behavioral therapy specifically developed for patients with borderline personality disorder (Linehan, 1993a, 1993b). Their protocol addressed "(the) neurobiology of ADHD, mindfulness, chaos and control, behavior analysis, emotion regulation, depression, medication in ADHD, impulse control, stress management, dependency, ADHD in relationship and self respect. ... In the last session the experiences in the therapy were summarized and the next steps were planned (transformation to a self-help group)" (pp. 179–80). It is unclear whether the patients were aware of the plans for the transformation of the therapy group into a self-help group, whether the self-help group was time limited or ongoing, or what effect

Table 23.1 Outcome studies using CBT in adults with ADHD

Study	Subjects	Therapy	Medications	Results
Wilens et al. (1999)	26 patients systematic chart review	Naturalistic cognitive therapy in an outpatient practice based on treatment guidelines as outlined by McDermott (2000)	"Patients generally had their medications stabilized early in treatment." 24 of 26 patients were on medications, which were antidepressants (predominantly SSRIs), benzodiazepines, and/or stimulants.	"Clinically significant improvement was found in retrospective and prospective measures for ADHD, depression and anxiety for medication treatment, and for cognitive therapy beyond the improvement seen from medications."
Hesslinger et al. (2002)	8 patients open trial	Structured skills training program (13 sessions) based on dialectic behavior therapy (DBT).	3 patients were on methylphenidate (20–50 mg/day) for the entire treatment period. 3 patients were on methylphenidate or desipramine for part of the treatment.	"All psychometric scales (ADHD Checklist [DSM-IV], 16 items of the SCL-90-R, Beck Depression Inventory, and visual analogue scale) improved with the treatment."
Stevenson et al. (2002)	43 patients randomized, controlled trial with 1 year follow-up	Cognitive remediation program targeting attention problems, poor motivation, poor organizational skills, impulsivity, reduced anger control, and low self-esteem	"Some patients were medicated in community treatment with medications stabilized prior to study, throughout the treatment and until the two-month follow up." 11 of 21 patients in the control group and 12 of 23 patients in the treatment group were taking medications. "Most medicated participants were taking only stimulants (n = 19), two were taking only antidepressants, and two were taking both medications."	"Reduced ADHD symptoms, improved organizational skills, and reduced level of anger.... Clinically significant improvements in ADHD symptoms and organizational skills were maintained after one year.... No differences between medicated and unmediated patients."
Stevenson et al. (2003)	35 patients randomized, controlled trial with 2- month follow-up	Cognitive remediation program described in Stevenson et al. (2002) modified as "a self-directed psychosocial intervention with minimal therapist contact"	"Participants were accepted either unmedicated or on medication stabilized at the participants' optimum dose." 11 of 17 patients in the treatment group and 12 of 18 patients in the control group were medicated. Types of medication were not listed. "Outcome was not significantly associated with (medication status)...suggesting no major influence...on treatment efficacy."	"The treatment group reported significantly reduced ADHD symptoms, improved organizational skills and self esteem, and better anger control compared to waiting list controls. Comorbid anxiety, depression, high levels of stress and learning problems, did not effect (sic) treatment outcome. Improvements in ADHD symptoms and organizational skills were maintained at a 2-month follow-up.'
Safren et al. (2005)	40 patients randomized to active CBT or med maintenance only, independently rated, controlled trial	A skills-building, CBT intervention targeting residual, core, and associated symptoms of ADHD	Patients were adults with ADHD with continued clinically significant symptoms (of at least "moderate" severity) despite stable medication treatment for 2 months. Participants were asked not	The CBT group had 56% treatment responders compared with 13% responders in the continued meds alone group. CBT resulted in lower independent-evaluator (IE) rated and self-reported ADHD

(cont.)

257

Table 23.1 (cont.)

Study	Subjects	Therapy	Medications	Results
			to change their existing medication dosages by more than 10% for 1 month. "Most patients were on a stimulant medication and/or bupropion (Wellbutrin), or venlafaxine (Effexor). Adequacy of psychopharmacotherapy was not formally assessed."	symptom severity scores and ADHD CGI-severity scores, anxiety scores, as well as significantly lower IE-rated Hamilton Depression scores with a trend for lower self-reported Beck Depression Inventory scores. Outcome analyses of ADHD and CGI ratings were robust against covarying out baseline depression and depression changes.
Rostain and Ramsay (2006)	A prospective open study of 43 adults with ADHD treated for 6 months with a combination of "carefully managed medication and (CBT) tailored for ADHD."	Sixteen 50-min individual psychotherapy sessions over 6 months comprised of psychoeducation about ADHD; conceptualizations of the patient's difficulties; review of coping strategies for ADHD symptoms (e.g., organization/time management); CBT modification of "patterns that interfere with effective coping (including medication compliance issues)"; and "identifying and using personal strengths and supportive resources." Based on Ramsay & Rostain (2003)	Mixed salts of amphetamine titrated to 20 mg bid over 3 weeks, which was used to determine the regular dose for the remainder of the study. Clinical effectiveness/side effects assessed at each visit, and medication adjustments were made by physician/patient mutual agreement. When mixed amphetamine salts side effects were intolerable, methylphenidate was substituted using a similar titration schedule.	ADHD symptoms were assessed pre- and post-treatment using the BADDS scale. The general level of patient functioning assessed using the Clinical Global Impression (CGI). The Clinical Global Impression for ADHD (CGI-A) was used to measure severity of current ADHD symptoms. Results for comorbid symptoms measured using standardized clinical outcome scales for depression (the Beck Depression Inventory-II and Hamilton Depression), anxiety (the Beck Anxiety Inventory and Hamilton Anxiety), and hopelessness (the Beck Hopelessness Inventory). Clinical measures indicated significant improvement on post-treatment measures of ADHD symptoms, depression, anxiety, and overall functioning compared to pre-treatment results.

this apparent lack of termination of the group (but ending of the therapy) had on outcomes, particularly measures of depression and overall well-being.

The authors described the therapy as follows:

The group was chaired by two psychotherapists being trained in DBT. Participants agreed to a setting with 13 sessions on a weekly base over a period of 3 months each session lasting 2 hours. There was no charge for the participants. Written material and daily exercises were distributed to the participants before and after each

session. Participants had the opportunity to ask for additional individual sessions and were allowed to contact therapists by phone in case of severe crisis" (pp. 178–9).

There was no assessment of the quality of the therapy, which is particularly important when one is using trainees in an outcome study. In the subsection, "Session with partners and family members" in the "Contents of the therapy" section, the authors wrote, "Arrangements were made to meet with partners or families of every participant separately. In these sessions patients and partners had the opportunity to present and discuss their specific problems" (p. 180). It is unclear if patients and their partners were offered one or more of these sessions and whether these sessions were considered part of the 13 sessions listed in the protocol. This lack of clarity, combined with the failure to report the number of "extra sessions" or phone contacts that patients were allowed in the protocol, makes the true number of sessions (much less other therapist/patient contacts) difficult to assess.

The control group was "clearly compromised by the high dropout rate" of four of seven patients over 3 months (Hesslinger et al., 2002). Some but not all of the patients were on stimulants or antidepressants:

In three patients of our control group, an adequate medical treatment of ADHD was introduced between baseline and follow-up assessment, while in our treatment group there was no overall change in medication. . . . Since there was no overall change in concomitant medication with stimulants in the treatment group, this change (i.e., improvement in psychometric scores from pre- to post-treatment) cannot be attributed to a medication effect (p. 182, parenthetical comment added by SPM).

However, there were no measures of medication treatment quality. Outcomes were measured using psychometric scales, all of which improved significantly: the ADHD Checklist (*DSM-IV*), 16 items of the SCL-90-R, the Beck Depression Inventory (BDI), and personal health status rated on a visual analogue scale (VAS).

Stevenson et al. (2002 and 2003)

Stevenson et al. (2002, 2003) developed their cognitive remediation program (CRP) comprised of a combination of cognitive remediation techniques (used for treating, among others, patients with head trauma) and CBT. The overall treatment was targeted to the psychosocial issues that can exacerbate ADHD in adults, such as skill deficits, disorganized and/or chaotic working environments, and poor stress management. CRP strategies were used to help patients develop essential learning skills, whereas CBT was employed to challenge cognitions that interfere with skills acquisition, as well as to improve self-esteem and anger management (Stevenson, personal communication, July 19, 2006).

In the 2002 report, Stevenson and her colleagues described a randomized controlled trial of CRP for

adult ADHD in 43 patients. They used "a three-pronged approach to reduce the impact of cognitive impairments: (i) retraining cognitive functions; (ii) teaching internal and external compensatory strategies; and (iii) restructuring the physical environment to maximize functioning" (pp. 610–11). The CRP had a small group format with three main components: (1) eight, weekly, 2-hour, therapist-led group sessions; (2) a workbook with exercises; and (3) a support person for each patient (Stevenson, personal communication, July 19, 2006). The support people acted as coaches "to aid participants with the acquisition of skills by having a cueing or prompting role . . . (and were trained to) (i) to remind their partner to attend sessions, (ii) to attend sessions and take notes as required, and (iii) to discuss problems with homework exercises" (p. 612). The support people were either provided by the participants or were college students recruited by the study. The authors reported no significant difference in treatment outcome between participants who provided their own support person compared with those who had a student support.

Some patients were medicated in community treatment, with medication selection and dose stabilized before entrance into the study. In "community treatment," patients are treated by their usual healthcare providers in the manner in which their clinicians typically treat these disorders (i.e., the patients are treated by non-research clinical staff as if they are not in a research study). No attempt is made by the researchers to influence in any way the treatment of the patient by their usual treaters (with the possible exception of sharing diagnostic material). Patients were asked to maintain the stable dose throughout the treatment and the 2-month follow up period (but not through the 1-year follow-up, which the authors noted "did not seem reasonable to request"; pp. 611–12). Patients were free to change their medicated/unmedicated status or medication dose during the period between the 2-month and the 1-year follow-up. The authors reported, "It is important to note that no differences were found between medicated and non-medicated participants on any assessment measure" (p. 612), though there were no measures of medication efficacy.

Patients reported reduced ADHD symptomatology, improved organizational skills, and reduced levels of anger, and the authors found that clinically significant improvements in ADHD symptomatology and organizational skills were maintained 1 year after the intervention. They found no differences between

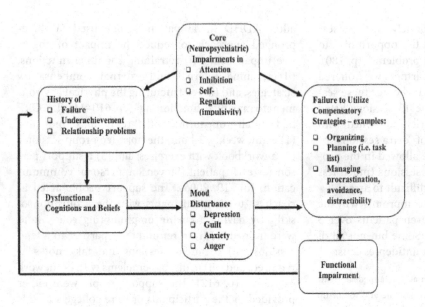

Figure 23.1 A cognitive-behavioral model of impairment in an adult ADHD. With permission from Safren, Sprich, Chulvick, & Otto (2004).

medicated and unmedicated patients at the end of treatment or 2 months or 1 year post-treatment. However, the authors noted, "Disappointingly, there were not more substantial gains in self-esteem and state and trait anger. There is no doubt that both self-esteem and anger management are important issues for adults with ADHD. However, separate interventions may be required to obtain more substantial improvements in these domains" (p. 615).

In the second study Stevenson et al. (2003) modified their original protocol to develop a randomized, controlled design for 35 adults using a self-directed psychosocial intervention with minimal therapist contact. They developed a self-help book that covered education about ADHD, listening and organizational skills, impulse control techniques, cognitive strategies for anger management and improved self-esteem, and strategies to overcome attention and motivational difficulties. The protocol provided one therapist-led session at the start, middle, and end of the program for a total of three sessions. These sessions were primarily used as review sessions, but also allowed the clinicians to monitor progress and provide motivation to participants to complete the program. In addition, participants were paired with a support person whose role was to remind them by weekly telephone contact to complete readings and exercises on a weekly basis. To measure compliance, the support people also recorded whether the self-help book had been read and whether set exercises had been completed. The self-help book was collected at the end of the program, and com-

pleted exercises were photocopied as a further measure of compliance.

The treatment group reported significantly reduced ADHD symptomatology, improved organizational skills and self-esteem, and better anger control post-treatment compared to waiting list controls. The authors noted, "Following the program, participants frequently expressed surprise at how simple strategies such as use of a diary, time management and reflective listening could improve their everyday functioning" (Stevenson et al., 2003, p. 99). Comorbid anxiety, depression, high levels of stress, and learning problems did not affect treatment outcome. As in the 2002 study, the authors reported that outcome was not significantly associated with medication status. Improvements in ADHD symptomatology and organizational skills were maintained at a 2-month follow-up.

Safren et al. (2004, 2005)

Safren and his colleagues took a different approach to the question of the usefulness of CBT and medications. They postulated that a history of failure experiences can enhance the negative affect and cognitive avoidance often seen in adults with ADHD, further impairing ADHD-related attentional and organizational difficulties (Safren et al., 2004). Their conceptualization is summarized in Figure 23.1 and in the following:

We reasoned that psychopharmacology may ameliorate many of the core symptoms of ADHD (attentional problems, high activity, impulsivity), but believe that it does not provide a patient with concrete strategies and skills for coping with associated functional impairment. Quality of life impairments such as underachievement, daily organizational and administrative goals (i.e., bills, mail, hassles), weekly work or school related tasks, and relationship difficulties associated with ADHD in adulthood require active problem-solving, which can be achieved with skills training over and above medication management (Safren et al., 2005, p. 832).

They devised a series of psychosocial interventions with two primary targets: improving organizational and attentional skills and addressing cognitive and behavioral patterns that increase demand-related distress and decrease avoidance of the use of these skills.

To test the efficacy of these interventions, the authors designed a randomized and controlled preliminary study in which participants were adults with ADHD with continued clinically significant symptoms (of at least "moderate" severity, as determined by an independent evaluator) despite being on stable medication treatment for ADHD for 2 months. Participants were asked not to change their existing medication dosages by more than 10% for 1 month (and were chosen, in part, because they had no plans to do so). All individuals were treated with a variety of psychopharmacological regimens for ADHD. Most patients were on a stimulant medication and/or bupropion (Wellbutrin) or venlafaxine (Effexor). The adequacy of psychopharmacotherapy was not formally assessed as part of this "small-scale study" (Safren et al., 2005, p. 839).

Safren and his colleagues devised a protocol of three core treatment modules (of ten sessions) and several optional modules (of up to five additional sessions), "formulating specific components to match specific problem areas. ... All modules contained elements of motivational interviewing, and practice, repetition and review of previously learned skills" (p. 834). The core treatment modules included training in the use of a specific structure (built around a calendar and notebook), problem solving, and cognitive restructuring skills to treat distractibility. Another core treatment module dealt "with the dysfunctional thoughts that increase negative affect and enhance avoidance of work-related topics ... (using) procedures for cognitive restructuring for ADHD ... adapted from the parent procedures outlined by (Judith) Beck (1995) and detailed further by McDermott (2000)" (Safren et al., 2004, p. 356). These techniques targeted, in part, the rapidly experienced downward spirals in

ADHD adults' perception and assessment of unattractive tasks, which can lead to negative self-evaluation and affect and subsequent avoidance of the task.

Three optional treatment modules (of up to an additional five sessions) were included to deal with other difficulties that are frequently associated with adults with ADHD. Patients were to complete the additional treatment modules only if they manifested clinically significant difficulties in these symptom domains. The optional modules were specific, focused applications of skills to cope with procrastination, anger and frustration management, and communication skills.

Safren and associates' (2005) study had some limitations. The pharmacotherapy provided to the patients by nonstudy clinicians was not tightly controlled by the researchers. Although patients were instructed not to change medications, three changed medicines during the study period. Upon discovery of these changes, Safren and colleagues adopted more active monitoring of medication changes throughout the rest of the study. They wrote, "Replication analyses, however revealed a similar pattern of results when excluding these individuals from analysis" (Safren et al., 2005, p. 839). Safren also noted limitations with a small sample size, the absence of a follow-up period to investigate the maintenance of gains, and lack of a placebo psychotherapy control instead of the no-additional treatment control. Despite these limitations, the results of this preliminary study were quite successful. Compared to the Continued Psychopharmacology Alone Group, the CBT group showed the following four gains:

1. The CBT group had more treatment "responders" (defined as a 2-point change in the CGI severity scale): 56% vs. 13%.
2. CBT resulted in lower independent evaluator (IE) rated ADHD Symptom Severity Scale scores (14.18 point vs. 5.2 point decrease) and IE-rated ADHD CGI-severity scores (1.69 vs. 0.54 point reduction).
3. CBT resulted in lower self-report ADHD Current Symptom Scale scores (14.94 vs. 2.53 point decrease).
4. CBT also resulted in significantly lower IE-rated Hamilton Anxiety scores and self-reported Beck Anxiety Inventory scores, as well as significantly lower IE-rated Hamilton Depression scores, with a trend for lower self-reported Beck Depression Inventory scores.

Of note, the authors showed that outcome analyses of ADHD and CGI ratings were robust when controlling for baseline depression and depression changes.

Safren and colleagues (2005) concluded that their protocol for CBT for residual ADHD symptoms in adults was feasible to administer (the principal investigator and three therapists learned how to deliver the intervention) and acceptable to patients (no participant dropped out of the intervention condition). They noted,

The present sample consisted of medication-treated individuals who had not achieved adequate control of their symptoms. The treatment therefore was successful in an otherwise treatment-refractory population. Despite the underlying neurobiological basis of ADHD, cognitive-behavioral therapy was successful as a next-step treatment approach in patients receiving medications. ... Accordingly, cognitive-behavioral therapy appears to be a useful component of treatment for adults with ADHD who do not fully respond to medications alone" (p. 839).

Rostain and Ramsay (2006)

Rostain and Ramsay (2006) reported a prospective study of 43 adults with ADHD treated for 6 months with a combination of "carefully managed medication and cognitive-behavioral treatment tailored for ADHD" (p. 151).

Patients were prescribed mixed salts of amphetamine titrated to 20 mg bid over 3 weeks. Based on the results of this 3-week trial, a regular dose was selected and maintained through the remainder of the study. Clinical effectiveness and side effects were assessed at each visit, and medication adjustments were made by mutual agreement of the physician and patient based on these assessments. When the side effects of mixed amphetamine salts were intolerable, methylphenidate was substituted using a similar titration schedule.

The CBT comprised sixteen 50-minute individual psychotherapy sessions scheduled during the course of 6 months. The 6-month duration was chosen

to allow for weekly skill acquisition sessions at the start of treatment and a subsequent gradual reduction of session frequency, encouraging participants to increasingly rely on their coping skills. ... Considering ADHD is a developmental disorder, a lengthier course of psychosocial treatment may be required to adequately develop adaptive coping skills, such as in the Wilens et al. (1999)

study in which the mean course of CBT was almost 12 months (Rostain & Ramsey, 2006, pp. 152–3).

A clinical psychologist at the University of Pennsylvania Adult ADHD Treatment and Research Program with experience in CBT and the assessment and treatment of adults with ADHD administered the CBT. The course of treatment was based on a model of CBT modified for adults with ADHD that was previously developed by the authors (Ramsay & Rostain, 2003). According to the authors, the "twofold goal of the CBT was to help participants (a) develop and implement individualized adaptive coping strategies to manage ADHD related symptoms and (b) identify and modify dysfunctional thoughts and beliefs that contribute to inefficient coping, emotional difficulties (e.g., mood, anxiety, anger), negative self-evaluation, and/or pessimism" (Rostain & Ramsey, 2006, p. 153).

The CBT interventions in Rostain and Ramsay (2006) included (1) psychoeducation about ADHD, (2) conceptualizations of the patient's difficulties, (3) review of coping strategies for ADHD symptoms (e.g., organization and time management), (4) CBT modification of "patterns that interfere with effective coping (including "medication compliance issues"; p. 153), and (5) "identifying and using personal strengths and supportive resources" (p. 153).

They assessed ADHD symptoms with the BADDS scale (Brown, 1996), a clinician-administered 40-item instrument that broadly measures ADHD symptoms in adults. The general level of functioning of the patient was assessed using the Clinical Global Impression (CGI). The Clinical Global Impression for ADHD (CGI-A) was used to measure the severity of current ADHD symptoms. The authors noted, "A separate clinician rating of ADHD symptoms was used to provide a measure of symptom change that might not be reflected in a rating of the general level of functioning" (p. 153).

Results were assessed for comorbid symptoms using standardized clinical outcome scales for depression – the Beck Depression Inventory-II (Beck & Steer, 1987) and Hamilton Depression (Hamilton, 1967); for anxiety – the Beck Anxiety Inventory (Beck & Steer, 1990) and Hamilton Anxiety (Hamilton, 1959); and for hopelessness – the Beck Hopelessness Inventory (Beck & Steer, 1989). Clinical measures indicated significant improvement on post-treatment measures of ADHD symptoms, depression, anxiety, and overall function-ing compared to pre-treatment results.

Discussion

Medications

To varying degrees, all six studies had two compo-nents: medications and CBT. One crucial issue with the use of medications in all the studies was the lack of measurement of their effectiveness, which limited the interpretation of the usefulness of medications in these treatment protocols.

The study of Wilens et al. (1999) was a natural-istic open trial of medications and a modified form of Beck's cognitive therapy based on treatment guide-lines developed by McDermott (2000). Based on clin-ical experience, McDermott (2000) concluded that patients required some (but not total) initial control of their core symptoms of ADHD to be able to use CBT, which in turn helped improve the patients' core symp-toms, comorbid disorders, and associated problems. McDermott hypothesized that medication would be more effective than CBT in dealing with ADHD core symptoms (at least initially) and that most patients would need it to effectively engage in the CBT. Yet in these guidelines (McDermott, 2000; Wilens et al., 1999), there was no expectation that medication would be sufficient to totally eliminate the core symptoms of ADHD without the CBT, based, in part, on the high proportion of patients in the treatment group (46%) who had failed previous medication trials.

Of the 26 patients reported in Wilens et al. (1999), only 2 had CBT without medication (albeit, with some success). This low number may be partly accounted for by the nature of the population being treated. As Weiss et al. (1999, p. 196) noted,

This population was heavily comorbid; 58 percent met the criteria for depression, 54 percent for generalized anxiety, and 46 percent for dysthymic disorder. Almost 70 percent of the patients were on SSRIs, 60 percent on stimulants, and 10 percent on tricyclics. Fifty-eight percent were on combinations of medications, and only 15 percent were on no medication at all. Although McDermott described this as a chronic, disabled and treatment-resistant population, it remains to be determined how this population will eventually compare to general clinic samples.

There are also data from child studies of behav-ior therapy and medication that suggest that medica-tion (with or without behavior therapy) is "clinically and statistically superior" (MTA Cooperative Group, 1999a, p. 1078) to treatments with no or poorly man-aged medication regimens (Greene & Ablon, 2001). (It should be noted that the generalizability of child stud-ies to adult treatments is uncertain.) No attempt was made in the study of Wilens et al. (1999) to determine the effectiveness of the medications separately from the rest of the treatment.

The study of Rostain and Ramsay (2006) was a prospective open trial of medications and modified cognitive therapy. Ramsay and Rostain hypothesized a more central role for medications in the treatment of adult ADHD, with CBT primarily providing augmen-tation of the effects of medication:

Whereas the stimulant medications are known to improve symp-toms of ADHD, the possible therapeutic effects of CBT are less clear. Perhaps participants' symptoms improved because their comorbid conditions were treated effectively rather than the core symptoms of ADHD per se. It could be that CBT augments pharmacother-apy by treating comorbid problems and/or residual ADHD symp-toms…thus allowing adults with ADHD to more effectively and consistently employ coping skills with which to manage the chronic difficulties associated with ADHD (Rostain & Ramsay, 2006, p. 157).

As with Wilens et al. (1999), no attempt was made to determine the effectiveness of medications separately from the rest of the treatment.

Safren and colleagues (2004) developed a modified form of CBT that was used as supplemental therapy in patients who had been stabilized on their medications. Their model is more balanced in the presumption of the relative effects of medication compared with CBT:

Physiologically, ADHD is a neuropsychiatric disorder that may be associated with decits in the prefrontal cortex and related subcor-tical systems.…These neurobiological decits can result in chronic cognitive and behavioral impairments, including impairments in attention, inhibition, and self-regulation.…Both core and associ-ated symptoms can result in a history of failures or underachieve-ment.…The result is that the cognitive and affective response to external demands may engender avoidance of some of the very com-pensatory strategies…which could help ameliorate some of the core decits of ADHD. The results…are cognitive–behavioral patterns that may foster rather than attenuate the impact of neuropsychi-atric decits on functional performance.…Psychopharmacology can ameliorate many of the core symptoms of ADHD: attentional prob-lems, high activity, and impulsivity. It does not intrinsically provide patients with concrete strategies and skills for coping with associated functional impairment, however (pp. 350–1).

A basic assumption underlying the Safren and colleagues (2004) study was that random assortment of patients with stable medication regimens (which patients agreed not to change) should produce no significant differences post-treatment due to medication effects (given a large enough patient sample). Therefore any change between the groups should be due primarily to the addition of the CBT research protocol. Again, no attempt was made to determine the effectiveness of the medications separately from the rest of the treatment.

The lack of measures of medication effectiveness perhaps had its greatest effect in the interpretation of the results of Stevenson et al. (2002, 2003) and of Hesslinger et al. (2002), who reported, "Following a naturalistic design medical treatment was left to the decision of the patients" (p. 179). One might assume that patients who chose to use medications were followed with no structured measures of medication effectiveness by their medical/mental health caregivers outside of the study (i.e., in what is often described as "community treatment").

Hesslinger and his colleagues (2002, p. 182) wrote, "Since there was no overall change in concomitant medication with stimulants in the treatment group, this change (i.e., improvement in psychometric scores from pre- to post-treatment) cannot be attributed to a medication effect" (parenthetical comment added by SPM). In essence, they suggested that medications are not necessary to produce improvement in patients who used their protocol. In both studies of Stevenson and co-workers, the authors reported no differences between their medicated and unmedicated patients. As with the Hesslinger study, patients were medicated in their communities, and no structured measures of medication efficacy were reported. In their 2003 study, Stevenson et al. wrote, "Participants were accepted either unmedicated or on medication stabilized at the participants' optimum dose" (p. 95). It is unclear who determined whether the participants were, in fact, on their optimum doses of medication. Was this assessment made by the study authors or the community treaters? Were the community treaters solely involved in this determination, or was it a collaboration with the clinical research staff? What criteria were used to define the "optimum dose" – the lack of change in the dose of medication over a specified time or some other

measure? To what extent were participants involved in the assessment of whether they were on their optimum dose?

Stevenson and associates (2002, p. 614) stated further,

A further question that this study addresses is whether medication status had any effect on treatment outcome. All the analyses reported in the "effect of treatment" section were repeated, but with one extra factor included in the ANOVA, that of medication status (Medicated vs Non-medicated). This factor had no significant effect on any outcome measure. Thus, medication status appeared to exert no obvious effect on the success or otherwise of the CRP.

Assessments by clinicians, researchers, and/or patients of medication effects (or the lack of effects) are rendered essentially meaningless without measures of medication effectiveness. This assertion is not hypothetical.

The questions – "How do long-term medication and behavioral treatments compare with one another? Are there additional benefits when they are used together? What is the effectiveness of systematic, carefully delivered treatments vs. routine community care"? – were at the core of the multicenter study, Multimodal Treatment Study of Children with ADHD (MTA Cooperative Group, 1999a, p. 1073; MTA Cooperative Group, 1999b; Taylor, 1999). In the decade since its first report the MTA "has provided a bewildering wealth of data (more than 70 peer-reviewed articles)" (Murray et al., 2008, p. 424). Although care must be taken generalizing the results of this (still-debated) study of children with ADHD (presumably) in the American health care system, its results may shed light on similar issues in adult ADHD studies.

The authors of the MTA concluded, "Combined treatment and medication management treatments were clinically and statistically superior to…community care in reducing children's (core) ADHD symptoms" (1999a, p. 1078; parenthetical comment added by SPM). Greene and Ablon (2001, p. 115) found that "medical management alone was found to be significantly more effective for the core symptoms of ADHD as compared to behavioral treatment alone and routine (community) care." Jenson et al. (2005, p. 1633) argued that the "less effective nature of community-delivered treatment" was related to "the substantially lower doses (of medications) used by community physicians for community-treated subjects, as well as the much less frequent monitoring (generally once per month for medication management versus two times per year for community care)."

Valid inferences about the role of medications and the use of CBT in ADHD adults can be drawn from the Hesslinger et al. (2002) and Stevenson et al. (2002, 2003) studies, but they must not only be accurate but also somewhat conservative in their interpretation and reporting. Note the differences between the conclusion of Hesslinger and colleagues (2002, p. 182) – "improvement in psychometric scores from pre- to post-treatment cannot be attributed to a medication effect" – and that of Stevenson and associates (2002, p. 614): "Thus, medication status appeared to exert no obvious effect on the success or otherwise of the CRP." The Hesslinger group's assertion is valid whether or not medication treatment was effective. They could reasonably counsel a patient that participation in this form of treatment does not require the use of medication to yield improvement in psychometric scales. However, they do not have data that could reasonably predict whether their treatment protocol would be more or less effective than medication or whether medication use might enhance or detract from the effectiveness of the treatment.

In contrast, the Stevenson group's assertion may be misinterpreted as suggesting that medication "would have no obvious effect" (i.e., beneficial or deleterious influence) on their protocol. This statement is only accurate to the extent that the medication treatments used in their studies were effective therapies – hypotheses that were not tested in their research.

Although Stevenson and her associates do not claim that their treatment protocol is equivalent or superior to medication treatment, care must be taken to prevent this clear misperception of their data by others. It is reasonable to imagine that some patients (or even relatively well-informed clinicians) might assume that if medications exerted no influence over the CRP treatment, then medication therapy must be inferior or at best equivalent to CRP treatment (unless the CRP protocol changed a more effective medication therapy into a less effective one).

Cognitive-Behavioral Therapy

The cognitive-behavioral therapy of ADHD in adults essentially has two components: establishing structure in the adult's life and teaching the patient the skills necessary to deal with impediments to establishing and maintaining structure. The therapies in all six studies

targeted behavioral changes, and all addressed cognitions that interfered with the desired behaviors.

At first consideration, it might not be apparent why a "cognitive" component seems to be required to make behavioral interventions effective. ADHD is a disorder that is defined by dysfunctional behaviors: hyperactivity, impulsivity, and distractibility (defined as the behavior of attending to stimuli other than those that are generally considered most important). Yet, although all of these therapies use behavioral techniques, none of the treatments is purely behavioral.

The cornerstone of most forms of CBT is the interplay among behaviors, emotions, and cognitions. Although ADHD is defined by dysfunctional behaviors, it also has strong emotional and cognitive/belief components. As Spencer and colleagues (1994, p. 333) noted, "This disorder is not benign.... Given the longer duration of psychopathology and the increased demands for independent functioning, the level of dysfunction may be even more severe in adults than in children. A lifetime of interpersonal, academic, and occupational failure may be qualitatively and quantitatively different than a limited experience in childhood in a more protected family setting."

McDermott's modification of standard Beckian cognitive therapy for use with adults with ADHD, while retaining the core of behavioral change common to all forms of CBT, also strongly emphasizes changing beliefs (accomplished to a large extent by change in cognitions). Belief change is used to ameliorate the sources of cognitions such as "I can't change my condition, so there's no point in trying." These beliefs and the cognitions to which they give rise interfere with standard CBT problem solving and structure building. The relatively greater emphasis on belief change in the modified form of Beck's CT may be different from the relatively greater focus on changing thoughts, feelings, and behaviors in specific situations that is the basis of the cognitive therapy of more acute disorders, such as anxiety or depression (in patients with relatively good intermorbid functioning).

The belief change in McDermott's treatment guidelines is much like Rostain and Ramsay's (2006, p. 153) second treatment goal of "identify(ing) and modify(ing) dysfunctional thoughts and beliefs that contribute to inefficient coping, emotional difficulties (e.g., mood, anxiety, anger), negative self-evaluation, and/or pessimism." It is important to note that all forms of Beck's CT require changes in all of these components to produce long-term improvement in the patient's condition.

Hesslinger et al.'s protocol also seems to be focused more broadly on the general aspects of the lives of adults with ADHD, such as mindfulness, chaos and control, emotion regulation, depression, stress management, dependency, ADHD in relationships, and self-respect. This is consistent with their use of their therapy group as a springboard to the establishment of a self-help group, which would be helpful, in part, by encouraging patients to maintain the gains they made in treatment, many of which were based on behavioral skills.

The protocol of Safren et al. and the two treatment regimens of Stevenson et al. revolve more centrally around the sustained use of behavioral tools such as notebooks and schedules. At the same time, they stress the importance of teaching patients the skills necessary to deal with issues like distractibility that can sidetrack their continued use and improvement of the tools they have learned. One major source of "distraction" for these patients are thoughts such as "Normal people don't need to keep notebooks like this, and I think I've finally conquered my ADHD, so I don't need to use my notebook anymore (so I won't feel so 'abnormal')." Often these thoughts arise from a core belief such as "I'm defective," which has built up over decades of experiences of failure (McDermott, 2000).

Thus the therapies vary in the relative importance given to behaviors and cognitions in the assessment and treatment of ADHD and comorbid disorders. Stevenson and Safren put more emphasis on behavioral interventions to develop a manageable structure, whereas Hesslinger, McDermott, and Rostain and Ramsay focus more on cognitive/belief change to deal with impediments to preserving that structure. These differences are probably relatively small, because ultimately the success of any CBT is defined by the behaviors it changes, no matter what methods are used to create the behavioral change.

In almost all CBTs, the basic theoretical context is important in determining not only which techniques are used but also in selecting and prioritizing treatment targets. Thus, the basic theory behind a treatment method is more than theoretical – it plays a central role in the therapy. This is because most CBTs stress the importance of teaching patients a new way of understanding how they perceive and interact with their world and how this understanding makes them feel and behave. Patients are often taught how to "be

their own therapists" (Beck, 1995); that is, after terminating therapy to learn to understand problems and develop ways to solve them as they have done with their therapists. To do this most effectively, patients need to be treated in (and therefore learn) a consistent therapeutic model.

The studies described in this chapter employed many of the same cognitive and behavioral techniques but used them differently because of their different conceptual systems (e.g., DBT, CRP, or more standard CBT). Thus, a DBT therapist might deal with a patient's repeated tardiness when coming to therapy as a "therapy-interfering behavior" (Linehan, 1993a, 1993b). A more behaviorally based therapist might explore new ways to structure the patient's day to make the time before leaving work less "jam-packed," whereas a more cognitively based therapist might explore the patient's cognitions before leaving work, such as "I'll feel less guilty about not staying late at work if I just get one task done before I leave."

Ultimately, all of these CBTs will help the patient define the problem; find its cognitive, behavioral, and affective determinants; and develop alternative behavioral and/or cognitive strategies to deal with issues in a new way. However, it is important that these similar approaches be done in a manner consistent with the therapeutic model in the treatment, instead of "cutting and pasting" different techniques from different models. If model consistency is not maintained, the confusion that ensues will thwart the patient in learning the model.

Although all of these treatments were CBTs, they had very different structures. Three were individual treatments: the studies of Safren et al. and Rostain and Ramsay were time-limited protocols and that by Wilens et al. was an open-ended, naturalistic treatment. Three studies – Hesslinger et al. and the two Stevenson et al. protocols – were group therapies using treatments originally developed for two populations that often present very differently: individuals with borderline personality disorder and persons with head trauma. Even Stevenson et al.'s two studies, which essentially had the same underlying theoretical core, had very different structures: eight weekly sessions with a therapist versus three sessions with a therapist over 8 weeks.

The treatments provided by all six studies have in common, however, reliance on outside "homework" assignments. As with most CBTs, all of these therapies are based to a large extent on teaching patients new skills. An individual with ADHD can no more learn a new technique for dealing with distractibility by practicing it only once or twice per week than a person can learn how to type or ride a bike by doing it once or twice per week. Burns and Nolan-Hoeksema (1991) showed that compliance with homework is the single best predictor of treatment success in a CBT for depression.

Because of the pervasive and relatively unremitting nature of their ADHD and comorbid disorders, these patients may need to acquire a set of skills even broader than those needed by patients with anxiety or depression. Stevenson and associates (2003, p. 93) noted, "Although the (CRP) program was successful, close adherence to the program was necessary for optimum treatment gains."

Yet, as Weiss and colleagues (1999, p. 196) wrote, "Application of this form of therapy to ADHD may also present special challenges. ... Some of the typical procedures of cognitive therapy may be difficult for particular patients with ADHD, including, for example, writing down lists of cognitions, as 'homework' assignments." Homework compliance is an important and often very fruitful (though neglected) area of intervention in any CBT.

Summary

The psychiatric literature on the use of psychotherapy for the treatment of adults with ADHD shows poor response to more traditional psychotherapies, but recent reports of outcome studies for newer CBTs are promising (Kolar et al., 2008). One group treatment adapted dialectic behavioral therapy (Hesslinger et al., 2002). The protocols for two studies were adapted from cognitive remediation therapy, which is often used for patients with head trauma (Stevenson et al., 2002, 2003). Another compelling study (Safren et al., 2005) used a protocol based on standard CBT techniques with a form of Beck's cognitive therapy specifically modified for this disorder (McDermott, 1995, 2000; Weiss et al., 1999; Wilens et al., 1999). A more recent study (Rostain & Ramsay, 2006) also investigated the combination of cognitive therapy and medications.

All these CBT models showed some effectiveness, although there were no head-to-head trials, so their relative effectiveness cannot be assessed. All the research studies were generally in the early phase of development of the therapies, with the methodological problems often seen in initial clinical studies. Therapy guidelines applying these models, based on recent research and my experience, are suggested.

Conclusion

The CBT of adults with ADHD is still in its infancy. Although all of the treatments discussed were forms of cognitive-behavioral therapy, other forms of psychosocial treatment are yet to be studied, and perhaps a different form of psychotherapy could add to the benefits these therapies attained.

Furthermore, psychotherapy studies in this population may need to be structured quite differently from psychotherapy studies for other disorders. For example, it may be more difficult to maintain a wait list control group for individuals with ADHD who may be impulsive and have a tendency to be too disorganized to seek treatment until a crisis occurs. In contrast, patients with major depression may lack the energy and motivation to seek alternative treatments.

One way to alleviate this problem would be to use control groups with essentially placebo treatments, but there needs to be a general consensus on what comprises a placebo psychotherapy for this population. A large portion of the ADHD population has comorbid anxiety and depression and may often feel an almost crushing sense of guilt and shame. The attention and acceptance of an empathic therapist may have powerful positive effects on ameliorating (at least, for a time) these potentially debilitating emotions. The encouraging stance most therapists maintain also may provide strong motivation (at least initially) to change long-held behaviors – regardless of whether the therapist is the active or placebo treater.

These nonspecific therapy effects may confound the short-term assessment of the effectiveness of a particular psychotherapeutic treatment. Rostain and Ramsay (2006) have raised the possibility that a lengthier course of psychosocial treatment may be beneficial for patients' development of stronger adaptive coping skills. Longer therapeutic trials also may eliminate some of the effects of this nonspecific, therapeutic-relationship-driven interference with assessment of the psychosocial treatment.

Even more important in separating nonspecific from protocol-specific outcomes is long-term follow-up of study patients. Teaching patients the skills to manage their chronic ADHD long after the end of treatment must be the ultimate goal of any therapeutic intervention for adult patients with ADHD. This makes post-treatment, long-term follow-up crucial in studies of any psychotherapy for adults with ADHD.

All of the reports discussed had positive outcomes, although most could be considered pilot studies to some extent. As such, their general applicability may be limited due to methodological issues. More controlled trials need to be completed examining the relative merits of each of these forms of CBT for adults with ADHD, thereby measuring their usefulness with general adult ADHD populations and with specific ADHD subpopulations and to determine further modifications.

Nonetheless, given the rather large cadre of patients with residual symptoms and/or dysfunction after even the most successful pharmacological interventions, these studies, taken individually or as a group, suggest that specific psychotherapies may play an important role in the treatment of adults with ADHD. The significant costs of this disorder to patients, their loved ones, and society in general strongly support further psychosocial treatment development and research.

References

Alpert J, Maddocks A, Nierenberg A, O'Sullivan R, Pava J, Worthington, J, et al. (1996). Attention deficit hyperactivity disorder in childhood among adults with major depression. *Psychiatry Res* 62:213–9.

Anderson J, Williams S, McGee R, Silva P. (1987). DSM III disorders in preadolescent children. *Arch Gen Psychiatry* 44:69–76.

Barkley R. (1990). *Attention Deficit Hyperactivity Disorder: A Handbook for Diagnosis and Treatment*. New York: Guilford Press.

Barkley R. (2002). Psychosocial treatments for attention-deficit/hyperactivity disorder in children. *J Clin Psychiatry* 63(suppl 12):36–43.

Bauermeister JJ, Canino G, Bird H. (1994). Epidemiology of disruptive behavior disorders. In: Greenhill L, ed. *Child and Adolescent Psychiatric Clinics of North America*. Philadelphia: W. B. Saunders: 177–94.

Beck AT, Steer RA. (1987). *Manual for the Revised Beck Depression Inventory*. San Antonio: Psychological Corporation.

Beck AT, Steer RA. (1989). *Manual for the Beck Hopelessness Scale*. San Antonio: Psychological Corporation.

Beck AT, Steer RA. (1990). *The Beck Anxiety Inventory: Manual*. San Antonio: Psychological Corporation.

Beck J. (1995). *Cognitive Therapy: Basics and Beyond*. New York: Guilford Press.

Bemporad J. (2001). Aspects of psychotherapy with adults with attention deficit disorder. *Ann N Y Acad Sci* 931:302–9.

Bemporad J, Zambenedetti M. (1996). Psychotherapy of adults with attention deficit disorder. *J Psychother* 5:228–37.

Biederman J, Faraone SV, Spencer T, Wilens TE, Norman D, Lapey KA, et al. (1993). Patterns of psychiatric comorbidity, cognition, and psychosocial functioning in adults with attention deficit hyperactivity disorder. *Am J Psychiatry* 150:1792–8.

Bockting CL, Spinhoven P, Koeter MW, Wouters LF, Schene AH. (2006). Prediction of recurrence in recurrent depression and the influence of consecutive episodes on vulnerability for depression: a 2-year prospective study. *J Clin Psychiatry* 67(5): 747–55.

Brown TE. (1996). *Brown Attention Deficit Disorder Scales*. San Antonio: Psychological Corporation.

Brown TE, ed. (2000). *Attention Decit Disorders and Comorbidities in Children, Adolescents, and Adults*. Washington, DC: American Psychiatric Press.

Burns D, Nolen-Hoeksema S. (1991). Coping styles, homework compliance, and the effectiveness of cognitive-behavioral therapy. *J Consult Clin Psychol* 59(2):305–11.

Davidson MA. (2008). ADHD in adults: a review of the literature. *J Atten Disord* 11(6):628–41.

DeRubeis RJ, Gelfand LA, Tang TZ, Simons AD. (1999). Medications versus cognitive behavior therapy for severely depressed outpatients: mega-analysis of four randomized comparisons. *Am J Psychiatry* 156(7):1007–13.

Dodson WW. (2005). Pharmacotherapy of adult ADHD. *J Clin Psychol* 61(5):589–606.

Greene RW, Ablon JS. (2001). What does the MTA study tell us about effective psychosocial treatment for ADHD? *J Clin Child Psychol* 30(1):114–21.

Hallowell E. (1995). Psychotherapy of adult attention deficit disorder. In: Nadeau KG, ed. *A Comprehensive Guide to Attention Deficit Disorder in Adults: Research, Diagnosis, and Treatment*. New York: Brunner/Mazel: 146–67.

Hamilton M. (1959). The assessment of anxiety states by rating. *Br J Med Psychol* 32:50–5.

Hamilton M. (1967). Development of a rating scale for primary depressive illness. *Br J Soc Clin Psychol* 6:278–96.

Hesslinger B, van Elst L, Nyberg E, Dykierek P, Richter H, Berner M, et al. (2002). Psychotherapy of attention deficit hyperactivity disorder in adults: a pilot study using a structured skills training program. *Eur Arch Psychiatry Clin Neurosci* **252**(4):177–84.

Hinshaw S, Erhardt D. (1991). Attention deficit hyperactivity disorder. In: **Kendall P**, ed. *Child and Adolescent Therapy: Cognitive-Behavioral Procedures*. New York: Guilford Press: 98–122.

Jensen PS, Garcia JA, Glied S, Crowe M, Foster M, Schlander M, et al. (2005). Cost-effectiveness of ADHD treatments: findings from the multimodal treatment study of children with ADHD. *Am J Psychiatry* **162**(9):1628–36.

Kadden RM, Cooney NL, Getter H, Litt MD. (1989). Matching alcoholics to coping skills or interactional therapies: posttreatment results. *J Consult Clin Psychol* **57**(6):698–704.

Kadden RM, Litt MD, Kabela-Cormier E, Petry NM. (2007). Abstinence rates following behavioral treatments for marijuana dependence. *Addict Behav*, **32**(6): 1220–36.

Kolar D, Keller A, Golfinopoulos M, Cumyn L, Syer C, Hechtman L. (2008). Treatment of adults with attention-deficit/hyperactivity disorder. *Neuropsychiatr Dis Treat* **4**(1):107–21.

Linehan M. (1993a). *Cognitive-Behavioral Treatment of Borderline Personality Disorder*. New York: Guilford Press.

Linehan M. (1993b). *Skills Training Manual for Treating Borderline Personality Disorder*. New York: Guilford Press.

Mannuzza S, Klein RG, Bessler A, Malloy P, LaPadula M. (1993). Adult outcome of hyperactive boys: educational achievement, occupational rank, and psychiatric status. *Arch Gen Psychiatry* **50**:565–76.

Mannuzza S, Klein RG, Bonagura N, Malloy P, Giampino, TL, Addalli KA. (1991). Hyperactive boys almost grown up. V. Replication of psychiatric status. *Arch Gen Psychiatry* **48**:77–83.

McDermott SP. (1995). *Treatment of adult ADHD with cognitive behavioral therapy*. Paper presented at: Annual Meeting of the American Academy of Child and Adolescent Psychiatry.

McDermott SP. (2000). Cognitive therapy of adults with attention-deficit/hyperactivity disorder. In: **Brown TE**, ed. *Attention Deficit Disorders and Comorbidities in Children, Adolescents, and Adults*. Washington, DC: American Psychiatric Press: 651–90.

McDermott SP, Wright FD. (1992). Cognitive therapy: long-term outlook for a short-term psychotherapy. In: **Rutan JS**, ed. *Psychotherapy for the 1990s*. New York: Guilford Press: 61–99.

MTA Cooperative Group. (1999a). A 14-month randomized clinical trial of treatment strategies for attention-deficit/hyperactivity disorder. Multimodal Treatment Study of Children with ADHD. *Arch Gen Psychiatry* **56**(12):1073–86.

MTA Cooperative Group. (1999b). Moderators and mediators of treatment response for children with attention-deficit/hyperactivity disorder: the Multimodal Treatment Study of children with attention-deficit/ hyperactivity disorder. *Arch Gen Psychiatry* **56**(12):1088–96.

Murphy K, Barkley R. (1996). Prevalence of DSM-IV symptoms of ADHD in adult licensed drivers: implications for clinical diagnosis. *J Atten Disord* **1**(3):147–61.

Murray DW, Arnold LE, Swanson J, Wells K, Burns K, Jensen P, et al. (2008). A clinical review of outcomes of the Multimodal Treatment Study of children with attention-deficit/hyperactivity disorder (MTA). *Curr Psychiatry Rep* **10**(5):424–31.

Najavits LM, Weiss RD. (1994). The role of psychotherapy in the treatment of substance-use disorders. *Harv Rev Psychiatry* **2**(2):84–96.

Ramsay JR, Rostain AL. (2003). A cognitive therapy approach for adult attention-decit/hyperactivity disorder. *J Cogn Psychother* **17**(4):319–34.

Ramsay JR, Rostain AL. (2005). Adapting psychotherapy to meet the needs of adults with attention-deficit/ hyperactivity disorder. *Psychother Theory, Res Pract Train* **42**(1):72–84.

Ratey JJ, Greenberg MS, Bemporad JR, Lindem KJ. (1992). Unrecognized attention-deficit hyperactivity disorder in adults presenting for outpatient psychotherapy. *J Child Adolesc Psychopharmacol* **2**(4):267–75.

Rostain AL, Ramsay JR. (2006). A combined treatment approach for adults with ADHD – results of an open study of 43 patients. *J Atten Disord* **10**(2): 150–9.

Safer DJ, Krager JM. (1988). A survey of medication treatment for hyperactive/inattentive students. *JAMA* **260**(15):2256–8.

Safren SA, Otto MW, Sprich S, Winett CL, Wilens TE, Biederman J. (2005). Cognitive-behavioral therapy for ADHD in medication-treated adults with continued symptoms. *Behav Res Ther* **43**(7):831–42.

Safren SA, Sprich S, Chulvick S, Otto MW. (2004). Psychosocial treatments for adults with attention-deficit/ hyperactivity disorder. *Psychiatr Clin North Am* **27**(2):349–60.

Shekim WO, Asarnow RF, Hess E, Zaucha K, Wheeler N. (1990). A clinical and demographic profile of a sample of adults with attention deficit hyperactivity disorder, residual state. *Compr Psychiatry* **31**:416–25.

Siev J, Chambless DL. (2007). Specificity of treatment effects: cognitive therapy and relaxation for generalized anxiety and panic disorders. *J Consult Clin Psychol* 75(4):513–22.

Spencer T, Biederman J, Wilens TE, Faraone SV, Li T. (1994). Is attention deficit hyperactivity disorder in adults a valid diagnosis? *Harv Rev Psychiatry* 1: 326–35.

Spencer T, Biederman J, Wilens TE, Harding M, O'Donnell D, Griffin S. (1996). Pharmacotherapy of attention deficit disorder across the life cycle. *J Am Acad Child Adolesc Psychiatr* 35(4):409–32.

Stevenson CS, Stevenson RJ, Whitmont S. (2003). A self-directed psychosocial intervention with minimal therapist contact for adults with attention deficit hyperactivity disorder. *Clin Psychol Psychother* 10:93–101.

Stevenson C, Whitmont S, Bornholt L, Livesey D, Stevenson R. (2002). A cognitive remediation programme for adults with Attention Deficit Hyperactivity Disorder. *Aust N Z J Psychiatry* 36(5):610–16.

Swanson J, Arnold L, Vitiello B, Abikoff H, Wells K, Pelham W, et al. (2002). Response to commentary on the Multimodal Treatment Study of ADHD (MTA): mining the meaning of the MTA. *J Abnorm Child Psychol* 30(4):327–32.

Taylor E. (1999). Development of clinical services for attention-deficit/hyperactivity disorder. *Arch Gen Psychiatry* 56(12):1097–9.

van Apeldoorn FJ, van Hout WJ, Mersch PP, Huisman M, Slaap BR, Hale WW, 3rd, et al. (2008). Is a combined therapy more effective than either CBT or SSRI alone? Results of a multicenter trial on panic disorder with or without agoraphobia. *Acta Psychiatr Scand* 117(4):260–70.

Weiss M, Hechtman LT, Weiss G. (1999). *ADHD in Adulthood: A Guide to Current Theory, Diagnosis, and Treatment*. Baltimore: Johns Hopkins University Press.

Weiss M, Murray C. (2003). Assessment and management of attention-deficit hyperactivity disorder in adults. *Can Med Assoc J* 168(6):715–22.

Weiss M, Safren SA, Solanto MV, Hechtman L, Rostain AL, Ramsay JR, et al. (2008). Research forum on psychological treatment of adults with ADHD. *J Atten Disord* 11(6):642–51.

Wilens TE, Biederman J, Spencer TJ. (2002). Attention deficit/hyperactivity disorder across the lifespan. *Annu Rev Med* 53:113–31.

Wilens TE, Biederman J, Spencer TJ, Frances R. (1994). Comorbidity of attention deficit hyperactivity disorder and the psychoactive substance use disorders. *Hosp Comm Psychiatry* 45:421–35.

Wilens TE, McDermott SP, Biederman J, Abrantes A, Hahesy A, Spencer TJ. (1999). Cognitive therapy in the treatment of adults with ADHD: a systematic chart review of 26 cases. *J Cogn Psychother* 13(3):215–26.

Wilens TE, Spencer TJ, Biederman J. (2001). A review of the pharmacotherapy of adults with attention-deficit/hyperactivity disorder. *J Atten Disord* 5(4):189–202.

Young S, Gudjonsson GH. (2008). Growing out of ADHD: the relationship between functioning and symptoms. *J Atten Disord* 12(2):162–9.

Chapter 24

Neurofeedback training for adult ADHD

Seija Sirviö and Ylva Ginsberg

Neurofeedback, also called EEG biofeedback, has been a nonpharmacological treatment for attention-deficit hyperactivity disorder (ADHD) since 1979 and has a growing scientific evidence base. It is an operant conditioning procedure whereby individuals learn to self-regulate bioelectrical activity in the brain. During neurofeedback training an electroencephalogram (EEG) is recorded, and the relevant training measures are extracted and fed back to the individual using audiovisual, online, real-time feedback. The overall goal of neurofeedback is to improve mental flexibility and so produce a mental state appropriate to situational requirements.

Short history of neurofeedback

Brain imaging technologies like fMRI, PET scans, and SPECT are developing quickly and make it possible to gather more information about the brain's structure and function. The EEG has a long history, beginning in the late 1880s when the German physicist H. Hertz discovered this way to measure the brain's electrical activity. R. Caton later showed that the brain's bioelectrical activity fluctuated according to mental processing demands. In the late 1960s J. Kamayia took the first step in training the voluntary production of brainwaves by giving a verbal response to a trainee each time a specific brainwave activity was produced. Kamayia was able to demonstrate that a human could gain control over brainwave activity with instrumental feedback.

As a researcher for NASA, B. Sterman came from another angle. He used cats in an experiment aimed at studying rocket fuels' relationship to seizure disorders. Ten of the 50 cats that were used in the research had previously been trained in a totally different setting to produce a specific brainwave – sensorimotor

rhythm (SMR). Very surprisingly the ten cats that had been trained to produce SMR were seizure resistant compared to the other cats. In a long series of studies Sterman and his colleagues thereafter demonstrated that both animals and humans were able to alter their amplitude of frequencies in the area of the sensorimotor cortex. Patients with epilepsy could reduce their seizure activity by increasing frequencies in the 12- to 15-Hz range (SMR) by operant conditioning (Sterman, 2000). These findings led to the use of neurofeedback for ADHD, after an observation by J. Lubar (Shousse & Lubar, 1979) that increased SMR activity resulted in decreased hyperactivity, such as that observed in cats while mousing.

Cortico-electrical activity as a measure of states of arousal and diagnostic evaluation

Imaging techniques like PET, fMRI, and SPECT show anatomical, structural, and electrophysiological changes in individuals with ADHD. The involved regions are areas controlling the core symptoms of ADHD/ADD, such as a lack of behavioral inhibition and attention (e.g., the basal ganglia, cerebellum, and areas in the corpus callosum, prefrontal cortex, anterior cingulated gyrus, and the caudate). There are also studies showing a relationship between EEG findings and those areas, suggesting that ADHD to a substantial degree is a result of underarousal (Monastra, 2005; Sowell et al., 2003) and that there are different subtypes of ADHD (Clarke et al., 2001a, 2001b, 2001c, 2002, 2003).

A quantitative EEG (QEEG) is obtained by using software to analyze different aspects of the brain's bioelectrical activity and then compare them to a normative database of EEGs in healthy controls. EEGs

ADHD in Adults: Characterization, Diagnosis and Treatment, ed. Jan Buitelaar, Cornelis Kan and Philip Asherson.
Published by Cambridge University Press. © Cambridge University Press 2011.

are recorded in one or multiple sites, showing spectral characteristics as the distribution of brainwave frequencies and amplitudes. Normal brainwave patterns have been found to correspond to various mental states. Slow-wave activities are divided into three categories: delta, 0–3 Hz; theta, 4–7 Hz; and alpha, 8–12 Hz. Delta is characterized by sleep; theta and alpha are characterized by drowsiness, relaxation, and internal orientation. States of focus and alertness have a frequency range from 12–20 Hz, whereas low beta ranging from 12–15 Hz, beta ranging from 16–20 Hz, and faster frequencies such as high beta ranging from 20–34 Hz usually correspond to ruminating and anxiety. Alpha rhythm is the dominant activity in healthy controls in rest; GABA release slows the alpha rhythm into slower theta frequencies, so that the brain gradually shuts down the sensory registration to the cortex and changes the state of the brain to enable sleep. Theta and delta are believed to originate from subcortical layers, the reticular activating system (RAS), and the thalamus and are more elevated in amplitude during sleep. The faster frequencies are thought to originate from localized cortico-cortical and thalamo-cortical areas and are more active while processing more specialized information (Hughes & Roy John, 1999; Monastra, 2005).

By using normative databases and QEEG measures, researchers have been able to identify and extract individuals with ADHD from nonclinical samples (Chabot & Serfontein, 1996; Clarke et al., 2001a, 2001b, 2001c, 2002, 2003; Janzen et al., 1995; Monastra, 2005; Monastra, Lubar, & Linden, 2001). According to these studies, by using QEEG measures, one can discriminate ADHD/ADD diagnosed children from normal children with a specificity of 80–90%. The majority of children diagnosed with ADHD display elevated frontal theta or alpha excess, decreased amplitudes of higher frequencies, hypercoherence, and also a high incidence of abnormal interhemispheric asymmetry. The findings are primarily located in the frontal, frontal-midline, and central midline cortical areas of the cortex. In a study including 482 subjects, aged 6–30, Monastra et al. (1999) found that all individuals with ADHD showed higher slow-wave activity compared to faster activity. The ratios of theta and beta frequency activity were even higher for the younger participants. QEEG measures had an 85% predictive power for behavior and academic performance. Monastra et al. (2001) later replicated these findings in a group of 129 subjects aged 6–20.

Among children diagnosed with ADHD, Clarke et al. (2001a, 2001b, 2001c, 2002, 2003) identified different subtypes of ADHD corresponding to three clusters: one group with excessive beta activity, another group showing elevated high-amplitude theta and decreased beta and delta activity, and a third group with a maturational lag showing increased slow-wave and deficiencies of fast-wave activity.

Bresnahan and colleagues (Bresnahan, Anderson, & Barry, 1999; Bresnahan & Barry, 2002) have suggested that changes in the EEG pattern of subjects with ADHD are due to increased age. Their 1999 study included 150 subjects aged 6–42. QEEGs were measured from midline sites and compared to those of normal healthy subjects. Elevated theta activity was consistent through all age groups of subjects with ADHD, but adults with ADHD did not show decreased beta activity, as was earlier reported for children and adolescents with ADHD. In the adult ADHD group the beta amplitude tended to be normal compared to healthy individuals. Similar results were presented in the 2002 study including 150 adults, who were divided into three groups – subjects with ADHD, subjects who were assessed for ADHD but did not meet diagnostic criteria for it, and healthy controls – with 50 subjects in each group. The adults with ADHD maintained excessive slow-wave activity, but not less beta activity. Findings of more normalized beta activity with increasing age are suggested to correlate with reduced hyperactivity, and findings of excessive slow-wave activity are thought to correlate with increased impulsivity.

What happens during neurofeedback?

There are several biofeedback training options, but all aim to teach an individual to gain control over physiological functions. For biofeedback addressing the peripheral nervous system (PNS), sensors are attached to different parts of the body to measure biological signals produced by muscles, sweat glands, body temperature, and heart rhythm. The registration instrument gives feedback when the individual produces the biological activity of interest, thereby enhancing learning and individual control over the trained function.

In contrast, neurofeedback is directed to the central nervous system (CNS) and uses the brain's bioelectrical activity as recorded by the EEG as the biofeedback medium. The EEG signal consists of tiny fluctuations of electricity in selected frequency bands that result from the summed activity of neurons in the cerebral

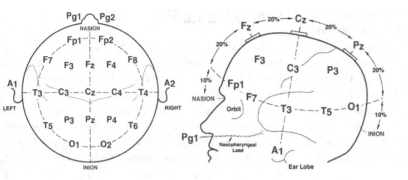

Figure 24.1 The International 10–20 Electrode Placement System. Courtesy of Grass Technologies, An Astro-Med, Inc. Product Group, West Warwick, RI, USA.

cortex. Electrodes passively conduct voltage potentials from columns of neurons in the brain and pick up microvolt signals. The voltages are measured in 1 millionth of a volt or microvolt. The frequency spectrum varies from 0 to 40 Hz or more (Hz, cycles per second).

Choosing electrode placements for neurofeedback training

The standard for locating electrodes on the scalp is the International 10–20 System (Fig. 24.1). This system uses certain landmarks, such as the nasion (front) and inion (rear) of the head, for the placement of electrodes to ensure their accurate relationship to the underlying brain tissue. The placement is guided by knowledge of how different brain areas control ways of mediating arousal, information processing, moods, and movements. Electrodes are attached to the scalp and the ear lobe or mastoid using conductive paste.

Training can be conducted during single, dual, or multiple recordings. Electrodes for training ADHD are usually placed on the sensorimotor-strip as C3, C4, and Cz (Fig. 24.1) and also at more frontal sites (i.e. Fz). The EEG measures the difference between the bioelectrical activity (amplitude) and the so-called active (placed at the selected placement on the skull) and the passive (usually placed on the ear lobe or mastoid) sensors. The computer software then converts this information into visual, auditory, or combined visual and auditory feedback; the type of feedback is chosen among the possibilities provided by different computerized hardware and software designed for neurofeedback. Feedback is the modality that gives individuals an opportunity to experience how their brains are reacting during different situations and to learn how to change or modulate their brainwave patterns.

ADHD is seen as producing dysregulated brainwave functioning, and neurofeedback training is commonly designed to inhibit low-wave activity (theta) and enhance faster activity (beta). For instance; if an individual shows high theta/beta ratios accompanied by concentration deficits, the training would place the sensor on Cz (perhaps C3, C4, or Fz) and set the training parameters to enhance beta activity (12–15 Hz or 15–20 Hz) in order to improve the ability to maintain focus. It is equally important to design the training to simultaneously inhibit production of lower frequencies, as theta, and inhibit brainwaves associated with stress and anxiety, as high beta. This kind of training is supposed to reduce the amplitude of slower waves and simultaneously increase target brainwave activity by only giving positive feedback or reward when all criteria are met. The rewards often consist of points earned, pictures moving, and/or sound pitch, based on the principle of operant conditioning.

Before the training starts, an assessment is usually made, involving the collection of background

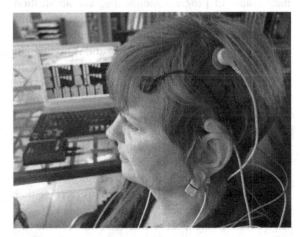

Figure 24.2 A client in neurofeedback training.

information, interviews with relatives, psychological testing, EEG measurements, determination of handedness, and the administration of rating scales and of computerized tests of attention. Conners' Rating Scales are often used to gather information about the behavior of the child at home and in the school setting; they cover a wide range of behavioral, emotional, social, and academic issues. The latest version (Conners, 1997) includes parent and teacher forms for ages 6–18 and self-report forms for ages 8–18.

To obtain more objective measurements, continuous performance tests (CPTs), which are computerized tests designed to assess attention, are used widely. CPTs include the Test of Variables in Attention (TOVA; Greenberg et al., 1993), Conners' CPT, and Conners' CPT II (Conners, 2000). A common factor in CPTs is that they present a repetitive and boring task and require both response accuracy and sustained attention over time. The person has to respond to a stimulus, either visual or auditory, but inhibit response to other stimuli, and this task is meant to measure aspects of impulsivity, inattention, and sustained attention.

Information from the assessment is used as guidelines for the training parameters, placements of the sensors, and the training program. Rating scales and tests of attention are also used in measuring treatment efficacy and as markers for possible adjustments to the training set-up during the training phase. During the training, thresholds for feedback are adjusted to maintain the client's motivation.

Each session lasts about 45 minutes, which results in at most 30 minutes of effective feedback training because of progress monitoring, the application of electrodes, etc. The trainee sits in front of a computer screen that displays the visual feedback and/or listens to audio feedback (Fig. 24.2) and is first taught the meaning of the feedback. Positive changes in psychophysiology, behavior, and/or cognitive performance have been seen to occur after a minimum of 20 sessions (Rossiter & LaVaque, 1995).

Neurofeedback training is also done with bipolar (sequential) montage, usually using single-channel recording in which the active and the passive sensors are placed on the skull and the reference sensor on the ear lobe or mastoids. The placements can be either intra- or interhemispheric, and the obtained EEG signal is a measurement of the difference between the two placements.

Controlled studies

Neurofeedback for ADHD has been compared to other treatments in several studies. Rossiter and LaVaque (1995) compared neurofeedback to stimulant therapy in 46 patients (aged 8–21) in an open, nonrandomized study. The medication-only group received either methylphenidate or dextroamphetamine, and the group receiving neurofeedback training got 20 sessions over a 3-month period. Both groups showed significant improvements in pre- and post testing. In 2004 the results were replicated in another open, nonrandomized study including 62 patients. This later study also showed that neurofeedback training produced the same outcome as the stimulant drugs (Rossiter & LaVaque, 2004). Linden, Habib, and Radojevic (1996) studied 18 patients who were randomly selected to neurofeedback or a wait-list control group. The neurofeedback group demonstrated significant pre- and post testing improvements in measurements of attention and cognitive performance. Neither group received medication. Another study by Fuchs et al. (2003) compared neurofeedback to methylphenidate (n = 34, children aged 8–12 years) in an open, nonrandomized study in which participants were assigned to either neurofeedback or methylphenidate according to their parents' preference. The study showed that both groups improved in pre- and post testing of different variables in attention and behavior.

A larger study was conducted by Monastra, Monastra, and George (2002), comparing effects of neurofeedback, Ritalin, and parenting styles. The subjects were 100 children aged 6–19. They participated for one year in the study that included the administration of Ritalin and the provision of parent counseling and academic support at school. Fifty-one of the children also received neurofeedback. Pre- and post testing with behavioral rating scales, TOVA, and QEEG recording at Cz while the subjects were completing reading, listening, and drawing tasks were done for all the 51 subjects while they were off Ritalin. The study showed significant improvement in cortical arousal on the QEEG, behavioral ratings, and TOVA in the group receiving neurofeedback while unmedicated, compared to the control group. The neurofeedback group also showed improvement on the QEEG measurement of neurophysiological changes. Two years later Monastra and Monastra conducted a follow-up study of 86 of the participants in the earlier study, showing a continuing effect in the neurofeedback group in reducing core symptoms of ADHD such as behavior and attention problems; these participants also showed improved levels of cortical activation as measured by QEEG. Furthermore, 34 of the subjects who received neurofeedback were able to decrease their stimulant medication by half (Monastra, 2005).

Criticism of neurofeedback's effectiveness points to the lack of studies controlled for bias (Loo & Barkley, 2005; Vernon, Frick, & Gruzelier, 2004). Double-blind, randomized, and more controlled studies have to be done to prove the efficacy of neurofeedback. In addition, sample sizes have to be larger, and long-term effects and side effects have to be studied. There is also a question whether neurofeedback is correlated to the obtained improvements. However, the base of evidence for neurofeedback keeps growing.

A recent study by Strehl et al. (2006) demonstrated that study participants (23 children with ADHD, aged 8–13) learned to regulate slow cortical potential (SCP) after 30 sessions and obtained significant improvements in behavior and attention. All the obtained improvements were stable 6 months after training. The results resembled those of an earlier study of SCP training (25 sessions) for children with ADHD by Heinrich (2004). Significant improvements in impulsivity were confirmed in this open, nonrandomized study comparing 11 children in the experimental group and 9 on a waiting list. SCP differs from frequency neurofeedback training, which adjusts the theta/beta ratio, by addressing low event-related direct-current shifts of the EEG beneath the frequencies described. However, both approaches share the general principle of giving feedback on the brain's electrical activity to obtain self-regulation. Leins et al. (2007) compared the efficacy of SCP and the theta/beta protocol. Subjects were blinded to group assignment, and each group consisted of 19 children (aged 8–13), who completed 30 sessions of training. They found equally significant improvements in cognition and behavior in both groups, and subjects also demonstrated the ability to intentionally regulate their cortical activity.

At present there are no controlled group studies with neurofeedback in adults with ADHD to the authors' knowledge.

Future perspectives

Given the findings of subtypes in ADHD and possible changes in EEG due to age and to deficiencies, such as hypercoherence and a high incidence of abnormal interhemispheric asymmetry reported in children with ADHD, there could be a need for other training options in addition to the theta/beta ratio and SCP training. The possibilities of detecting, localizing, and obtaining specific localizations of abnormal EEGs could be of importance in addressing individual EEG anomalies. Real-time fMRI neurofeedback has been able to demonstrate individuals' abilities to gain control over activation in specific deep-structured brain areas (i.e. deCharms et al., 2004; Rota et al., 2008). Low-resolution electromagnetic tomography (LORETA) provides a three-dimensional image of localized brain functions and, when used as a neurofeedback medium, allows training to be targeted to specific subcortical areas such as the anterior cingulate cortex (Congedo, Lubar, & Joffe, 2004). The recently introduced Z-score neurofeedback training, an instantaneous and ongoing comparison of a client's EEG to a database of normal subjects' EEGs, addresses not only the amplitude but also the connectivity (i.e. hypercoherence, asymmetry) of the brain's bioelectrical activity. Although in an experimental phase, these approaches could be of interest in the future, enabling the possibility of individualizing bioelectrical feedback to target training.

Summary and conclusions

Neurofeedback can be an interesting choice of treatment for ADHD in conjunction with other treatments or when other treatments fail. It has been shown that both animals and humans can learn to control their brainwaves by operant conditioning. Furthermore, it has been documented that different electro-cortical activities reflect different states of arousal and that a number of disorders, including ADHD, can be discriminated by characteristic patterns on the QEEG. The studies conducted so far have shown that neurofeedback addresses the core symptoms of ADHD. The majority of the research has been done with children and adolescents, and although research shows encouraging results there is a need for further controlled and larger group studies of children and particularly of adults with ADHD.

Recommended reading

Demos JN. (2005). *Getting Started with Neurofeedback*. New York: W. W. Norton.

Thompson M, Thompson L. (2003). *The Neurofeedback Book – An Introduction to Basic Concepts in Applied Psychophysiology*. Wheat Ridge, CO: Association for Applied Psychophysiology and Biofeedback.

Links for more information

SAN (Society of Applied Neuroscience) is a European organization aimed to enhance research as knowledge within the area of neuroregulation: www.applied-neuroscience.org

ISNR (International Society of Neuro Regulation) is the international organization of Neurofeedback: www.isnr.org

References

Bresnahan SM, Anderson JW, Barry RJ. (1999). Age-related changes in quantitative EEG in attention-deficit/hyperactivity disorder. *Biol Psychiatry* **46**(12):1690–7.

Bresnahan SM, Barry RJ. (2002). Specificity of quantitative EEG analysis in adults with attention deficit hyperactivity disorder. *Psychiatry Res* **112**(2): 133–44.

Chabot RJ, Serfontein G. (1996). Quantitative electroencephalographic profiles of children with attention deficit disorder. *Biol Psychiatry* **40**: 951–63.

Clarke AR, Barry RJ, McCarthy R, Selikowitz M. (2001a). Age and sex effects in the EEG: differences in two subtypes of attention-deficit/hyperactivity disorder. *Clin Psychophysiol* **112**(5):815–25.

Clarke AR, Barry RJ, McCarthy R, Selikowitz M. (2001b). Electroencephalogram differences in two subtypes of attention-deficit/hyperactivity disorder. *Psychophysiology* **38**(2): 212–21.

Clarke AR, Barry RJ, McCarthy R, Selikowitz M. (2001c). Excess beta activity in children with attention-deficit/hyperactivity disorder: an atypical electrophysiological group. *Psychiatry Res* **103**(2–3):205–18.

Clarke AR, Barry RJ, McCarthy R, Selikowitz M, Brown CR. (2002). EEG evidence for a new conceptualisation of attention deficit hyperactivity disorder. *Clin Neurophysiol* **113**(7):1036–44.

Clarke AR, Barry RJ, McCarthy R, Selikowitz M, Clarke DC, Croft RJ. (2003). EEG activity in girls with attention-deficit/hyperactivity disorder. *Clin Neurophysiol* **114**(2):319–28.

Congedo M, Lubar JF, Joffe D. (2004). Low-resolution electromagnetic tomography neurofeedback. *IEEE Trans Neural Syst Rehabil* **12**(4):386–97.

Conners CK. (1997). *Conners Rating Scales – Revised; Technical Manual*. North Tonawande, NY: Multi-Health System.

Conners CK. (2000). *Conners CPT-II: Continuous Performance Test-II*. Toronto, ON: Multi-Health System.

deCharms RC, Christoff K, Glover GH, Pauly JM, Whitfield, S, Gabrieli, JD. (2004). Learned regulation of spatially localized brain activation using real-time fMRI. *Neuroimage* **21**(1):436–43.

Fuchs T, Birbaumer N, Lutzenberger W, Gruzelier JH, Kaiser J. (2003). Neurofeedback treatment for attention-deficit/hyperactivity disorder in children: a comparison with methylphenidate. *Appl Psychophysiol Biofeedback* **20**:1–12.

Greenberg LM, Dupuy TR. (1993). *Interpretation Manual for the Test of Variables of Attention*. Los Alamitos, CA: Universal Attention Disorders.

Heinrich H. (2004). Training of slow cortical potentials in ADHD: evidence for positive behavioral and neurophysiological effects. *Biol Psychiatry* **55**:772–5.

Hughes MD, Roy John E. (1999). Conventional and quantitative electroencephalography in psychiatry. *J Neuropsychiatry Clin Neurosci* **11**:190–208.

Janzen T, Graap K, Stephanson S, Marshall W, Fitzsimmons G. (1995). Differences in baseline EEG measures for ADD and normally achieving preadolescent males. *Biofeedback Self-Regul* **20**:65–82.

Linden M, Habib T, Radojevic V. (1996). A controlled study of the effects of EEG biofeedback on cognition and behavior of children with attention deficit disorders and learning disabilities. *Biofeedback Self-Regul* **21**:35–49.

Leins U, Goth G, Hinterberger T, Klinger C, Rumpf N, Strehl U. (2007). Neurofeedback for children with ADHD: a comparison of SCP and Theta/Beta protocols. *Appl Psychophysiol Biofeedback* **32**(2):73–88.

Loo SK, Barkley RA. (2005). Clinical utility of EEG in attention deficit hyperactivity disorder. *Appl Neuropsychol* **12**(2):64–76.

Monastra VJ. (2005). EEG biofeedback (neurotherapy) as a treatment for attention-deficit/hyperactivity disorder: rationale and empirical foundation. *Child Adolesc Psychiatr Clin North Am* **14**(1):55–82.

Monastra VJ, Lubar JF, Linden M. (2001). The development of a quantitative electroencephalographic scanning process for attention deficit-hyperactivity disorder: reliability and validity studies. *Neuropsychology* **15**(1):136–44.

Monastra VJ, Lubar JF, Linden M, VanDeusen P, Green G, Wing W. (1999). Assessing attention deficit hyperactivity disorder via quantitative electroencephalography: an initial validation study. *Neuropsychology* **13**(3):424–33.

Monastra VJ, Monastra DM, George S. (2002). The effects of stimulant therapy, EEG biofeedback and parenting style on the primary symptoms of attention deficit/hyperactivity disorder. *Appl Psychophysiol Biofeedback* 27(4):231–49.

Rossiter TR, LaVaque T. (1995). A comparison of EEG biofeedback and psychostimulants in treating attention deficit hyperactivity disorders. *J Neurother* 1:48–59.

Rossiter TR, LaVaque T. (2004). The effectiveness of neurofeedback and stimulant drugs in treating ADHD. Part II: replication. *Appl Psychophysiol Biofeedback* 29(4):233–43.

Rota G, Sitaram R, Veit R, Erb M, Weiskopf N, Dogil G, Birbaumer N. (2009). Self-regulation of regional cortical activity using real-time fMRI: the right inferior frontal gyrus and linguistic processing. *Hum Brain Mapp* 30(5):1605–14.

Shousse MN, Lubar JF. (1979). Sensorimotor rhythm (SMR) operant conditioning and methylphenidate in the treatment of hyperkinesis. *Biofeedback Self-Regul* 4:299–311.

Sowell ER, Thompson PM, Welcome SE, Henkenius AL, Toga AW, Peterson BS. (2003). Cortical abnormalities in children and adolescents with attention-deficit hyperactivity disorder. *Lancet* 362:1699–707.

Sterman MB. (2000). Basic concepts and clinical findings in the treatment of seizure disorders with EEG operant conditioning. *Clin EEG* 31:45–55.

Strehl U, Leins U, Goth G, Klinger C, Hinterberger T, Birbaumer N. (2006). Self-regulation of slow cortical potentials: a new treatment for children with attention-deficit/hyperactivity disorder. *Pediatrics* 118(5): e1530–40.

Vernon D, Frick A, Gruzelier J. (2004). Neurofeedback as a treatment for ADHD: a methodological review with implications for future research. *J Neurother* 8(2): 53–81.

Chapter

25

Alternative and complementary treatments for ADHD

Lacramioara Spetie and L. Eugene Arnold

The recent boxed warnings for stimulants have added impetus to the increasing interest in finding alternatives to pharmacological and behavioral treatment for attention-deficit hyperactivity disorder (ADHD). Many parents and adults with ADHD have already turned to alternative treatments or to adjunctive (complementary) treatments that might reduce the need for medication. In this chapter, alternative/complementary treatments (Tx) are defined as any treatment other than those endorsed by the professional associations: prescription psychoactive drugs, standard behavioral treatments, and special educational support.

Most treatments for ADHD were first documented in children, followed by later and less extensive documentation in adults (e.g. stimulants, antidepressants, and behavioral treatments). Alternative/complementary treatments have generally inadequate documentation even in children and even less research in adults with ADHD. Most studies have serious methodological flaws, including small sample sizes, questionable diagnostic rigor, heterogeneous samples, lack of control or comparison groups, and limited measurements of behavioral and cognitive outcomes. Because the studies in adults are so few, we summarize the child literature and make comments about extrapolation to adults. Most alternative treatments are etiologically targeted, and therefore scientific evaluation and clinical use of such treatments require more etiological depth of diagnosis than the phenomenological criteria of *DSM-IV-TR* (American Psychiatric Association, 2000).

Nutritional supplementation

Nutritional supplementation treatments are based on the assumption that certain nutrients that are crucial for normal brain functioning are either lacking in the diet in optimal amount or are required by some individuals in higher than ordinary amounts and should therefore be added. Both macronutrients (amino acids, lipids, and carbohydrates) and micronutrients (vitamins and minerals) have been proposed as treatment for ADHD.

Amino acid supplementation

Amino acid supplementation is the alternative treatment that has perhaps been the most studied in adults. Amino acids are the precursors of neurotransmitters such as catecholamines and serotonin that have been shown to be implicated in the pathophysiology of ADHD. Studies have found low CNS levels of amino acids in patients with ADHD (Baker et al., 1991; Bornstein et al., 1990). Stein and Sammaritano (1984) reported that, compared to matched normals with similar dietary intake, 8- to 10-year-old hyperkinetic boys excreted more nitrogen and showed different distribution patterns of excretion, flux, and protein synthesis. Recent studies have found a significant association between certain variants of the catechol o-methyltransferase (COMT) gene and behavioral and cognitive deficits in children with ADHD (Bellgrove et al., 2005; Thapar et al., 2005). Studies done in adults (see Table 25.1) found some short-term improvement in symptoms but no lasting benefit beyond 2–3 months. Therefore, amino acid supplementation may have a role in providing temporary relief while arranging or initiating other interventions, but does not seem to be a promising area for long-term treatment. Importantly, it may carry some risk (Pakes, 1978; Sidransky, 1997; Sternberg, 1996). Although the eosinophilia/myalgia syndrome reported in the 1980s seems to have been either spurious or associated with manufacturing impurities (Sidransky, 1997;

Table 25.1 Adult studies of amino acid supplementation

Study	Amino acid	Results
Wood et al., 1985a (double-blind crossover design)	dl-phenylalanine	Short-term improvement ($p < 0.09$); all benefit was lost after 3 months
Wood et al., 1985b (double- blind crossover design)	l-phenylalanine	No short- or long-term improvement
Wood et al., 1985b (placebo washout, open trial)	l-tyrosine	Short-term improvement that was lost after the 10th week of treatment
Reimherr et al., 1987 (open trial)	l-tyrosine	Marked response at 2 weeks that was lost at 8 weeks of treatment
Shekim et al., 1990 (open trial)	S-adenosyl-l-methionine	Significant improvement at 4 weeks; no longer term trial
DeFrance et al., 1997	commercial mixture (Kantroll) of amino acids	Significant improvement in cognitive processing speed in normal volunteer young adults

Williamson et al., 1998), there may be other risks associated with this "supply side" approach to neurotransmission; for example, the post-reuptake breakdown products of the monoamine neurotransmitters may be toxic to the cell.

L-Carnitine

Carnitine is essential for fatty acid metabolism, transporting lipids across the microsomal inner membrane as acylcarnitine (Arduini et al., 1994) and supporting elongation of essential fatty acids (Ricciolini et al., 1998). Humans synthesize only one-quarter of their needed supply of carnitine, making it a partially essential nutrient. Some theorize that abnormalities in energy production and fatty acid oxidation may affect at least some ADHD cases. A Dutch study reported that supplementing the diet with L-carnitine significantly improved the cognitive and behavioral symptoms of ADHD (Van Oudheusden & Scholte, 2002), but two subsequent American trials (Arnold et al., 2007) failed to demonstrate its value for combined-type ADHD. It remains investigational for inattentive-type ADHD.

Essential fatty acid supplementation

Certain polyunsaturated fatty acids play a key role in the axonal myelinization process and form the neuronal membrane scaffolding for receptors and other cell-surface structures. Neuronal membranes are composed of phospholipids containing large amounts of the n-3 and n-6 (or omega-3 and omega-6) acids (the first unsaturated bonds 3 or 6 carbons, respectively, from the noncarboxyl "tail" of the molecule).

Human metabolism cannot manufacture these fatty acids de novo, and hence they are "essential" (needed in the diet). Essential fatty acids (EFA) are also metabolized to prostaglandins and other eicosanoids, which modify many metabolic processes, activate eicosanoid receptors, and interact with proinflammatory cytokines (Lands, 1998; Maes, 1998). In general, the eicosanoids from omega-6 acids tend to be more pro-inflammatory, whereas those from omega-3 tend to suppress inflammation. Lab animal behavior can be manipulated by varying the quantity and quality of EFA. Juvenile and young adult monkeys with long-term n-3 fatty acid deficiency show increased activity, and both human and monkey infants show changes in visual attention with n-3 deficiency (Neuringer, 1998).

A diet that does not provide the necessary intake of such fatty acids may impair brain function and induce symptoms of inattention, distractibility, poor impulse control, and the like (Richardson, 2004).

Essential fatty acids claimed to be helpful include EPA eicosapentaenoic acid (EPA) and docosahexaenoic acid (DHA) of the omega–3 series and gamma-linolenic acid (GLA) of the omega–6 series. A related nutrient, vitamin E (alpha and gamma tocopherol) has also been implicated. In summary, the two studies using only omega-6 (GLA) and the two using only omega-3 (DHA) failed to demonstrate convincing results, but those using a combination of GLA, EPA, and DHA reported modest to moderate benefit (see Table 25.2). Further controlled trials in patients are necessary. Essential fatty acid supplementation may be more effective in selected patients with low serum levels of the specific EFA supplemented.

Table 25.2 Studies of essential fatty acid supplementation

Study & Dx	Essential fatty acid	Design	Results
Aman et al., 1987 ADHD	Gamma-linolenic acid (n-6 series, evening primrose oil)	Double blind, placebo controlled, crossover	Equivocal results for ADHD
Arnold et al., 1989 ADHD	Efamol (evening primrose oil containing gamma-linolenic acid and linoleic acid: n-6)	Placebo controlled double blind, crossover with random assignment	Equivocal results for ADHD
Voigt et al., 2001 ADHD	Docosohexaenoic acid (n-3)	Double blind, placebo controlled, randomized	Some decrease in impulsivity, otherwise no improvement
Richardson & Puri, 2002 (pilot study) 41 children ADHD with and without dyslexia	8 daily capsules containing EPA, DHA, GLA, vitamin E, cis-linoleic acid, AA, thyme oil	Double blind, placebo controlled, randomized	Mild improvement in inattention
Richardson, 2003 (preliminary data) on 102 children aged 8–12 with dyslexia	Daily doses as follows: EPA, 186 mg; DHA, 480 mg; GLA, 96 mg; vitamin E, 60 IU; cis-linoleic acid, 864 mg; AA, 42 mg; and thyme oil, 8 mg	Double blind, placebo controlled, randomized	Preliminary results showed improvement in reading abilities in most of the children who completed the study
Stevens et al., 2003 Hyperactivity	480 mg DHA, 80 mg EPA, 40 mg arachidonic acid (AA), 96 mg GLA, and 24 mg alpha-tocopherol acetate for 4 months	Double blind, placebo controlled, randomized	Some improvement in conduct and attention symptoms
Hirayama et al., 2004 ADHD	DHA	Double blind, placebo controlled, randomized	No significant improvement
Richardson & Montgomery, 2005 Developmental coordination disorder with or without comorbid ADHD	Supplement containing 80% fish oil and 20% evening primrose oil (558 mg EPA; 174 mg DHA; 60 mg GLA; 9.6 mg alpha-tocopherol (vitamin E)	Randomized, double blind placebo controlled involving treatment in parallel groups for 3 months	Significant improvement in measures of reading, spelling, and behavior in the active treatment group
Sinn & Bryan, 2007 ADHD	PUFA (polyunsaturated fatty acid), micronutrient supplements	Randomized, placebo controlled, double blind over 15 weeks.; survey data collection, with 104 returned	Significant medium to large treatment effects on parent ratings of core ADHD symptoms in both PUFA treatment groups compared to placebo; no additional effects with micronutrients

Abbreviations used: DHA = docosahexaenoic acid; EPA = eicosapentaenoic acid; GLA = gamma-linolenic acid; AA = arachidonic acid.

Choline supplementation

Dean and Morgenthaler (1990) advocated choline supplementation as choline is one of the building blocks of acetylcholine, a neurotransmitter involved in memory. Another study found lower concentrations of choline-containing compounds in the brains of children with memory deficits (Yeo et al., 2000). Choline supplementation could conceivably be a "supply side" route to the benefit demonstrated by nicotine in some adults with ADHD. No controlled trial of choline as a treatment could be found.

Dimethylaminoethanol (DMAE) has several accepted names in the literature, including deanol and dimethylethanolamine. It is the immediate precursor of choline (trimethylaminoethanol) and is claimed to increase production of acetylcholine. DMAE was originally marketed as a prescription drug (Deaner[(R)]) for hyperactivity/minimal brain dysfunction, but was withdrawn from the market as only "possibly effective" in the early 1980s, after the US Food and Drug Administration (FDA) began requiring efficacy evidence as well as safety evidence. It is now marketed as a nonprescription nutrient for ADD and learning problems. It is one of the better studied alternative treatments, with about 10 double-blind, placebo-controlled small trials.

Some studies showed encouraging enough results to be considered promising pilot data. In 1958 an open study in 108 children with behavioral problems suggestive of minimal brain injury disorder without epilepsy and 17 children with behaviors suggesting minimal brain injury with epilepsy were treated with Deanol at a maintenance dose ranging between 20 and 200 mg daily, with most of them receiving an average dose of 50 mg (Oettinger, 1958): 48% percent experienced good improvement and 20% experienced fair improvement in the symptoms of overactivity, short attention span, and poor academic performance. Probably the best study was Lewis and Young's (1975) three-group parallel comparison, which showed placebo-controlled effect sizes (ESs) of 0.1 to 0.6 on various measures, compared to methylphenidate placebo-controlled ESs of 0.8–1.3 in the same study. Both quality and quantity of effect seem highly dose dependent, with a suspicion that higher doses have a catecholamine effect. A global estimate of ES considering all the positive studies (disregarding the negative) would be 0.2 to 0.5 if the dose were 500 mg a day or higher, but there are enough flaws in the published studies that the FDA did not consider it approvable as efficacious.

Glyconutritional supplements

Glyconutritional supplements contain basic saccharides necessary for cell communication and formation of glycoproteins and glycolipids: glucose, galactose, mannose, N-acetylneuraminic acid, fucose, N-acetylgalactosamine, and xylose. Only the first two are abundant in the ordinary diet. In an open trial of glyconutritional and phytonutritional (flash freeze-dried fruits and vegetables) supplementation with 17 ADHD children, Dykman and Dykman (1998) found significant ($p < 0.05$–$p < 0.001$) reductions in parent SNAP-IV ratings of inattention, hyperactivity-impulsivity, and oppositional symptoms, with similar trends on teacher ratings. In a second open trial of the same supplements in 18 children, Dykman and McKinley (1997) found reductions in parent inattention ratings from 2.47 to 2.05 ($p < .006$) and in hyperactivity-impulsivity ratings from 2.23 to 1.54 ($p < -.003$), sustained for 6 weeks. However, a third open trial reportedly failed to duplicate such results. No trials have been reported in adults, but if glyconutritional supplements were ever found effective in controlled trials, there is no

reason to believe they would not work as well in adults as in children. However, this is not a promising treatment.

Supplementation with vitamins and minerals

Vitamins and minerals act as cofactors in important steps in neurotransmitter synthesis and energy metabolism. Three strategies for vitamin supplementation are (1) recommended daily allowance/recommended daily intake (RDA/RDI) multivitamin preparations, (2) megavitamin multiple combinations, and (3) mega-doses of specific vitamins.

A randomly assigned double-blind, placebo-controlled trial of RDA vitamin and mineral supplementation in 47 6-year-old children not selected for ADHD (Benton & Cook, 1991) found an 8.3-point IQ advantage ($p < 0.001$), mainly in nonverbal ability, an increase in concentration, decreased fidgeting on a frustrating task ($p < 0.05$), and advantage on a reaction time task interpreted to reflect sustained attention (ES = 1.3, $p < 0.05$). More controlled studies are needed. If shown effective for ADHD in controlled trials, RDA supplementation should work as well for adults as children because vitamin need seems to be lifelong. Megavitamin multiple combinations have not been found effective in double-blind, placebo-controlled trials and do not seem worth pursuing for children or adults. They carry some risk.

The use of single vitamins in mega-doses to alter neural metabolism in specific ways has not been adequately explored, despite some encouraging early reports (e.g. Brenner, 1982; Coleman et al., 1979).

Zinc

Zinc is an important cofactor for 100 enzymes. One study suggested that evening primrose oil (a supplement rich in gamma-linolenic acid – GLA) was most effective in children who had borderline zinc nutritional status (Arnold et al., 2000). In two Middle Eastern samples, zinc sulfate monotherapy was superior to placebo in reducing ADHD symptoms, and children treated with methylphenidate experienced more improvement in symptoms when they also took daily zinc supplements compared to those who only took methylphenidate and placebo (Akhonzadeh, Mohammadi, & Khademi, 2004; Bilici et al., 2004). Zinc as potential monotherapy and as adjunct to stimulant is currently being explored in an American sample at Ohio State University. Whether zinc is critical in ADHD may depend highly on the routine diet in a particular region or culture; the Middle East, where the positive trials were carried out, is an area of endemic zinc deficiency. If found effective, the results with zinc (and other supplements) should apply also to adults with ADHD.

Magnesium

Magnesium (Mg) is another important mineral that may be low in some patients with ADHD. Supplementation with magnesium improved hyperactivity in Polish children with documented low blood magnesium (Starobrat-Hermelin & Kozielec, 1997). Supplementation with magnesium and vitamin B6 seemed helpful in another open study from France (Mousain-Bosc et al., 2004). However, two American samples failed to find Mg deficiency by blood test. Mg can be toxic in too high doses and should not be supplemented in high doses without tests indicating need.

Iron

Iron supplementation appeared helpful in reducing ADHD symptoms in children with ADHD and documented iron deficiency (Konofal et al., 2004, 2006), although the difference between iron supplement and placebo was not significant at the small sample size used in the pilot trial. In a double-blind, placebo-controlled trial in 73 teenage nonanemic but iron-deficient girls, Bruner et al. (1996) found improvements in verbal learning and memory. In a trial of gastro-protected ferritin in 33 iron-deficient children, Burattini et al. (1990) found a decrease in hyperactivity. Iron status could be an important consideration for menstruating women with ADHD. Indeed, it is interesting to speculate whether this factor could partially account for the more equal sex distribution in adult ADHD compared to prepubertal children, where it is predominantly a male problem.

Deleading therapy

It has been shown that exposure to heavy metals could have adverse effects on children's cognitive functioning. In those patients with ADHD who are found to have elevated levels of heavy metals (such as lead or cadmium) chelation therapy may significantly

improve their ADHD symptoms (David et al., 1976, 1983).

Dietary eliminations

There is some evidence that in some cases the etiology of ADHD symptoms is related to environmental and food allergies, and therefore certain dietary modifications such as additive-free or oligoantigenic diets may lead to symptom improvement. A respectable number of studies have convincing placebo or other controls, but the results of many studies have been questioned on diagnostic or sampling grounds (see Table 25.3). Dietary sensitivities seem to be a real issue for a minority of children with ADHD. Because the evidence points to more effect in preschoolers than older children, this issue probably does not have much application to adults unless they have obvious food allergies/sensitivities. In contrast to the respectable evidence for other dietary sensitivities, the studies of sugar elimination have been generally negative.

Homeopathic treatments

Homeopathic treatments have been studied as alternatives to pharmacological treatments in various medical conditions. Several open studies have reported a decrease in ADHD symptoms in children treated with homeopathic remedies (Frei & Thurneysen, 2001, 2006; Jacobs et al., 2005; Strauss, 2000). However, without a placebo comparison, it is not possible to consider their findings an evidence base for treatment. If such treatment were proven in controlled studies, it would probably apply also to adults.

Herbal treatments

Certain Chinese traditional herbs (ginseng, ginkgo biloba) with antioxidant and vessel-relaxing properties can improve blood flow to the brain, theoretically improving brain functioning. An open study in 36 children aged 3–17 reported that the herbal extract combination Panax quinquefolium and ginkgo biloba improved the symptoms of ADHD in most cases (Lyon et al., 2001). Again, placebo-controlled studies are needed, but if found effective, antioxidants should work as well with adults as with children.

Grapine is a powerful antioxidant derived from grape seeds and maritime pine bark that has been found to protect various cells against various potentially damaging agents and pathophysiological

Table 25.3 Dietary intervention clinical trials

Author	Type of dietary intervention	Sample (N, Dx, age)	Design	Results
Conners et al., 1976	Kaiser-Permanente Diet or control for 4 weeks; crossover to other arm for 4 weeks	15 children aged 6–12 with *DSM-II* hyperkinetic reaction of childhood	Double blind, crossover	Improved teacher ratings on the Kaiser Permanente diet compared to controls; improved parent and teacher ratings compared to baseline
Goyette et al., 1978	Challenge (50% adult RDA of FDA-approved artificial colors) and placebo chocolate cookies for 8 weeks	16 children aged 4–11 who had symptom reduction of at least 25% on elimination diet	Double-blind, counter-balanced, crossover challenge	No difference in parent or teacher ratings; three children who were deemed "dye sensitive" had worse visual tracking performance 1 hour after challenge
Goyette et al., 1978	Challenge (50% adult RDA of FDA-approved artificial colors) and placebo chocolate cookies 2/day × 2 weeks	13 children aged 3–10 who had at least 25% symptom reduction on elimination diet or were borderline responders	Double-blind, crossover challenge	Worse parent-rated behavioral symptoms 3 hours after challenge
Harley, Matthews, et al., 1978	Random assignment to Kaiser Permanente diet or control diet for 3–4 weeks; crossover to the other arm for 3–4 weeks	36 boys aged 6–12 and 10 boys aged 3–5 with hyperkinetic disorder	Double-blind, crossover challenge	No improvement in behavioral observations or neuropsychological tests; some improvement on parent ratings; no improvement on teacher ratings
Harley, Ray, et al., 1978	Entire family on elimination diet for 4 weeks; crossover challenges with active cookies and candy bars (50% adult RDA of FDA-approved artificial colors) or placebo for 9 weeks	9 boys who were responsive to elimination diet	Double-blind, placebo controlled, crossover challenge	No significant difference on any of the ratings (behavioral observations, parent and teacher measures, neuropsychological measures)
Levy et al., 1978	Elimination diet for 4 weeks, followed by challenge with five tartrazine cookies or placebo for 2 weeks, then crossover for 2 weeks, then washout elimination diet for 4 weeks	22 children aged 4–8 diagnosed with hyperactivity	Double-blind, placebo-controlled, crossover challenge	Improved parent behavior ratings for the first 4 weeks on elimination diet; no differences on parent or teacher ratings or neuropsychological testing between challenge and placebo
Levy & Hobbes, 1978	Elimination diet for 4 weeks, followed by challenge with five tartrazine cookies or placebo for 2 weeks, then crossover for 2 weeks, then washout elimination diet for 4 weeks	8 children aged 4–8	Double-blind, placebo-controlled, crossover challenge	No significant differences
Williams & Cram, 1978	Modified Feingold diet for 5 weeks Randomization to one of following Tx: stimulants with challenge cookies (with mixture of colorings), stimulants with control chocolate cookies, placebo with control cookies, placebo with challenge cookies Crossover to next arm until all four arms completed	26 children aged 6–14 diagnosed with hyperactivity who had responded to at least 3 months of stimulant therapy	Double-blind, placebo-controlled, crossover challenge	Improved teacher and parent ratings on stimulant phases; mixed scores with challenge cookies

(cont.)

Table 25.3 (cont.)

Author	Type of dietary intervention	Sample (N, Dx, age)	Design	Results
Swanson & Kinsbourne, 1980	Feingold diet × 3 days; capsules of nine food dyes vs. placebo sugar, one daily for 3 days	40 children aged 6–12; 20 had had good response to stimulants and 20 had had no response to stimulants	Double-blind, placebo-controlled challenge	No difference in ratings between dye and placebo; more errors during neuropsychological testing 2–3 hours after challenge
Weiss et al., 1980	Elimination diet; challenge drink (seven colors and cranberry coloring) vs. placebo, once daily for 77 days (one challenge drink on 8 separate days randomly during study period)	22 children aged 2.5–7	Double-blind, placebo-controlled, repeated crossover challenge	No difference in ratings 3.5 and 24 hours after challenge drink
Mattes & Gittelman, 1981	Feingold diet Randomized to challenge (13 mg mixture of all FDA-approved food colorings) vs. placebo cookies for 1 week, then crossover and 1 week washout in between	11 children aged 4–12 maintained on Feingold diet whose symptoms worsened consistently when exposed to artificial food colorings	Double-blind, placebo-controlled, crossover challenge	No significant changes on challenge vs. placebo on any of the ratings
Egger et al., 1985	4 weeks of oligoantigenic diet; double-blind, placebo-controlled crossover gradual reintroduction of excluded foods to responders	76 children with hyperactivity; only 28 completed the entire study	Open double trial followed by double-blind placebo-controlled, crossover challenge in 28 of the children who had improved the most in the 4 weeks of oligoantigenic diet	62 of 76 improved with oligoantigenic diet; improved parent ratings with placebo
David, 1987	Additive elimination diet Tartrazine challenges – 50 mg followed by 250 mg tartrazine 2 hours later – or challenge with benzoic acid (same doses as tartrazine)	24 children aged 1–12	Double-blind, placebo-controlled challenge trial	No changes on ratings on challenge versus placebo
Rowe, 1988	Feingold diet for 6 weeks; gradual transition to regular diet over next 3–6 months; challenge with carmoisine 50 mg or tartrazine 50 mg or placebo (lactose) capsules once daily for 1 week at a time for a total of 2 weeks	55 children aged 3–15	Double-blind, placebo-controlled crossover challenge trial	40/55 improved on parent ratings; 26/40 remained improved after stopping Feingold diet; 14/55 had difficulties when reintroducing the regular diet; 2/9 showed changes on ratings following challenge
Wilson & Scott, 1989	Additive-free diet Randomized to one of three arms: control drink/control drink plus tartrazine and sunset yellow/ control drink plus sodium metabisulphite and sodium benzoate	29 children aged 2–13	Double-blind, placebo-controlled challenge	6/19 had no difference in symptoms; 13/19 repeated trial and only 6/13 had no significant changes with challenge drinks; 3/13 showed worse symptoms following challenge drinks

Table 25.3 (cont.)

Author	Type of dietary intervention	Sample (N, Dx, age)	Design	Results
Kaplan et al., 1989	3 weeks of baseline diet (regular food as prepared by families); 3 weeks of equivalent diet (same nutrients as baseline diet, but prepared by hospital kitchen); and 4 weeks of Alberta Children's Hospital diet (all food dyes, food flavors, preservatives, monosodium glutamate, chocolate, and caffeine were eliminated and the amount of simple sugars was decreased); for 15 children other foods they were sensitive to were eliminated (such as milk and dairy products)	24 children diagnosed with hyperactivity aged 3.5–6	Double-blind placebo-controlled; only the data from the last 2 weeks were included in the data analyses	More than half of the subjects had significant improvement in behavioral ratings on the experimental diet; night awakenings and latency to sleep onset also improved
Pollock & Warner, 1990	Additive-free diet maintained; challenge with food color capsules (tartrazine, sunset yellow, carmoisine, amaranth) daily during 2 separate weeks; placebo capsules for 3 weeks in between	39 children aged 2–15 recruited from pediatric allergy clinic	Double-blind, placebo-controlled challenge	Significant increase (worsening) in parent ratings during challenge weeks
Egger et al., 1992	4 weeks of oligoantigenic diet; reintroduction of foods; three intradermal injections of betaglucuronidase and mixed food additives and antigens, each 2 months apart versus placebo; reintroduction of provoking foods	185 children with *DSM-III-R* hyperkinetic syndrome; 40 children who responded to oligoantigenic diet continued with phases 3 and 4 (enzyme-potentiated desensitization)	Double-blind, placebo-controlled trial of enzyme-potentiated desensitization; 4 phases	116 responders to oligoantigenic diet; 15/20 children on enzyme-potentiated desensitization (EPD) diet and 7/20 on placebo tolerated the reintroduction of provoking foods; 16/20 children on EPD and 4/20 placebo reported improvement at end of trial
Carter et al., 1993	Oligoantigenic diet for 3–4 weeks followed by open reintroduction of additives, then placebo controlled double blind challenge protocol	78 children with *DSM-III* ADHD	Open diet, then open challenge, then crossover, double-blind placebo-controlled challenge	59/78 had improved parent ratings; 47 responders completed open reintroduction of provoking foods and additives; 19 responders completed crossover trial; 14/19 showed worse behavioral ratings after reintroduction of additives
Schmidt et al., 1997	9 days each of oligoantigenic diet (OAD) and control diet (common foods with similar appearance). Random assignment to order, with assessment at days 3 and 8 for each diet; then 3 days washout and reassessment; 37 of 49 children treated with methylphenidate (MPH)	49 children age 6–12 with *DSM-III-R* ADHD	Crossover, double-blind placebo-controlled randomized trial	12/49 responded to (OAD); 2/49 worsened with OAD; 16/36 responded to MPH compared to control diet; 4/36 worsened with MPH; 8/36 responded to OAD compared to MPH

(cont.)

Table 25.3 (cont.)

Author	Type of dietary intervention	Sample (N, Dx, age)	Design	Results
Dengate & Ruben, 2002	Open phase elimination diet for 3 weeks; then challenge with bread containing maximum dose calcium propionate versus preservative-free bread (four slices daily for 3 days with crossover the following week)	Open phase: 56 children aged 4–12 Crossover challenge: 27/33 of those completing open phase	Double-blind, placebo-controlled challenge crossover trial	Improved scores with elimination diet; 14/27 had worse rating with challenge compared to placebo; 8/27 had no changes with challenge; 5/27 improved with challenge
Bateman et al., 2004	Diet free of artificial colorings and sodium benzoate during the study; challenge with 300 cc fruit juice with 20-mg artificial colorings (sunset yellow, tartrazine, carmoisine, ponceau) versus placebo fruit juice daily for one week during second and fourth weeks of study	397 three-year-olds, both ADHD and normal	Double-blind, placebo-controlled crossover challenge trial	No significant changes in performance on neuropsychological tests in challenge versus placebo weeks; significant increase in parent hyperactivity ratings during challenge periods No significant difference by ADHD Dx vs. not

processes. Homeopaths also prescribe it to improve memory, concentration, and attention and it has been recommended in the treatment of ADHD (Anderson & Peiper, 1996; Bell & Peiper, 1997; Greenblatt, 1999). Unfortunately, the data supporting its effectiveness in ADHD are anecdotal at best. If ever found effective in controlled studies, it should apply as well to adults as children.

Hypericum (St. John's wort) may be especially worth investigating for adults. It is used in Europe anecdotally for treating ADHD without the benefit of supporting research. Some European studies for depression found it more effective than placebo, and because most standard prescription antidepressants also help in ADHD, especially in adults, we might well expect Hypericum to benefit patients with comorbid ADHD and mild depression. Hypericum is not standard treatment at this time, but merits controlled study in adult ADHD; if used, it requires caution regarding sun exposure. There are also several case reports of improvement in ADHD symptoms with Vitex (vitex agnus castus; Hueneke, 2004), but this herb must be considered investigational.

Important caution: Herbs, if they work, are crude drugs and can carry the same risks as refined prescription drugs, including interactions with other herbs and drugs. Physicians should ask about herb use before prescribing medication for ADHD, and if the physician does not ask, the adult with ADHD should volunteer any such use and ask about possible interactions.

EEG biofeedback (neurofeedback)

Electroencephalographic (EEG) biofeedback involves induction of sensorimotor (12–15 Hertz) or higher (15–18 Hertz) beta band EEG rhythms and suppression of theta rhythms by visual and auditory feedback (see Chapter 24). The theory is based on data showing that many patients with ADHD have more slow-wave (especially theta, 3.5–8 Hertz) power in their EEG spectral analysis than normal controls and conversely less beta (12–20 Hz) power (Monastra et al., 2002, 2005). The lower beta frequencies (12–15 Hertz) are associated with calm immobility in experimental animals and are called sensorimotor rhythm (SMR). The higher beta frequencies (>15 Hz) are associated with focusing on a task or other situations requiring attention.

During tasks that require focused attention and sustained mental effort, increased arousal, evidenced by higher beta (16–20 Hz and higher), is noted over prefrontal, frontal, and central midline regions. Positron emission tomography (PET) and single photon emission computed tomography (SPECT) in patients with ADHD have noted lower blood flow/metabolism suggesting underarousal in these regions, and this underarousal is evident in EEG studies. Many patients with ADHD have more slow-wave (theta) activity in these regions than normal controls and conversely less beta power (Monastra, 2002, 2005). Theoretically, this slow-wave activity or underarousal

Table 25.4 Controlled studies of EEG biofeedback (neurofeedback) in ADHD

Study	Results
Rossiter & La Vaque, 1995 (comparison of EEG biofeedback vs. stimulant)	Improvement on TOVA, CPT, and parent BASC compared with baseline by both treatments. No significant difference; uninterpretable.
Linden et al., 1996 (randomized controlled trial of EEG biofeedback vs. wait list control)	Improvement on K-BIT IQ composite and parent Conners rating greater than wait list
Carmody, 2001 (clinical trial of EEG biofeedback vs. wait list controls)	Decreased impulsivity on TOVA; improved teacher ADDES ratings of impulsivity compared to controls
Monastra et al., 2002 (clinical trials of comprehensive clinical care, CCC vs. CCC plus EEG biofeedback). Self-selected, not randomized.	Sustained improvement on TOVA and ADDES without stimulant 1 year after biofeedback training
Fuchs et al., 2003 (clinical trial of neurofeedback vs. MPH)	Improvement on TOVA and Conners with both treatments. No significant difference between groups; uninterpretable.
Heywood & Beale, 2003 (placebo-controlled crossover trial)	No significant differences compared to placebo
Greco, 2004 (randomized, single-blind controlled clinical trial)	Significant improvement by Conners parent rating scale compared to placebo
deBeus et al., 2006 (double-blind, crossover design)	Significant improvement in symptoms during biofeedback, not placebo
Beauregard & Levesque, 2006 (randomized trial, controlled against a wait list group)	Significant improvement in symptoms of inattention and hyperactivity; increased activation of right anterior cingulate cortex during selective tasks on fMRI

Abbreviations used: ADDES = Attention Deficit Disorders Evaluation Scale; BASC = Behavior Assessment System for Children; CPT = Continuous Performance Test; K-BIT = Kaufman Brief Intelligence test; TOVA =Test of Variables of Attention; CCC = Comprehensive Clinical Care; MPH = Methylphenidate; fMRI = functional MRI.

is associated with the core ADHD symptoms of inattention, hyperactivity, and impulsivity. Neurophysiologists have examined whether laboratory animals and humans could learn to increase SMR to reduce hyperactivity and enhance beta while suppressing theta to diminish inattention. This learned control of cortical frequencies has formed the theoretical and clinical application of neurofeedback (EEG biofeedback) in the treatment of ADHD.

A combination of videogame feedback with EEG monitoring is based on technology used by NASA astronauts and US Air Force pilots to improve their ability to stay attentive in the cockpit. A strap helmet with EEG sensors monitors brainwaves and provides real-time feedback to the videogame controls, modifying the ability to control speed, steering, and other elements needed to score in the videogame (deBeus et al., 2006). Several studies (see Table 25.4) found encouraging evidence and should be replicated to confirm neurofeedback's effectiveness. The data for neurofeedback look promising and it appears safe, but this expensive treatment still lacks a convincing published well-controlled double-blind study to justify the expense and effort involved. So far the studies have been done with children, but when it is adequately proven, it should apply as well to adults as children, given the fact that adults respond well to biofeedback in other domains and disorders.

Channel-specific perceptual training

In a single-blind prevention paradigm, Arnold et al. (1977) randomly assigned matched trios and quads of first graders selected for vulnerability on a perceptual screening battery to either 6 months of channel-specific perceptual training (n = 23), 6 months of regular academic tutoring (n = 23), or no-contact control (n = 40); at 1-year follow-up, the trained group surpassed both control groups in blinded teacher Conners ratings (ES = 1.0, $p < 0.01$), Wide Range Achievement Test (WRAT) reading achievement (12.6 standard points difference, $p < 0.01$), and Wechsler IQ (8 points difference, $p < 0.05$), though baseline measures were not different. The sample was not selected for having ADHD, and it is not clear whether what seemed to work for prevention in early development would work as treatment later on, after symptoms are fully developed.

Vestibular stimulation

Previc (1993) has suggested that the utricles/otoliths produce noradrenergic sympathetic brain stimulation, whereas the semicircular canals produce cholinergic parasympathetic brain stimulation. In a case report (Bhatara et al., 1978) a 5-year-old boy demonstrated improvement in symptoms of hyperkinetic behavior after a 4-week regime of controlled semicircular canal stimulation. It was postulated that the behavioral improvement resulted from an increase in task-relevant arousal in the reticular formation, accompanied by increased cortical inhibition. In a subsequent study (Bhatara et al., 1981) 18 hyperkinetic children were treated with eyes-open rotational vestibular stimulation. After eight sessions of rotational stimulation over a 4-week period they scored better on teacher ratings than after eight control sessions. In a single-blind crossover study with 12 children identified through teacher scale screening, Arnold et al. (1985) found an ES of 0.5 between vestibular rotational stimulation alone and two control conditions (missing significance at the sample size), compared to an ES of 0.2 between visual rotational stimulation alone and the same control conditions in a similar group of 18 children (randomized from the same sample).

An open trial of the comprehensive motion apparatus (CMA), which provides motion stimulation to otoliths and somewhat to semicircular canals, in 14 dyslexic children (mean age,12 + 2.6 yr.) showed pre-post improvement in parent rating of attention (ES = 1.5, $p < 0.003$) and objective cognitive/achievement tests (ES = 0.4–1.2, $p = 0.05 - 0.001$; Ferrara et al., 1999; Stillman, 1998, personal communication). However, a controlled trial of the CMA in children with diagnosed ADHD failed to find a difference from placebo in ADHD symptoms for combined-type ADHD without learning disorder. It is not clear whether the CMA could be useful for those with inattentive-type ADHD or those with comorbid learning disorder.

Other perceptual stimulation/training

The Interactive Metronome (Koomar et al., 2001) provides perceptual-motor concentration training with biofeedback about accuracy from motion sensors as the child taps to the beat provided by the program; open trials showed improvements in timing that correlate at 0.2–0.4 with teacher ratings of attention. In a three-group randomized trial (Shaffer et al., 2001), 56 boys aged 6–12 with ADHD were randomly assigned to the Interactive Metronome, videogames, or no intervention. Of 58 pre–post measures, the metronome group improved on 53, the videogame group on 40, and the no-intervention group on 28. The pattern was statistically significant. If confirmed by peer-reviewed replication, this treatment would probably be more effective in children than in adults.

In general, although stimulation and training of specific perceptual channels merit further research in controlled trials, especially targeting subgroups that test for deficiencies in the particular perceptual modality, they are not as likely to help adults as children, given their developmental focus and the preliminary data suggestion of greater benefit at younger ages.

Massage

Massage's effects on well-being are well known. Several studies have found it confers a significant improvement in mood and ADHD symptoms in children and adolescents. In a massage trial directly targeting ADHD, Field et al. (1998) randomly assigned 28 adolescent boys with *DSM-III-R* ADHD to ten 15-minute sessions of either massage or relaxation therapy (on consecutive school days). Massage consisted of 30 10-second moderate-pressure back-and-forth strokes in each of three body regions: neck, from neck to shoulders and back, and the thoracolumbar vertebral column. The control relaxation training condition targeted the same three body regions. After the 10 sessions, teachers rated the massaged group as showing less hyperactivity and spending more time on task than the relaxation group (77% vs. 51%, compared to 43% and 40% at baseline). On the Conners 10-item scale, the massaged boys improved from 28 at baseline to 11.3, whereas the controls deteriorated from 19.6 to 28.5. The massaged adolescents also rated themselves happier after the sessions (Field et al., 1998). In another study (Khilnani et al., 2003) 30 students between ages 7 and 18 were randomly assigned to a massage group or a wait list control group, with the massage group receiving massage therapy for 20 minutes twice a week for a month. The students who received massage therapy showed improved short-term mood state and longer term improvement in classroom behavior. This treatment shows promise in view of its safety and inexpensive application by trained family members. If confirmed by larger controlled trials, it is likely to be as effective in adults as in children, although no controlled adult study was found.

Acupuncture

There are no published systematic data in ADHD. Loo (1998), in unpublished preliminary pre–post single-blind data from students in grades K–3, found improvements in Conners 10-item scores by teachers (n = 7) from 17.0 to 12.0 and in analogous parent scores (n = 6) from 23.1 to 15.5. She noted that children with the most severe ADHD could not cooperate with the treatment. Presumably, adults with ADHD would be better able to cooperate, regardless of the severity of disorder, so this treatment, if shown effective in double-blind controlled trials, may be more applicable to adults than to children.

Yoga

Yoga has gained in popularity in recent years because of its perceived benefits in reducing stress and improving concentration. One open study reported that children who participated in yoga training regularly showed a significant improvement in emotional and behavioral problems (Jensen & Kenny, 2004). If these findings are confirmed by well-designed controlled studies, this treatment would seem at least as applicable to adults as to children.

Tai chi

Tai chi is a Chinese martial art of slow-moving exercise that in one open study significantly improved ADHD symptoms, mood, and anxiety in 13 adolescents with a diagnosis of ADHD (Hernandez-Reif, Field, & Thimas, 2001). This should have been a controlled study and, if upheld by peer-reviewed evidence, might apply as well to adults as to children.

Meditation

Kratter (1983) randomly assigned 24 children aged 7–12 with *DSM-III* ADD-H to either meditation training or progressive relaxation with 4 weeks of twice-weekly sessions or a wait list control group. Both active treatments but not being on the wait list reduced impulsivity and improved scores on parent behavior scales, but not teacher scales; only meditation training showed significant improvement on a test assessing selective attention. Moretti-Altuna (1987) randomly assigned 23 boys aged 6–12 with ADD-H to meditation

training, medication, or standard therapy; meditation showed significant advantage in classroom behavior, but not in parent ratings or psychological tests. Thus meditation warrants further study for both children and adults. It should theoretically be as good (or better) for adults as for children.

EMG biofeedback, relaxation training, and hypnosis

These three related treatment modalities are typically used in some combination. The few published data on hypnotherapy alone for ADHD are discouraging: for example, Calhoun and Bolton (1986) were unsuccessful in three attempts to hypnotize 10 of the 11 hyperactive children they tried it with. Possibly adults with ADHD would be better able to cooperate with hypnosis, and an adult pilot study may be worth a try. Breathing control alone, used not only in hypnosis but also in meditation and relaxation, showed no difference from sham training in six hyperactive, intelligent 6–8-year-olds (Simpson & Nelson, 1974). However, the hypnotic techniques of imagery and progressive relaxation have often been incorporated into successful EMG biofeedback protocols. EMG biofeedback-facilitated relaxation training merits further study for patients with ADHD who do not benefit from stimulants or who object to them. Though trials in adults were not found, it should theoretically work as well in adults as in children.

Mirror feedback

Mirrors have been proposed as a way of increasing self-control and attentional focus by increasing self-focus in children with ADHD (Zentall, Hall, & Lee, 1998). In a single-blind randomized trial in 16 hyperactive-inattentive (HI) and 27 normal middle school students, a word puzzle that differentiated the HI from the control subjects with an effect size of 0.75 ($p < 0.05$) in the no-mirror condition showed a between-groups ES of only 0.2 (n.s.) with a mirror in front of the child as he or she worked. The mirror condition improved the performance of the HI children by half the no-mirror difference between groups. With no instruction about the mirror, the HI children who actually looked in the mirror scored equal to the no-mirror scores of the controls. This intervention carries a risk associated with diagnostic validity: the normal controls showed a trend of performance decrement with the mirror, especially if they looked in it (Zentall et al., 1998). This intervention may have more possibilities for adults than for children. Though not easily applicable to a regular classroom, it may be useful for adults with ADHD who work at desk jobs in cubicles or in individual offices and deserves further trials in that application.

Green outdoor settings

Environmental psychology literature suggests that exposure to natural environments may improve cognitive functioning. One uncontrolled survey study looked at the benefits of exposure to natural green outdoor settings in children with ADHD and found significant improvement in symptoms following time spent outside in natural environments (Kuo & Taylor 2004). The study has been criticized for several reasons, including a heterogeneous sample, lack of independent validation of the ADHD diagnosis, and lack of a comparison group. If it were proven valid, this intervention could probably be applied to adults. Even if it provided only placebo benefit, however, there seems little risk in it. In view of its safety, low expense, and ease of implementation, it probably does not need to meet a high standard of proof: a walk in the park on the way to work might be good for the soul even if it does not help ADHD.

Immune therapy

Food-borne allergy may not be the only immunological consideration for etiological subgroups of ADHD. In 50 children (mean age 9) with pediatric autoimmune neuropsychiatric disorders associated with streptococcal group A beta-hemolytic infection (PANDAS), Swedo et al. (1998) found a 40% rate of ADHD. It is not clear what proportion of an unselected ADHD sample would have PANDAS. However, Hagerman and Falkenstein (1987) reported twice the rate of otitis media in hyperactive children compared to controls, suggesting either immune problems or greater exposure to infectious agents. Perlmutter et al. (1999) tried two kinds of immune therapy in 30 children with PANDAS in a placebo-controlled parallel design, with 10 randomly assigned to each condition. Obsessive-compulsive symptoms improved impressively with either plasma exchange or intravenous immunoglobulin; tics also improved with plasma exchange. Unfortunately, Perlmutter et al. (1999) did not report the effect on ADHD symptoms.

Immunological therapy targeting Candida (Palacios, 1976, 1977) might be a logical alternative to the antifungal therapy discussed later, but apparently has not been proposed for ADHD. For food sensitivities, Egger et al. (1992) have reported significant ($p < 0.001$) benefit from enzyme-potentiated desensitization in a double-blind, placebo-controlled trial. Immune therapy, if shown effective for ADHD, should have some application to adults, because immune dysfunctions can persist through adulthood.

Antifungal treatment

Treatment with antifungal agents such as nystatin (in combination with sugar restriction and other measures) was advocated by Crook (1985, 1989, 1991) and others based on the hypothesis that repeated antibiotic use for otitis media changes intestinal flora, allowing yeast overgrowth, which compromises immune function and changes the gut mucosal barrier to allow absorption of food antigens. Several components of this hypothesis are supported by collateral documentation from other fields (e.g. Hagerman & Falkenstein, 1987; Nsouli et al., 1994; Vargas et al., 1993). This hypothesis, though, is not supported by any systematic prospective trial data in ADHD. A trial of nystatin alone for fatigue, premenstrual tension, gastrointestinal symptoms, and depression associated with Candida vaginitis had negative results (Dismukes et al., 1990). A systematic randomly assigned trial in ADHD should be carried out; preferably it should be a double-blind, placebo-controlled trial accompanied by sugar restriction and other supportive measures recommended by the advocates of this treatment. If found effective, it should theoretically work as well in adults as in children, provided they are selected for recent antibiotic use, fungal metabolites, or other risk factors.

Thyroid treatment

Some studies have found a rate of thyroid dysfunction in ADHD ranging from 2–5% (Valentine et al., 1997; Weiss et al., 1993), and the rate may be higher in those with comorbid mood disorder (West et al., 1996). In children and adults with thyroid dysfunction, thyroid status seems to be related to attentional and hyperactive-impulsive symptoms (Hauser et al., 1997; Rovet & Alvarez, 1996). In a double-blind, placebo-controlled, crossover trial of thyroid supplementation, only one of nine children with ADHD and normal thyroid function improved compared to five of eight with ADHD and resistance to thyroid hormone (Weiss & Stein, 2000). The original report of improvement in ADHD from treatment of thyroid hormone resistance included adults with ADHD and resistance to thyroid hormone (Hauser et al., 1997). Thus thyroid treatment does not seem promising in ADHD patients with normal thyroid function, but would seem to be the treatment of choice for those with thyroid dysfunction. Therefore all patients with ADHD should be screened for historical and physical exam signs of possible thyroid dysfunction (Weiss & Stein, 2000). This possibility is at least as relevant for adults as for children with ADHD.

Approach to selecting treatment

The best approach to treatment should start with a good history and physical exam that will check for signs of thyroid dysfunction; a history of allergies, dietary balance/deficiency, and lead or other heavy metal exposure; and general medical problems. As indicated by the history and physical, a complete blood count and electrolytes are desirable as a general screen and to pick up mineral deficiencies. In areas with high rates of subclinical lead poisoning or when there is a history of recent lead exposure, a serum lead should be done. Although not routine at this point, more complete screening for all minerals (e.g., iron, zinc) could be justified if there is any question from the dietary history and especially for menstruating girls or women with ADHD. Because alternative treatments are mostly targeted to specific etiologies, it would be reasonable to consider implementing them first (rather than alternatively) *when etiologies amenable to specific treatment are diagnosed*. After ruling out such etiologies one could implement the standard generic treatments (psychotropic medication and behavioral treatment) as the main therapeutic thrust. In questionable cases, a therapeutic trial may be indicated.

Recommendations for future research

Future research efforts should (1) mount definitive trials and replications of promising treatments that may have some advantage over the standard treatments if proven effective, (2) mount controlled clinical trials of treatments for which a controlled trial is easy and cheap (Arnold, 1995), (3) mount open pilot trials of well-considered hypotheses for which there are no pilot data and for which a controlled trial would

be expensive or difficult, and (4) define subgroups (characteristics and proportion of diagnosed ADHD patients) appropriate for treatments for which efficacy has been demonstrated in a controlled manner. For all categories, it will be important to emphasize effect sizes to assess the clinical importance.

Practical clinical conclusions

While awaiting further research, the following ideas are compatible with good clinical practice. Apply the "safe, easy, cheap" (SEC) rule to evaluating possible treatments. A treatment that is obviously SEC does not require as much scientific evidence of efficacy to justify trying it as a treatment that is risky, difficult, or expensive. For example, a RDI/RDA multivitamin/mineral tablet, a mirror on the workspace, time in an open green space, meditation, and systematic relaxation appear SEC even though they do not have conclusive evidence of efficacy. Some of them might be good for the individual's general health even if ineffective for ADHD. Remember that delay of established treatment can be a risk in itself. Herbs carry risk and should be treated as crude drugs, with attention to their side effects and interactions.

When any treatment is tried, it is important to establish a baseline assessment (e.g., rating scale by a person familiar with patient) for comparison to later status after the treatment is tried. Try only one new treatment at time, and give it adequate time to determine whether it makes a difference. Many of the alternative and complementary treatments take longer to show effect than FDA-approved medication. A patient who is having good results from any treatment should not lightly abandon it to pursue a novel alternative.

References

Akhonzadeh S, Mohammadi M-R, Khademi, M. (2004). Zinc sulfate as an adjunct to methylphenidate for the treatment of attention deficit hyperactivity disorder in children: a double blind, randomized trial. *BMC Psychiatry* 4(9).

Aman MG, Mitchell EA, Turbott SH. (1987). The effects of essential fatty acid supplementation by Efamol in hyperactive children. *J Abnorm Child Psychol* 15:75–90.

American Psychiatric Association. (2000). *Diagnostic and Statistical Manual of Mental Disorders*. 4th ed. text. rev. Washington, DC: American Psychiatric Association.

Anderson N, Peiper H. (1996). *ADD: The Natural Approach*. East Canaan, CT: Safe Goods.

Arduini A, Denisova N, Virmani A, Avrova N, Federici G, Arrigoni-Martelli E. (1994). Evidence for the involvement of carnitine-dependent long-chain acyltransferases in neuronal triglyceride and phospholipid fatty acid turnover. *J Neurochem* 62:1530–8.

Arnold LE. (1995). Some nontraditional (unconventional and/or innovative) psychosocial treatments for children and adolescents: critique and proposed screening principles. *J Abnormal Child Psychol* 23(1): 125–40.

Arnold LE, Barnebey N, McManus J, Smeltzer D, Conrad A, Winer G, Desgranges L. (1977). Prevention by specific perceptual remediation for vulnerable first–graders: controlled study and follow–up of lasting effects. *Arch Gen Psychiatry* 34:1279–94.

Arnold LE, Bozzolo H, Amato A, Holloway J, Cook A, Ramadan Y, et al. (2007). Acetyl-l-carnitine (ALC) in attention-deficit/hyperactivity disorder (ADHD): a multi-site placebo-controlled pilot trial. *J Child Adolesc Psychopharmacol* 17(6):791–801. 2007.

Arnold LE, Clark DL, Sachs LA, Jakim S, Smithies C. (1985). Vestibular & visual rotational stimulation as treatment for attention deficit and hyperactivity. *Am J Occup Ther* 39(2):84–9l.

Arnold LE, Kleykamp D, Votolato NA, Taylor WA, Kontras SB, Tobin K. (1989). Gamma-linolenic acid for attention-deficit hyperactivity disorder: placebo-controlled comparison to D-amphetamine. *Biol Psychiatry* 25:222–8.

Arnold LE, Pinkham SM, Votolato N. (2000). Does zinc moderate essential fatty acid and amphetamine treatment of attention-deficit/hyperactivity disorder? *J Child Adolesc Psychopharmacol* 10(2):111–17.

Baker GB, Bornstein RA, Rouget AC, Therrien S, van Muyden J. (1991). Phenylethylaminergic mechanisms in attention-deficit disorder. *Biol Psychiatry* 29:15–22.

Bateman B, Warner JO, Hutchinson E, et al. (2004). The effects of a double blind, placebo controlled, artificial food colourings and benzoate preservative challenge on hyperactivity in a general population sample of preschool children. *Arch Dis Child* 89:506–11.

Beauregard M, Lévesque J. (2006). Functional magnetic resonance imaging investigation of the effects of neurofeedback training on the neural bases of selective attention and response inhibition in children with attention-deficit/hyperactivity disorder. *Appl Psychophysiol Biofeedback* 31(1):3–20.

Bell R, Peiper H. (1997). *The ADD and ADHD Diet*. East Canaan, CT: Safe Goods.

Bellgrove MA, Domschle K, Hawi Z, Kirley A, Mullins C, Robertson IH, Gill M. (2005). The methionine allele of the COMT polymorphism impairs prefrontal cognition in children and adolescents with ADHD. *Exp Brain Res* 163:352–60.

Benton D, Cook R. (1991). Vitamin and mineral supplements improve the intelligence scores and concentration of six-year-old children. *Pers Individ Diff* 12:1151–8.

Bhatara V, Clark DL, Arnold LE. (1978). Behavioral and nystagmus response of a hyperkinetic child to vestibular stimulation. *Am J Occup Ther* 32(5):311–16.

Bhatara V, Clark DL, Arnold LE, Gunsett R, Smeltzer DJ. (1981). Hyperkinesis treated by vestibular stimulation: an exploratory study. *Biol Psychiatry* 16(3): 269–79.

Bilici M, Yildirim F, Kandil S, Bekaroglu M, Yildirmis S, Deger O, et al. (2004). Double blind, placebo controlled study of zinc sulfate in the treatment of attention deficit hyperactivity disorder. *Prog Neuropsychopharmacol Biol Psychiatry* 28:181–90.

Bornstein RA, Baker GB, Carroll A, King G, Wong JT, Douglass AB. (1990). Plasma amino acids in attention deficit disorder. *Psychiatry Res* 33:301–6.

Brenner A. (1982). The effects of megadoses of selected B complex vitamins on children with hyperkinesis; controlled studies with long-term follow-up. *J Learn Disabil* 15:258–64.

Bruner AB, Joffe A, Duggan AK, Casella F, Brandt J. (1996). Randomized study of cognitive effects of iron supplementation in non-anemic iron-deficient girls. *Lancet* 347:992–6.

Burattini MG, Amendola F, Aufierio T, Spano M, Di Bitonto G, Del Vecchio GC, De Mattia D. (1990). Evaluation of the effectiveness of gastro-protected proteoferrin in the therapy of sideropenic anemia in childhood. *Minerva Pediatr* 42:343–7.

Calhoun G, Jr, Bolton JA (1986). Hypnotherapy: a possible alternative for treating pupils affected with attention deficit disorder. *Percept Mot Skills* 63:1191–5.

Carmody D. (2001). EEG biofeedback training and ADHD in an elementary school setting. *J Neurother* 4: 5–27.

Carter CM, Urbanowicz M, Hemsley R, et al. (1993). Effects of a few food diet in attention deficit disorder. *Arch Dis Child* 69:564–8.

Coleman M, Steinberg G, Tippett J, Bhagavan HN, Coursin DB, Gross M, Lewis C, DeVeau L. (1979). A preliminary study of the effect of pyridoxine administration in a subgroup of hyperkinetic children: a double-blind crossover comparison with methylphenidate. *Biol Psychiatry* 14:741–51.

Conners C, Goyette C, Southwick D, et al. (1976). Food additives and hyperkinesis: a controlled double-blind experiment. *Pediatrics* 58:154–66.

Crook WG. (1985). Pediatricians, antibiotics, and office practice. *Pediatrics* **76**(1).

Crook WG. (1989). *The Yeast Connection*. 3rd ed. Jackson, TN: Professional Books.

Crook WG. (1991). A controlled trial of nystatin for the candidiasis hypersensitivity syndrome [letter]. *New Engl J Med* **324**(22):1592-4.

David OJ, Hoffman SP, Clark J, Grad G, Sverd J. (1983). The relationship of hyperactivity to moderately elevated lead levels. *Arch Environ Health* **38**(6):341-6.

David OJ, Hoffman SP, Sverd J, Clark L, Voeller K. (1976). Lead and hyperactivity. Behavioral response to chelation: a pilot study. *Am J Psychiatry* **133**(10):1155-8.

David TJ. (1987). Reactions to dietary tartrazine. *Arch Dis Child* **62**:119-22.

Dean J, Morgenthaler J. (1990). *DMAE. Smart Drugs and Nutrients*. Menlo Park, CA: Health Freedom Publications.

deBeus R, Ball JD, et al. Progress in efficacy studies of EEG biofeedback for ADHD. Paper presented at: Annual Meeting of American Psychiatric Association; May 2006; Toronto.

DeFrance JF, Hymel C, Trachtenberg MC, Ginsberg LD, Schweitzer FC, Estes S, et al. (1997). Enhancement of attention processing by Kantroll in healthy humans: a pilot study. *Clin EEG* **28**:68-75.

Dengate S, Ruben A. (2002). Controlled trial of cumulative behavioural effects of a common bread preservative. *J Paediatr Child Health* **38**:373-6.

Dismukes WE, Wade JS, Lee Jy, Dockery BK, Hain JD. (1990). A randomized double-blind trial of nystatin therapy for the candidiasis hypersensitivity syndrome. *New Engl J Med* **323**:1717-23.

Dykman KD, Dykman RA. (1998). Effect of nutritional supplements on attentional-deficit hyperactivity disorder. *Integr Physiol Behav Sci* **33**:49-60.

Dykman, KD, McKinley R. (1997). Effect of glyconutritionals on the severity of ADHD. *Proc Fisher Inst Med Res* **1**(1):24-5.

Egger J, Carter CM, Graham PJ, et al. (1985). Controlled trial of oligoantigenic treatment in the hyperkinetic syndrome. *Lancet* **1**:540-5.

Egger J, Stolla A, McEwen LM. (1992). Controlled trial of hyposensitisation in children with food-induced hyperkinetic syndrome. *Lancet* **339**:1150-3.

Ferrara M, Davis R, Taylor S, Daniel L, Treloar J, Peterson C. (1999). The use of continuous automated passive motion on improving the symptoms of developmental dyslexia in children. Paper presented at: 12th International Symposium of Adapted Physical Activity; Barcelona.

Field TM, Quintino O, Hernandez-Reif M, et al. (1998). Adolescents with attention deficit hyperactivity disorder benefit from massage therapy. *Adolescence* **33**:103-8.

Frei H, Thurneysen A. (2001). Treatment for hyperactive children: homeopathy and methylphenidate compared in a family setting. *Br Homeopath J* **90**:183-8.

Fuchs T, Birbaumer N, Lutzenberger W, et al. (2003). Neurofeedback treatment for attention-deficit/hyperactivity disorder in children: a comparison with methylphenidate. *Appl Psychophysiol Biofeedback* **28**:1-12.

Goyette GH, Connors CK, Petti TA, et al. (1978). Effects of artificial colors on hyperkinetic children: a double-blind challenge study [proceedings]. *Psychopharmacol Bull* **14**:39-40.

Greco D. (2004). A randomized, double-blind clinical trial of EEG neurofeedback treatment for attention-deficit/hyperactivity disorder. Paper presented at: Annual Meeting of the International Society for Neuronal Regulation; August 2004; Fort Lauderdale, FL.

Greenblatt J. (1999). Nutritional supplements in ADHD [letter]. *J Am Acad Child Adolesc Psychiatry* **38**(10):1209-10.

Hagerman RJ, Falkenstein AR. (1987). An association between recurrent otitis media in infancy and hyperactivity. *Clin Pediatr* **26**:253-7.

Harley J, Matthews C, Eichman P. (1978). Synthetic food colors and hyperactivity in children: A double-blind challenge experiment. *Pediatrics* **62**:975-83.

Harley J, Ray R, Tomasi L, et al. (1978). Hyperkinesis and food additives: testing the Feingold hypothesis. *Pediatrics* **61**:818-8.

Hauser P, Soler R, Brucker-Davis F, Weintraub BD. (1997). Thyroid hormones correlate with symptoms of hyperactivity but not inattention in ADHD. *Psychoneuroendocrinology* **22**:107-14.

Hernandez-Reif M, Field TM, Thimas E. 2001. Attention Deficit Hyperactivity Disorder: benefits from Tai Chi. *J Bodywork Move Ther* **5**(2):120-3.

Heywood C, Beale I. (2003). EEG biofeedback vs. placebo treatment for attention-deficit/hyperactivity disorder: a pilot study. *J Atten Disord* **7**:43-55.

Hirayama S, Hamazaki T, Terasawa K. (2004). Effect of docosahexaenoic acid-containing food administration on symptoms of attention-deficit/hyperactivity disorder: a placebo-controlled double-blind study. *Eur J Clin Nutr* **58**:467-73.

Hueneke P. (2004). Clinical observations on Vitex and ADHD. *J Aust Trad Med Soc* **10**(1): 7-8

Jacobs J, Williams AL, Girard C, Yanchou-Njike V, Katz D. (2005). Homeopathy for Attention Deficit

Hyperactivity Disorder: a pilot randomized–controlled study. *J Altern Complement Med* **11**(5*)*: 799–806.

Jensen PS, Kenny DT. (2004). The effects of yoga on the attention and behavior of boys with attention-deficit/hyperactivity disorder (ADHD). *J Atten Disord* 7:205–16.

Kaplan B, McNicol J, Conte RA, Moghadam HK. (1989). Dietary replacement in preschool aged hyperactive boys. *Pediatrics* **83**(1):7–17.

Khilnani S, Field T, Hernandez-Reif M, et al. (2003). Massage therapy improves mood and behavior of students with attention-deficit/hyperactivity disorder. *Adolescence* 38:623–38.

Konofal E, Cortese S, Lecendreux M. (2006). Effectiveness of iron supplementation in children with ADHD. Symposium presentation at: 53rd Annual Meeting of the American Academy of Child & Adolescent Psychiatry; Oct. 26, 2006.

Konofal E, Lecendreux M, Arnulf I, Mouren MC. (2004). Iron deficiency in children with ADHD. *Arch Pediatr Adolesc Med* **158**(12):1113–5.

Koomar J, Burpee JD, DeJean V, Frick S, Kawar J, Fischer DM. (2001). Theoretical and clinical perspectives on the Interactive Metronome: a view from occupational therapy practice. *Am J Occup Ther* 55(2):163–6.

Kratter J. (1983). The use of meditation in the treatment of attention deficit disorder with hyperactivity. *Dissertation Abstracts International* 44:1965.

Kuo FE, Taylor AF. (2004). A potential natural treatment for attention-deficit/hyperactivity disorder: evidence from a national study. *Am J Clin Nutr* 94:1580–6.

Lands WEM. (1998). Overview and Equatins predicting plasma concentrations from dietary intake: metabolic consequences for prostaglandin, leukotriene, and thromboxane production. Paper presented at: NIH Workshop on Omega-3 Essential Fatty Acids and Psychiatric Disorders; Sept. 2–3, 1998; Bethesda, MD.

Levy F, Dumbrell S, Hobbes G, et al. (1978). Hyperkinesis and diet: a double-blind crossover trial with a tartrazine challenge. *Med J Aust* 1:61–4.

Levy F, Hobbes G. (1978). Hyperkinesis and diet: a replication study. *Am J Psychiatry* 135:1559–60.

Lewis JA, Young R. (1975). Deanol and methylphenidate in minimal brain dysfunction. *Clin Pharmacol Ther* 17:534–40.

Linden M, Habib T, Radojevic V. (1996). A controlled study of the effects of EEG biofeedback on cognition and behavior of children with attention deficit disorder and learning disabilities. *Biofeedback Self Regul* 21:35–49.

Lyon M, Cline J, Zepetnek JT, Shan JJ, Pang P, Benishin C. (2001). Effect of the herbal extract combination Panax quinquefolium and Ginkgo biloba on attention deficit hyperactivity disorder: a pilot study. *J Psychiatry Neurosci* 26(3): 221–8.

Maes M. (1998). Essential fatty acids as determinants of cytokine immunoneuroendocrine interactions in major depression. Paper presented at: NIH Workshop on Omega-3 Essential Fatty Acids and Psychiatric Disorders; Sept. 2–3, 1998; Bethesda, MD.

Mattes JA, Gittelman R. (1981). Effects of artificial food colorings in children with hyperactive symptoms: A critical review and results of a controlled study. *Arch Gen Psychiatry* 38: 714–18.

Monastra VJ, Monastra DM, George S. (2002). The effects of stimulant therapy, EEG biofeedback, and parenting style on the primary symptoms of attention-deficit/hyperactivity disorder. *Appl Psychophysiol Biofeedback* 27: 231–49.

Moretti–Altuna G. (1987). The effects of meditation versus medication in the treatment of Attention Deficit Disorder with Hyperactivity. *Dissertation Abstracts International* 47:4658

Neuringer M. (1998). Overview of omega-3 fatty acids in infant development: visual, cognitive, and behavioral outcomes. Paper presented at: NIH Workshop on Omega-3 Essential Fatty Acids and Psychiatric Disorders; Sept. 2–3; Bethesda, MD.

Nsouli TM, Nsouli SM, Linde RE, O'Mara F, Scanlon RT, Bellanti JA. (1994). Role of food allergy in serous otitis media. *Ann Allergy* 73:215–19.

Oettinger L. (1958). The use of Deanol in the treatment of behavior in children. *J Pediatr* 5:671–5.

Pakes GE. (1978). Death and liquid protein. *Am Pharmacy* 18:4–5.

Palacios HJ. (1976). Hypersensitivity as a cause of dermatologic and vaginal moniliasis resistant to topical therapy. *Ann Allergy* 37:110–13.

Palacios HJ. (1977). Desensitization for monilial hypersensitivity. *Virginia Med J* June:393–5.

Perlmutter SJ, Leitman SF, Garvey MA, Hamburger S, Feldman E, Leonard HL, Swedo SE. (1999). Therapeutic plasma exchange and intravenous immunoglobulin for obsessive-compulsive and tic disorders in childhood. *Lancet* 354(9185):1153–8.

Pollock I, Warner JO. (1990). Effect of artificial food colours on childhood behaviour. *Arch Dis Child* 65:74–7.

Previc FH. (1993). Do the organs of the labyrinth differentially influence the sympathetic and parasympathetic systems? *Neurosci Biobehav Rev* 17:397–404.

Reimherr FW, Wender PH, Wood DR, Ward M. (1987). An open trial of l-tyrosine in the treatment of attention deficit disorder, residual type. *Am J Psychiatry* 144:1071–3.

Ricciolini R, Scalibastri M, Kelleher JK, Carminati P, Calvani M, Arduini A. (1998). Role of acetyl-l-carnitine in rat brain lipogenesis: implications for polyunsaturated fatty acid synthesis. *J Neurochem* 71:2510–7.

Richardson AJ. (2003). Clinical trials of fatty acid supplementation in dyslexia and dyspraxia. In: Glen AIM, Peet M, Horrobin DF, eds. *Phospholipid Spectrum Disorder in Psychiatry and Neurology*. Carnforth: Marius Press: 491–500.

Richardson AJ. (2004). Long chain polyunsaturated fatty acids in childhood developmental and psychiatric disorders. *Lipids* 39(11):1–8.

Richardson AJ, Montgomery P. (2005). The Oxford Durham Study: a randomized, controlled trial of dietary supplementation with fatty acids in children with developmental coordination disorder. *Pediatrics* 115(5):1360–6.

Richardson AJ, Puri BK. (2002). A randomized double blind, placebo-controlled study of the effects of supplementation with highly unsaturated fatty acids on ADHD-related symptoms in children with specific learning difficulties. *Prog Neuropsychopharmacol Biol Psychiatry* 26:233–9.

Rossiter TR, La Vaque TJ. (1995). A comparison of EEG biofeedback and psychostimulants in treating attention deficit/hyperactivity disorders. *J Neurother* 1:48–59.

Rovet J, Alvarez M. (1996). Thyroid hormone and attention in school-age children with congenital hypothyroidism. *J Child Psychol Psychiatry* 37:579–85.

Rowe KS. (1988). Synthetic food colourings and 'hyperactivity': a double-blind crossover study. *Aust Paediatr J* 24:143–7.

Schmidt MH, Mocks P, Lay B, et al. (1997). Does oligoantigenic diet influence hyperactive/conduct-disordered children: a controlled trial. *Eur Child Adolesc Psychiatry* 6:88–95.

Shaffer RJ, Jacokes LE, Cassily JF, Greenspan SI, Tuchman RF, Stemmer PJ. (2001). Effect of Interactive Metronome training on children with ADHD. *Am J Occupat Ther* 55:155–62.

Shekim WO, Antun F, Hanna GL, McCracken JT. (1990). S-adenosyl-L-methionine (SAM) in adults with ADHD, RS: preliminary results from an open trial. *Psychopharmacol Bull* 26:249–53.

Sidransky H. (1997). Tryptophan and carcinogenesis: review and update on how tryptophan may act. *Nutr Cancer* 29:181–94.

Simpson DD, Nelson AL. (1974). Attention training through breathing control to modify hyperactivity. *J Learn Disabil* 7:15–23.

Sinn N, Bryan J. (2007). Effect of supplementation with polyunsaturated fatty acids and micronutrients on ADHD-related problems with attention and behaviour. *J Dev Behav Pediatr* 28(2): 82–91.

Starobrat-Hermelin B, Kozielec T. (1997). The effects of magnesium physiological supplementation on hyperactivity in children with ADHD. Positive response to magnesium oral loading test. *Magnes Res* 10(2):149–56.

Stein TP, Sammaritano AM. (1984). Nitrogen metabolism in normal and hyperkinetic boys. *Am J Clin Nutr* 39:520–4.

Sternberg EM. (1996). Pathogenesis of L-tryptophan eosinophilia-myalgia syndrome. *Adv Exp Med Biol* 398:325–30.

Stevens L, Zhang W, Peck L, et al. (2003). EFA supplementation in children with inattention, hyperactivity, and other disruptive behaviors. *Lipids* 38:1007–21.

Strauss L. (2000). The efficacy of a homeopathic preparation in the management of attention deficit hyperactivity disorder. *Biol Ther* 18:197–201.

Swanson JM, Kinsbourne M. (1980). Food dyes impair performance of hyperactive children on a laboratory learning test. *Science* 207:1485– 7.

Swedo SE, Leonard HL, Garvey M, Mittleman B, Allen AJ, Perlmutter S, et al. (1998). Pediatric autoimmune neuropsychiatric disorders associated with streptococcal infections: clinical description of the first 50 cases. *Am J Psychiatry* 155:264–71.

Thapar A, Langley K, Fowler T, Rice F, Turic D, Whittinger N, et al. (2005). Cathecol o-methyltransferase gene variant and birth weight predict early-onset antisocial behavior in children with attention deficit hyperactivity disorder. *Arch Gen Psychiatry* 62:1275–8.

Valentine J, Rossi E, O'Leary P, Parry TS, Kurinczuk JJ, Sly P. (1997). Thyroid function in a population of children with ADHD. *J Pediatr Child Health* 33: 117–20.

Van Oudheusden LJ, Scholte HR. (2002). Efficacy of carnitine in the treatment of children with attention deficit hyperactivity disorder. *Prostaglandins Leukot Essent Fatty Acids* 67(1): 33–8.

Vargas SL, Patrick CC, Ayers GD, Hughes WT. (1993). Modulating effect of dietary carbohydrate supplementation on Candida albicans colonization and invasion in a neutropenic mouse model. *Infect Immun* 61:619–26.

Voigt RG, Llorente AM, Jensen CL, et al. (2001). A randomized, double blind, placebo-controlled trial of docosahexaenoic acid supplementation in children with attention-deficit/ hyperactivity disorder. *Disabil Rehabil* 139: 189–96.

Weiss B, Williams JH, Margen S, et al. (1980). Behavioral responses to artificial food colors. *Science* 207:1487–9.

Weiss RE, Stein MA. (2000). Thyroid function and attention deficit hyperactivity disorder. In: Accardo P, Blondis TA, Whitman BY, Stein MA, eds. *ADHD in Children and Adults.* New York: Marcel Dekker: 419–30.

Weiss RE, Stein MA, Trommer B, Refetoff S. (1993). Attention-deficit hyperactivity disorder and thyroid function. *J Pediatr* 123:539–45.

West SA, Sax KW, Stanton SP, Keck PE, Jr, McElroy SL, Strakowski SM. (1996). Differences in thyroid function studies in acutely manic adolescents with and without ADHD. *Psychopharmacol Bull* 32(1):63–6.

Williams JI, Cram DM. (1978). Diet in the management of hyperkinesis: a review of the tests of Feingold's hypotheses. *Can Psychiatr Assoc J* 23:241–8.

Williamson BL, Tomlinson AJ, Mishra PK, Gleich GJ, Naylor S. (1998). Structural characterization of contaminants found in commercial preparations of melatonin: similarities to case-related compounds from L-tryptophan associated with eosinophilia-myalgia syndrome. *Chem Res Toxicol* 11:234–40.

Wilson N, Scott A. (1989). A double-blind assessment of additive intolerance in children using a 12 day challenge period at home. *Clin Exp Allergy* 19:267–72.

Wood DR, Reimherr FW, Wender, PH. (1985a). Amino acid precursors for the treatment of attention-deficit disorder, residual type. *Psychopharm Bull* 21: 146–9.

Wood DR, Reimherr FW, Wender, PH. (1985b). Treatment of attention-deficit disorder with dl-phenylalanine. *Psychiatry Res* 16:21–6.

Yeo RA, Hill D, Campbell R, Vigil, J, Brooks VM. (2000). Developmental instability and working memory ability in children: a magnetic resonance spectroscopy study. *Dev Neuropsychol* 17(2):143–59.

Zentall SS, Hall AM, Lee DL. (1998). Attentional focus of students with hyperactivity during a word-search task. *J Abnorm Child Psychol* 26:335–43.

Afterword: ADHD in adults – toward a new definition in *DSM-V*

Jan K. Buitelaar

Introduction

The current definition of ADHD in *DSM-IV* (American Psychiatric Association, 1994) has been developed exclusively on the basis of field trial data in a clinically referred sample of children and adolescents (Lahey et al., 1994). Key elements of this definition are the distinction between two separate dimensions of nine inattentive symptoms and of nine hyperactive-impulsive symptoms; the three clinical subtypes of ADHD (predominantly hyperactive-impulsive type, predominantly inattentive type, and combined type), which could be distinguished by the degree of deviance on these separate dimensions; and requirements that some symptoms causing impairment should be present prior to age 7 years and that some impairment from these symptoms should be present in two or more settings. Furthermore, the precise wordings of the single symptoms are strongly adapted to children and are not always suitable for adolescents or adults. Take, for example, symptoms such as "often loses things necessary for tasks or activities (e.g. toys, school assignments, pencils, books, or tools)" or "often leaves seat in classroom or in other situations in which remaining seated is expected."

In the years after the introduction of *DSM-IV*, ADHD in adults has become an undeniable clinical reality. Prospective longitudinal studies indicate that childhood ADHD persists into young adulthood in 15–65% of cases (Faraone, Biederman, & Mick, 2006). About 15% of children and adolescents with ADHD show persistence into adult age, when ADHD in adulthood is defined as still meeting full childhood criteria. Persistence rises to 65% when residual symptoms and functional impairment are also taken into account (Faraone, Biederman, & Mick, 2006). Increasing evidence exists for the validity of ADHD as an adult disorder, including a similar configuration into 2- and 3-factor models of hyperactive-impulsive and inattentive symptoms as found in children and adoles-

cents (Kooij et al., 2004), as well as patterns of comorbidity, family-genetic and molecular-genetic factors, neuropsychological deficits, brain imaging abnormalities, and responses to medications that are very similar to those in children and adolescents with ADHD (Faraone, 2005; Faraone et al., 2000).

Because the ADHD criteria have never been validated or adapted for use in adults, many diagnostic issues remain that should be considered when revising the definition of ADHD for the *DSM-V* (McGough & Barkley, 2004). They include the following: many of the current childhood symptoms are developmentally inappropriate for adults, the psychometric and distributional properties of the symptoms in adult populations are unknown, the diagnostic threshold of six or more of nine symptoms may be too restrictive for adults, the age-of-onset criterion is unvalidated when making an adult ADHD diagnosis, and impairment of functioning criteria should be adapted to the context of adulthood (Buitelaar, 2009; McGough & Barkley, 2004). In this chapter, each of these issues is discussed in more detail.

Modifying the diagnostic criteria for adult ADHD

Reading the *DSM-IV* criteria of ADHD with an adult patient in mind will immediately reveal the developmentally inappropriateness of some criteria. Many focus on the classroom context in which the child is expected to remain seated until receiving permission to do otherwise and is expected to be mentally engaged in schoolwork that has to be finished in a defined period of time. This is far from representative of the situation at work or at home where the average adult will have much more opportunities and degree of freedom to set his or her own expectations in terms of behavior and output. In addition, a criterion such as "runs about or climbs excessively" is not readily applicable to the adult context. Systematic study is required to map how the diagnostic criteria for adult AHD should be modified to take account of age-dependent developmental changes.

A first step in examining the appropriateness and validity of the current ADHD symptoms for the definition of ADHD in adults is to study the distribution in the general population of the inattention and hyperactivity-impulsivity items that currently define the condition under *DSM-IV*. In the Netherlands, we have collected self-report data on *DSM-IV* symptoms of ADHD using a modified ADHD-DSM-IV rating scale from a population-based sample of 1813 adults (Kooij et al., 2004). The composition of the sample by gender and age was as follows: men 44.7%, women 55.3%; 18–29 years, 14.9%; 30–44 years, 37.5%; 45–59 years, 30.0%; and 60–75 years, 17.7%. There appeared to be a marked variation between symptoms being endorsed "never," with relatively high rates of more than 50% for the inattention symptoms of "fails to finish tasks," "difficulty organizing tasks," and "avoids academic work" and for the hyperactive-impulsive symptoms of "leaves seat," "difficulty engaging in leisure activities," and "talks excessively." Symptoms rated as present "often" or "very often" also varied widely, with some rated to be present in more than 10% of the general population ("careless mistakes," "easily distracted," "forgetful," "fidgeting and squirming," "runs and climbs," and "always on the go") and others being present in less than 5% of the population ("leaves seat"). These marked differences in distribution of the individual symptoms items suggest that specific symptoms make a different contribution to the clinical diagnosis, with very frequently endorsed symptoms probably being less specific for ADHD, and rarely endorsed symptoms having low sensitivity.

To further explore whether the contribution of individual symptoms varies depending on the total number of ADHD symptoms present, the sample was broken down by total symptom level and separately for inattention and hyperactivity-impulsivity. All symptoms were categorized as present or absent. Then we looked at whether the presence of each symptom was significantly above or below chance level (see Fig. 1).

In subjects with nine symptoms, by definition each symptom is present. Because very few subjects had eight symptoms, we combined subjects with seven and eight symptoms. For example, in subjects with four symptoms, each symptom has an a priori probability to be present of 0.44 (i.e. 4 times 0.11). We found that

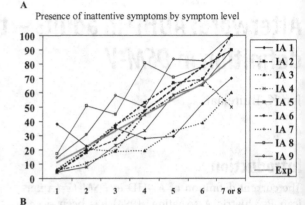

A

Presence of inattentive symptoms by symptom level

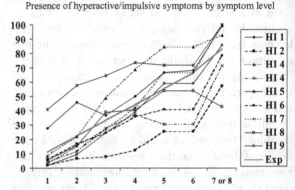

B

Presence of hyperactive/impulsive symptoms by symptom level

Figure 1 These graphs show whether the presence of each inattentive (IA) or hyperactive-impulsive (HI) symptom was significantly above or below chance level, depending on the total number of symptoms of a subject. In subjects with nine symptoms, by definition each symptom is present. Because very few subjects had eight symptoms, we combined subjects with seven and eight symptoms. For example, in subjects with four symptoms, each symptom has an a priori probability to be present of 0.44 (i.e. 4 times 0.11).

two inattentive items, "easily distracted" and "forgetful," were present significantly more often in subjects with lower (i.e. 0, 1, and 2 symptoms) and subthreshold (i.e., 4 and 5 symptoms) levels of symptoms than can be expected by chance. Two other symptoms, "careless mistakes" and " does not listen," were present at chance level at lower symptom levels, but were endorsed significantly less often when the symptom level increased. These symptoms therefore appear to be rather unspecific and characterize many subjects in the populations who do not meet threshold criteria for ADHD in adults. In contrast, the symptoms "fails to finish tasks" and "difficulty organizing tasks" were underrepresented in subjects with lower levels of symptoms and characterized subjects with higher and threshold level of symptoms. These symptoms appear to mark the severity of ADHD in adults and may be more specific to the disorder. A similar logic can be followed for hyperactive-impulsive symptoms. The symptoms "always on the go" and "fidgeting and squirming" were overly present at low and intermediate symptom levels and thus appear to be less specific for establishing ADHD. In contrast, "leaves seat" was not scored unless there were very high symptom levels and thus seems to be a marker of greater severity and specificity for ADHD in adults.

A complementary approach has been to compare the frequency of self-reported *DSM-IV* symptoms of ADHD among a clinical sample of adults with ADHD (N = 142), a clinical control group (N = 97), and a community control group (N = 109) in the United States (Barkley, 2008b). The two most common symptoms of inattention in the ADHD group, "difficulties sustaining attention to tasks" and "easily distracted," were endorsed by 97% of the adults with ADHD, but were also the most commonly endorsed symptoms in the clinical control group (82–87%), but not in the community control group. In a similar way, the two hyperactive symptoms most often endorsed in the ADHD group, "fidgeting with hand or feet or squirming in seat" and "feeling restless," were endorsed rather frequently in the clinical control group and less often in the community control group. Thus, both inattention and hyperactive-impulsive symptoms of ADHD were relatively common in clinical samples of adult patients, whether they had ADHD or not, thereby suggesting that although they are sensitive to the diagnosis they lack specificity.

Although the frequencies of these symptoms were much lower in the community sample, some symptoms of ADHD were found to occur in well above 10% of adults in the community sample, just as they did in the Dutch sample. Inattentive symptoms were quite prevalent in 5–19% and hyperactive-impulsive symptoms in 6–22% of a US community sample (Murphy & Barkley, 1996b). Many ADHD symptoms thus seem to be unspecific and reflect a more general state of restlessness and attentional problems rather than the presence of the distinct syndrome of ADHD.

This leads to the next issue, which is to examine whether it is possible to identify specific ADHD *DSM-IV* symptoms that best predict the presence of ADHD in adults. Using the Dutch population-based data, we performed analyses on those subjects with four or more current ADHD criteria, because there

were too few subjects with five and six current symptoms (Buitelaar, 2009). We ran these analyses twice, both with and without taking into account the presence of ADHD symptoms in childhood. As expected, for all individual ADHD symptoms, the presence of a symptom raised the odds of meeting criteria for four or more current ADHD symptoms in either of the two symptom domains (inattention and hyperactivity-impulsivity), and this effect was stronger when childhood criteria were not taken into account. However, there was much variance among symptoms in their predictive value. Among the inattentive symptoms, "making careless mistakes in work" showed little predictive value, whereas the item "difficulty organizing tasks" was highly predictive, in particular when childhood symptoms were also taken into account. To a lesser extent "difficulty sustaining attention," "difficulty following through on instructions," and "often losing things" were indices of the presence of an ADHD syndrome. Among the hyperactive-impulsive symptoms "running about," "blurting out answers," and "often interrupting others" were rather often associated with the presence of at least four current ADHD symptoms.

Barkley et al. (2008b) performed univariate and multivariate analyses to examine which individual symptoms and subset of ADHD symptoms were best at accurately discriminating those with ADHD from clinical and community controls. The diagnoses of ADHD and psychiatric disorder other than ADHD were established by clinical interviews. For the inattention symptoms, "easily distracted" performed best and accurately classified 97% of the ADHD cases and 98% of the community controls. Using three additional symptoms (poor sustained attention, being poorly organized, and being forgetful) further increased the classification accuracy up to 99% for each group. Four hyperactive-impulsive symptoms (fidgeting/squirming, feelings of restlessness, blurting out answers, difficulty awaiting turn) led to accurate classification of 94% of the ADHD and 91% of the community control cases.

The next analysis focused on the discrimination between ADHD and the clinical controls. The following three inattentive symptoms – "failure to pay attention to details," "difficulty sustaining attention," and "failing to follow through on instructions" – correctly classified 87% of the ADHD group but just 44% of the clinical controls. For the hyperactive-impulsive symptoms, "fidgeting/squirming," "leaving seat," "difficulty engaging in leisure activity," and "interrupting others" accurately classified 76% of ADHD cases and 49% of clinical control cases. These findings suggest good sensitivity but poor specificity for clinical diagnosis.

These analyses lead to two main conclusions. First, among both the inattentive and hyperactive-impulsive symptoms there is a strong redundancy, meaning that we do not need all the symptoms to accurately classify ADHD in adults. Second, the current symptoms have insufficient discriminatory power in the comparison between adults with ADHD and those with other psychiatric disorders.

The final issue is then whether it is possible to propose new symptoms for ADHD in adults that are better able to discriminate between ADHD and other psychiatric disorders and facilitate making the differential diagnosis. To this end, a list was developed of 91 new symptoms that could be relevant for diagnosing ADHD in adults (Barkley, 2008a). These symptoms were all considered to reflect behaviors related to executive functioning (i.e. aspects of self-control and self-regulation). Information about the presence of these new symptoms was collected by a structured interview in the same sample of adults with ADHD, clinical controls, and community controls used in the studies outlined earlier. Nine symptoms were found to discriminate strongly between adults with ADHD and clinical and community controls and therefore to be potential new symptoms with improved sensitivity and specificity for ADHD in adulthood:

- Make decisions impulsively
- Have difficulty stopping my activities or behavior when I should do so
- Start a project or task without reading or listening to directions carefully
- Poor follow-through on promises or commitments I may make to others
- Have trouble doing things in their proper order or sequence
- More likely to drive a motor vehicle much faster than others
- Prone to daydreaming when I should be concentrating on something
- Have trouble planning ahead or preparing for upcoming events
- Can't seem to persist at things I do not find interesting

These symptoms merit further study in independent datasets.

Modifying the diagnostic threshold for adult ADHD

A problem in the study of ADHD in adults is the choice of the diagnostic threshold. Under the *DSM-IV* algorithm the threshold of six out of nine symptoms in either of the inattention or hyperactivity-impulsivity domains is required for the diagnosis during childhood, and there are no separate or age-adjusted criteria for ADHD in adults. However, children are normally more active and have more difficulty in concentrating than adults, leading to a higher base rate of symptom levels in children than in adults. Therefore, one may argue that the threshold should be set lower in adults, who might experience impairment at a lower level of symptoms.

We used the data of the Dutch population study to estimate the diagnostic threshold in adults (Kooij et al., 2004) by plotting the number of inattentive and hyperactive-impulsive symptoms against the aggregated measure of impairment, while using a general measure of mental health (the GHQ-28) as a covariate. Analyses of covariance (ANCOVAs) – using the between-subjects factor "number of symptoms" in seven levels (6 or more symptoms, 5, 4, 3, 2, 1, and 0 symptoms) and GHQ-28 as the covariate – indicated that subjects with four or more inattentive symptoms had impairment scores that were significantly increased compared to those with two, one, and no inattentive symptoms. In a similar analysis of covariance, subjects with four or more hyperactive-impulsive symptoms were significantly more impaired than subjects with three, two, one, and no hyperactive-impulsive symptoms. Subsequent ANCOVAs that included gender and age in addition to GHQ-28 as covariates and ANCOVAs for men and women and for young and old subjects separately replicated the finding of a cut-off of four symptoms (Kooij et al., 2004).

These findings are consistent with the results of other analyses. In the dataset collected by Barkley et al. (2008) and discussed earlier, all adult ADHD subjects had three or more inattention symptoms, and 72% had three or more hyperactive symptoms. In contrast, 98% of the community group had three or fewer symptoms of inattention and 100% had three or fewer symptoms of hyperactive-impulsive behavior. Thus, a threshold of four or more symptoms would lead to a nearly perfect discrimination between adult ADHD and community controls, whereas a threshold of six symptoms would appear to be too stringent and would misclassify a subsample of ADHD subjects as normal. In addition, an earlier US study indicated that a threshold of four of either inattentive or hyperactive-impulsive symptoms would represent the 93rd percentile in that general population sample. This percentile is often used in clinical practice to establish someone as clinically deviant or developmentally inappropriate in his or her symptoms (Murphy & Barkley, 1996a, 1996b). A threshold of six symptoms would statistically represent the 98th percentile of the normal distribution and lead to defining only the most extreme subjects as having ADHD.

However, inconsistent findings also exist. Subjects with subthreshold ADHD symptoms, defined as never having met *DSM-IV* criteria for ADHD and reporting a chronic history of three or more inattentive symptoms or three or more hyperactive-impulsive symptoms, had milder impairments of functioning and a lower different familial loading compared to patients with full ADHD and patients with late-onset ADHD (Faraone, Biederman, Spencer, et al., 2006). The key point is here that in the Faraone study the subthreshold group had not met full ADHD criteria earlier in childhood, whereas in the studies of Buitelaar et al. and Barkley et al. (2008) they had. Thus lowering the diagnostic threshold to four symptoms would still require the presence of full ADHD earlier in development.

Of course, not all these analyses bear on the discrimination between ADHD in adults and psychiatric controls. The threshold of four or more symptoms would lead to classifying ADHD in a number of patients with other psychiatric disorders. Whether this is a meaningful way to describe comorbid ADHD in these patients requires further study, because it may be that having defined ADHD in childhood using the criteria of six or more items and then having four or more current symptoms may indeed reflect persistence of ADHD even in the presence of co-occurring conditions such as anxiety and depression.

Modifying the age-of-onset criterion for adult ADHD

The current *DSM-IV* age-of-onset criterion of ADHD requires that some symptoms and related impairment of functioning be present prior to age 7 years. This criterion was first set for the definition of ADHD in

DSM-III in 1980. At that time, no empirical data were available to support it. Furthermore, the validity of this criterion was not evaluated in the field trial for the *DSM-III-R* definition of ADHD in 1987. When developing the definition of ADHD for the *DSM-IV*, a larger field trial was performed, but the *DSM-IV* definition was established and published before analyses on the age-of-onset criterion were completed (Barkley & Biederman, 1997). The results of these analyses indicated that 18% of those having the combined type of ADHD, 2% of those having the hyperactive-impulsive type, and 43% of those having the inattentive type had their onset of impairment after age 7 years (Applegate et al., 1997). The key point is that both empirical and conceptual reasons exist for viewing ADHD as a disorder that typically has its onset of symptoms during childhood, yet no empirical data exist to establish the age-of-onset criterion at age 7 rather than at later ages such as 12 or 15 years.

It has been argued that the age-of-onset criterion at age 7 year is overly restrictive and would result in many adults and some older children with ADHD not receiving the diagnosis (Barkley & Biederman, 1997). Children with well-developed cognitive abilities or living in supportive and structured environments may function adequately in childhood, despite the presence of some symptoms of ADHD. Only until later in life, when the demands of the school or work environment or of the more complex social world of adolescents and young adults exceed their self-control and executive skills would higher levels of symptoms and associated impairments occur. Clinically, many patients first diagnosed with ADHD at an adult age report the first onset of their symptoms and impairment of functioning during their late childhood, teens, or even early adulthood (Faraone & Biederman, 2005). Yet there are also data that adolescents and adults who have been carefully diagnosed with ADHD in childhood report their age of onset to be approximately 5 years later than the known age of onset (Barkley, 2008b).

Evidence for changing the age-of-onset criterion has been provided by recent studies. Its validity was examined by comparing subjects with full ADHD who met all *DSM-IV* criteria for childhood-onset ADHD, subjects with late-onset ADHD who met all criteria except the age-at-onset criterion, and subjects without ADHD who did not meet any criteria (Faraone, Biederman, Spencer, et al., 2006). Subjects with late-onset and full ADHD appeared to have similar patterns of psychiatric comorbidity, functional impairment, and familial transmission. This finding suggested that late-onset ADHD in adults is a valid category and that the age-of-onset criterion as set in *DSM-IV* is too stringent. However, this study was limited by sampling only clinically referred patients.

We attempted to replicate and extend this finding relating to the age-of-onset criterion for adult ADHD by sampling from our Dutch population database. We selected adults with at least four current symptoms of ADHD of any subtype and who met criteria for ADHD in childhood (early-onset, N = 56), adults with at least four current symptoms of ADHD of any subtype but who did not meet criteria for ADHD in childhood (late-onset, N = 122), and a random sample of age- and gender-matched normal controls who did not meet current and childhood criteria for ADHD (N = 98). When comparing these three groups, the late-onset adult ADHD group was similar to the early-onset ADHD group in terms of severity of current ADHD symptoms, indices of impairment of functioning, and GHQ scores for comorbid anxiety, depression, and somatization. Both ADHD groups differed on all indices significantly from the normal controls (Buitelaar, 2009).

These data lead to the proposal that age 15 is a more useful and valid age-of-onset for ADHD, taking into account the substantive sample of patients with adult ADHD with rather minimal symptoms and impairment during childhood and increasing levels of symptoms and impairment in late adolescence and early adulthood.

Specifying impairment of functioning criteria

The *DSM-IV* definition of ADHD requires symptoms and impairment of functioning in more than one setting. Defining impairment of functioning in adults with ADHD is more complicated than in children and adolescents. On the one hand, adults are expected to assume responsibility in various roles in adult life, such as spouse and parent, employer, or co-worker. These roles may require complex skills and a differentiated behavioral repertoire, and other persons may be dependent on the adequate performance of the individual in any of these roles. This creates numerous opportunities for inadequate functioning and thus impairment. On the other hand, adults have more opportunities than children and adolescents to create their own environment and to avoid tasks and

roles they do not like or find difficult to perform. These opportunities may therefore hide impairment of functioning.

One way to improve the measurement of impairment in adults with ADHD is to develop standardized instruments. These instruments should tap into all relevant adult roles and include queries about school outcome, job performance, relationship history, functioning in leisure time, legal infractions, lifestyle and health behavior, and driving performance. For example the Weiss impairment scales cover impairments in multiple domains including family, work, education, life skills, self-concept, social behavior, and risky behaviors.

Another complementary way to improve measurement is to examine in detail the relationship between symptoms and impairment. Which symptoms of ADHD are more impairing, and in whom and when? Using the Dutch epidemiology dataset described earlier, we performed multiple regression analyses with the aggregated impairment score as the dependent variable, and inattentive symptoms and hyperactive-impulsive symptoms as the independent variables. Inattentive symptoms predicted 14% of the variance in the overall impairment measure. Three inattentive items were particularly associated with greater impairment of functioning: "difficulty sustaining attention," "avoids mental efforts," and "forgetful." The contribution of other inattentive symptoms was minor or even absent, after controlling for the presence of all other symptoms. Hyperactive-impulsive symptoms predicted 19% of the variance in the impairment score. The strongest contribution came from three items – "leaves seat," "running about," and "difficulty engaging in leisure time" – that were each independently from other symptoms associated with greater impairment of functioning.

Concluding remarks

Using our Dutch adult population sample of self-report data for current and childhood ADHD symptoms we were able to address several issues relating to the diagnostic validity and utility of individual symptoms. First, we were able to replicate the 2- and 3-factor models of the symptoms of ADHD that had been tested and confirmed in earlier studies in children and adolescents. This shows that the symptoms that define ADHD cluster together in an characteristic way throughout the life span.

In terms of their distribution in the general population, several *DSM-IV* symptoms proved to be problematic for their use in the diagnostic algorithm for ADHD in adults. The symptoms "careless mistakes," "easily distracted," "forgetful," "fidgeting and squirming," "runs and climbs," and "always on the go" were endorsed by 10% of more of the population and seem to be rather general and not specific to ADHD. The symptoms "easily distracted," "forgetful," "always on the go," and "fidgeting and squirming" were present significantly more often in subjects with lower and subthreshold levels of symptoms. This subset of self-rated ADHD symptoms therefore seem to reflect a broader and more general dimension of inattention and restlessness that is not specific to the disorder in adults.

In contrast, the symptoms "fails to finish tasks" and "difficulty organizing tasks" mark higher levels of ADHD symptoms, index the severity of ADHD, and are therefore more specific to the clinical condition. The symptom "difficulty organizing tasks" was strongly predictive of the presence of the ADHD syndrome in adults, particularly when childhood symptoms were also taken into account. This symptom, in combination with three other symptoms – "difficulty sustaining attention," "difficulty following through on instructions," and "often losing things" – could form the basis for a smaller, less redundant, and more effective set of symptoms with greater sensitivity and specificity to be used for a new diagnostic algorithm for ADHD in adults.

Concerning hyperactive-impulsive symptoms, "running about," "blurting out answers," and "often interrupting others" would be good candidates for a modified set of symptoms. Two of these symptoms, "difficulty sustaining attention" and "running about," were also among the most impairing symptoms. However, the analysis of the impact of individual symptoms on impairment of functioning put the spotlight on a partly different set of symptoms, including "avoids mental efforts," "forgetful," "leaves seat," and "difficulty engaging in leisure time".

In contrast to a recent study in clinical samples (Faraone, Biederman, Spencer, et al., 2006), we found that subjects with four and five current symptoms (that is, at subthreshold levels following current diagnostic criteria) in the general population were about equally impaired in functioning as subjects with six or more (i.e. threshold or above) symptoms. We also replicated the finding that subjects with an early onset and late onset of ADHD were very similar in external indices such as impairment of functioning and patterns of comorbid psychopathology.

One limitation of our analyses is the use of self-report rating scale data alone, which may give rise to different results from investigator-based interviews or informant data. Although these self-reported ADHD symptoms show predicted relationships with various external variables, our analyses should be replicated using ADHD symptom scores obtained by investigator-rated symptoms following standardized interview protocols such as the Conners Adult ADHD Diagnostic Interview.

Overall we conclude that ADHD as currently measured in adults is a valid diagnosis that predicts, as reviewed elsewhere in this book, important associations with comorbid conditions, impairments, treatment response, and genetic, neurobiological, and environmental factors. However, further work is required to clarify the full extent of the symptoms and impairments associated with ADHD in adults and to delineate properly age-adjusted methods of diagnosis that are both sensitive and specific to the disorder and its associated impairments.

References

American Psychiatric Association. (1994). *Diagnostic and Statistical Manual of Mental Disorders*. 4th ed. Washington, DC: American Psychiatric Association.

Applegate B, Lahey BB, Hart EL, Biederman J, Hynd GW, Barkley RA, et al. (1997). Validity of the age-of-onset criterion for ADHD: a report from the DSM-IV field trials. *J Am Acad Child Adolesc Psychiatry* **36**(9): 1211–21.

Barkley RA. (2008a). Identifying new symptoms for ADHD in adulthood. In: Barkley RA, Murphy KR, Fischer M, eds. *ADHD in Adults: What the Science Says*. New York: Guilford Press:

Barkley RA. (2008b). Symptoms and age of onset. In: Barkley RA, Murphy KR, Fischer M, eds. *ADHD in Adults: What the Science Says*. New York: Guilford Press:

Barkley RA, Biederman J. (1997). Toward a broader definition of the age-of-onset criterion for attention-deficit hyperactivity disorder. *J Am Acad Child Adolesc Psychiatry* **36**(9):1204–10.

Barkley RA, et al. (2008). ADHD in Adults: What the Science Says. New York: Guilford Press.

Buitelaar JK. (2009). ADHD in adults – Towards a new definition in DSM-V. In: Shaffer D, Leibenuft E, Rohde L, Sirovatka P, Rogier DA, eds. *Externalizing Disorders of*

Childhood: Refining the Research Agenda for DSM-V. Arlington, VA: American Psychiatric Association:

Faraone SV. (2005). The scientific foundation for understanding attention-deficit/hyperactivity disorder as a valid psychiatric disorder. *Eur Child Adolesc Psychiatry* **14**(1):1–10.

Faraone SV, Biederman J. (2005). What is the prevalence of adult ADHD? Results of a population screen of 966 adults. *J Atten Disord* **9**(2):384–91.

Faraone SV, Biederman J, Mick E. (2006). The age-dependent decline of attention deficit hyperactivity disorder: a meta-analysis of follow-up studies. *Psychol Med* **36**(2):159–65.

Faraone SV, Biederman J, Spencer T, Mick E, Murray K, Petty C, et al. (2006). Diagnosing adult attention deficit hyperactivity disorder: are late onset and subthreshold diagnoses valid? *Am J Psychiatry* **163**(10):1720–9.

Faraone SV, Biederman J, Spencer T, Wilens T, Seidman LJ, Mick E, Doyle AE. (2000). Attention-deficit/hyperactivity disorder in adults: an overview. *Biol Psychiatry* **48**(1):9–20.

Kooij JJS, Buitelaar JK, Van Den Oord EJ, Reijnders C, Hodiamont P. (2004). Attention-Deficit/Hyperactivity Disorder in a primary care sample of adults: confirmatory factor models, gender and age differences, and prevalence. *Psychol Medicine*.

Lahey BB, Applegate B, McBurnett K, Biederman J, Greenhill L, Hynd GW, et al. (1994). DSM-IV field trials for attention deficit hyperactivity disorder in children and adolescents. *Am J Psychiatry* **151**(11):1673–85.

McGough JJ, Barkley RA. (2004). Diagnostic controversies in adult attention deficit hyperactivity disorder. *Am J Psychiatry* **161**(11):1948–56.

Murphy K, Barkley RA. (1996a). Attention deficit hyperactivity disorder adults: comorbidities and adaptive impairments. *Compr Psychiatry* **37**(6): 393–401.

Murphy K, Barkley RA. (1996b). Prevalence of DSM-IV symptoms of ADHD in adult licensed drivers: Implications for clinical diagnosis. *J Atten Disord* **3**:147–61.

Appendix 1: Patient organizations for ADHD (countries in alphabetical order)

Austria	Anne Tischlinger Verein Adapt Landstr.Hauotstr.84/4 1030 Vienna Austria Tel: 43 676 516 5687 Fax: 43 1879 75 48 verein_adapt@yahoo.com www.adapt.at
Belgium (Dutch speaking)	centrum ZitStil Ria Van Den Heuvel Heistraat 321 B-2610 Wilrijk info@zitstil.be www.zitstil.be
Belgium (English speaking)	ADHD family support group Brussels Donnalea Barber home: Rue de la Prison 22 B-1310 La Hulpe simon.barber@skynet.be
Belgium (English speaking)	English-speaking Adult Group Belgium Brussels Stephanie Clark Huisadres: Puttestraat 42 B-3080 Leuven stephanie.clark@pandora.be anglophonebags.blogspot.com/
Belgium (French speaking)	TDAH Belgique Rue Fond du Village, 26–1315 Piétrebais 010.84.54.45–0472.27.76.04 info@tdah.be www.forumhyper.net/scarlett/
Canada	CADDRA 40 Wynford Drive, Suite 304A Toronto, Ontario M3C 1J5 www.caddra.ca
Canada	CHADD Canada CHADD Canada Inc. P.O. Box 23043 Citadel RPO St. Albert, AB T8N 6Z9 chaddcanada@hotmail.com www.chaddcanada.org

Cyprus	ADD-ADHD SUPPORT Cyprus Susan J. Chrysostomou sue@add-adhd.org.cy www.add-adhd.org.cy
Denmark	ADHD-Foreningen Birgit Christiansen Kongensgade 68 DK-5000 Odense C bc@adhd.dk www.adhd.dk
Germany	BV AUK, e.v. Detlev Boeing Brusselsesteenweg 151 B-3080 Tervuren boeing@pandora.be www.bv-auek.de
Germany	BV-AD Germany Bundesvereinigung Aufmerksamkeitsstörung Deutschland Esther Rohde-Köttelwesch Ben-Gurion-Ring 161 60437 Frankfurt estherrohde@t-online.de Verein.zFwK@t-online.de info@wahrnehmungsstoerung.com www.wahrnehmungsstoerung.com
Germany	BV-AH e.V. Bundesverband Aufmerksamkeitsstörung/Hyperaktivität e.V. Dr. Myriam Menter Postfach 60 D-91291 Forchheim info@bv-ah.de www.bv-ah.de
France	Hypersupers Christine Gétin 37 Rue des Paradis F-95410 Groslay christine.getin@tdah-france.fr www.tdah-france.fr
Hungary	POSITIV Hajdu Józsefné kisbagi@freemail.hu vardai@axelero.hu www.pozitiv-osze.freeweb.hu
Ireland	Hadd Ierland Stefanie Mahony North Brunswick Street IE-Dublin 7 mahony@eircom.net hadd@eircom.net
Italy	Aifa Astrid Gollner Via Sabotino 4 I-21046 Malnate (VD) amonetti@libero.it referente.varese@aifa.it www.aifa.it

Norway	ADHD-Foreningen Knut Bronder Arnstein Arnebergsvei 30 1366 Lysaker post@adhd-foreningen.no www.adhd-foreningen.no
Spain	Federacion Espanola de Asociaciones de Ayuda al Deficit de Atencion e Hiperactividad Fulgencio Madrid Plaze de la Universidad 2/1F ES-30001 Murcia penchom@cesmurcia.es
Spain	Fundacion Adana Patricia Negre Calle Muntaner 250, principal 1' Barcelona, 08021 patinegre@yahoo.com www.f-adana.org
Sweden	Riksförbrudet Attention Ann-Kristin Sandberg Förmangsvägen 2 SE-11743 Stockholm aks@attention-riks.se www.attention-riks.se
The Netherlands	Balans (parents association) Arga Paternotte / Ids Terpstra De Kwinkelier 39 NL 3722 AR Bilthoven Arga.Paternotte@balansdigitaal.nl Ids.Terpstra@balansdigitaal.nl www.balansdigitaal.nl
The Netherlands	Impuls (adults association) Impuls/ADHD Regina Van Criekinge Huisadres:Treilerstraat 89 NL-1503 JD Zaandam huis: 31 75 6141264 Fax 31 75 6141266 regina@ADHD-global.org www.impulsdigitaal.nl
United Kingdom	Addiss Andrea Bilbow 10 Station Road Mill Hill London NW7 2JU andrea@addiss.co.uk
United Kingdom	Adult Attention Deficit Disorder UK Information on meetings of ADHD adult support groups. www.aadd.org.uk/
United States	CHADD 8181 Professional Place – Suite 150 Landover, MD 20785 Tel: 301-306-7070 Fax: 301-306-7090 www.chadd.org

Appendix 2: Useful websites for ADHD (in alphabetical order)

http://www.addcoach4u.com	Comprehensive list of websites on adult attention-deficit disorder
http://www.additudemag.com	Site sponsored by ADDitude magazine, a national monthly magazine for the ADHD community. Monthly articles by doctors suggest treatment for ADD ADHD children and adults
http://www.adhdbijvolwassenen.nl	Dutch treatment program for adults with ADHD
http://adhddriving.ca	Allows clinicians to gather information about their patients' driving history and current driving profiles. It consists of the Jerome Driving Questionnaire (JDQ), the World Health Organization Adult ADHD Self-Report Scale of symptoms of Inattention and Impulsivity (ASRS), and the Driving Behavior Survey (DBQ) by Professor Russell Barkley
http://www.attentiondeficit-info.com	Informative source and reference for those interested in better understanding this disorder and an additional help for health professionals
http://www.cdc.gov/ncbddd/ADHD/	Centers for Disease Control and Prevention
http://www.cmeonadhd.com	Online continuing medical education (CME) presentations given by local and international experts
http://doctor.webmd.com/physician_finder/home.aspx?sponsor=core	List of physicians in the United States who treat adults with ADHD created and maintained by Shire
http://en.wikipedia.org/wiki/Attention-deficit_hyperactivity_disorder	Entry from Wikipedia, the free encyclopedia
http://familydoctor.org/online/famdocen/home/children/parents/behavior/118.html	Health information for the whole family
http://www.help4adhd.org/	The National Resource Center on AD/HD: A Program of CHADD is a clearinghouse for science-based information about all aspects of AD/HD
http://helpguide.org/mental/adhd_add_adult_symptoms.htm	Nonprofit resource
http://www.mayoclinic.com/health/adhd/DS00275/	Website by Mayo Clinic Staff
http://www.nimh.nih.gov/health/topics/attention-deficit-hyperactivity-disorder-adhd/index.shtml	Information from the National Institute of Mental Health
http://www.psychiatrienet.nl/links/1886_ADHD_bij_volwassenen	Describes relevant sites selected by psychiatrists

Index

Printed in the United States
By Bookmasters